Fluorescence-Guided Surgery of Cancer

Fluorescence-Guided Surgery of Cancer

Editor: Jaime Allison

AMERICAN
MEDICAL PUBLISHERS
www.americanmedicalpublishers.com

AMERICAN
MEDICAL PUBLISHERS
www.americanmedicalpublishers.com

Cataloging-in-Publication Data

Fluorescence-guided surgery of cancer / edited by Jaime Allison.
p. cm.
Includes bibliographical references and index.
ISBN 979-8-88740-124-9
1. Cancer--Surgery. 2. Cancer--Intraoperative radiotherapy. 3. Fluorescence.
4. Radiosurgery. 5. Computer-assisted surgery. I. Allison, Jaime.
RD651 .F58 2023
616.994 059--dc23

American Medical Publishers,
41 Flatbush Avenue,
1st Floor, New York,
NY 11217, USA

ISBN 979-8-88740-124-9 (Hardback)

Contents

Preface IX

Chapter 1 **Usefulness and Prospects of Sentinel Lymph Node Biopsy for Patients with Breast Cancer Using the Medical Imaging Projection System** 1
Yuki Nakamura, Masahiro Takada, Michiko Imamura, Akane Higami, He Jiaxi, Makoto Fujino, Rie Nakagawa, Yukiko Inagaki, Yoshiaki Matsumoto, Kosuke Kawaguchi, Masahiro Kawashima, Eiji Suzuki and Masakazu Toi

Chapter 2 **5-Aminolevulinic Acid Multispectral Imaging for the Fluorescence-Guided Resection of Brain Tumors** 7
Patra Charalampaki, Phileas Johannes Proskynitopoulos, Axel Heimann and Makoto Nakamura

Chapter 3 **Spray Fluorescent Probes for Fluorescence-Guided Neurosurgery** 17
Yosuke Kitagawa, Shota Tanaka, Yugo Kuriki, Kyoko Yamamoto, Akira Ogasawara, Takahide Nejo, Reiko Matsuura, Tsukasa Koike, Taijun Hana, Satoshi Takahashi, Masashi Nomura, Shunsaku Takayanagi, Akitake Mukasa, Mako Kamiya, Yasuteru Urano and Nobuhito Saito

Chapter 4 **Quantitative Modulation of PpIX Fluorescence and Improved Glioma Visualization** 21
Michael Reinert, Deborah Piffaretti, Marco Wilzbach, Christian Hauger, Roland Guckler, Francesco Marchi and Maria Luisa D'Angelo

Chapter 5 **Pelvic Reconstruction with a Novel Three-Dimensional-Printed, Multimodality Imaging Based Endoprosthesis Following Enneking Type I + IV Resection** 30
Zeping Yu, Wenli Zhang, Xiang Fang, Chongqi Tu and Hong Duan

Chapter 6 **Current Trends for Improving Safety of Stereotactic Brain Biopsies: Advanced Optical Methods for Vessel Avoidance and Tumor Detection** 45
Serik K. Akshulakov, Talgat T. Kerimbayev, Michael Y. Biryuchkov, Yermek A. Urunbayev, Dara S. Farhadi and Vadim A. Byvaltsev

Chapter 7 **Confocal-Assisted Multispectral Fluorescent Microscopy for Brain Tumor Surgery** 54
Patra Charalampaki, Makoto Nakamura, Dimitrios Athanasopoulos and Axel Heimann

Chapter 8 **Receptor-Targeted Fluorescence-Guided Surgery with Low Molecular Weight Agents** 63
Servando Hernandez Vargas, Christie Lin, Hop S. Tran Cao, Naruhiko Ikoma, Solmaz AghaAmiri, Sukhen C. Ghosh, Adam J. Uselmann and Ali Azhdarinia

Chapter 9 **Blood-Brain Barrier, Blood-Brain Tumor Barrier and Fluorescence-Guided Neurosurgical Oncology: Delivering Optical Labels to Brain Tumors** 78
Evgenii Belykh, Kurt V. Shaffer, Chaoqun Lin, Vadim A. Byvaltsev, Mark C. Preul and Lukui Chen

Chapter 10 **Survival Outcomes Among Patients with High-Grade Glioma Treated with 5-Aminolevulinic Acid–Guided Surgery** 105
Sirin Gandhi, Ali Tayebi Meybodi, Evgenii Belykh, Claudio Cavallo, Xiaochun Zhao, Masood Pasha Syed, Leandro Borba Moreira, Michael T. Lawton, Peter Nakaji and Mark C. Preul

Chapter 11 **Novel Visualization Methods Assisted Transurethral Resection for Bladder Cancer** 118
Honglin Li, Yubin Cao, Pingchuan Ma, Zhongkai Ma, Chunjie Li, Wenbin Yang and Lingyun Zhou

Chapter 12 **Clinical Benefits of Combining Different Visualization Modalities in Neurosurgery** 129
Karl-Michael Schebesch, Katharina Rosengarth, Alexander Brawanski, Martin Proescholdt, Christina Wendl, Julius Höhne, Christian Ott, Hans Lamecker and Christian Doenitz

Chapter 13 **Photodynamic Therapy for the Treatment of Glioblastoma** 140
Samuel W. Cramer and Clark C. Chen

Chapter 14 **Near-Infrared Fluorescence Imaging and Photodynamic Therapy for Liver Tumors** 151
Masaki Kaibori, Hisashi Kosaka, Kosuke Matsui, Morihiko Ishizaki, Hideyuki Matsushima, Takumi Tsuda, Hidehiko Hishikawa, Tadayoshi Okumura and Mitsugu Sekimoto

Chapter 15 **Acridine Orange: A Review of Novel Applications for Surgical Cancer Imaging and Therapy** 162
Vadim A. Byvaltsev, Liudmila A. Bardonova, Naomi R. Onaka, Roman A. Polkin, Sergey V. Ochkal, Valerij V. Shepelev, Marat A. Aliyev and Alexander A. Potapov

Chapter 16 **Application of Indocyanine Green During Arteriovenous Malformation Surgery: Evidence, Techniques and Practical Pearls** 169
Chase H. Foster, Peter J. Morone, Samuel B. Tomlinson and Aaron A. Cohen-Gadol

Chapter 17 **Efficacy of Indocyanine Green Fluorescence Angiography in Preventing Anastomotic Leakage After McKeown Minimally Invasive Esophagectomy** 177
Rao-Jun Luo, Zi-Yi Zhu, Zheng-Fu He, Yong Xu, Yun-Zheng Wang and Ping Chen

Chapter 18 **Applications of Microscope-Integrated Indocyanine Green Videoangiography in Cerebral Revascularization Procedures** 183
Claudio Cavallo, Sirin Gandhi, Xiaochun Zhao, Evgenii Belykh, Daniel Valli, Peter Nakaji, Mark C. Preul and Michael T. Lawton

Chapter 19 **Application of Fluorescein Fluorescence in Vascular Neurosurgery** 193
Xiaochun Zhao, Evgenii Belykh, Claudio Cavallo, Daniel Valli, Sirin Gandhi, Mark C. Preul, Peter Vajkoczy, Michael T. Lawton and Peter Nakaji

Chapter 20 **Optical Characterization of Sodium Fluorescein *In Vitro* and *Ex Vivo*** 205
Ran Xu, Wanda Teich, Florian Frenzel, Katrin Hoffmann, Josefine Radke, Judith Rösler, Katharina Faust, Anne Blank, Susan Brandenburg, Martin Misch, Peter Vajkoczy, Julia Sophie Onken and Ute Resch-Genger

Chapter 21 **Intraoperative Confocal Laser Endomicroscopy *Ex Vivo* Examination of Tissue Microstructure During Fluorescence-Guided Brain Tumor Surgery** 213
Evgenii Belykh, Xiaochun Zhao, Brandon Ngo, Dara S. Farhadi, Vadim A. Byvaltsev, Jennifer M. Eschbacher, Peter Nakaji and Mark C. Preul

Permissions

List of Contributors

Index

Preface

The world is advancing at a fast pace like never before. Therefore, the need is to keep up with the latest developments. This book was an idea that came to fruition when the specialists in the area realized the need to coordinate together and document essential themes in the subject. That's when I was requested to be the editor. Editing this book has been an honour as it brings together diverse authors researching on different streams of the field. The book collates essential materials contributed by veterans in the area which can be utilized by students and researchers alike.

Surgery is an important treatment option for cancer patients. Fluorescence-guided surgery (FGS) of cancer is an intraoperative medical technique that produces real time fluorescence image of the surgical region which helps the surgeons in performing the surgical procedure. Till now, various types of cancers such as head and neck cancer, breast cancer, lung cancer, esophagus cancer, hepatocellular carcinoma, gastric cancer, and melanoma have been treated with the help of FGS. Conventional imaging techniques such as CT and MRI are expensive and difficult and cannot be used at the time of surgery. On the other hand, FGS provides real-time imaging during surgery and it is less costly and easier to use. It is significant to achieve a negative tumor margin for a successful cancer resection as the presence of residual tumor cells after surgery may cause tumor recurrence that leads to poor prognosis. This book is compiled in such a manner, that it will provide an in-depth knowledge about the theory and practice of fluorescence-guided surgery of cancer. It aims to present researches that have transformed this discipline and have aided in its advancement. This book will help the readers in keeping pace with the rapid changes in this field.

Each chapter is a sole-standing publication that reflects each author´s interpretation. Thus, the book displays a multi-facetted picture of our current understanding of application, resources and aspects of the field. I would like to thank the contributors of this book and my family for their endless support.

Editor

1

Usefulness and Prospects of Sentinel Lymph Node Biopsy for Patients with Breast Cancer Using the Medical Imaging Projection System

Yuki Nakamura[1], *Masahiro Takada*[1*], *Michiko Imamura*[2], *Akane Higami*[1], *He Jiaxi*[1], *Makoto Fujino*[1], *Rie Nakagawa*[1], *Yukiko Inagaki*[1], *Yoshiaki Matsumoto*[1], *Kosuke Kawaguchi*[1], *Masahiro Kawashima*[1], *Eiji Suzuki*[1] *and Masakazu Toi*[1]

[1] *Department of Surgery (Breast Surgery), Kyoto University Hospital, Kyoto, Japan,* [2] *Department of Breast and Endocrine Surgery, Hyogo College of Medicine, Hyogo, Japan*

Correspondence:
Masahiro Takada
masahiro@kuhp.kyoto-u.ac.jp

Background: The Medical Imaging Projection System (MIPS) projects indocyanine green (ICG) fluorescence images directly on the surgical field using a projection mapping technique. We conducted an observational study of sentinel lymph node (SLN) biopsy using the prototype MIPS; we found a high identification rate. However, the number of SLN-positive cases was small, and the sensitivity could not be evaluated. The aim of this study was to investigate the clinical usefulness of the MIPS assisted ICG fluorescence method using commercially available equipment.

Methods: This was a retrospective observational study. Patients with primary breast cancer who underwent SLN biopsy using the MIPS at Kyoto University Hospital from April to December 2020 were included in the study. The primary endpoints were the identification rate of SLNs and detection of positive SLNs by the MIPS. The secondary endpoint was the number of SLNs excised using the MIPS per patient. We also conducted a questionnaire survey focused on the utility of the MIPS; it involved doctors with an experience in using the MIPS.

Results: Seventy-nine patients (84 procedures) were included in the study. In 60 (71%) procedures, both the radioisotope (RI) method and MIPS were used. At least one SLN could be detected by the MIPS in all the procedures, with an identification rate of 100% (95% confidence interval 95.6–100%). A total of 19 (7%) positive SLNs were removed, which were identifiable by the MIPS. Among 57 patients in whom the MIPS and RI methods were used, there was no positive SLN only identified by the RI method. The results of the questionnaire survey showed that the MIPS enabled the operator and assistant to share the ICG fluorescence image in the surgical field and to communicate with each other easily.

Conclusion: The current study demonstrated that the identification rate of SLNs using the MIPS was high, and the MIPS can be used for detecting positive SLNs. It was suggested that the MIPS will be useful in learning SLN biopsy procedures.

Keywords: breast cancer, sentinel lymph node biopsy, indocyanine green fluorescence method, projection mapping, identification rate

INTRODUCTION

Sentinel lymph node (SLN) biopsy is the standard of care for patients with clinically node-negative breast cancer. In addition to the radioisotope (RI) and blue dye methods, SLN identification with indocyanine green (ICG) fluorescence was first reported in 2005 (1). From a prior meta-analysis, the SLN identification rates using the ICG fluorescence method and RI method were similar (2).

The Medical Imaging Projection System (MIPS) is a novel near infrared (NIR) fluorescence imaging system that projects ICG fluorescence images directly on the surgical field using a projection mapping technique. The MIPS assisted ICG fluorescence method involves an accurate and continuous projection of ICG fluorescence signals, which enables a real-time navigation surgery for SLN biopsy without shifting the visual focus from the surgical field. It does not require operating lights. In 2018, we conducted an observational study of SLN biopsy using the prototype MIPS in 56 patients (59 procedures) at our institution; the identification rate was comparable to that obtained with the ICG fluorescence method using a conventional NIR system. However, the low percentage of patients with SLN metastasis led to insufficient evaluation of detection of positive SLNs by the MIPS (3).

The aim of this study was to assess SLN identification and detection of positive SLNs using the commercial-type MIPS. We also conducted a questionnaire survey on the utility of the MIPS.

PATIENTS AND METHODS

Patients

The eligibility criteria included: histologically confirmed breast cancer, clinically node-negative tumor, and patients who underwent SLN biopsy using the MIPS. Patients with a previous history of axillary surgery were excluded. Patients who received preoperative systemic therapy (PST) were included.

The study protocol was approved by the institutional review board of Kyoto University Hospital.

Methods

This was a retrospective observational study. Data on age, body mass index (BMI), tumor size, tumor histology, subtype, with or without PST, number of SLNs, and combined use of the RI method were extracted from the medical records. We also conducted a questionnaire survey involving doctors at Kyoto University Hospital and the Hospital of Hyogo College of Medicine with experience in using the MIPS.

Detailed features of MIPS and its surgical procedures have been reported previously (4). The commercial-type MIPS was used in this study, in which flexibility of the projection head was improved by introducing the same arm control technology as the surgical microscope; surgeons were able to adjust the projection angle freely during the procedures (**Figures 1** and **2**).

Endpoints

The primary endpoints included the identification rate of SLNs and detection of positive SLNs by the MIPS. The identification rate was calculated as the percentage of all patients in whom at least one SLN was detected using the MIPS. The detection of positive SLNs was evaluated using the percentage of positive SLNs among all the excised SLNs.

The secondary endpoints included: the number of SLNs excised by the MIPS per patient, relationship between clinical factors and number of detected SLNs, and the detection of SLNs by the MIPS and the RI method among patients after PST. All statistical analyses were performed using JMP® Pro (ver. 15.2.0; SAS Institute, Inc. Cary, NC, USA).

RESULTS

A total of 79 patients (74 and 5 with unilateral and bilateral tumors, respectively) underwent SLN biopsy using the MIPS from April to December 2020. The analysis was based on 84 procedures. The median age was 59 (range 35–84) years, and the median BMI was 21.1 (range 16.4–32.6) kg/m^2. More than half of the procedures were performed for T1 tumors (55%), and 15 (18%) procedures were performed for ductal carcinomas *in situ*. Of the 15 patients with DCIS, 13 patients underwent mastectomy and 2 patients were suspected of having invasive carcinoma by imaging findings. Of the 84 procedures, 11 (13%) were performed after PST and all of these patients were clinical node negative. The RI and MIPS methods were both used in 60 (71%) procedures of 57 patients (**Table 1**).

The identification rate of the MIPS was 100% (84/84: 95% confidence interval [CI] 95.6–100%). Macrometastases were found in 19 (7%) of the 256 SLNs, detected by the MIPS.

Of 185 SLNs excised among the patients who underwent SLN biopsy using both the MIPS and RI methods, 90 (49%) SLNs were identified by both the MIPS and RI methods, 91 (49%) only by the MIPS, 2 (1%) only by the RI method, and 2 (1%) by neither the MIPS nor RI method. The number of positive SLNs detected by both the MIPS and RI methods was 8, that only by the MIPS was 1, that only by the RI method and by neither the MIPS nor RI method were 0 (**Table 2**).

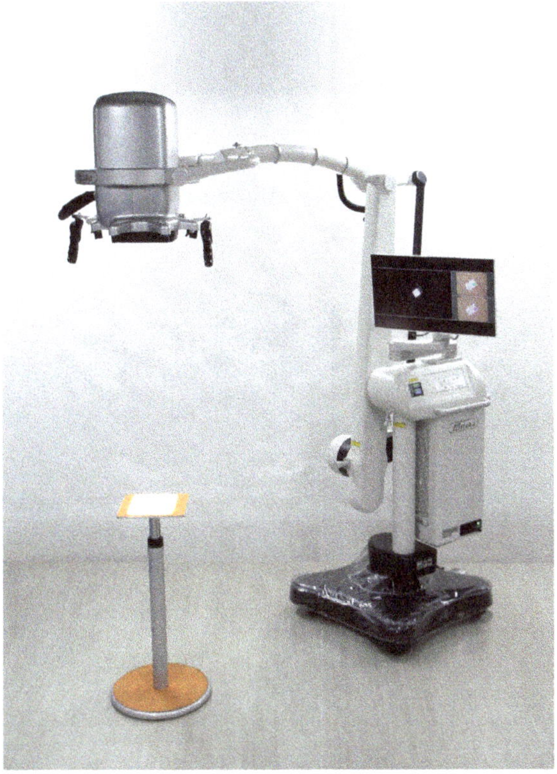

FIGURE 1 | The Medical Imaging Projection System (MIPS). Photograph of the commercial-type MIPS used in this study.

TABLE 1 | Patient and tumor characteristics.

Factors	N	%
All procedures	84	
Age, median (range)	59 (35–84)	
Body Mass Index, median (range)	21.1 (16.4-32.6)	
Tumor stage		
Tis	15	18
T1a	6	7
T1b	10	12
T1c	30	36
T2	21	25
T3	1	1
Histology		
Ductal Carcinoma in situ	15	18
Invasive carcinoma (no special type)	60	71
Invasive lobular carcinoma	5	6
Others	4	5
Subtype		
Hormone-receptor-positive and HER2-negative	53	63
Hormone-receptor-positive and HER2-positive	6	7
Hormone-receptor-negative and HER2-positive	2	2
Triple negative	8	10
Unknown	15	18
Histological grade		
1	16	19
2	30	36
3	23	27
Unknown	15	18
Preoperative systemic therapy		
Yes	11	13
No	73	87
Combined use of radioisotope method		
Yes	60	71
No	24	29

HER2, human epidermal growth factor receptor 2.

The median number of SLNs detected by the MIPS per patient was 3 (range, 1–6). The median number of SLNs identified by the MIPS among patients with a high BMI (≥ 22 kg/m^2) was almost equal to that of patients with a low BMI (<22 kg/m^2) (P = 0.09). Of the procedures performed after PST, the median number of SLNs identified by the MIPS was 3 (range, 2–5) (**Table 3**).

Among patients who underwent SLN biopsy after PST, the identification rate of the MIPS was 100% (95% CI 74.1-100%) and that of the RI method was 100% (95% CI 70.1-100%). The median number of SLNs identified by the RI method was 1 (range, 1-3). The number of positive SLNs was one, which was detected by both the MIPS and RI methods.

The results of the questionnaire survey are shown in **Table 4**. Regarding the clinical advantage of the MIPS, 69% of the doctors answered that operators could perform the procedures easily by confirming the ICG fluorescence image directly in the surgical field; 54% answered that operators could perform the procedures without disrupting the surgical workflow since the MIPS did not require operating lights during the procedures; 62% answered that operators could operate smoothly without holding the NIR camera, and 62% answered that both the operator and assistant could communicate with each other easily by sharing the ICG fluorescence image in the surgical field during the surgery. Regarding the relationship between the MIPS and procedure difficulty including duration of surgery, 38% of the doctors felt that the MIPS led to a shorter duration of surgery, 31% did not feel so, and 31% were indifferent.

DISCUSSION

The current study showed the reproducibility of the MIPS for SLN identification and the feasibility of detection of positive SLNs by the MIPS.

It has been reported that the SLN identification rate ranged from 89–100%, and the mean number of removed SLNs was 1.5–3.4, using the ICG fluorescence method (2). In the current study, the SLN identification rate was 100% (95% CI: 95.6–100%), and the median number of SLNs detected by MIPS was 3 (range 1–6), and our results were comparable to those of the ICG fluorescence method using a conventional NIR system.

In this study, 17% of the patients had positive SLNs, which was higher than that in our previous study; however, it was lower than those in previous reports (5). Preoperative examination of axillary lymph nodes in our institution includes palpation, ultrasonography, and contrast-enhanced magnetic resonance imaging (CE-MRI). If nodal involvement is suspected, ultrasound-guided fine-needle aspiration biopsy (US-FNA) is also performed. CE-MRI and US-FNA increase the accuracy of

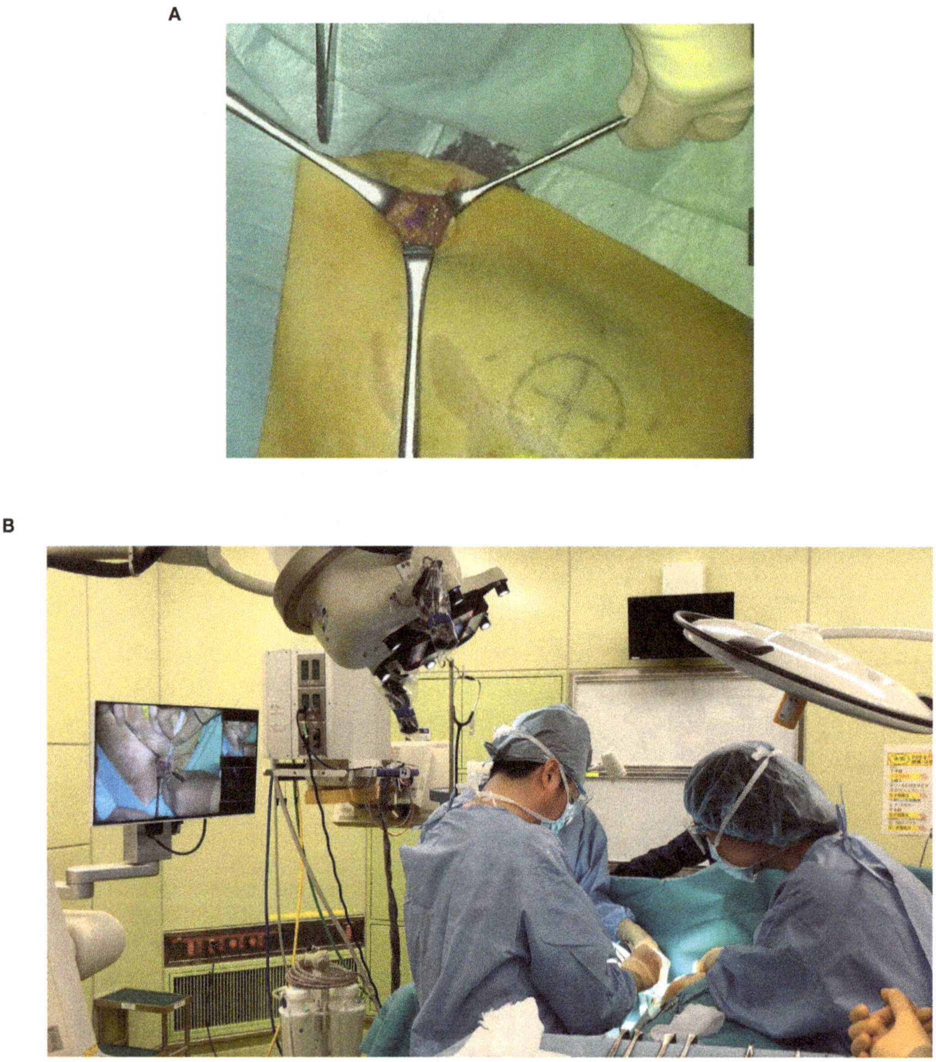

FIGURE 2 | Intraoperative photograph of using the MIPS. **(A)** Operator can confirm the ICG fluorescence image directly in the surgical field. **(B)** Both the operator and assistant can share the ICG fluorescence image in the surgical field.

TABLE 2 | The number of SLNs among cases using MIPS and RI.

SLN biopsy procedures	Identified SLNs (total N=185)	Positive SLNs (total N=9)
MIPS and RI	90	8
MIPS only	91	1
RI only	2	0
Neither MIPS nor RI (Palpation)	2	0

SLN, sentinel lymph node; MIPS, medical imaging projection system; RI, radioisotope.

TABLE 3 | Number of SLNs identified by the MIPS according to patient characteristics.

Characteristics	N	Median	Range	P value
All procedures	84	3	1-6	
BMI				
<22 kg/m^2	46	3	1-6	0.09
≧22 kg/m^2	38	2.5	1-5	
PST				
Yes	11	3	2-5	0.75
No	73	3	1-6	

SLN, sentinel lymph node; BMI, body mass index; PST, preoperative systemic therapy.

preoperative axillary staging (4, 6); the involvement of these examinations may have contributed to the low proportion of positive SLNs in our study. In this study, there was no positive SLN that was identified only by the RI method, and the MIPS identified all the positive SLNs in the patients in whom both the RI method and the MIPS were used. It is suggested that the detection of positive SLNs by the MIPS is comparable to detection by the RI method.

TABLE 4 | Results of the questionnaire survey for doctors with an experience in using MIPS.

Questionnaire survey	Number of 'yes'	% (total 13)
Which do you consider to be a clinical advantage of MIPS?		
Operators can perform the procedures easily by confirming the ICG fluorescence image directly in the surgical field.	9	69
Operators can perform the surgery without disruption of the surgical workflow since MIPS does not require operating lights.	7	54
Operators can operate smoothly without holding the NIR camera.	8	62
The operator and assistant can communicate with each other easily due to the possibility of sharing the ICG fluorescence image.	8	62
Do you feel the MIPS leads to shorter surgery duration?		
Yes	5	38
No	4	31
Neither	4	31

MIPS, medical imaging system projection system; ICG, indocyanine green.

It has been reported that the number of detected SLNs decreases as the BMI increases (7). However, in our study, the number of SLNs excised from patients with a high BMI was almost equal to that from patients with a low BMI. The MIPS may be useful in identifying SLNs among patients with a high BMI. We used BMI 22 as cutoff value, following the domestic standard value in Japan. There was no statistically significant difference in the number of sentinel lymph node identified, when we used the cutoff value of 25, 28 and 30 (p value 0.33, 0.75 and 0.62, respectively).

SLN biopsy after PST is feasible for patients with clinically node-negative cancer at baseline (8, 9). However, SLN biopsy after PST for patients with clinically node-positive cancer has a low identification rate and a high false-negative rate (10–12). Removal of three or more SLNs has been reported to reduce the false-negative rate to below 10% in patients with clinically node-positive cancer (13). In the present study, SLN biopsies after PST were performed in 11 (13%) procedures. Although this is a small number of cases, the identification rate by the MIPS among them was 100% (95% CI 74.1–100%), and the median number of excised SLNs was 3 (range 2–5).

The main clinical advantage of the MIPS is the ease of communication between the operator and assistant due to the possibility of sharing the ICG fluorescence image in the surgical field. From the results of the questionnaire survey, more than half of the doctors confirmed this advantage. The percentage of doctors who considered the communication between operator and assistant as a clinical advantage of the MIPS was 100%, 25%, and 67% among doctors who graduated ≤5 years, 6–10 years, and ≥11 years prior to the procedures. This tendency indicated that the communication between the operator and assistant would be useful in teaching the procedures to doctors willing to learn. We also expected a shorter duration of surgery with the MIPS, but the percentage of doctors who felt that using the MIPS shortened the duration of surgery was only 38%.

There are several limitations to the present study. First, our sample size was relatively small; however, it did not hinder the clinical utility of the MIPS, as shown by the lower limit of the 95% CIs, which was above 90%. Second, the retrospective nature of the study; however, our results were comparable to those of our previous prospective observational study. Third, the small number of SLN biopsies after PST; we need to investigate the utility of the MIPS in more cases after PST. Forth, the evaluation of the MIPS in learning procedures was not objective; we need to evaluate the learning curve of SLN biopsy procedures using the MIPS.

In conclusion, this study demonstrated that the identification rate of SLNs using the MIPS was high and the MIPS can be used for the detection of positive SLNs. The MIPS enabled an ease of communication between the operator and assistant. It was suggested that this advantage of the MIPS will be useful in learning SLN biopsy procedures.

ETHICS STATEMENT

The studies involving human participants were reviewed and approved by Kyoto University Graduate School and Faculty of Medicine, Ethics Committee. Written informed consent for participation was not required for this study in accordance with the national legislation and the institutional requirements.

AUTHOR CONTRIBUTIONS

YN contributed to data collection and analysis and wrote this manuscript. MTa made important corrections to the manuscript. MI, AH, HJ, MF, RN, YI, YM, KK, MK, ES, and MTo answered the questionnaire survey and checked the final version of the manuscript. All authors contributed to the article and approved the submitted version.

ACKNOWLEDGMENTS

The authors thank doctors of Department of Breast and Endocrine Surgery of Hyogo College of Medicine for answering the questionnaire survey.

REFERENCES

1. Kitai T, Inomoto T, Miwa M, Shikayama T. Fluorescence Navigation With Indocyanine Green for Detecting Sentinel Lymph Nodes in Breast Cancer. *Breast Cancer* (2005) 12:211–5. doi: 10.2325/jbcs.12.211
2. Sugie T, Ikeda T, Kawaguchi A, Shimizu A, Toi M. Sentinel Lymph Node Biopsy Using Indocyanine Green Fluorescence in Early-Stage Breast Cancer: A Meta-

Analysis. *Int J Clin Oncol* (2017) 22:11–7. doi: 10.1007/s10147-016-1064-z
3. Takada M, Takeuchi M, Suzuki E, Sato F, Matsumoto Y, Torii M, et al. Real-Time Navigation System for Sentinel Lymph Node Biopsy in Breast Cancer Patients Using Projection Mapping With Indocyanine Green Fluorescence. *Breast Cancer* (2018) 25:650–5. doi: 10.1007/s12282-018-0868-2
4. Houssami N, Ciatto S, Turner RM, Cody HS III, Macaskill P. Preoperative Ultrasound-Guided Needle Biopsy of Axillary Nodes in Invasive Breast Cancer: Meta-Analysis of its Accuracy and Utility in Staging the Axilla. *Ann Surg* (2011) 254:243–51. doi: 10.1097/SLA.0b013e31821f1564
5. Krag DN, Anderson SJ, Julian TB, Brown AM, Harlow SP, Ashikaga T, et al. Technical Outcomes of Sentinel-Lymph-Node Resection and Conventional Axillary-Lymph-Node Dissection in Patients With Clinically Node-Negative Breast Cancer: Results From the NSABP B-32 Randomised Phase III Trial. *Lancet Oncol* (2007) 8:881–8. doi: 10.1016/S1470-2045(10)70207-2
6. Liang X, Yu J, Wen B, Xie J, Cai Q, Yang Q. MRI and FDG-PET/CT Based Assessment of Axillary Lymph Node Metastasis in Early Breast Cancer: A Meta-Analysis. *Clin Radiol* (2017) 72:295–301. doi: 10.1016/j.crad.2016.12.001
7. Goyal A, Newcombe RG, Chhabra A, Mansel REALMANAC Trialists Group. Group at. Factors Affecting Failed Localisation and False-Negative Rates of Sentinel Node Biopsy in Breast Cancer—Results of the ALMANAC Validation Phase. *Breast Cancer Res Treat* (2006) 99:203–8. doi: 10.1007/s10549-006-9192-1
8. Classe JM, Bordes V, Campion L, Mignotte H, Dravet F, Leveque J, et al. Sentinel Lymph Node Biopsy After Neoadjuvant Chemotherapy for Advanced Breast Cancer: Results of Ganglion Sentinelle Et Chimiotherapie Neoadjuvante, a French Prospective Multicentric Study. *J Clin Oncol* (2009) 27:726–32. doi: 10.1200/JCO.2008.18.3228
9. van Deurzen CH, Vriens BE, Tjan-Heijnen VC, van der Wall E, Albregts M, van Hilligersberg R, et al. Accuracy of Sentinel Node Biopsy After Neoadjuvant Chemotherapy in Breast Cancer Patients: A Systematic Review. *Eur J Cancer* (2009) 45:3124–30. doi: 10.1016/j.ejca.2009.08.001
10. Boughey JC, Suman VJ, Mittendorf EA, Aherndt GM, Wilke LG, Taback B, et al. Sentinel Lymph Node Surgery After Neoadjuvant Chemotherapy in Breast Cancer Patients: A Systematic Review. *Eur J Cancer* (2009) 45:3124–30. doi: 10.1016/j.ejca.2009.08.001
11. Boileau JF, Poirier B, Basik M, Holloway CM, Gaboury L, Sideris L, et al. Sentinel Node Biopsy After Neoadjuvant Chemotherapy in Biopsy-Proven Node-Positive Breast Cancer: The SN FNAC Study. *J Clin Oncol* (2015) 33:258–64. doi: 10.1200/JCO.2014.55.7827
12. Kuehn T, Bauerfeind I, Fehm T, Fleige B, Hausschild M, Helms G, et al. Sentinel-Lymph-Node Biopsy in Patients With Breast Cancer Before and After Neoadjuvant Chemotherapy (SENTINA): A Prospective, Multicentre Cohort Study. *Lancet Oncol* (2013) 14:609–18. doi: 10.1016/S1470-2045(13)70166-9
13. El Hage Chehade H, Headon H, El Tokhy O, Heeney J, Kasem A, Mokbel K. Is Sentinel Lymph Node Biopsy a Viable Alternative to Complete Axillary Dissection Following Neoadjuvant Chemotherapy in Women With Node-Positive Breast Cancer at Diagnosis? Updated Meta-Analysis Involving 3,398 Patients. *Am J Surg* (2016) 212:969–81. doi: 10.1016/j.amjsurg.2016.07.018

2

5-Aminolevulinic Acid Multispectral Imaging for the Fluorescence-Guided Resection of Brain Tumors

Patra Charalampaki [1,2†], Phileas Johannes Proskynitopoulos [1†], Axel Heimann [3] and Makoto Nakamura [1,2]*

[1] *Department of Neurosurgery, Cologne Medical Center, Cologne, Germany,* [2] *Witten-Herdecke University, Witten, Germany,* [3] *Institute for Neurosurgical Pathophysiology, Medical University Mainz, Mainz, Germany*

Correspondence:
Patra Charalampaki
charalampaki@yahoo.de

† *These authors have contributed equally to this work*

Fluorescence-guided surgery with five-aminolevulinic acid (5-ALA) is the state-of-the-art treatment of high-grade gliomas. However, intraoperative visualization of 5-ALA under blue light remains challenging, especially when blood covers the surgical field and thereby fluorescence. To overcome this problem and combine the brightness of visible light with the information delivered with fluorescence, we implemented multispectral fluorescence (MFL) in a surgical microscope, a technique that is able to project both information in real-time. We prospectively examined 25 patients with brain tumors. One patient was operated on two different lesions in the same setting. The tumors comprised: six glioblastomas, four anaplastic astrocytomas, one anaplastic oligodendroglioma, two meningiomas, 11 metastatic tumors, one acoustic neuroma, and one ependymoma. The MFL technique with a real-time overlay of fluorescence and white light was compared intraoperatively to the classic blue filter. All lesions were clearly visible and highlighted from the surrounding tissue. The pseudocolor we chose was green, representing fluorescence, with the surrounding brain tissue remaining in its original color. When blood was covering the surgical field, orientation was easy to maintain. The MFL technique opens the way for precise and clear visualization of fluorescence in real-time under white light. It can be easily used for the resection of all tumors accumulating 5-ALA. Drawbacks of classic PpIX fluorescence such as hidden fluorescence, intraoperative changes could be overcome with the presence of additional white light in MFL technique.

Keywords: brain tumor, 5-ALA = 5-aminolevulinic acid, microscopic surgery, neurological surgery, fluorescence guided surgery

INTRODUCTION

Malignant brain tumors and especially high-grade gliomas (HGG) are characterized by their aggressiveness and incurability. An influential phase III trial was able to show that mean survival of patients diagnosed with glioblastoma (GBM) is only 14.6 months when treated with radiotherapy and temozolomide (1) and that a mere 9.8% survived for 5 years (2). Apart from the use of radio- and chemotherapy, survival, neurological function, and the patients' quality of life highly depend on the extent and safety of neurosurgical resection (3, 4).

For the neurosurgical treatment of HGG, total resection of the tumor while not causing new neurological deficits is the primary goal (4, 5). For this matter, the use of five-aminolevulinic acid (5-ALA) (6) in fluorescence-guided surgery (FGS) has significantly improved HGG therapy (7).

Since the first observational study of 5-ALA fluorescence-guided surgery for the resection of HGG (8) followed by a promising prospective study (9), a prospective phase III trial was able to show that its use significantly improved progression-free survival with 41% in the 5-ALA and 21.1% in the white light group at 6 months (10). Furthermore, 5-ALA has also been **used** for the visualization of other entities like meningiomas and/or metastases, although more appealing and strong evidence for its use in these lesions is needed (11, 12).

Nonetheless, some disadvantages exist. Blue light is used for excitation of the protoporphyrin IX (PpIX) fluorescence and is strongly absorbed by blood cells, as it has a strong attenuation to hemoglobin (6, 13). Even a single layer of erythrocytes can absorb the light and make the underlying PpIX fluorescence invisible to the surgeon. In the literature, this fact is described as a minor problem during surgery when continuous rinsing is applied (6). However, at final inspection of the surgical cavity, coagulated blood can easily masque malignant tumor tissue (6, 14). Hence, the surgeon needs to repeatedly switch between white and blue light in order to both detect bleeding sites and remove the tumor. Furthermore, if blood is lying above the tissue the view under blue light becomes dark and it gets more difficult to remove any blood or remaining tumor. If one does so, there is a high risk of destroying more vulnerable blood vessels existing in malignant tumor tissue when trying to treat bleeding with coagulation. Also, it is easier and more intuitive for the surgeon to pay attention to the total visual field under white light as opposed to blue light. Apart from that, there is an ergonomic problem when it is essential to repeatedly switch between white and blue light especially if heavy bleeding occurs. Hence, one could argue that it would be necessary to combine the advantages of both white and blue light in the setting of brain surgery with 5-ALA in order to diminish their disadvantages.

To do so, the multispectral fluorescence microscopy (MFL) was incorporated into a commercially available microscope (ARveo, Leica Microsystems, Wetzlar, Germany). We have already investigated its use for the combination of indocyanine green (ICG) fluorescence and white light images in the therapy of vascular anomalies of the brain in both an animal model, and on a human cadaver model as well as in clinical use for vascular and tumor applications (15–17). Such a microscope also allows simultaneous visualization of PpIX fluorescence and white light. After merging, this combined image is then delivered via the ocular and shows both the fluorescent properties of the inspected field and the anatomical details as visualized under white light (13, 17).

To the best of our knowledge, no other observational study has used MFL for the intraoperative visualization of brain tumors accumulated with PpIX fluorescence. As the MFL mode uses the information obtained from the blue light image, we hypothesized that the intraoperative assessment of the fluorescence quality and contrasts in the MFL mode would match the fluorescence under blue light. Thus, outcome parameters of this study were the matching information of both fluorescent pictures and intraoperative usability of the MFL mode when assessing and resecting a brain tumor. With this study, we want to get first insights into the use of MFL as a possible tool that could diminish the technological and ergonomical disadvantages of the visualization of PpIX fluorescence under blue light for fluorescence-guided surgery of brain tumors.

MATERIALS AND METHODS

The present study was approved by the ethics committee of the University of Witten/Herdecke, Germany (Nr: 35/2017). All patients participating in this prospective observational study gave written informed consent and were recruited in the Department of Neurosurgery of the Cologne Medical Center, Cologne, Germany. The follow-up was performed in the usual manner for every patient that is treated because of a brain tumor in our clinic.

Inclusion criteria for this study were:

- Primary or secondary brain tumor on an MRI, regardless of WHO grading
- no contraindication for the administration of 5-ALA
- histopathological confirmation of a brain tumor (primary and secondary)
- Written informed consent
- Age 18–75 years although we included also elderly patients if the Karnofsky index higher than 80%.

Exclusion criteria were:

- Severe comorbid diseases that could negatively influence the participation in this study
- Therapeutically uncontrollable arterial hypertension (i.e., systolic pressure above 200 mmHg and diastolic pressure above 120 mmHg)
- Lung diseases that are related to complications during narcosis and anesthesia (such as cystic fibrosis, alpha-1-antitrypsin-deficiency, sarcoidosis, allergic alveolitis, tuberculosis, etc.)
- Patient that received an attenuated vaccine 14 days or the influenza vaccination 7 days prior to their participation in this study
- All comorbid diseases that could influence the participation in this study.

In total, we examined 25 patients (11 women and 14 men) that were operated over the course of 22 months (**Table 1**) between 2018 and 2019. A total of 26 lesions were extirpated and assessed with the novel technique (one patient was operated on two different regions and had two different craniotomies in the same setting). The average age at operation was 62.29 years. The underlying diagnoses that we summarized as HGG were glioblastoma ($n = 6$), anaplastic astrocytoma ($n = 4$), and anaplastic oligodendroglioma ($n = 1$). Apart from that, we investigated the off-label use of 5-ALA in metastases from bronchial carcinoma ($n = 5$), metastasis from colon carcinoma ($n = 3$), metastases from breast carcinoma ($n = 1$), meningioma ($n = 2$), ependymoma (WHO grade II, $n = 1$), acoustic neurinoma

TABLE 1 | List of patients operated on with the additional use of the MFL-technique.

Patient-Nr.	Gender	Age at operation	Tumor entity	Tumor location	Primary tumor or mutation status	Fluorescence quality	Postoperative new neurological deficit	MRI- contrast enhanced resection
1	F	71	Metastasis	Left parietal	Adeno-ca lung	Capsule intensive, content barely	None	Complete
2	F	59	Metastasis	Right temporal	Sigma-ca GI tract	Very intensive	None	Complete
			Metastasis	Right parietal	Sigma-ca GI tract	Very intensive	None	Complete
3	F	83	Metastasis	Right cerebellar	Adeno-ca lung	Intensive but inhomogeneous	None	Complete
4	M	63	Metastasis	Right parietal	Large cell ca lung	Very intensive	None	Complete
5	M	41	Anaplastic Astrocytoma	Right parietal	IDH-mutate, MGMT +	Very intensive	None	Minimal rest near postcentral
6	F	72	GBM cystic	Right temporal	IDH-mutate, MGMT +	Cyst very intensive, content barely	None	Minimal ependymal rest around the ventricle wall
7	F	75	Meningioma WHO I	Left frontal		Very intensive	None	Complete
8	M	50	Anaplastic Oligodendroglioma	Right frontal	MGMT +	Very intensive	None	Complete
9	M	56	Metastasis	Right frontal	Adeno-ca lung	Very intensive	None	Complete
10	M	53	GBM	Right temporal	IDH-wild type, MGMT +	Very intensive	None	Complete
11	M	77	Metastasis	Right frontal	Sigma-ca GI tract	Very intensive	None	Complete
12	F	77	Meningioma WHO I	Right parietal		Very intensive	None	Complete
13	F	51	Acoustic Neuroma	Right cerebelo-pontine angle		Intensive but inhomogeneous	Hypakusis	Complete
14	M	73	GBM	Right frontal	MGMT –	Very intensive	None	Complete
15	M	62	GBM	Right parieto-occipital	IDH-wild type, MGMT –	Very intensive	None	Minimal rest in the calcarine sulcus
16	M	44	Anaplastic Astrocytoma	Left trigonum, thalamus, midbrain	IDH-wild type, MGMT –	Very intensive	None	Incomplete resection due to midbrain thalamus infiltration
17	M	63	Metastasis	4th ventricle	Adeno-ca lung	Very intensive	Diziness	Complete
18	M	73	GBM	right frontal	IDH-wild type, MGMT –	Very intensive	None	No MRI postop
19	M	50	Ependymoma WHO II	4th ventricle		Very intensive	None	Complete
20	M	51	Metastasis	Spinal	Myxoid liposarcoma	Intensive but inhomogeneous	None	Complete
21	F	78	Metastasis	Left temporal	Squamous tongue ca	Very intensive	None	Complete
22	F	32	Anaplastic Astrocytoma	Left frontal precentral	IDH-mutate, MGMT +	Very intensive	None	Complete
23	M	65	Anaplastic Astrocytoma	Left frontal precentral	IDH-mutate, MGMT +	Very intensive	None awake surgery	Complete
24	F	76	GBM	Right frontal precentral	IDH-wild type, MGMT +	Very intensive	Hemiparesis arm 4/5	Minimal rest precentral, intraoperative monitoring + + +
25	F	63	Metastasis	Right frontal	Breast-ca	Very intensive	None	Complete

Ca = Carcinoma, GBM = Glioblastoma, GI = gastrointestinal, IDH = isocitrate dehydrogenase, M = male, MGMT = O^6-methylguanine DNA methyltransferase, F = female.
In patient number 2, two different craniotomies had to be performed as the tumor was metastasized into both the temporal and parietal lobe. Patient 10 in this table is described in case vignette #1, patient 23 in case vignette #2 and patient 21 in case vignette #3.

($n = 1$), metastasis from a myxoid liposarcoma ($n = 1$), and metastasis from tongue carcinoma ($n = 1$) (**Table 1**).

All patients received an oral dosage of 20 mg 5-ALA per kilogram body weight at least 3 h before the surgical procedure. Post-operatively, all patients were treated on the operative intensive care unit of our clinic before being moved to the general ward and kept in an area with low light exposition due to the phototoxic properties of 5-ALA.

Technical Considerations

The MFL system, mounted on a conventional microscope (ARveo, Leica Microsystems, Wetzlar, Germany), consists out of a fluorescence excitation filter covering the absorption spectrum of PpIX in broad range around 405 nm, but blocking the PpIX emission peak at 635 nm to acquire the red fluorescence signal with a separate fluorescence camera. The PpIX fluorescence signal is processed into a pseudo color image with high contrast to the operative field (e.g., green) and transparently overlaid to the stereoscopic, optical view in the eyepieces (Leica Captiview). In addition, the pseudo color fluorescence image can be recorded and observed as embedded information in the white light image on the monitor. The microscope control allowed switching directly from white to blue light or MFL mode or from blue light to MFL mode and vice versa for surgical workflow support and comparison purposes.

Operative Procedure

Following the craniotomy, we continued with a sharp surgical incision of the dura mater. Once the brain parenchyma was visualized macroscopically, we started to continue the procedure under the operation microscope (ARveo, Leica microsystems, Wetzlar Germany). If according to the MRI and intraoperative neuronavigation (Stealth Station, Medtronic, USA) the lesion was on the surface of the brain we continued under blue light in order to assess PpIX fluorescence and coherently visualize and identify the tumor. If the tumor was exposed, we changed to MFL-mode and observed the operation field and evaluated if the fused MFL image matched the different properties of the white light and blue light images. In tumors lying more deeply in the brain parenchyma we first operated under white light until the lesion was exposed. Then, we continued in the same fashion as described before.

When we suspected slight bleeding inside the surgical field during resection under blue light we changed to white light and assessed bleeding. After that, we turned to the MFL-mode in order to evaluate both the fluorescent properties of the tumor tissue and the bleeding. To achieve hemostasis, we switched back to white light. We evaluated the surgical field in the MFL-mode only in the case of slight bleedings that masked the fluorescence under blue light in order to not jeopardize the patient. Larger bleedings were immediately treated under white light. We repeated this procedure in the cases where small bleedings occurred while meticulously resecting the lesion under blue light.

During final inspection of the cavity under blue light we changed to white light to do a final assessment of coagulated blood or small bleeding that both could conceal tumor tissue. Then we switched to the MFL-mode to assess if the bleeding sites were matching the ones identified under white light. After that, we turned to blue light again. If any previously masked lesions were then identified we resected them accordingly until no fluorescent tissue was visible. Following the final inspection, we continued with sufficient hemostasis and closure of the surgical wound under white light. At the end of the operation, we assessed the resected tumor *ex vivo* under blue light and then changed to MFL-mode for the assessment of its fluorescent properties and if the characteristics of both images match. After each operation, the operating surgeon (CC) assessed the raw data (green fluorescence in a black picture, similar to what one sees when using the blue light in the classical way), which is calculated based upon the blue light fluorescence data. This was then compared to the MFL picture regarding matching fluorescence areas and shades.

RESULTS

As the software was installed in a surgical microscope the operative use of the MFL technique was easy to implement in the clinical setting. To correlate the overlay of fluorescence between the traditional blue light mode and the MFL mode the surgeon did an intraoperative assessment. Before switching to the MFL mode, the PpIX fluorescence under blue light was assessed for correspondence to the MFL picture.

In all 26 surgeries, we were able to correlate the pink fluorescence under blue light with the "green" fluorescence in the MFL-mode. The intensity of the green indicated fluorescence was always similar to the intensity of pink seen under blue light. In contrast to the conventional blue mode, under the MFL mode bleeding did not cause any problem as the sources of bleeding were immediately identifiable and were treated accordingly. Thus, periodic switching back to the white light was not necessary during the resection under the MFL fluorescence mode, which facilitated resection and surgical convenience especially in the situations that were ergonomically or surgically challenging (such as when larger bleedings occurred or at the final inspection).

Postoperatively, we reviewed the raw fluorescence signal video recordings and MFL video. Again, the perceived intensities and locations of pseudo colored green fluorescence overlay in the MFL mode corresponded perfectly with the single channel fluorescence recordings in all 26 surgeries. There was no instance when the natural color of the surgical field of view, reflections from the brain tissue or cerebrospinal fluid would impede fluorescence overlay visualization or create a false positive pseudocolored green fluorescence overlay.

In three cases, PpIX fluorescence using the MFL technique was intensive but inhomogeneous (see **Table 1**). In one metastasis from a bronchial carcinoma, the capsule fluorescence was very intense while its content lacked fluorescent intensity. In one GBM case, the cyst capsule displayed a strong fluorescent while the content only slightly fluoresced. In the remaining 20/25, the fluorescence quality was very intensive, while different shades of fluorescence were observed depending on the tumor site, i.e., center vs. periphery. The quality of the fluorescence signal displayed in the MFL mode was subjectively similar to the fluorescence under blue light using the traditional filter. Hence the different fluorescent shades representing different tumor areas were displayed correctly (**Supplementary Video 1**). This is the case because the data used to generate the MFL picture is taken from the visual information under blue light while simultaneously combining this information with the white light picture.

In 3/25 cases a new neurological deficit was found after the procedure. One patient was operated during awake surgery. In one patient, the intraoperative monitoring was positive and thus the surgeon decided to leave a minimal tumor residual in the precentral region. This patient then presented with a new hemiparesis of the left arm (muscle strength 4/5).

Regarding the degree of resection, postoperative MRI confirmed complete resection in 20/26 lesions. The extent of resection was determined using postoperative T1 weighted MRI scans with contrast. Those were compared with the preoperative MRI scans for residual contrast enhancement. In five lesions, a minimal residual was still present on the MRI. For one patient no postoperative imaging study was available.

Case 1: Glioblastoma (Figure 1)

A 53-year-old male reported to our clinic with persisting headaches, amnesia, concentration deficits, confusion, and coordination deficits on the left side. This was accompanied by a tendency to fall to the left and insecure gait. The initial CT scan obtained showed a lesion in the right temporal-parietal region with significant surrounding edema. The cranial MRI scan revealed a lesion highly suspicious for GBM. We, therefore, scheduled the patient for the resection of the lesion. Prior to the intervention the patient received 20 mg per kilogram bodyweight of 5-ALA. Microsurgical resection of the tumor was performed with the modified microscope and concurring sonographic navigation and neuronavigation. The use of the MFL mode showed a coherent fusion of both white light and blue light images of the highly fluorescent tumor tissue and allowed for easy assessment of any bleedings occurring throughout resection. A tissue sample of the resected tumor was sent to the affiliated department of neuropathology and revealed a GBM. After the operation at the final neurological examination the patient presented himself with no neurological deficits and was totally mobile. Postoperative MRI showed a complete resection of the tumor.

Supplementary File shows a short segment of the operation of this patient.

Case 2: Anaplastic Astrocytoma WHO Grade III (Figure 2)

A 65-year-old male initially presented himself with temporary hemiparesis of the right side accompanied by nausea. An initial MRI showed a hyperintense lesion on T2 in the left medial cingulate gyrus. We scheduled the patient for a biopsy of the lesion, which revealed an anaplastic astrocytoma (IDH-mutation, MGMT+, WHO grade III). After being discharged to his home prior to the elective surgery the patient presented himself through our emergency room with focal epileptic seizures of the right leg, namely the thigh region, causing local pain and cramps. We then decided to resect the lesion as soon as possible. Prior to the intervention the patient received 20 mg per kilogram bodyweight of 5-ALA. We planned neurophysiological monitoring of the right arm and leg during the operation to secure neurological function of the nearby supplementary motoric cortex. Microsurgical resection of the tumor was performed following by neurophysiological monitoring and neuronavigation. After the lesion was identified in the depth of the longitudinal fissure the use of the MFL mode showed a coherent fusion of both the white light and blue light images of the highly fluorescent tumor tissue and was able to assess bleedings occurring throughout resection. The resection was finished without any complications. After the operation, neurological examination revealed a light right leg hemiparesis, which was in remission on the day of discharge. Postoperative MRI showed a complete resection of the tumor.

Case 3: Metastases From a Squamous Carcinoma of the Tongue (Figure 3)

A 78-year-old female suffering from a known squamous carcinoma of the tongue came via the emergency room of our clinic because of a decline in her general condition accompanied by confusion and dizziness for the previous 3 weeks. The conducted MRI showed a necrotic and cystic lesion in the left temporal region with a midline shift. We, therefore, planned resection of the symptomatic temporal lesion. A CT scan obtained for disease staging showed several pulmonary lesions and potential lymph node metastases in the mediastinum as well as a lesion in the left gluteal region and inguinal lymph nodes, all highly suspicious of metastases. The patient received 5-ALA. The use of the MFL mode showed a coherent fusion of both the white light and blue light images of the highly fluorescent metastatic lesion tissue and was able to assess bleedings occurring throughout resection. The resection was finished without any complications and at the end no fluorescence was detected. The histological diagnosis revealed metastatic cells of the squamous carcinoma of the tongue. Postoperative MRI showed a complete resection of the tumor.

DISCUSSION

Even though the use of 5-ALA in neurosurgical patients was reported for the first time almost 20 years ago, fluorescence-guided surgery is, on the one hand, standard of care for brain tumor surgery, while on the other hand, still a developing field, especially in the improvement of fluorescence visibility from the technical point of view. This is highlighted by the fact that 5-ALA has only recently been approved by the FDA (18) and that it is currently used mainly for resection of HGG. Although 5-ALA has improved the outcomes of oncological neurosurgery, it comes with several technical disadvantages that need to be overcome.

To the best of our knowledge, the present observational study is the first investigation that describes a promising new technique that could help to improve PpIX fluorescence-guided tumor surgery while being easy to implement in the operation

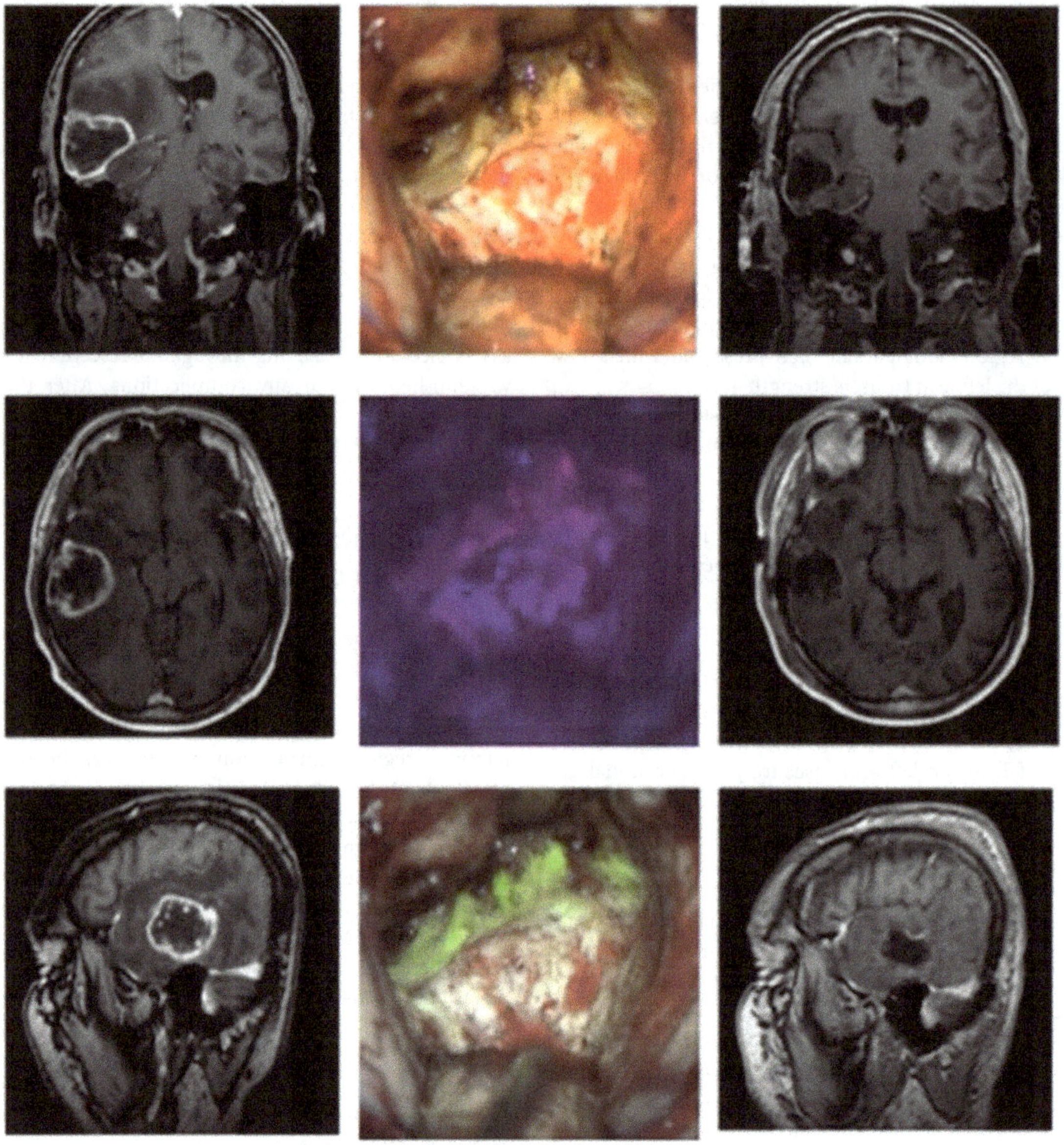

FIGURE 1 | Glioblastoma in a 53-year-old patient. The left column shows the MRI images (T1 weighted with contrast, from top to bottom: coronary, axial, sagittal) before the operation, the right column the postoperative MRI. In the middle column, the top picture shows the surgical field under white light, below it under blue light, and at the bottom the fusion of both images in the MFL-mode.

room. As hypothesized, intraoperative blue light images matched the MFL images while the new visualization technique did not violate operation ergonomics. On the contrary, as we have shown in **Supplementary Video 1**, drawbacks of the traditional blue filter such as blood covering the surgical field were more easily controllable. As we have illustrated in great detail through our small sample and the three illustrative cases, the MFL technique is able to visualize and combine both the picture generated under blue light as well as the white light picture in real-time. Thereby it enables the surgeon to assess the tumor and the surrounding neuroanatomy under white light. Through this, the ergonomic problem of switching between the different light modes and the need to continuously rinse the operation in order to prevent slight bleeding from covering the operation site could be solved. Most importantly, the ability to assess bleeding sites while also operating tumor tissue enables the surgeon to identify regions in real-time that could masque tumor tissue when blood coagulation has happened. Apart from that, learning to resect tumors in this augmented reality setting could prove to be more intuitive as opposed to the traditional way under blue light.

Furthermore, previously to this study we made the observation that this mode is able to sufficiently differentiate

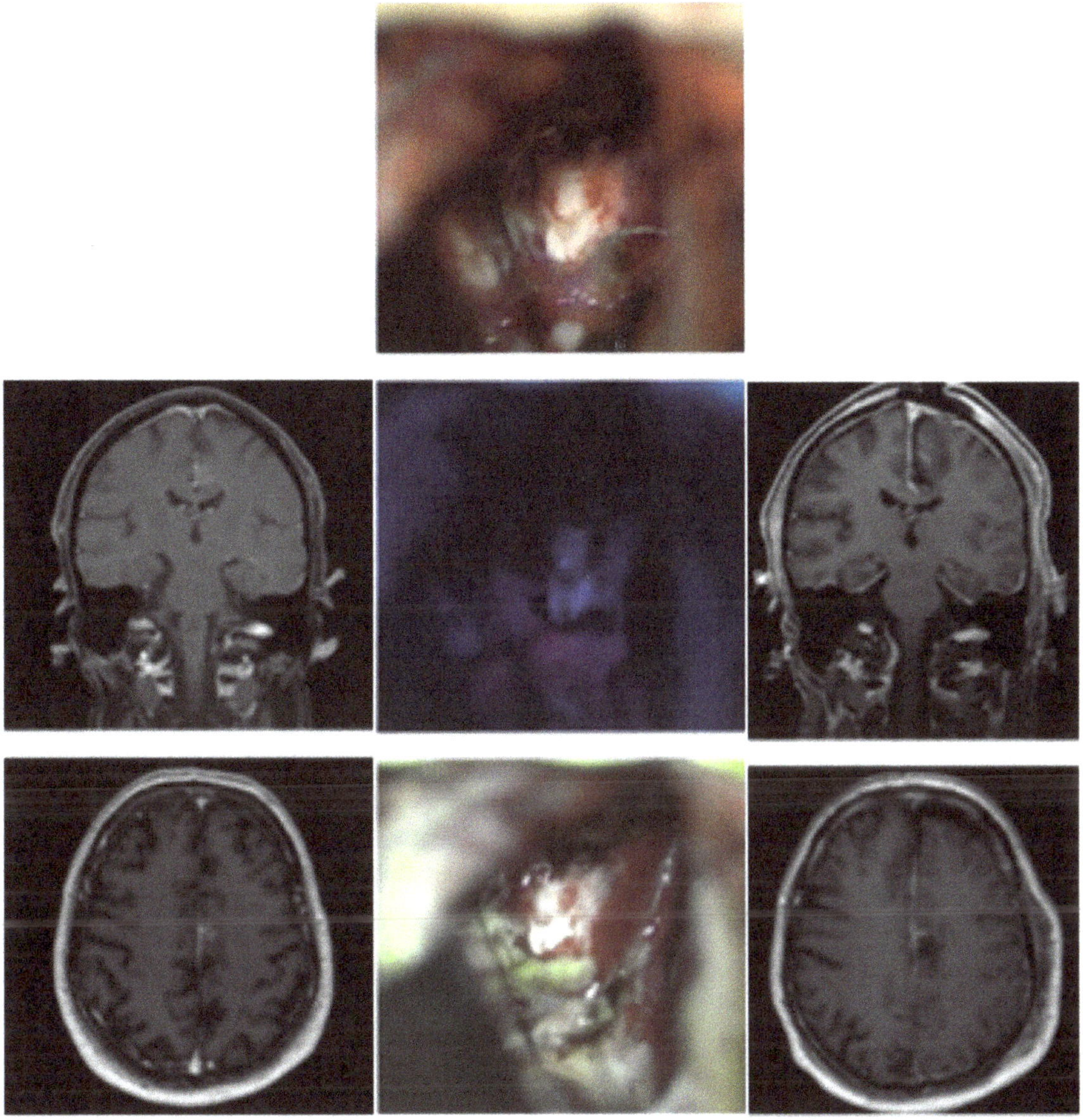

FIGURE 2 | Anaplastic astrocytoma in a 65-year-old patient. The left side shows the preoperative MRI (contrast-enhanced), while the right column shows the early 48 h-postoperative MRI. In the middle column the operative cavity shows the field under white light, below it under blue light, and at the bottom the fusion of both images in the MFL-mode.

between the brain's physiological color and the artificial color chosen (15). This led us to believe that in the clinical setting of tumor surgery it would be easier to identify and resect tumor tissue in this augmented reality setting as opposed to operation under blue light were brain tissue is pretty much dark. We also made the same observation in a previous implementation of the MFL-mode for surgery of vascular malformations as well as tumors with indocyanine green (16).

In a recent paper, it was shown that the intensity of the PpIX fluorescence is related to the light source used, which, according to the authors, could have implications for surgery (19). This is further highlighted by the fact that various surgical microscopes can exhibit "considerably different illumination optical power levels at identical system settings" (20). According to Belykh et al. (20), this is the case because of several factors that are related to [1] the excitation light, as microscopes have variations in excitation light power which are related to several factors, [2] the detection of the emitted light, depending on optical parameters such as the distance between object and objective, sensitivity of the camera chip/eye, etc., and [3] factors related to the tissue itself, such as blood or light scatter, to name a few (21). Being aware of the effect of the light source upon the fluorescence properties of PpIX, we have tried to minimize this effect by undertaking several measures. All operations were

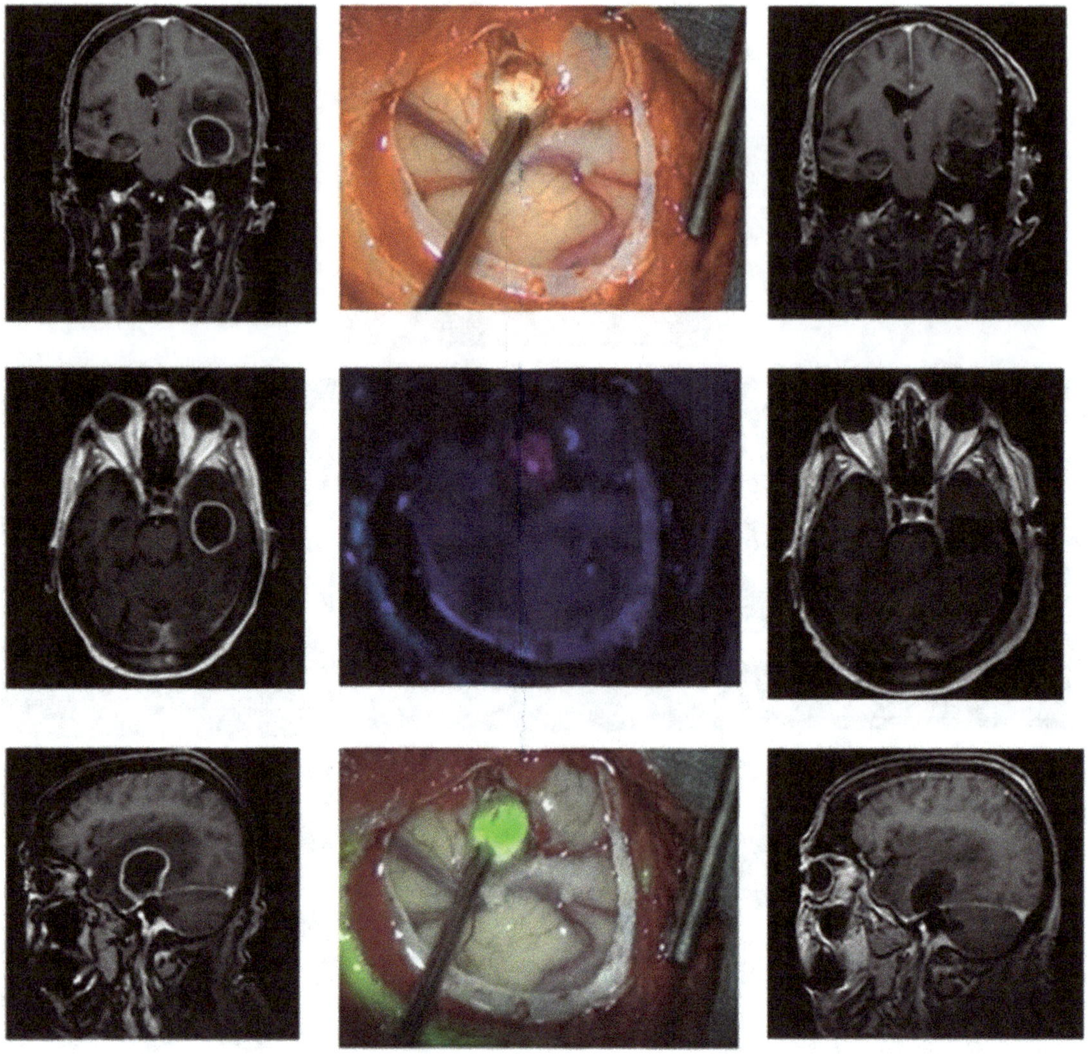

FIGURE 3 | Metastasis from a squamous tongue carcinoma in a 78 old patient. Preoperative (left side) and postoperative MRIs (right side) showing the lesion and the total resection zone, respectively. In the middle column, the operative cavity is seen. The top picture shows the exposed tumor under white light, below it under blue light with pink nuances, and at the bottom the fusion of both images in the MFL-mode ("green" is the tumor in pseudo-color mode).

performed by the same surgeon (CC), the microscope used was always identical, the angle between the light source and the surface of interest was always tried to be kept at 90° for the best illumination effect. Apart from that, the parameters that influence the fluorescence (namely illumination, magnification, and working distance) were tried to be kept as constant as possible. Only if operative challenges had to be met, the surgeon changed them accordingly to her needs.

Apart from the means used by the surgeon to cope with the problem of light intensity depending on the light source used, some technical points have to be mentioned and discussed. PpIX is excited with blue light of a narrow spectral range around 405 nm. Illuminated with such light the healthy tissue can be observed as a blue image. With increasing tumor cell density, the red fluorescence marking is added to the reflected blue light and colorizes the observed tissue detail from pinkish blue to strong pink (tissue with low up to strong PpIX fluorescence).

This color shift is generally independent of the excitation intensity, allowing the interpretation for surgical resection as long as the color visibility is given, but with further decrease of excitation intensity the visibility of the observed color signal becomes too dark and recognition of the faint fluorescence in the resection area is more or less impossible.

Comparing the PpIX MFL-white light fluorescence illumination used in the present study to the blue light fluorescence, the excitation of white light fluorescence is broad and comprising the wavelengths shorter than 400 nm up to

700 nm, excluding the PpIX emission peak around 635 nm for the detection of the PpIX fluorescence.

Because the detected fluorescence intensity is related to the light source excitation level in the absorption range of PpIX and the optical parameters, the MFL system allows the control of the related effects as much as possible to provide correct fluorescence intensity and visibility for the combined digital anatomical white light and fluorescence image on the monitor and for the fluorescence image overlay in the eyepieces.

In this observational study, we also report tumors other than HGG that showed PpIX fluorescence even though we applied 5-ALA in an “off-label” setting. Such lesions were different metastatic processes, meningiomas, acoustic neurinoma as well as ependymoma. Although in the literature, mainly HGGs are regarded as tumors that express the highly fluorescent PpIX and hence have fluorescent properties under blue light evidence exists that other brain lesions can also be visualized with 5-ALA, such as brain metastases (22). Of note, this seems to be only the case in approximately 50% of metastases while, interestingly, in one recent study, neither the primary site of the metastases nor their histologic subtype correlated with fluorescence behavior (22). Hence, we believe that with more knowledge about the different metastases and their 5-ALA metabolism this drug will eventually become more important for the field of neurosurgical oncology. Therefore, s it is crucial to address well-evaluated and documented disadvantages of 5-ALA regarding operation ergonomics and bleeding complications. The described novel MFL technology is able to bring light back to the operating field during the 5-ALA guided surgery, similarly to what we have previously described for fluorescence guided surgery using other fluorophores like ICG even for vascular pathologies (15) or brain tumor treatment (16). For that matter, the presented real time augmented reality setting combined with a commercially available microscope could be a promising tool to improve surgical therapy.

Nonetheless, the present study bears a few limitations. Being an observational study, we were only able to get the first insight into the way the MFL-mode could be used in neurosurgery. All pictures obtained in the MFL-mode were matching the fluorescence pictures under blue light while, however, the fluorescence and its contrast to the surrounding brain tissue was subjectively perceived stronger in the MFL-mode as opposed to the blue light pictures. In other words, we did not include any objective data such as quantitative assessment of fluorescence intensities or histopathological analysis of the tumor zones and the areas that showed different fluorescence intensity. Hence, future studies would need to quantitatively compare blue light and white light pictures to the generated MFL-mode picture regarding factors such as fluorescence intensity, discrimination of different tissues in real-time, or/and simultaneously identification of anatomically relevant structures such as blood vessels, to name a few. Apart from that, it is on our next steps to compare the traditional way of operating with both blue and white light to the sole use of the MFL-mode toward clinical endpoints such as progression-free survival, neurological function, or degree of tumor resection.

CONCLUSION

The MFL technique embedded on a classic surgical microscope opens the way for precise and clear visualization of brain tissue PpIX fluorescence in real-time under white light. It can be easily implemented in the resection of all brain lesions accumulating 5-ALA and producing PpIX. Drawbacks of classic PpIX fluorescence visualization techniques such as difficulty in identification of bleeding sources, operating in dark environment and the necessity to regularly switch off the fluorescence mode could be overcome with the presence of additional white light which allows for clear simultaneous visualization of the exposed brain in natural colors and PpIX fluorescence in green pseudocolor.

ETHICS STATEMENT

The studies involving human participants were reviewed and approved by University of Witten/Herdecke, Germany (Nr: 35/2017). The patients/participants provided their written informed consent to participate in this study. Written informed consent was obtained from the individual(s) for the publication of any potentially identifiable images or data included in this article.

AUTHOR CONTRIBUTIONS

PP and PC drafted the manuscript. PC and AH designed the manuscript. All operations were carried out by PC and MN. All authors read and approved the final manuscript.

SUPPLEMENTARY MATERIAL

Supplementary Video 1 | Intraoperative video as recorded with the operative microscope. The video was recorded during resection of the glioblastoma described in the case vignette #1. The video shows in the beginning the classic blue fluorescence while later on the multispectral fluorescence (MFL) mode is visible. The fluorescent tissue appears in the pseudo-color green. In this video, the different fluorescent shades are clearly visible, which helps identifying different areas of the lesion. It also shows that any blood covering the surgical field is immediately visible and can then be removed without losing focus of the tissue of interest. Finally, coagulated blood can be identified during dissection and then be removed while immediately seeing any underlying fluorescent tissue.

REFERENCES

1. Stupp R, Mason WP, van den Bent MJ, Weller M, Fisher B, Taphoorn MJ, et al. Radiotherapy plus concomitant and adjuvant temozolomide for glioblastoma. *N Engl J Med.* (2005) 352:987–96. doi: 10.1056/NEJMoa043330
2. Stupp R, Hegi ME, Mason WP, van den Bent MJ, Taphoorn MJ, Janzer RC, et al. Effects of radiotherapy with concomitant and adjuvant temozolomide versus radiotherapy alone on survival in glioblastoma in a randomised phase III study: 5-year analysis of the EORTC-NCIC trial. *Lancet Oncol.* (2009) 10:459–66. doi: 10.1016/S1470-2045(09)70025-7

3. Almenawer SA, Badhiwala JH, Alhazzani W, Greenspoon J, Farrokhyar F, Yarascavitch B, et al. Biopsy versus partial versus gross total resection in older patients with high-grade glioma: a systematic review and meta-analysis. *Neuro Oncol.* (2015) 17:868–81. doi: 10.1093/neuonc/nou349
4. D'Amico RS, Englander ZK, Canoll P, Bruce JN. Extent of resection in glioma–a review of the cutting edge. *World Neurosurgery.* (2017) 103:538–49. doi: 10.1016/j.wneu.2017.04.041
5. Goldbrunner R, Ruge M, Kocher M, Lucas CW, Galldiks N, Grau S, et al. The treatment of gliomas in adulthood. *Dtsch Arztebl Int.* (2018) 115:356–64. doi: 10.3238/arztebl.2018.0356
6. Stepp H, Stummer W. 5-ALA in the management of malignant glioma. *Lasers Surg Med.* (2018). 50:399–419. doi: 10.1002/lsm.22933
7. Hadjipanayis CG, Widhalm G, Stummer W. What is the surgical benefit of utilizing 5-aminolevulinic acid for fluorescence-guided surgery of malignant gliomas? *Neurosurgery.* (2015) 77:663–73. doi: 10.1227/NEU.0000000000000929
8. Stummer W, Stocker S, Wagner S, Stepp H, Fritsch C, Goetz C, et al. Intraoperative detection of malignant gliomas by 5-aminolevulinic acid-induced porphyrin fluorescence. *Neurosurgery.* (1998) 42:518–26. doi: 10.1016/S0303-8467(97)81684-8
9. Stummer W, Novotny A, Stepp H, Goetz C, Bise K, Reulen HJ. Fluorescence-guided resection of glioblastoma multiforme by using 5-aminolevulinic acid-induced porphyrins: a prospective study in 52 consecutive patients. *Neurosurg.* (2000) 93:1003–13. doi: 10.3171/jns.2000.93.6.1003
10. Stummer W, Pichlmeier U, Meinel T, Wiestler OD, Zanella F, Reulen HJ, et al. Fluorescence-guided surgery with 5-aminolevulinic acid for resection of malignant glioma: a randomised controlled multicentre phase III trial. *Lancet Oncol.* (2006) 7:392–401. doi: 10.1016/S1470-2045(06)70665-9
11. Ferraro N, Barbarite E, Albert TR, Berchmans E, Shah AH, Bregy A, et al. The role of 5-aminolevulinic acid in brain tumor surgery: a systematic review. *Neurosurg Rev.* (2016) 39:545–55. doi: 10.1007/s10143-015-0695-2
12. Motekallemi A, Jeltema HR, Metzemaekers JD, van Dam GM, Crane LM, Groen RJ, et al. The current status of 5-ALA fluorescence-guided resection of intracranial meningiomas-a critical review. *Neurosurg Rev.* (2015) 38:619–28. doi: 10.1007/s10143-015-0615-5
13. Roberts DW, Olson JD, Evans LT, Kolste KK, Kanick SC, Fan X, et al. Red-light excitation of protoporphyrin IX fluorescence for subsurface tumor detection. *J Neurosurg.* (2018) 128:1690–7. doi: 10.3171/2017.1.JNS162061
14. Stepp H, Schnell O. Brain tumor imaging with ALA. In: Hamblin MR, Huang Y, editors. *Imaging in Photodynamic Therapy. 1st ed.* Boca Raton: CRC Press. (2017). p. 369–406.
15. Athanasopoulos D, Heimann A, Nakamura M, Kakaletri I, Kempski O, Charalampaki P. Real-time overlapping of indocyanine green—video angiography with white light imaging for vascular neurosurgery: technique, implementation, and clinical experience. *Oper Neurosurg.* (2020) opaa050. doi: 10.1093/ons/opaa050
16. Charalampaki P, Nakamura M, Athanasopoulos D, Heimann A. Confocal-assisted multispectral fluorescent microscopy for brain tumor surgery. *Front Oncol.* (2019) 9:583. doi: 10.3389/fonc.2019.00583
17. Nickele C, Nguyen V, Fisher W, Couldwell W, Aboud E, David C, et al. A pilot comparison of multispectral fluorescence to indocyanine green videoangiography and other modalities for intraoperative assessment in vascular neurosurgery. *Operat Neurosurg.* (2019) 17:103–9. doi: 10.1093/ons/opy237
18. Hadjipanayis CG, Stummer W. 5-ALA and FDA approval for glioma surgery. *J Neuro-Oncol.* (2019). 141:479–86. doi: 10.1007/s11060-019-03098-y
19. Kamp MA, Knipps J, Neumann LM, Mijderwijk HJ, Dibue-Adjei M, Steiger HJ, et al. Is the intensity of 5-aminolevulinic acid-derived fluorescence related to the light source? *World Neurosurg.* (2019) 131:e271–e6. doi: 10.1016/j.wneu.2019.07.136
20. Belykh E, Miller EJ, Patel AA, Bozkurt B, Yagmurlu K, Robinson TR, et al. Optical characterization of neurosurgical operating microscopes: quantitative fluorescence and assessment of PpIX photobleaching. *Sci Rep.* (2018) 8:12543. doi: 10.1038/s41598-018-30247-6
21. Belykh E, Nelson LY, Seibel EJ, Preul MC. Factors that influence quantification of fluorescent signal during the 5-ALA-guided surgery. Letter to the editor regarding the paper "Is the Intensity of 5-Aminolevulinic Acid Derived Fluorescence Related to the Light Source? *World Neurosurg.* (2020)
22. Kamp MA, Fischer I, Buhner J, Turowski B, Cornelius JF, Steiger HJ, et al. 5-ALA fluorescence of cerebral metastases and its impact for the local-in-brain progression. *Oncotarget.* (2016). 7:66776–89. doi: 10.18632/oncotarget.11488

3

Spray Fluorescent Probes for Fluorescence-Guided Neurosurgery

Yosuke Kitagawa [1], Shota Tanaka [1], Yugo Kuriki [2], Kyoko Yamamoto [3], Akira Ogasawara [2], Takahide Nejo [1], Reiko Matsuura [1], Tsukasa Koike [1], Taijun Hana [1,4], Satoshi Takahashi [1], Masashi Nomura [1], Shunsaku Takayanagi [1], Akitake Mukasa [5], Mako Kamiya [3], Yasuteru Urano [2,3] and Nobuhito Saito [1]*

[1] Department of Neurosurgery, Graduate School of Medicine, The University of Tokyo, Tokyo, Japan, [2] Laboratory of Chemistry and Biology, Graduate School of Pharmaceutical Sciences, The University of Tokyo, Tokyo, Japan, [3] Laboratory of Chemical Biology and Molecular Imaging, Graduate School of Medicine, The University of Tokyo, Tokyo, Japan, [4] Genome Science Division, Research Center for Advanced Science and Technology, The University of Tokyo, Tokyo, Japan, [5] Department of Neurosurgery, Graduate School of Medical Sciences, Kumamoto University, Kumamoto, Japan

***Correspondence:**
Shota Tanaka
tanakas-tky@umin.ac.jp*

Keywords: fluorescent probe, glioma surgery, hydroxymethyl rhodamine green, topical, 5-aminolevulinic acid

Surgery is the initial and most important mode of treatment for glioma, the most common primary brain tumor. The greatest possible extent of resection and preservation of neurological functions are both the primary goals, although they tend to be in the trade-off relationship. Several surgical adjuncts have been developed for maximal safe resection, which include electrophysiological monitoring, navigation system, intraoperative imaging, and fluorescent probes. Intraoperative imaging such as MRI and ultrasound tend to overcome inacuracy due to brain shift during tumor resection. However, these devices tend to be costly. In contrast, fluorescent probes can be implemented to surgery by simply attaching an excitation and emission filters to a preexisting microscope, achieving high versatility with low cost. Fluorescence-guided surgery has been proven effective for radical tumor resection; fluorescent probes effectively visualize the tumor intraoperatively.

Fluorescence probes are useful indicators for biologically relevant targets, being sensitive, rapidly responsive, and capable of affording high spatial resolution via microscopic imaging without destroying structures (1). In surgery, many different types of fluorescent probes have been investigated in preclinical and clinical studies. They are classified based on the mechanisms of their actions into "always-on" probes and activatable probes (2). "Always-on" probes, administered with intravenous injection, readily reveal hypervascularized areas, differentiating the tumor from the normal brain parenchyma. These probes have several disadvantages in their use. They do not necessarily accumulate selectively in tumor tissues (3). Even if they do, they show high background signals, which makes it difficult to identify tumor tissues. On the contrary, activatable probes are efficient in identifying the tumor specifically either with its high substance accumulation or with its metabolic activation, although they often require a considerable time up to several hours in clinical use (4). One such example is activatable cell-penetrating peptide (ACPP) (5). The ACPP probe is a fluorescently labeled, polycationic cell-penetrating peptide coupled with a cleavable linker. When the probe is exposed to a protease being active in the tumor, the linker is cleaved and the inhibitory peptide is dissociated. Then it binds to and enters the tumor cells.

Three types of fluorescent probes are in use in neurosurgical procedures: 5-aminolevulinic acid (5-ALA), indocyanine green (ICG), and fluorescein sodium (6).

ICG and fluorescein sodium are classified as "always-on" probes (7), whereas 5-ALA is classified as an activatable probe. It induces the production of protoporphyrin IX (PpIX), which preferentially accumulates in glioma tissues. It reaches its peak 6 h after 5-ALA administration (8).

A randomized controlled study conducted by Stummer et al. assessed the efficacy of fluorescence-guided resection with 5-ALA in patients with malignant gliomas amenable to complete resection of contrast-enhancing tumor (9). The primary endpoints were the number of patients without contrast-enhancing tumor in early postoperative MRI and 6-month progression-free survival. Secondary endpoints were volume of residual tumor on postoperative MRI, overall survival, neurological deficit, and toxic effects. Patients assigned to fluorescence-guided surgery had a higher 6-month progression-free survival than did those assigned to conventional surgery (41.0 vs. 21.1%, $p = 0.0003$). The complete resection rate of contrast enhancing tumor in the fluorescence-guided surgery group compared favorably with that in the conventional surgery group (65 vs. 36%, $p < 0.0001$). They have shown that the use of 5-ALA resulted in a higher complete resection rate and a longer progression-free survival. Of note, no significant differences in overall survival, neurological deficit, or toxic effects were noted between the two groups. 5-ALA is now routinely used in clinical practice for high-grade glioma surgery. On the contrary, it fails to identify low-grade gliomas. There are some limitations in its use as well, which would include false positivity, false negativity, the need for preoperative oral administration, and the inability for re-administration (10).

We have previously reported on hydroxymethyl rhodamine green (HMRG) probes as activatable fluorescent probes for rapid cancer detection with topical spray (11). They are comprised of HMRG as fluorescent scaffold combined with various types of amino acids or dipeptides. Their fluorescence are completely quenched by spirocyclic caging but are activated rapidly with a one-step enzymatic reaction in the presence of specific aminopeptidase enzymes within a few to tens of minutes (**Figure 1**). Dipeptidylpeptidase IV and γ-glutamyltransferase (GGT) are some examples of dipeptidyl peptidases and aminopeptidases that are known to be expressed at the elevated levels in various types of cancers, such as hepatic cancer, esophagus cancer, ovarian cancer, and glioma as well, as compared to normal tissues (11–15). GGT is present on the plasma membrane and catalyzes the transfer of the N-terminal gamma-glutamyl group of substrates to acceptor molecules. When it encounters GGT on the surface of a cancer tissue, it is hydrolyzed by the enzymatic reaction to yield the highly fluorescent product, HMRG. *In vitro*, when red fluorescent protein was used as a reference for location of a cell of the ovarian cancer cell line SHIN3, sensitivity and specificity of detecting SHIN3-RFP tumors with gGlu-HMRG 10 min after injection were 100 and 100%, respectively. *In vivo*, after establishing the intraperitoneal dissemination mouse model using SHIN3, minute tumors <1 mm in diameter in the peritoneum could be readily identified as early as 30 s after spraying the gGlu-HMRG probe under fluorescence-guided endoscopy and they could be removed easily with forceps. Without fluorescent probes, confirming the completeness of resection would be difficult with naked eyes, and therefore would have to be ascertained by postoperative histological confirmation (16–18).

These HMRG probes can be applied for the detection of a brain tumor. Some probes fluorescence glioma tissue more than the surrounding normal brain tissue after their topical application (**Figure 2**). The biggest advantages of these activatable probes would be that they start to react immediately after spray and can be administered repeatedly during surgery with potentially high specificity and sensitivity. Topical application of spray probes can be performed with a much lower dose than systemic administration, and thus they are deemed safer. On the other hand, one caveat would be that the efficacy of spray fluorescent probes may be diminished by being washed away by active bleeding at the resection cavity before they provoke fluorescence in the tumor. Another concern would be that the surrounding brain tissue may overhang the resection cavity, which makes it difficult to efficiently apply fluorescent probes to the cavity and to accurately evaluate the degree of fluorescence.

We believe that these novel fluorescent probes have a potential as probes complementary to 5-ALA in high-grade glioma surgery. As discussed earlier, 5-ALA is highly effective and routinely administered for resection of high-grade gliomas, but these probes would be worth a try

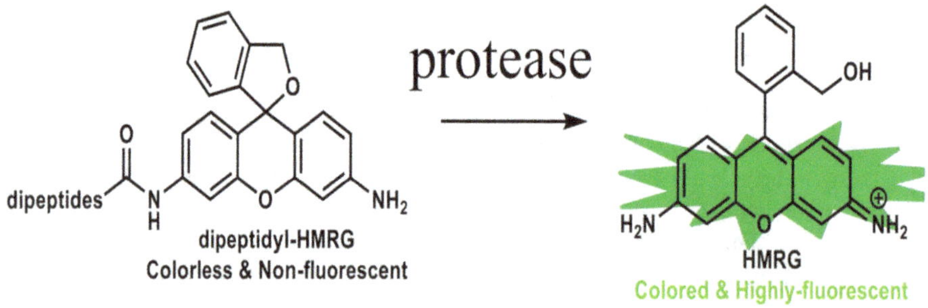

FIGURE 1 | Chemical structures of HMRG-based fluorescent probes. These probes are completely quenched due to spirocyclic caging but are activated with protease reaction.

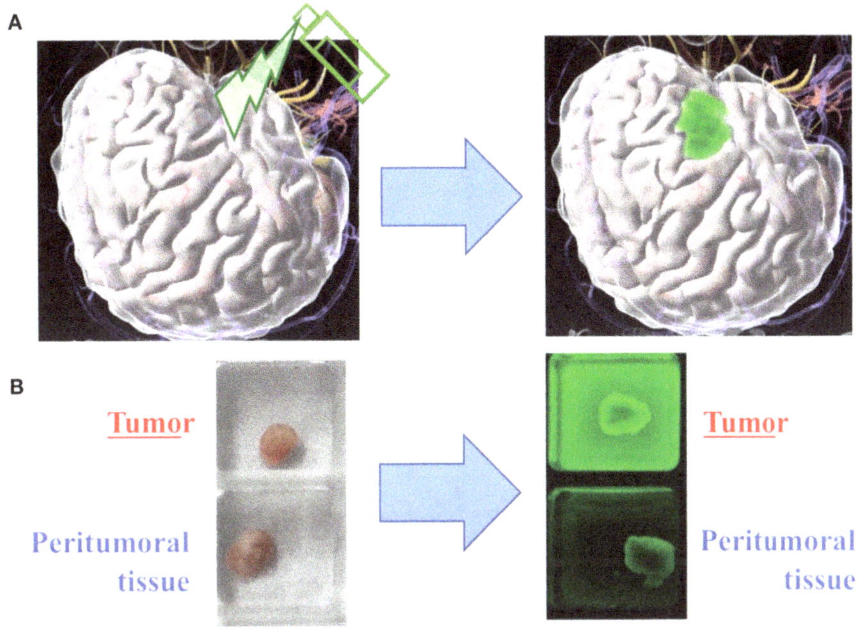

FIGURE 2 | Proof of concept in spray fluorescent probes. **(A)** The conceptual image of tumor detection with topical application of a fluorescent probe. **(B)** In a representative case of glioma, the fresh tumor tissue exhibits significantly stronger fluorescence as compared to the peritumoral tissue.

when the tumor does not fluorescence with 5-ALA or when 5-ALA fluorescence has significantly diminished at the end of tumor resection. In addition, they would be a breakthrough in low-grade glioma surgery, where 5-ALA is largely ineffective. Moreover, they are potentially applicable to virtually all types of brain tumors including malignant lymphoma and brain metastasis, which are the top differential diagnoses of glioma. Novel HMRG probes which specifically detect malignant lymphoma or brain metastasis are currently under investigation. Last but not the least, a larger clinical study is warranted to assess the clinical utility of our probes in brain tumor surgery.

AUTHOR CONTRIBUTIONS

YKi, ShoT, MK, and YU wrote the manuscript. YKu, KY, AO, TN, RM, TK, TH, SatT, MN, ShuT, AM, and NS carefully reviewed the manuscript.

REFERENCES

1. Tsien RY. Fluorescent and photochemical probes of dynamic biochemical signals inside living cells. In: Czarnik AW, editor. *American Chemical Society*. Washington, DC (1993). p. 130–46.
2. Kobayashi H, Ogawa M, Alford R, Choyke PL, Urano Y. New strategies for flourescent probe desogn in medical diagmpstic imaging. *Chem Rev.* (2011) 110:2620–40. doi: 10.1021/cr900263j
3. Diaz RJ, Dios RR, Hattab EM, Burrell K, Rakopoulos P, Sabha N, et al. Study of the biodistribution of fluorescein in glioma-infiltrated mouse brain and histopathological correlation of intraoperative findings in high-grade gliomas resected under fluorescein fluorescence guidance. *J Neurosurg.* (2015) 122:1360–9. doi: 10.3171/2015.2.JNS132507
4. Kobayashi H, Choyke PL. Target-cancer-cell-specific activatable fluorescence imaging probes: rational design and *in vivo* applications. *Acc Chem Res.* (2011) 44:83–90. doi: 10.1021/ar1000633
5. Nguyen QT, Olson ES, Aguilera TA, Jiang T, Scadeng M, Ellies LG, et al. Surgery with molecular fluorescence imaging using activatable cell-penetrating peptides decreases residual cancer and improves survival. *Proc Natl Acad Sci USA.* (2010) 107:4317–22. doi: 10.1073/pnas.0910261107
6. Belykh E, Martirosyan NL, Yagmurlu K, Miller EJ, Eschbacher JM, Izadyyazdanabadi M, et al. Intraoperative fluorescence imaging for personalized brain tumor resection: current state and future directions. *Front Surg.* (2016) 3:55. doi: 10.3389/fsurg.2016.00055
7. Eyupoglu IY, Hore N, Fan Z, Buslei R, Merkel A, Buchfelder M, et al. Intraoperative vascular DIVA surgery reveals angiogenic hotspots in tumor zones of malignant gliomas. *Sci Rep.* (2015) 5:1–7. doi: 10.1038/srep 07958
8. Stummer W, Stepp H, Moller G, Ehrhardt A, Leonhard M, Reulen HJ. Technical principles for protoporphyrin-ix-fluorescence guided microsurgical resection of malignant glioma tissue. *Acta Neurochir.* (1998) 140:995–1000. doi: 10.1007/978-3-319-93698-7_49
9. Stummer W, Pichlmeier U, Meinel T, Wiestler OD, Zanella F, Reulen HJ. Fluorescence-guided surgery with 5-aminolevulinic acid for resection of malignant glioma: a randomised controlled multicentre phase III trial. *Lancet Oncol.* (2006) 7:392–401. doi: 10.1016/S1470-2045(06)70665-9
10. Ferraro N, Barbarite E, Albert TR, Berchmans E, Shah AH, Bregy A, et al. The role of 5-aminolevulinic acid in brain tumor surgery: a systematic review. *Neurosurg Rev.* (2016) 39:545–55. doi: 10.1007/s10143-015-0695-2
11. Urano Y, Sakabe M, Kosaka N, Ogawa M, Mitsunaga M, Asanuma D, et al. Rapid cancer detection by topically spraying a γ-glutamyltranspeptidase-activated fluorescent probe. *Sci Transl Med.* (2011) 3:110ra119. doi: 10.1126/scitranslmed.3002823
12. Stremenova J, Krepela E, Mares V, Trim J, Dbaly V, Marek J, et al. Expression and enzymatic activity of dipeptidyl peptidase-IV in human astrocytic tumours are associated with tumour grade. *Int J Oncol.* (2007) 31:785–92. doi: 10.3892/ijo.31.4.785
13. Onoyama H, Kamiya M, Kuriki Y, Komatsu T, Abe H, Tsuji Y, et al. Rapid and sensitive detection of early esophageal squamous cell carcinoma with

fluorescence probe targeting dipeptidylpeptidase IV. *Sci Rep.* (2016) 6:1–7. doi: 10.1038/srep26399
14. Fujii T, Kamiya M, Urano Y. *In vivo* imaging of intraperitoneally disseminated tumors in model mice by using activatable fluorescent small-molecular probes for activity of cathepsins. *Bioconjug Chem.* (2014) 25:1838–46. doi: 10.1021/bc5003289
15. Liu Y, Tan J, Zhang Y, Zhuang J, Ge M, Shi B, et al. Visualizing glioma margins by real-time tracking of γ-glutamyltranspeptidase activity. *Biomaterials.* (2018) 173:1–10. doi: 10.1016/j.biomaterials.2018.04.053
16. Braun S, Vogl FD, Naume B, Janni W, Osborne MP, Coombes RC, et al. A pooled analysis of bone marrow micrometastasis in breast cancer. *N Engl J Med.* (2005) 353:793–802. doi: 10.1056/NEJMoa050434
17. Cote RJ, Rosen PP, Lesser ML, Old LJ, Osborne MP. Prediction of early relapse in patients with operable breast cancer by detection of occult bone marrow micrometastases. *J Clin Oncol.* (1991) 9:1749–56. doi: 10.1200/JCO.1991.9.10.1749
18. Lugo TG, Braun S, Cote RJ, Pantel K, Rusch V. Detection and measurement of occult disease for the prognosis of solid tumors. *J Clin Oncol.* (2003) 21:2609–15. doi: 10.1200/JCO.2003.01.153

4

Quantitative Modulation of PpIX Fluorescence and Improved Glioma Visualization

Michael Reinert[1,2,3,4], Deborah Piffaretti[1,5], Marco Wilzbach[6], Christian Hauger[6], Roland Guckler[6], Francesco Marchi[1,2] and Maria Luisa D'Angelo[1]*

[1] Laboratory for Biomedical Neurosciences, Neurocenter of Southern Switzerland, Ente Ospedaliero Cantonale, Torricella-Taverne, Switzerland, [2] Department of Neurosurgery, Neurocenter of Southern Switzerland, Ente Ospedaliero Cantonale, Lugano, Switzerland, [3] Faculty of Biomedical Neurosciences, Università Della Svizzera Italiana, Lugano, Switzerland, [4] Medical Faculty, University of Bern, Bern, Switzerland, [5] Faculty of Medicine, Graduate School for Cellular and Biomedical Sciences, University of Bern, Bern, Switzerland, [6] Carl Zeiss Meditec AG, Oberkochen, Germany

***Correspondence:**
Michael Reinert
michael.reinert@eoc.ch

5-Aminolevulinic acid (5-ALA) induced fluorescence to augment surgical resection for high grade glioma has become a standard of care. Protoporphyrin IX (PpIX) visibility is however subject to the variability of the single tumor expression and to the interobserver interpretation. We therefore hypothesized that in different glioma cell lines with variable 5-ALA induced fluorescence, the signal can be pharmacologically increased. We therefore analyzed in three different GBM cell lines, with different expression of epidermal growth factor receptor (EGFR), the variability of 5-ALA induced PpIX fluorescence after the pharmacological blockade at different steps of PpIX breakdown and influencing the outbound transport of PpIX. Using flow cytometry, fluorescence microplate reader, and confocal microscopy the PpIX fluorescence was analyzed after exposure to tin protoporphyrin IX (SnPP), deferoxamine (DFO), and genistein. We furthermore constructed a microscope (Qp9-microscope) being able to measure quantitatively the concentration of PpIX. These values were compared with the extraction of PpIX in tumor biopsy taken during the GBM surgery. Although all three cell lines showed an increase to 5-ALA induced fluorescence their baseline activity was different. Treatment with either SnPP, DFO and genistein was able to increase 5-ALA induced fluorescence. Qp9-microscopy of tumor sample produced a color coded PpIX concentration map which was overlaid on the tumor image. The PpIX extraction from tumor sample analyzed using the plate reader gave lower values of the concentration, as compared to the expected values of the Qp9-microscope, however still in the same decimal range of μg/mL. This may be due to homogenization of the values during extraction and cell disaggregation. In conclusion pharmacological augmentation in GBM cell lines of PpIX signal is possible. A quantitative PpIX map for surgery is feasible and may help refine surgical excision. Further correlations of tumor tissue samples and Qp9-microscopy is needed, prior to develop an intraoperative surgical adjunct to the already existing 5-ALA induced surgery.

Keywords: GBM—glioblastoma multiforme, 5-ALA=5-aminolevulinic acid, protoporphyin IX, quantification, breakdown, visualization, microscope

INTRODUCTION

It is widely accepted that the extent of surgical resection plays an important role in overall survival in patients with glioma, both in IDH wild type and IDH mutated, and both in high grade and low-grade glioma (1, 2). In high-grade glioma, the extent of resection is guided by MRI and directed to the contrast-enhancing portion of the lesion, while in low-grade glioma the resection is decided based on the tumor infiltration shown by T2 sequence alteration (3, 4). New techniques as fluorescence have become a standard of care for intraoperative resection of high grade glioma (4). Nowadays, however, growing evidence support the use of these detection techniques also in low grade glioma (5). PpIX fluorescence and its concentration in tumor cells depends on the balance between its synthesis, catabolism and outflow. The amount of PpIX in tumor cells is favored by both the activity of cytosolic porphobilinogen deaminase (PBGD) during the replication phase, and by the down-regulation of ferrochelatase (FECH) (6). However, other factors such as protein transporters, tyrosine kinase activity and its downstream effect on hemoxygenase-1 (HO-1), availability of free Fe^{2+}-ions and its effect on FECH, are related with PpIX fluorescence (7, 8). Because of the above mentioned factors, the final enhancing results are highly variable and difficult to predict both in clinical and laboratory setting, and might also depend on EGFR expression status in glioma cell lines (7). Proteins transporters such as ATP-binding cassette subfamily G member 2 (ABCG2) regulate intracellular concentration of PpIX. These proteins may also be differently expressed or activated in relation with the epigenetic status of GBM (9) (**Figure 1**).

Further well-known factors such as 5-ALA patient administration concentration, exposure time and tumor cell concentration influence the concentration of PpIX at the local level (4, 10). Furthermore, fading requires also consideration during light exposure. Also, 5-ALA fluorescence may vary spatially from one area to another of GBM (11). Lastly, two further factor that limit the validation of PpIX fluorescence consist in the inter-observer variability and in the different signal imaging obtained by the microscopic view or by the video screen. Based on all above mentioned limitations, there is an urgent need to go beyond the visual capacity of the human eye by measuring more accurately the tumor borders with quantitative pixel based method, and possibly by establishing a definite threshold for tumor activity presence.

The overall purpose of the study was to better understand the metabolic pathway of PpIX, and thereafter to augment pharmacologically its signal in different GBM cell lines in order to increase its visibility. This achievement might be exploited in the future also in photodynamic therapy. We thus selected three compounds: tin protoporphyrin IX (SnPP) a HO-1 blocker, deferoxamine (DFO) an iron chelator, and genistein. Genistein is a natural product (Isoflavone) (12), known as an angiogenesis inhibitor and as an inhibitor of ABCG2 transporter protein, thus influencing the outbound cell traffic of PpIX. All compounds are either FDA approved or previously described in human use. In order to avoid the limit of inter-observer variability and to capture also low concentrations of fluorescence tracer, barely visible by naked eye, a quantification of PpIX during surgical resection is required. We therefore developed a quantitative PpIX microscope (Qp9) according to previously described setup (13–15) aiming to correlate, for the first time, the color coded matrix images with the effective concentration of PpIX is to correlate these matrix images with the effective extraction concentration of PpIX.

METHODS

Cell Culture

Human GBM cell line U87MG obtained from American Type Culture Collection (89081402-1VL, Sigma-Aldrich) was maintained in Dulbecco's Modified Eagle Medium (DMEM, 61965, Gibco® Life technologies Europe), GlutaMAX cell culture medium supplemented with 10% fetal bovine serum (FBS, 10270, Gibco® Life technologies Europe), 1% non-essential amino acids (MEM NEAA, 11140, Gibco® Life technologies Europe), 1 mM sodium pyruvate (S8636, Sigma-Aldrich), penicillin 10,000 units/mL and streptomycin 10,000 μg/mL (15140, Gibco® Life technologies Europe).

The human GBM cell line U87wtEGFR overexpressing the EGFR gene, was generously provided by Prof. Dr. Frank Furnari (Laboratory of Tumor Biology, Ludwig Institute for Cancer Research, University of California-San Diego) and was cultured in DMEM GlutaMAX, 10% FBS and 1% penicillin-streptomycin, supplemented with 100 μg/mL of G418 disulfate salt (A1720, Sigma-Aldrich). U87MG vIII 4.12 cells stably expresses high level of the mutant EGFR variant III (deletion of exons 2-7) (CL 01004-CLTH, Tebu-bio) were maintained in DMEM GlutaMAX, 10% FBS, 1% penicillin-streptomycin and 0.2% of gentamicin 10 mg/mL (15710049, Thermo Fisher Scientific, Life Technologies Europe), enriched with 100 μg/mL of G418. All cells were kept at 37°C, 5% CO_2 atmosphere, in static conditions. Cells were harvested by incubation for 5 min at 37°C with 500 μL TrypLE™ Express Enzyme (1X), no phenol red (12604021, Gibco® Life technologies Europe) and blocked with DMEM supplemented with 10% FBS. During the time of the experiment, the cells were plated and after 24 h the medium was replaced with serum-free DMEM, high glucose, HEPES, no phenol red (21063045, Gibco® Life technologies Europe) for at least 24 h before starting the treatment (16).

Drug Treatment

5-ALA (Fagron DAC 2011), was freshly dissolved in milli-Q water at an intermediate concentration of 1 M and then diluted in serum free medium at a final concentration of 1 mM. DMSO 0.5% (vol/vol) (D2650, Sigma-Aldrich), was added to 5-ALA to increase its permeability into the cells as previously demonstrated by Lawrence et al. (17). Deferoxamine mesylate (492880, Desferal®, DFO, Novartis) was dissolved in milli-Q water. SnPP (sc-203452, Santa Cruz Biotech) and genistein (sc-3515, Santa Cruz Biotechnology) were dissolved in DMSO (16).

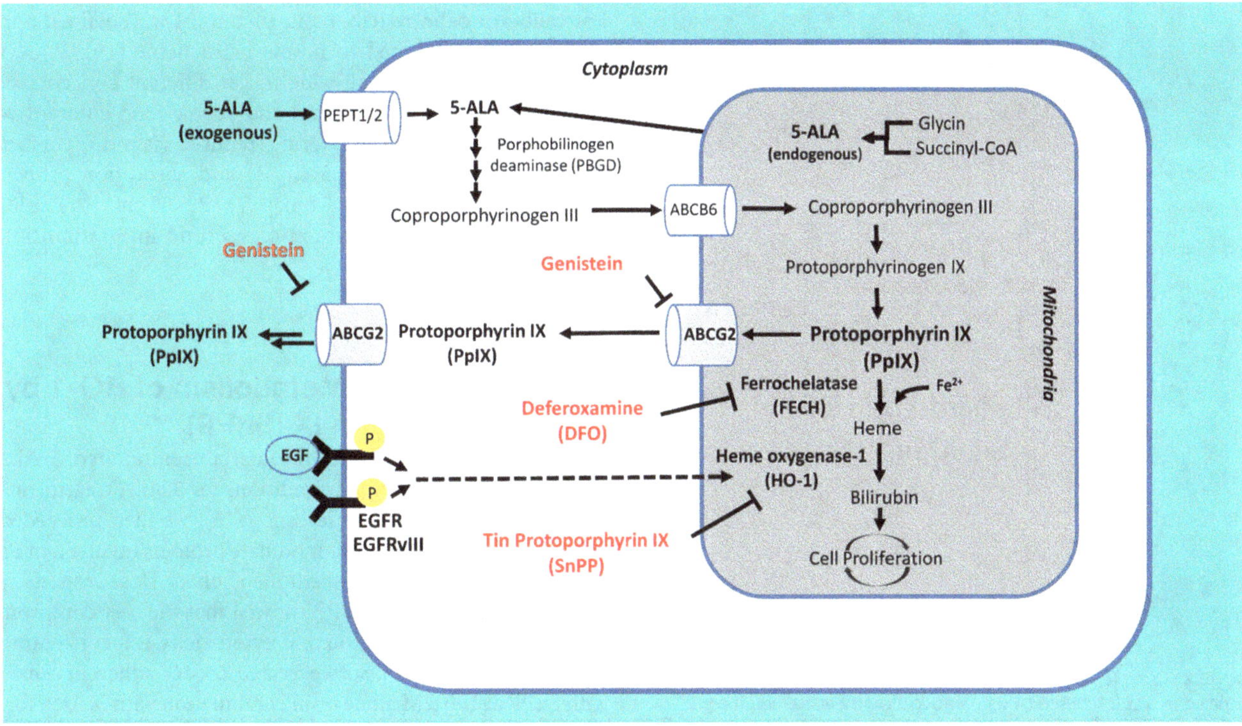

FIGURE 1 | PpIX metabolism. Exogenous 5-aminolevulinic acid (5-ALA) is internalized by tumor cells through the peptide transporter 1 and 2 (PEPT1/2), it is then converted into the fluorescent tracer protoporphyrin IX (PpIX) inside the mitochondrion. The accumulation of PpIX is antagonized by its active conversion through ferrochelatase (FECH) and heme oxygenase-1 (HO-1) and its efflux through ATP-binding cassette sub-family G member 2 (ABCG2). These proteins could be blocked by the action of deferoxamine (DFO), tin protoporphyrin IX (SnPP), and genistein.

PpIX Evaluation by Flow Cytometric Analysis

U87 cells were plated in a 6-well plate and treated with DFO 100 μM, SnPP 100 μM, or genistein 25 μM alone or in combination with 5-ALA at 1 mM or with all combinations of these treatments. After 8 h of treatment, cells were harvested, washed twice with phosphate buffered saline (PBS, 10010056, Gibco® Life technologies Europe) and centrifuged at 2,000 rpm for 5 min. The pellet was resuspended in 100 μL of PBS and the single cells suspension was analyzed by flow cytometry (excitation 408 and emission 630/38; CytoFLEX S, flow cytometry-Beckman Coulter) (16).

Confocal Microscopy

Cells were plated into Ibidi μ-slides VI0.4 (80606, Ibidi). After 24 h in FBS-free medium, cells were treated with DFO 100 μM, SnPP 100 μM, or genistein 25 μM alone or in combination with 5-ALA at 1 mM or with all combinations of these treatments. After 8 h of treatment, cells were washed twice with PBS, fixed with 4% paraformaldehyde for 10 min, washed with PBS. Slides were examined with a confocal line scanning microscope (LSM) Leica TCS SP5 equipped with the objective HCX PL APO lambda blue 40.0 × 1.25 OIL UV and an excitation of 405 nm and an emission of 620–650 nm (16).

Operative Microscope and Quantitative PpIX Microscope

For our tumor resection and cryosectioned slice of GBM xenograft mouse model, an operating microscope (OPMI) Pentero 900 (Carl Zeiss Meditec, AG, Oberkochen, Germany) with a BLUE-400 mode was used for imaging (8-bit RGB, 1,920 × 1,080 pixels) at a 20-cm distance from the target (18). Operative video was registered on BrainLab Buzz for later analysis (**Figure 4**, **Video S1**). For the quantification of the tumor samples taken during the surgery we constructed our custom-made microscope (Qp9) (**Figure 2**) its basic functionality described previously by Valdes et al. (13–15). The Qp9 microscope was calibrated to brain tissue mimicking phantoms with different known PpIX concentrations. The tumor samples were taken (**Video S1**) and then frozen at −80°C for later analysis with color matrix images obtained with Qp9. The sample was processed to trypLE lysis for cell disaggregation, as previously described in cell culture section, and then PpIX was extracted for TECAN analysis, for comparison with the Qp9 microscope.

Qp9 Microscope Setup

Tissue samples and cell cultures are imaged with a hyperspectral camera setup and a color camera attached to a microscope (OPMI pico, Carl Zeiss Meditec) with a fixed working distance of 200 mm. The image is divided by a beam splitter between the

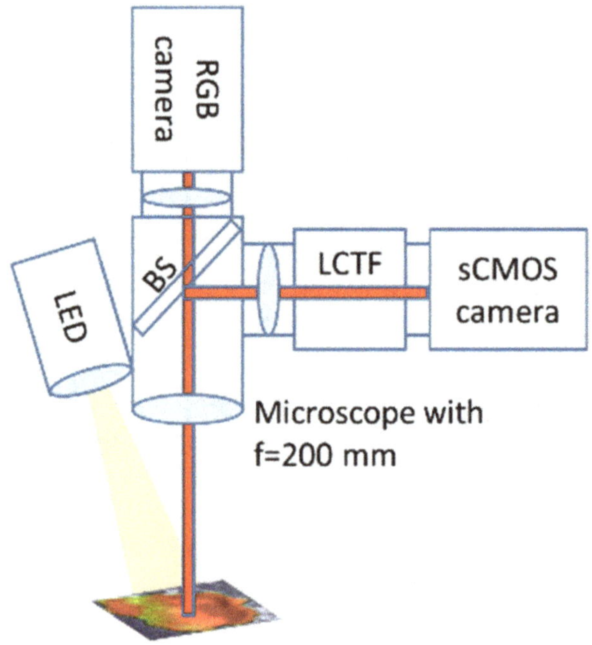

FIGURE 2 | Quantitative PpIX microscope. A tissue sample or cell culture is illuminated by a LED light source with white light or light at 405 nm. The microscope collects the reflected and fluorescent light with an objective lens with f = 200 mm. A beam splitter (BS) splits the light into two paths. One path is imaged with a hyperspectral camera setup. For an overview the second path is imaged on a color camera (RGB camera). The hyperspectral setup consists of a scientific CMOS camera (sCMOS) and a liquid crystal tunable filter (LCTF).

two imaging paths. The LED light source is capable to produce white light and violet light (405 nm) with an intensity of up to 30 mW/cm^2 at the sample.

The hyperspectral setup consists (13) of a scientific CMOS (pco.edge 4.2, PCO AG) camera and a liquid crystal tunable filter (LCTF, Meadowlark Optics, Inc.) (13–15).

The LCTF can be tuned between 420 and 730 nm in one nanometer steps. A typical full width at half maximum (FWHM) of a passband is 12 nm with a transmittance in the range of 5–30%. Outside the passband the transmittance is smaller than 1%.

A standard color camera (uEye CP with IMX252, IDS imaging GmbH) is connected to generate overview images.

With the hyperspectral setup one can record hyperspectral image stacks. The reflectance of the sample can be recorded using white light from the LED light source and fluorescence hyperspectral image stacks can be recorded using 405 nm light from the LED light source. For each pixel a white light reflectance and fluorescence spectrum is available.

These spectra are used to calculate absolute PpIX concentrations (15). So far, the system is calibrated to PpIX brain mimicking phantoms. The fluorescence spectrum is spectrally unmixed, so the pure PpIX signal can be separated from autofluorescence and other background signals such as ambient light. Then the white light spectrum is used to normalize for different tissue properties (different scattering and absorption). We get a PpIX concentration map of the measured samples overlaid on the image of the sample.

Calibration

For calibrating the system, tissue phantoms with defined optical properties were created to mimic brain tissue (19). PpIX was dissolved in dimethyl sulfoxide to get different concentrations (10 ng/ml–5 µg/ml), intralipid and yellow food colorant were used to generate varying scattering (reduced scattering coefficient at 635 nm, μ'_{sm} = 8.7–14.5 cm^{-1}) and absorption properties (absorption coefficient at 405 nm, μ_{ax} = 20–60 cm^{-1}). The lower detection limit of the system at one second integration time is 10 ng/ml of PpIX.

RESULTS

Inhibition of PpIX Metabolism of HO-1 by Tin Protoporphyrin IX (SnPP)

Having previously established the final concentration of 5-ALA at 1 mM for 8 h as the optimal conditions for 5-ALA treatment and quantification of PpIX fluorescence (16), we then proceeded to study the effect of drugs that modulate proteins involved in PpIX conversion into non-fluorescent metabolites. Dose response and cytotoxicity analysis for SnPP showed that the best compromise between PpIX accumulation and cytotoxicity is a concentration of SnPP at 100 µM (16). So, we treated 2 × 10^5 adherent cells/well with SnPP at 100 µM alone or in combination with 5-ALA for 8 h and then determined the mean cellular PpIX fluorescence by flow cytometry for biological duplicates. Based on two independent experiments performed by flow cytometry, we showed that the HO-1 inhibitor SnPP is able to significantly improve 5-ALA-induced PpIX fluorescence in U87MG and U87vIII, alone or in combination with 5-ALA. SnPP and 5-ALA co-treatment augmented the mean PpIX fluorescence by 81% for U87MG cells, by 39% for U87wtEGFR cells and by 48% for U87vIII cells compared to cells treated with 5-ALA alone, set as 100% (**Figure 3A**). The SnPP treatment alone showed an increment of PpIX fluorescence by 358% for U87MG cells, 252% for U87wtEGFR cells and 198% for U87vIII compared to untreated cells, set as 100% (**Figure 3A**) (16).

Inhibition of PpIX Synthesis by Fe^{2+}-Chelation and Inhibitory Effect on FECH

Based on our previous studies on cell cytotoxicity, we selected DFO at 100 µM to test the effect of FECH inhibition for 8 h in the presence or absence of exogenous 5-ALA (16). The treatment with DFO alone compared to control untreated cells showed a non-significant variation in PpIX fluorescence. In contrast, in the presence of exogenous 5-ALA, DFO significantly improved 5-ALA-induced PpIX fluorescence in all the three cell lines. In detail, the increase was of 16% for U87MG, of 6% for U87wtEGFR and of 22% for U87vIII cells when compared to cells incubated with 5-ALA alone, set as 100% (**Figure 3B**) (16).

Inhibition of PpIX Efflux by Genistein Acting on ABCG2

To retain the PpIX accumulated inside the cells, we tested the effect of inhibiting the main PpIX efflux transporter ABCG2 with genistein. Based on our previous cytotoxicity and

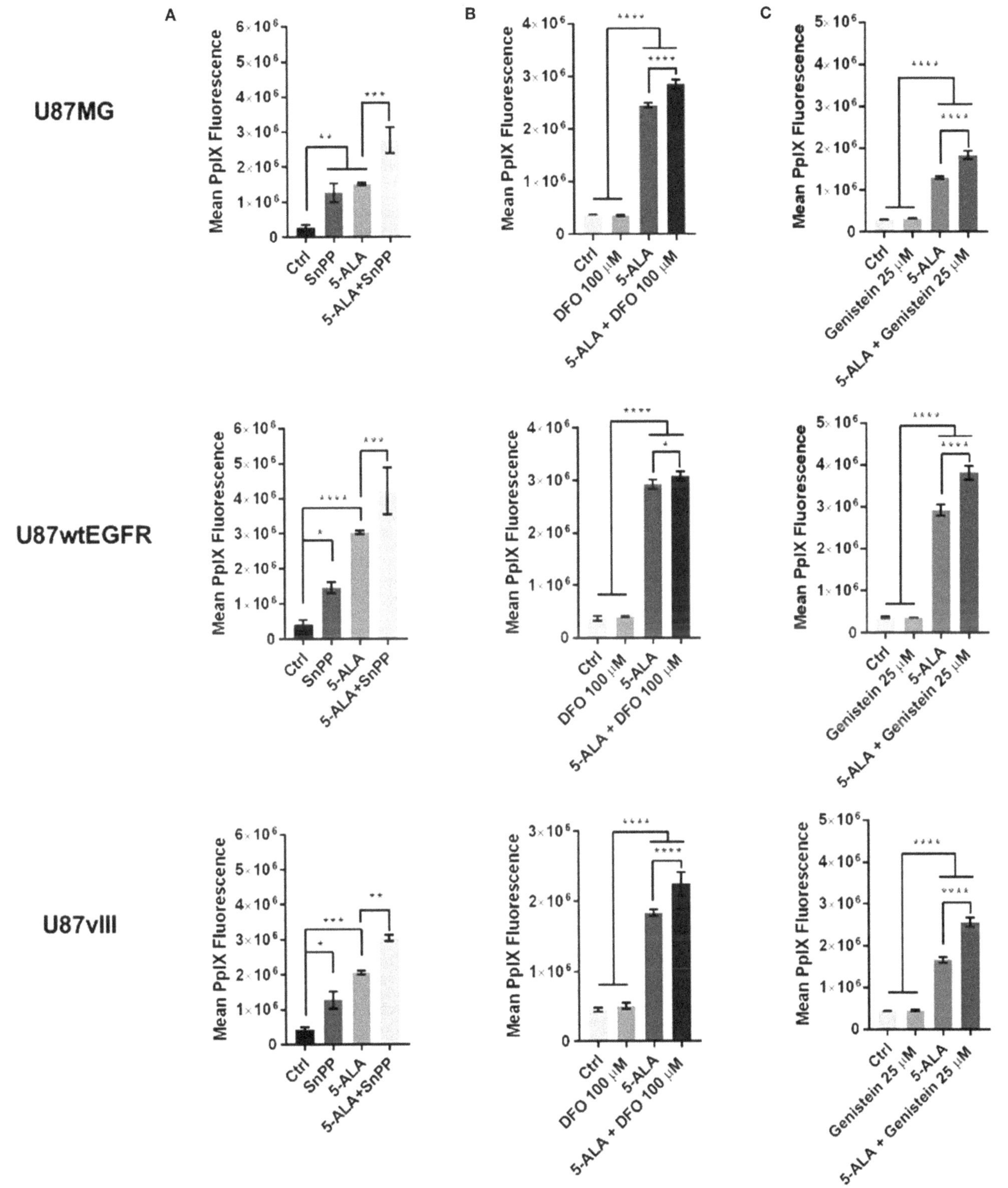

FIGURE 3 | Effect of single treatments on U87 GBM cell lines. Effect of **(A)** tin protoporphyrin IX (SnPP), **(B)** deferoxamine (DFO), and **(C)** genistein on three U87 cell lines differing for EGFR expression. Control untreated cells are compared with cells treated with the selected compound alone and cells treated with 5-ALA alone or with combination of 5-ALA and the indicated drug. Graphs show that all the three treatments in combination with 5-ALA significantly induce the fluorescence compared to 5-ALA alone. Results are expressed as mean ± SD (one-way ANOVA, Sidak's multiple comparison test $^{*}p < 0.05$; $^{**}p < 0.01$; $^{***}p < 0.001$; $^{****}p < 0.0001$). Where not specified the difference is not significant.

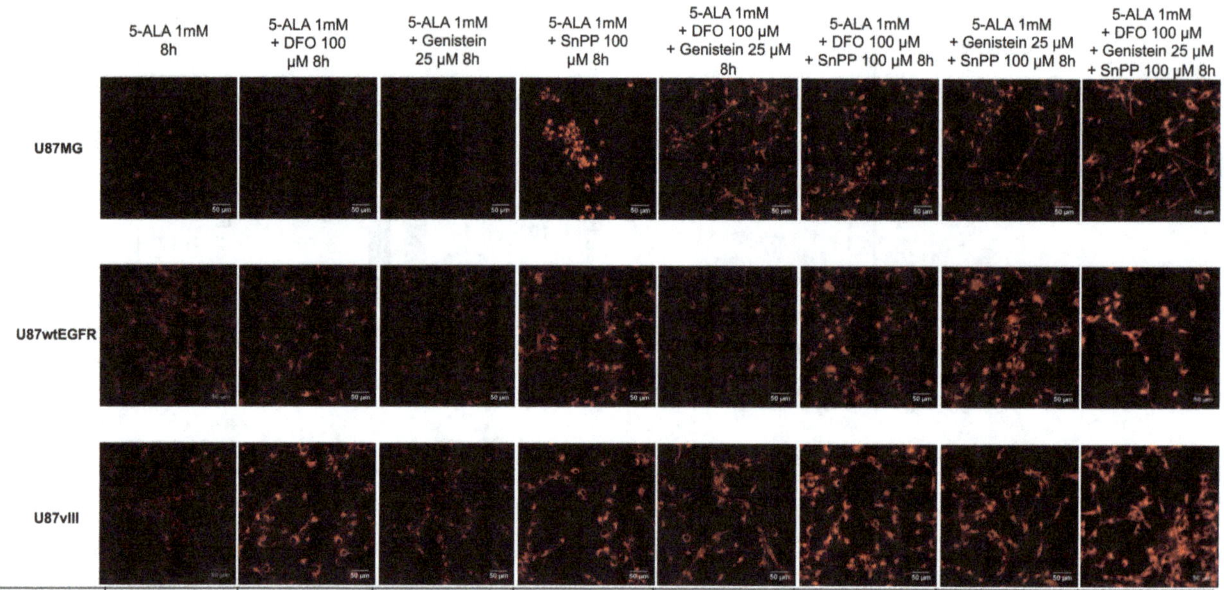

Cell line	5-ALA (alone)	DFO 100 µM	Genistein 25 µM	SnPP 100 µM	DFO 100 µM + Genistein 25 µM	DFO 100 µM + SnPP 100 µM	Genistein 25 µM + SnPP 100 µM	DFO 100 µM Genistein 25 µM SnPP 100 µM
U87MG	0 %	23 %	25 %	48 %	61 %	64 %	75 %	147 %
U87wtEGFR	0%	11%	48%	27%	83%	56%	140%	172%
U87vIII	0 %	26 %	79 %	42 %	161 %	78 %	136 %	228 %

FIGURE 4 | PpIX fluorescence accumulation after single and combined treatments. Confocal images showing the increment in PpIX fluorescence (represented in red, excitation 405 nm and emission 635 nm) in GBM cells after single and combined treatment with two or three drugs compared to 5-ALA alone (represented as 0%). Scale bars represent 50 µm. Table summarizes the increment of PpIX fluorescence in percentage. DFO (deferoxamine), SnPP (tin protoporphyrin IX).

pharmacological studies, we selected a genistein concentration of 25 µM (16). With the selected concentration we performed a more detailed analysis in biological triplicates of PpIX fluorescence by flow cytometry in the absence or presence of exogenous 5-ALA. Endogenous PpIX fluorescence was not affected by the blockade of the ABCG2 transporter in presence of genistein, whilst this was the case when 5-ALA was added to the culture medium for the three cell lines. In fact, the combined treatment with genistein and 5-ALA compared to 5-ALA alone (set as 100%) increased PpIX fluorescence by 42% for U87MG cells, by 31% for U87wtEGFR cells and by 54% for U87vIII cells (**Figure 3C**) (16).

Combined Treatments Improves PpIX Accumulation in U87 Glioblastoma Cell Lines

Detailed flow cytometric analysis led to the identification of combined treatments composed of two drugs leading to significantly increased mean PpIX fluorescence. For all three cell lines, the combination of reduced PpIX metabolism and impaired PpIX efflux resulted in augmented 5-ALA-induced fluorescence. Whilst SnPP and genistein is the best combination for U87MG (75% increase compared to 25% with genistein alone or 48% for SnPP alone) and U87wtEGFR cells (140% increase compared to 48% for genistein and 27% for SnPP), U87vIII cells responded better to DFO combined with genistein (161% increase compared to 79% with genistein and 26% for DFO) in the presence of exogenous 5-ALA, set as 0%. Maximal PpIX fluorescence is observed for the three lines with the combination of all three drugs, indicating that neither SnPP nor DFO, when tested alone, are able to completely block PpIX metabolism. In the presence of the three drugs the increment in PpIX fluorescence reached 147% for U87MG cells, 172% for U87wtEGFR cells and 228% for U87vIII cells as reported in the table of **Figure 4**. These data were confirmed by qualitative confocal microscopy analysis (**Figure 4**). Overall, these data indicated that inhibition of PpIX metabolism coupled to inhibition of PpIX efflux is expected to improve the visualization of GBM cells. Nevertheless, the optimal drug combination may depend on the genotype of the GBM cell, in particular considering the presence of defined gene mutations.

Intraoperative PpIX Fluorescence Guided Tumor Resection and Postoperative Quantification of PpIX Fluorescence of Tumor Samples and Comparison With PpIX Extraction

Figure 5 and **Video S1** show the intraoperative resection of GBM and the tissue which has been taken for later analysis with the Qp9-microscope. **Figure 6A** shows the color-coded image of the tumor samples with the concentration values for PpIX. The color-coded image represents areas of high and low PpIX concentration on its surface. The automated area of investigation of the Qp9

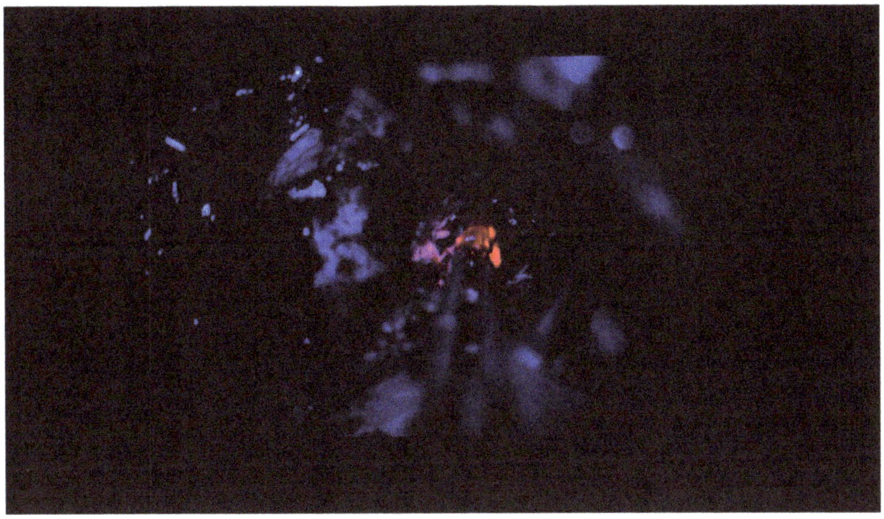

FIGURE 5 | 5-ALA guided surgery with OPMI PENTERO 900. Image of video showing the surgical intervention of glioblastoma removal. Under the blue light the tumor bulk is red, the fluorescence in the tumor margin is pink and more vague.

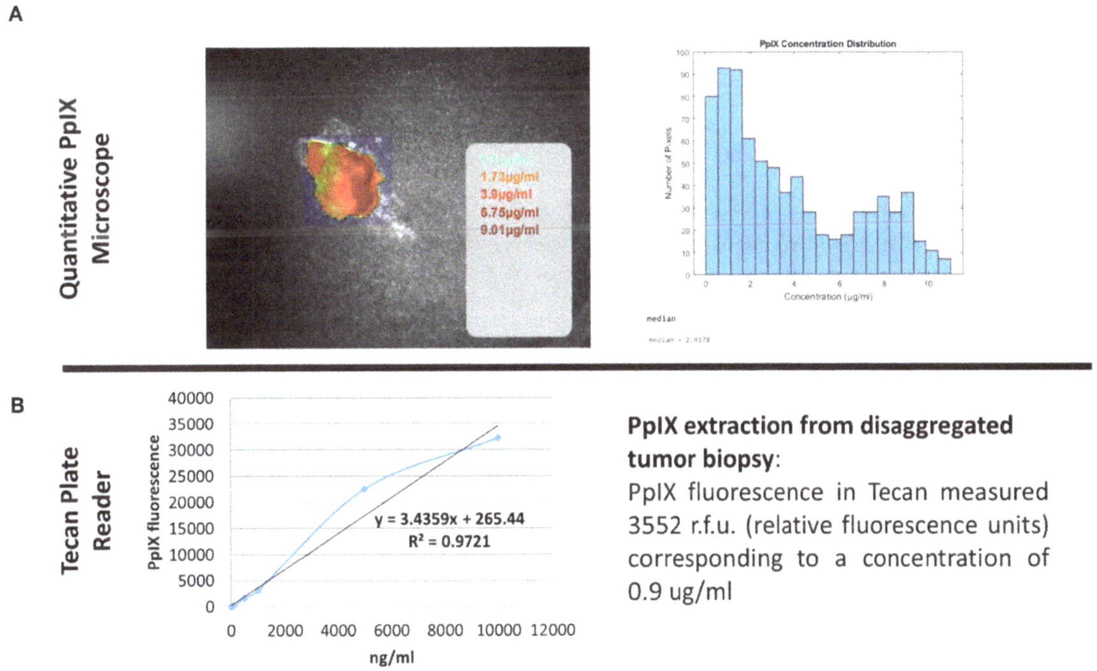

FIGURE 6 | Quantitative PpIX measurement. Comparison of two different methods able to quantitatively measure the accumulated PpIX in tissue biopsy. **(A)** Shows quantitative measurement performed with the Qp9 Zeiss microscope whereas **(B)** shows results obtained after methanolic-perchloric acid extraction from the whole biopsy.

microscope (**Figure 6A**) contains areas outside or at the margin of the tumor specimen and such are practically reported as very low or absence of PpIX (<0.1 µg/ml). This however does not affect the correlation as these very low values are not considered in the sample extraction. Tumor sample has thereafter been disaggregated and analyzed for its PpIX concentration (**Figure 6B**). The values of the disaggregated tumor tissue show concentration below the expected values measured by the Qp9 microscope yet in the same decimal.

DISCUSSION

There is no doubt that 5-ALA induced fluorescence has an impact on augmentation of the surgical resection in GBM surgery (20).

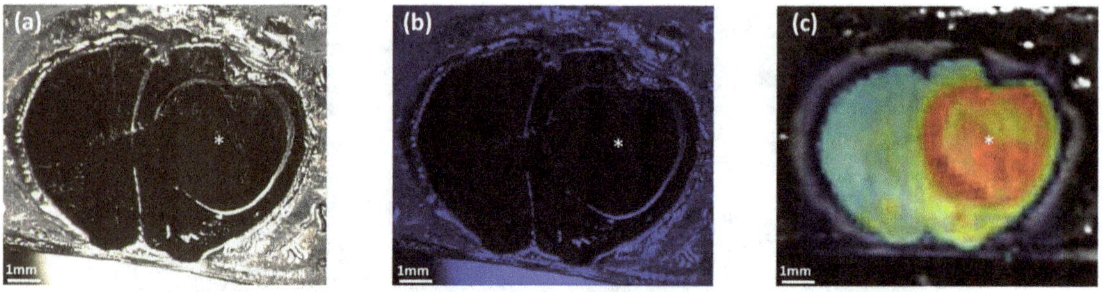

FIGURE 7 | Comparison between OPMI PENTERO 900 and Qp9 Zeiss microscopes. The figures show cryosectioned slice of GBM xenograft mouse model. In **(a,b)** visualization under OPMI PENTERO 900 with white light source and UV laser Blue 400, respectively. **(c)** Shows the color coded matrix image obtained after the PpIX quantification by Qp9. *tumor region. Scale bars = 1 mm.

Additionally, 5-ALA induced fluorescence harbors the potential for photodynamic therapy. For both treatments, a selective and controlled augmentation and especially quantification of the PpIX fluorescence signal is crucial for developing the technologies further. Therefore, we studied, in three different cell lines, the optimal conditions and pharmacological possibilities to augment the signal by influencing the balance of production, consumption and outbound transportation of PpIX. We also identified that different GBM cell lines have different PpIX signal, a phenomenon which has been also observed in the clinical situation (21). The evaluation of PpIX fluorescence positivity during the surgical operation of GBM is especially subjective to the surgeon's eye, limiting the usefulness and thus the impact on resection. Hence user independent evaluation of the operation situs will become necessary. Different groups in the past have described offline imaging techniques or online probes to interpret the quantitative values of PpIX (22). Yet the verification of microscopic arbitrary values as measured in the past and as in our study by the Qp9 microscope need to be further verified by selective tumor tissue analysis and quantitative PpIX extraction.

The values measured after extraction of PpIX from tumor samples were lower than what the values were in the Qp9 analysis. Reasons for that may be divers, resulting from extraction dilution or the disaggregation process. Although approximation of the effective PpIX concentration might technically be possible in the real surgical resection situation, these quantitative values will probably have no effect on the decision making for the tumor resection itself. Furthermore, during surgery of human GBM different factors may influence the visibility, respectively, the detection of PpIX fluorescence both with the naked eye or with the Qp9 microscope. Factors such as bleaching or different focus distance or even fluid covering may influence the signal intensity. Therefore, a sensible detection technique such as Qp9 or a mechanism enhancing the signal intensity such as heme oxygenase-1 blocker, iron chelating agents or PpIX transporter protein blocker may possibly be combined in the future for more sensible detection of different fluorescenting GBM or maybe even lower grade glioma. These findings will however need to be correlated with effective tumor cell infiltration in brain tumor. We have previously demonstrated that different GBM cell lines may have different PpIX signal intensity when treated with the same parameters (7, 16), a phenomenon also described *in vivo* (21). This phenomenon can be also seen in our mice GBM tumor model, as demonstrated in **Figure 7**, where tumor not visible to the naked eye with the conventional blue light of the operation microscope, can be made visible with color coded matrix under the Cp9 microscope. Belykh et al. have previously analyzed three different techniques (Scanning fiber endoscope (SFE), blue light and confocal scanning microscope) and concluded that SFE provides new endoscopic capability to visualize PpIX positivity at cellular levels (18, 23). We agree with Belykh et al. (18) that a more refined technique for visualization of PpIX such as SFE or now Qp9 are necessary. Techniques are complementary and probably cannot replace one with the other. The advantage of Qp9 over SFE may be that it can give the surgeon a faster overall picture of where remaining tumor is to be searched for and resected, however at the fate of more artifacts such as fluids, bleaching and focus distance. SFE will probably result more locally precise. Therefore, possibly a combination of both techniques may prove to be even more effective. Our next steps are passing from the cell cultures and offline tumor samples to immediate intraoperative monitoring first of tumor samples and analyzing the quantitative PpIX matrix color coded images with the effective tumor cell invasion.

ETHICS STATEMENT

The Ethic Committee of the Canton Ticino approved animal experiments in the animal application TI-05-19 Numero e-TV: 27255.

AUTHOR CONTRIBUTIONS

MR conceived the idea and wrote and edited the manuscript. DP performed experimental work and manuscript editing and reviewing. MW, CH, and RG performed Cp9 design and manuscript revision. FM and MD performed experimental work and manuscript editing and reviewing.

REFERENCES

1. Peng Q, Warloe T, Berg K, Moan J, Kongshaug M, Giercksky KE, et al. 5-Aminolevulinic acid-based photodynamic therapy: clinical research and future challenges. *Cancer.* (1997) 79:2282–308.
2. Stummer W, Pichlmeier U, Meinel T, Wiestler OD, Zanella F, Reulen HJ, et al. Fluorescence-guided surgery with 5-aminolevulinic acid for resection of malignant glioma: a randomised controlled multicentre phase III trial. *Lancet Oncol.* (2006) 7:392–401. doi: 10.1016/S1470-2045(06)70665-9
3. Fujii Y, Muragaki Y, Maruyama T, Nitta M, Saito T, Ikuta S, et al. Threshold of the extent of resection for WHO Grade III gliomas: retrospective volumetric analysis of 122 cases using intraoperative MRI. *J Neurosurg.* (2018) 129:1–9. doi: 10.3171/2017.3.JNS162383
4. Stummer W, Stepp H, Wiestler OD, Pichlmeier U. Randomized, prospective double-blinded study comparing 3 different doses of 5-aminolevulinic acid for fluorescence-guided resections of malignant gliomas. *Neurosurgery.* (2017) 81:230–9. doi: 10.1093/neuros/nyx074
5. Jaber M, Wölfer J, Ewelt C, Holling M, Hasselblatt M, Niederstadt T, et al. The value of 5-aminolevulinic acid in low-grade gliomas and high-grade gliomas lacking glioblastoma imaging features: an analysis based on fluorescence, magnetic resonance imaging, 18F-fluoroethyl tyrosine positron emission tomography, and tumor molecular factors. *Neurosurgery.* (2016) 78:401–11; discussion 411. doi: 10.1227/NEU.0000000000001020
6. Kim S, Kim JE, Kim YH, Hwang T, Kim SK, Xu WJ, et al. Glutaminase 2 expression is associated with regional heterogeneity of 5-aminolevulinic acid fluorescence in glioblastoma. *Sci Rep.* (2017) 7:12221 doi: 10.1038/s41598-017-12557-3
7. Fontana AO, Piffaretti D, Marchi F, Burgio F, Faia-Torres AB, Paganetti P, et al. Epithelial growth factor receptor expression influences 5-ALA induced glioblastoma fluorescence. *J Neurooncol.* (2017) 133:497–507. doi: 10.1007/s11060-017-2474-0
8. Ogino T, Kobuchi H, Munetomo K, Fujita H, Yamamoto M, Utsumi T, et al. Serum-dependent export of protoporphyrin IX by ATP-binding cassette transporter G2 in T24 cells. *Mol Cell Biochem.* (2011) 358:297–307. doi: 10.1007/s11010-011-0980-5
9. Oberstadt MC, Bien-Möller S, Weitmann K, Herzog S, Hentschel K, Rimmbach C, et al. Epigenetic modulation of the drug resistance genes MGMT, ABCB1 and ABCG2 in glioblastoma multiforme. *BMC Cancer.* (2013) 13:617. doi: 10.1186/1471-2407-13-617
10. Suero Molina E, Wölfer J, Ewelt C, Ehrhardt A, Brokinkel B, Stummer W. Dual-labeling with 5-aminolevulinic acid and fluorescein for fluorescence-guided resection of high-grade gliomas: technical note. *J Neurosurg.* (2018) 128:399–405. doi: 10.3171/2016.11.JNS161072
11. Parker NR, Khong P, Parkinson JF, Howell VM, Wheeler HR. Molecular heterogeneity in glioblastoma: potential clinical implications. *Front Oncol.* (2015) 5:55. doi: 10.3389/fonc.2015.00055
12. Taylor CK, Levy RM, Elliott JC, Burnett BP. The effect of genistein aglycone on cancer and cancer risk: a review of *in vitro*, preclinical, and clinical studies. *Nutr Rev.* (2009) 67:398–415. doi: 10.1111/j.1753-4887.2009.00213.x
13. Valdes PA, Jacobs VL, Wilson BC, Leblond F, Roberts DW, Paulsen KD. System and methods for wide-field quantitative fluorescence imagingduring neurosurgery. *Opt Lett.* (2013) 38:2786–8. doi: 10.1364/OL.38.002786
14. Valdés PA, Leblond F, Kim A, Harris BT, Wilson BC, Fan X, et al. Quantitative fluorescence in intracranial tumor: implications for ALA-induced PpIX as an intraoperative biomarker. *J Neurosurg.* (2011) 115:11–7. doi: 10.3171/2011.2.JNS101451
15. Valdés PA, Leblond F, Kim A, Wilson BC, Paulsen KD, Roberts DW. A spectrally constrained dual-band normalization technique for protoporphyrin IX quantification in fluorescence-guided surgery. *Opt Lett.* (2012) 37:1817–9. doi: 10.1364/OL.37.001817
16. Piffaretti D, Burgio F, Thelen M, Kaelin-Lang A, Paganetti P, Reinert M, et al. Protoporphyrin IX tracer fluorescence modulation for improved brain tumor cell lines visualization. *J Photochem Photobiol B.* (2019).
17. Lawrence JE, Patel AS, Rovin RA, Belton RJ Jr, Bammert CE, Steele CJ, et al. Quantification of protoporphyrin IX accumulation in glioblastoma cells: a new technique. *ISRN Surg.* (2014) 2014:405360. doi: 10.1155/2014/405360
18. Belykh E, Miller EJ, Hu D, Martirosyan NL, Woolf EC, Scheck AC, et al. Scanning fiber endoscope improves detection of 5-aminolevulinic acid-induced protoporphyrin IX fluorescence at the boundary of infiltrative glioma. *World Neurosurg.* (2018) 113:e51–69. doi: 10.1016/j.wneu.2018.01.151
19. Valdés PA, Leblond F, Jacobs VL, Wilson BC, Paulsen KD, Roberts DW. Quantitative, spectrally-resolved intraoperative fluorescence imaging. *Sci Rep.* (2012) 2:798. doi: 10.1038/srep00798
20. Stummer W. Fluorescence-guided resection of malignant gliomas. In: Moliterno Gunel J, Piepmeier J, Baehring J, editors. *Malignant Brain Tumors: State-of-the-Art Treatment.* Springer International Publishing (2017). p. 81–101. doi: 10.1007/978-3-319-49864-5_6
21. Hauser SB, Kockro RA, Actor B, Sarnthein J, Bernays RL. Combining 5-aminolevulinic acid fluorescence and intraoperative magnetic resonance imaging in glioblastoma surgery: a histology-based evaluation. *Neurosurgery.* (2016) 78:475–83. doi: 10.1227/NEU.0000000000001035
22. Richter JCO, Haj-Hosseini N, Hallbeck M, Wårdell K. Combination of hand-held probe and microscopy for fluorescence guided surgery in the brain tumor marginal zone. *Photodiagnosis Photodyn Ther.* (2017) 18:185–92. doi: 10.1016/j.pdpdt.2017.01.188
23. Belykh E, Miller EJ, Patel AA, Bozkurt B, Yağmurlu K, Robinson TR, et al. Optical characterization of neurosurgical operating microscopes: quantitative fluorescence and assessment of PpIX photobleaching. *Sci Rep.* (2018) 8:12543. doi: 10.1038/s41598-018-30247-6

5

Pelvic Reconstruction with a Novel Three-Dimensional-Printed, Multimodality Imaging Based Endoprosthesis Following Enneking Type I + IV Resection

*Zeping Yu†, Wenli Zhang†, Xiang Fang, Chongqi Tu and Hong Duan**

West China School of Medicine/West China Hospital, Sichuan University, Chengdu, China

***Correspondence:**
Hong Duan
duanhong1970@126.com

†These authors have contributed equally to this work and share first authorship

Background and Purpose: Pelvic tumor involving Type I + IV resections are technically challenging, along with various reconstructions methods presenting unsatisfactory outcomes and high complication rates. Since predominating studies preferred adopting pedicle screw-rod system (PRSS) to address this issue, we designed a novel three-dimensional-printed, multimodality imaging (3DMMI) based endoprosthesis with patient-specific instrument (PSI) assistance to facilitate the surgical reconstruction of pelvic tumor involving Enneking Type I + IV resection. We aimed to investigate the clinical effectiveness of this novel endoprosthesis and compare it with PRSS in Type I + IV reconstruction.

Methods: We retrospective studied 28 patients for a median follow-up of 47 months (range, 10 to 128 months) in this study with either 3D-printed endoprosthesis reconstruction (n = 10) or PRSS reconstruction (n = 18) between January 2000 and December 2017. Preoperative 3DMMI technique was used for tumor evaluation, PSI design, virtual surgery, and endoprosthesis fabrication. Clinical, oncological outcomes, functional assessments, and complications were analyzed between the two groups.

Results: Minor surgical trauma with mean operative duration of 251 ± 52.16 minutes ($p = 0.034$) and median intraoperative hemorrhage of 2000ml (range, 1600, 4000ml) ($p = 0.032$) was observed in endoprosthesis group. Wide margins were achieved in 9 patients of the endoprosthesis group compared with 10 in the PRSS group ($p = 0.09$). The 1993 version of the Musculoskeletal Tumor Society score (MSTS-93) was 23.9 ± 3.76 in endoprosthesis group, which was higher than PRSS group ($p = 0.012$). No statistical significance was found in relapse between two groups ($p = 0.36$). Complications were observed in two patients in endoprosthesis group compared with 12 patients in PRSS group ($p = 0.046$).

Conclusion: The novel design of this 3D-printed endoprosthesis, together with 3DMMI and PSI assisted, is technically accessible with favorable clinical outcomes compared with PRSS. Further study is essential to identify its long-term outcomes.

Keywords: Sacroiliac joint, pelvic tumor, hemipelvic reconstruction, pedicle screw-rod system, 3D-printed endoprosthesis

INTRODUCTION

Pelvic bone tumors invading sacroiliac joint are rare, and its reconstruction after wide resection still remains one of the most technically challenging procedures (1, 2). In contrast to the anatomical characteristics of extremities, pelvic tumors with occult symptoms are frequently not diagnosed until considerable tumor size (3, 4). Wide oncological resection combined with adjuvant therapies has shown its therapeutic advantage over hindquarter amputation in terms of expected survival, local tumor control, and quality of life (5, 6). With the advancements of multi-modality fusion imaging, adjuvant therapies, and three-dimensional printing technologies, various researchers have illustrated limb preservations are feasible for selected cases (1, 2, 4, 7–9). The main concern in reconstruction is to re-establish the continuity of the pelvic girdle and prevent the subsequent collapses or rotations of residual ilium under weight-bearing conditions and retain favorable limb functions in the long term. Though various surgical reconstructions after wide resection have been proposed, complications such as infection, implant loosening, breakage, and limb length discrepancy after limb-salvage procedures, staying at a high level, cannot be ignored (7, 10–12).

Some studies have adopted 3D-printed endoprosthesis, on the strength of a single or two image modalities, to accommodate the unique defect in the reconstruction of pelvis defect after wide resection (13, 14).However, solitary modality of image has its limitations in revealing complex structures because different modality images exhibit distinctive advantages and disadvantages for revealing different anatomical structures with various purposes (15). Surgeons rely on comprehensive analysis and clinical experience to integrate different and complex imaging information to form a stereoscopic image, which is subjective among individuals and may contribute to inaccurate resection and reconstruction. 3D-multimodality image (3DMMI) has fully exploited the strengths of different imaging technologies by integrating different modality images to a single visualized 3D model with both comprehensive informativeness and precision, which has been first applied in complex neurosurgery and has yielded satisfactory outcomes but less reported in orthopedics field (16–18). Since the application of 3DMMI in the pelvic girdle reconstruction, especially in type I+IV reconstruction, are rare. Studies either focus on PRSS reconstruction (1, 4) or 3D-printed endoprosthesis reconstruction for periacetabular region invading sacroiliac joint with a single modality of the image used (8, 10, 19). The purpose of this retrospective study was to present our experience that adopting the 3DMMI technique in reconstruction of type I+IV resection and describe the clinical outcomes, as well as complications compared with PRSS reconstruction.

PATIENTS AND METHODS

Patients Eligibility and Demographics

This is a retrospective case-control study of patients who had undergone iliosacral resection (Enneking Type I + IV) with reconstruction in our institution between January 2000 and December 2017. Data on demographics, tumor evaluations, operative duration, intraoperative hemorrhage, functional and oncological outcomes, as well as postoperative complications were collected (**Table 1**). The inclusion criteria for eligible participants were summarized as follows: (1) bone neoplasms classified as Enneking Type I + IV; (2) discontinuity of posterior pelvic ring after surgical resection; (3) anticipated surgical margin with a width of 20 mm for malignancies and 10mm for benign tumors as preoperatively evaluated; and (4) without major neurovascular structures involved. Exclusion criteria: patients underwent previous surgery at other institutions, recurrent tumor, pelvic neoplasms classified as any other Enneking Type, as well as hematologic malignancies were excluded from the study. To minimize surgical technique heterogeneity, all the surgeries were performed by two senior surgeons (Dr. Hong Duan and Dr. Chongqi Tu) from a single subdivision in orthopedic department

A total of 28 patients matching the study criteria were identified, of whom 18 patients received pedicle rod-screw system reconstruction (PRSS) and 10 patients were reconstructed with a novel 3D-printed endoprosthesis. There were six males and 4 females who underwent endoprosthesis reconstruction with a mean age of 32.7 years (range, 19 to 45 years). In the PRSS group, there were nine males and 9 females with a mean age of 39 years (range, 19 to 64 years). All patients diagnosed with osteosarcoma were administrated a two cycle neo-adjuvant chemotherapy (doxorubicin and cisplatin) before surgery, and another two-cycle protocol (vincristine, doxorubicin, ifosfamide, and etoposide) were applied in two patients with Ewing sarcoma. Three patients diagnosed with metastatic tumor received corresponding chemotherapy at the oncology department in our institution. Preoperative radiotherapy was not a routine procedure in our department and was only applied in patients with inadequate margin and recurrences after operation.

Endoprosthesis Design With 3DMMI Technique

In this study, a complete preoperative radiological examination was administrated for a detailed evaluation of the involvements and implementation of 3DMMI. Preoperative radiography assessments including a chest computed tomography (CT) and total-skeleton technetium-99 bone scanning were performed to confirm the distal metastasis sites of bone. X-ray was performed to evaluate the general condition of the bone and define whether a bone deformity exists. Contrast-enhanced CT (SOMATOM Emotion CT scanner) and magnetic resonance imaging (MRI) (Siemens Trio Tim 3.0T MRI scanner) of the pelvis were administrated to assess the extent of involvements in bony structures and soft tissue (**Figures 1A–C**). Vascular involvements were evaluated by computed tomography angiography (CTA), while neural involvements were evaluated by magnetic resonance water imaging (MRWI). MRI images were mapped to CT images through affine and diffeomorphic registration algorithm, which were all implemented in open-

TABLE 1 | Demographics, clinical outcomes, and complications of the patients in this study.

Patient number	Gender	Age (years)	Diagnosis	Enneking stage	Reconstruction	Surgical margin	Intraoperative blood loss (ml)	Operation time (min)	Follow-up (month)	Oncological outcome		Limb discrepancy (cm)	MSTS-93	Complications
										Local recurrence	survival status			
1	Male	38	Osteosarcoma	IIB	3D-printed endoprosthesis	Wide	1800	150	10		DOD	2	15	
2	Male	52	Osteosarcoma	IIB	Pedicle rod-screw, cement	Wide	3100	330	28		DOD	2	19	Implant breakage
3	Male	34	Ewing sarcoma	IIB	3D-printed endoprosthesis	Wide	2000	280	29		NED	0	21	
4	Male	21	Osteosarcoma	IIB	Pedicle rod-screw	Wide	1600	290	53		NED	0	21	
5	Female	64	Osteosarcoma	IIB	Pedicle rod-screw	Intralesional	5400	420	48	Yes	DOD	0	16	
6	Female	39	Chondrosarcoma	IIB	3D-printed endoprosthesis	Wide	2600	280	22		DOD	0	28	
7	Male	32	Ewing sarcoma	IIB	3D-printed endoprosthesis	Wide	3200	260	46		NED	2	26	Delayed wound union, deep infection
8	Male	50	Giant cell tumor	3	Pedicle rod-screw, cement	Marginal	2800	320	58		AWD	1.5	20	Implant breakage, delayed wound union,
9	Female	19	Chondrosarcoma	IIB	Pedicle rod-screw	Wide-contaminated	4200	380	78	Yes	NED	4	21	Delayed wound union, implant loosening
10	Female	37	Aneurysmal bone cyst	3	Pedicle rod-screw, bone graft	Wide	1800	170	52		NED	2	21	
11	Female	43	Malignant giant cell tumor	IIB	Pedicle rod-screw, bone graft	Marginal	2800	340	128		NED	0	21	Delayed wound union, deep infection
12	Female	22	Osteosarcoma	IIB	Pedicle rod-screw, bone graft	Wide	1800	220	48		DOD	3.5	26	
13	Male	45	Metastatic renal cancer	III	3D-printed endoprosthesis	Wide	2200	250	28		NED	1	25	Delayed wound union
14	Female	26	Osteosarcoma	IIB	Pedicle rod-screw, bone cement	Wide-contaminated	3200	360	60		DOD	3	20	Implant breakage, deep infection
15	Male	34	Chondrosarcoma	IIB	3D-printed endoprosthesis	Wide	1600	220	26		NED	1	26	
16	Female	37	Chondrosarcoma	IIB	Pedicle rod-screw, cement	Wide	2200	270	50		NED	2.5	25	Implant loosening,
17	Male	35	Chondrosarcoma	IIB	Pedicle rod-screw, cement	Intralesional	7700	310	30	Yes	DOD	0	10	Delayed wound union, deep infection
18	Male	26	Osteosarcoma	IIB	Pedicle rod-screw,	Wide	2600	360	100		AWD	2	18	Delayed wound union

(Continued)

TABLE 1 | Continued

Patient number	Gender	Age (years)	Diagnosis	Enneking stage	Reconstruction	Surgical margin	Intraoperative blood loss (ml)	Operation time (min)	Follow-up (month)	Oncological outcome		Limb discrepancy (cm)	MSTS-93	Complications
										Local recurrence	survival status			
					cement, bone graft									
19	Male	37	Osteosarcoma	IIB	Pedicle rod-screw, bone graft	Intralesional	4100	320	52	Yes	NED	0	21	Pulmonary embolism, delayed wound union
20	Female	57	Chondrosarcoma	IIB	Pedicle rod-screw, bone graft	Wide	2900	230	22	Yes	NED	2	26	
21	Female	24	Osteosarcoma	IIB	3D-printed endoprosthesis	Wide	2000	270	36		NED	0	23	Delayed wound union
22	Male	40	Chondrosarcoma	IIB	Pedicle rod-screw	Wide	3100	280	60		DOD	2.5	19	
23	Female	33	Chondrosarcoma	IIB	3D-printed endoprosthesis	Wide	1600	230	27		NED	0	25	
24	Male	58	Metastatic lung cancer	III	Pedicle rod-screw, cement	Intralesional	4300	430	28	Yes	DOD	3.5	20	
25	Female	29	Osteosarcoma	IIB	3D-printed endoprosthesis	Wide	1700	220	48		NED	0	27	
26	Male	52	Metastatic lung cancer	III	Pedicle rod-screw, bone graft	Wide	3600	290	10		NED	3	16	
27	Female	26	Osteosarcoma	IIB	Pedicle rod-screw, cement	Wide	2000	220	72		DOD	1	17	Implant loosening, deep infection
28	Male	19	Osteosarcoma	IIB	3D-printed endoprosthesis	Wide-contaminated	4000	350	29	Yes	AWD	0	23	Delayed wound union,

MSTS-93, 1993 version of Musculoskeletal Tumor Society function assessment score; DOD, died of disease; NED, no evidence of disease; AWD, alive with disease.

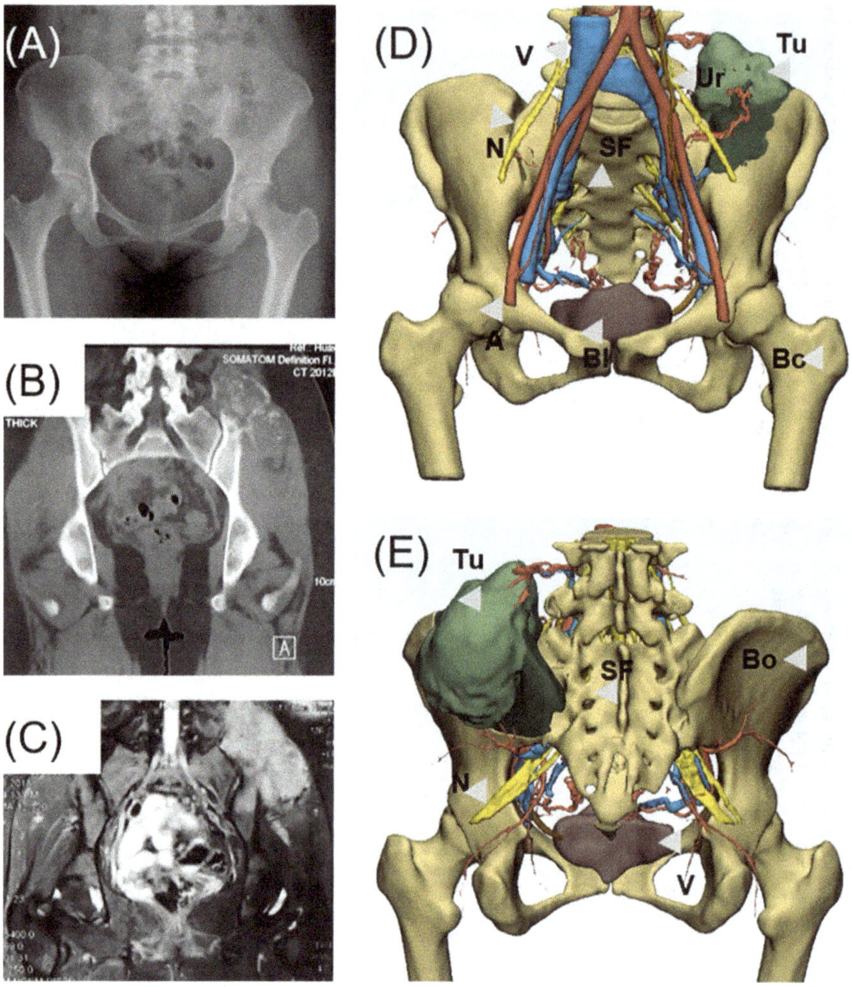

FIGURE 1 | **(A)** Preoperative X-ray shows the bone destruction invading the left ilium and sacroiliac region. **(B)** Computed tomography shows the chondrogenic bone destruction in left sacroiliac region with soft tissue mass. **(C)** Magnetic resonance imaging shows an extensive soft tissue involvement invading sacroiliac region. **(D)** Anterior view of 3D-multimodality image of tumor model of various structures presented. **(E)** Posterior view of 3D-multimodality image of tumor model. 3DMMi, 3D-multimodality image; A, artery; Bl, bladder; Bo, bone; Bc, bone cortex; Ki, kidney; N, nerve; SF, sacral foramina; Tu, tumor; Ur, ureter; V, vein.

source software named Advanced Normalization Tools (ANTS). Bony structures and nerves were segmented from CT and MRI respectively using a level-set based segmentation algorithm implemented in open-source software ITK-SNAP (20). Quality assurance and manual correction were performed after automatic segmentation (accuracy of registration >95%, maximum segmentation error <2 mm compared with the raw DICOM data). The 3DMMI of tumor model based on 3DMMI technique was then accomplished (**Figures 1D, E**) and then exported to stereolithographic (STL) format and opened in a workstation running Reverse Engineering (RE) software Creo Parametric 2.0 (Parametric Technology Co., USA) to identify the characteristics for the resection margin and cut plane. In this study, the minimum tumor-free margin of 20 mm in bone were regarded as sufficient as indicated by a series of studies reporting the satisfactory tumor-free margin ranging from 5 to 15 mm and 20 mm for chondrosarcoma (21–23) and osteosarcoma with sensitive response to neoadjuvant chemotherapy (24). The cut plane was then designed with a minimum 20-mm margin to the tumor with comprehensive consideration of surgical approach, tumor-free requirement, avoidance of neurovascular injury and viscera organs, feasibility to the installation of the patient-specific instrument (PSI). Virtual PSI was added to the 3DMMI model once the cut plane was defined (**Figures 2A, B**).

The endoprosthesis design was then designed to match the bony defect after resection, with several screw channels on the sacral lateral and iliac lateral. The length of cancellous bone screws was required to reach or exceed the cancellous bone screw for enhanced stabilization in implant-sacrum conjunction (**Figures 2C, D**). On the iliac side, conjunction was achieved through a T-shaped design with crossed screw fixation. Polyaxial screw was designed for extra stabilization and intraoperative adjustments in case of unexpected failure during the surgery. Furthermore, the polyaxial screw can be either fixed to the

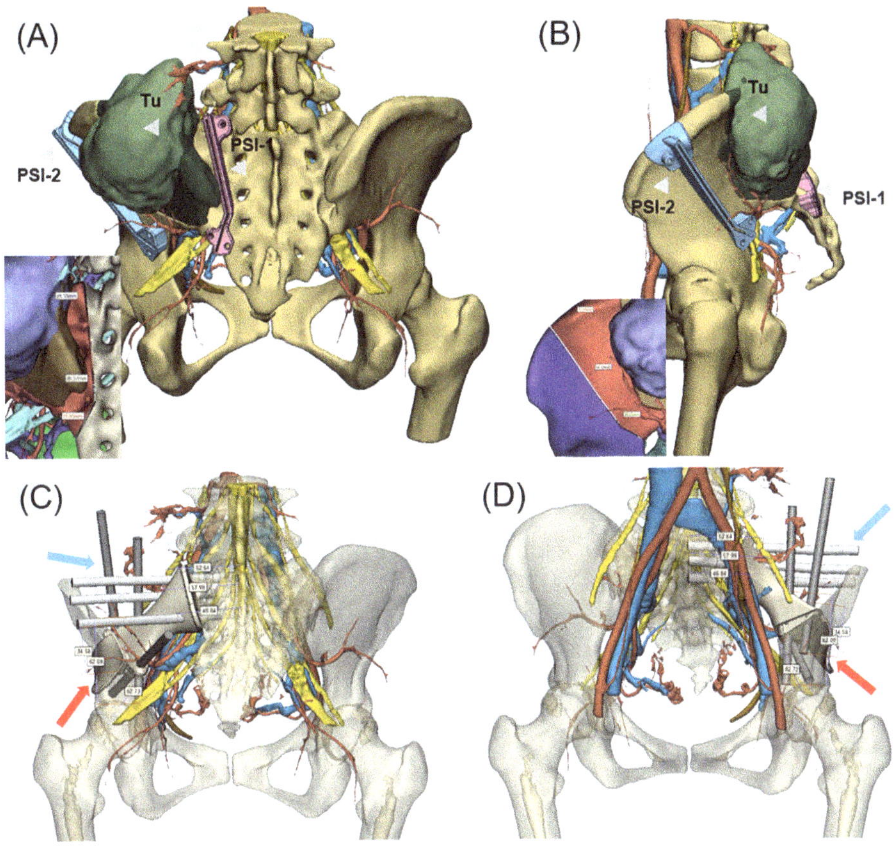

FIGURE 2 | **(A, B)** 3D-multimodality image of tumor model with PSI and surgical margin designed. The PSI-1 was placed on the sacral ala adjacent to sacral foramina and PSI-2 was placed on ilium with a adequate margin designed. The neurovascular structure were clearly shown to avoid intraoperative damage. In the left bottom, the purple region represented tumor, and the brown region represented the tumor edema with details of neurovascular structures, which guaranteed the accuracy of the resection. **(A)** (Posterior view), **(B)** (Lateral view). **(C, D)** The endoprosthesis and screw fixation design with the length of screws shown on the 3DMMI of the patient after tumor resection. The screws in the sacral side was expected to reach the middle line of sacrum and the residual ilium was crossed fixed with the screws of the ilium side. The blue arrow indicated the screws and the red arrow indicated the endoprosthesis. PSI, patient-specific instrument; Tu, tumor.

sacroiliac joint or designed to be a PRSS connecting vertebra and ilium. Finally, a rudimentary endoprosthesis (ChunLi Co, Beijing, China) was manufactured after streamlined modification for virtual operation on the printed tumor model (**Figures 3A, B**).

Surgical Techniques

The patients were placed in a lateral position on the contralateral side for patients who underwent endoprosthesis reconstruction. A posterior iliac incision extended with a posterior longitudinal midline approach was applied as previously reported in similar resections (25, 26). On the endopelvic side, abdominal muscles were detached from the iliac crest for exposure and protection of the external iliac vessels, femoral vessels, and nerves. On exoplevic side, gluteus muscles were detached from their origins to form a myocutaneous flap with superior gluteal neurovascular structures preserved. Subsequently, the dissection was performed on the endopelvic side down to the anterior cortex of the sacrum and identify the L4/L5 roots. Then, expose on the exopelvic side of ilium to the posterior aspect of sacrum. The exposure should be complete on previously located sites of PSI for the feasibility of PSI fixation and subsequent osteotomies. The PSIs were fixed with several 2-mm Kirschner wires (**Figures 3C–E**) and the osteotomies were performed in a straightforward manner using a swing saw on the sites of the ilium and sacral wing. If osteotomy was required to the sacral midline, osteotome would be applied on the anterior aspect. The tumor (**Figures 3F, G**) could be removed after dissection of sacrotuberous and sacrospinal ligaments. Since the endoprosthesis was a unique match to the defect, the reconstruction process, which has been described in the prosthesis design section, was carried on feasibly as preoperatively designed (**Figures 3H, 4A, B**).

The reconstruction method in PRSS (Medtronic, Inc., USA) group was performed in the same surgical approach. Two pedicle screws were implanted in the lateral side of L5 vertebral bodies and sacrum while another two screws were placed in the supraacetabular regions. Two titanium rods were used to connect the screws (**Figure 4C**). Technological process of how 3DMMI, PSI and endoprosthesis were implemented in this study has been presented in **Video S1**.

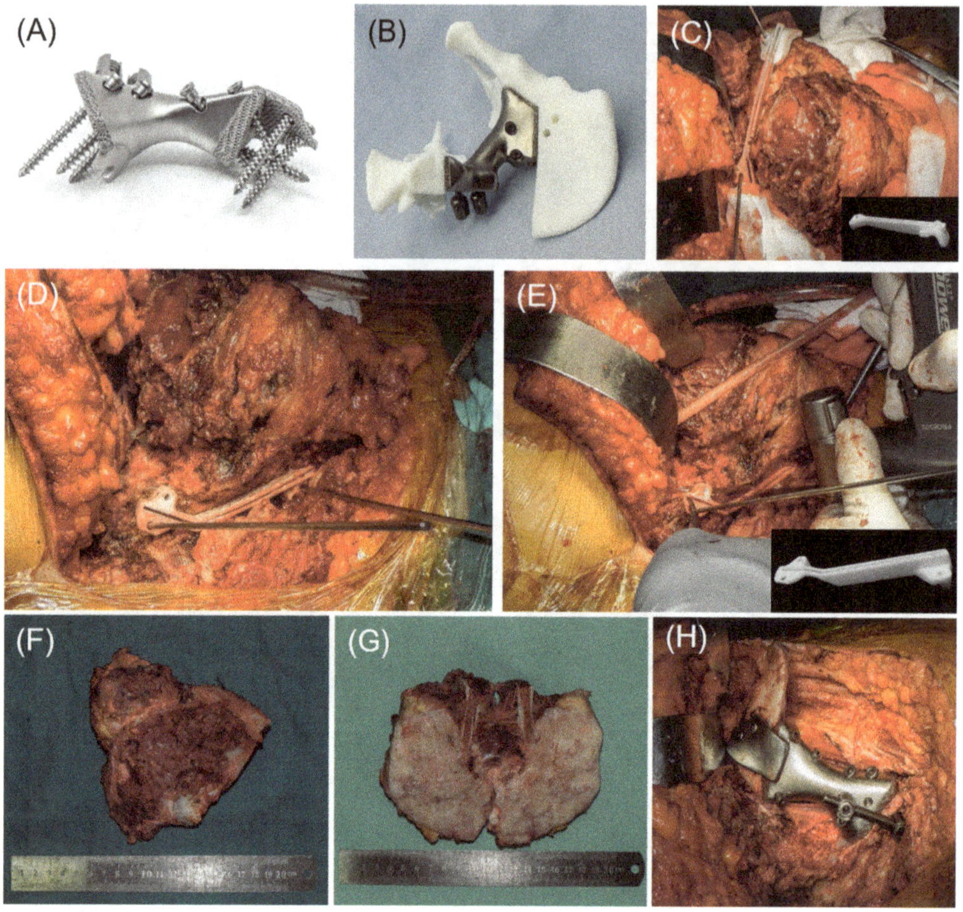

FIGURE 3 | **(A)** The 3D-printed endoprosthesis with screws fixed on. Extra pedicle screw design was added in case of unsatisfactory implantation of the endoprosthesis. The contact interface of endoprosthesis-iliosacral region was modified as porous hydroxyapatite design to facilitate bone ingrowth and osseointegration. **(B)** The virtual surgery on printed model with 3D-printed endoprosthesis implantation. **(C)** The resection of the ilium side and tumor exposure with complete capsule. The PSI was fixed on the ilium with Kirschner wire. **(D)** The resection of the sacrum side. **(E)** The resection was done in a straightforward manner with swing saw through the groove designed in the PSI. **(F)** The resected tumor. **(G)** Section view of the resected tumor. **(H)** The endoprosthesis has been implanted precisely.

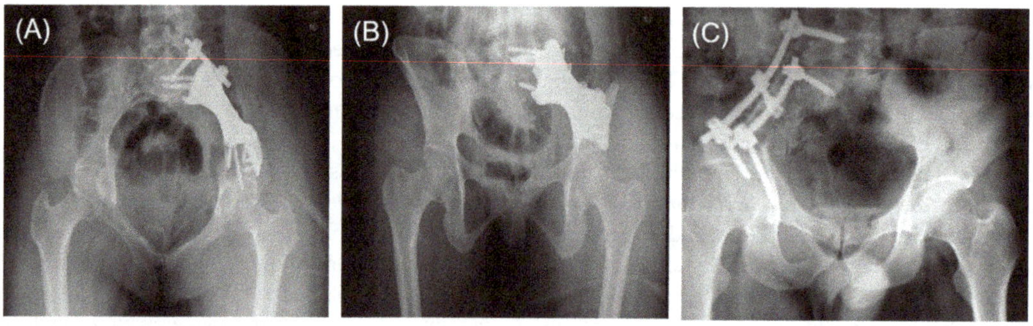

FIGURE 4 | **(A, B)** Anteroposterior view of postoperative plain film of the patient underwent 3D-printed endoprosthesis. **(C)** An example of patient received pedicle screw-rod fixation.

Postoperative Management

Customized lumbar pelvic hip braces were placed on all patients after surgery with the affected leg in a rotary neutral, 15° - 25°abduction, and 15°hip-flexion position. Three patients in the PRSS group presented with hemodynamic instability were admitted to the surgical intensive care unit (SICU) in our institution. The remaining patients were encouraged to early rehabilitation on the first day after surgery. Quadriceps isometric exercise and ankle flexion-extension exercises were executed during the first three days. Later on, active hip flexion not exceed 90° was executed to patents with a walking aid in the following two weeks. Partial weight-bearing was administrated since the third week and was gradually increased until normal weight-bearing status. The patients in the PRSS group started active hip flexion after 4 weeks and partial weight-bearing at 6 weeks timepoint. The adjuvant chemotherapy regimen was administrated in all patients with osteosarcoma and Ewing sarcoma. The follow-up regimen including physical examination and radiological tests were conducted monthly for the first three months and every 3 months thereafter in the first two years. After that, the follow-up was performed every 6 months. The function was evaluated by the Musculoskeletal Tumor Society (MSTS-93) score[13].

Statistical Analysis

Continuous data with normal distribution were expressed as the mean ± standard deviation and data with non-normal distribution were expressed as median and range. Student's t-test was used for continuous data with normal distribution, otherwise, Mann–Whitney U test was used. Overall survival (OS) was defined as death due to any cause. Disease-free survival (DFS) was defined as the time to relapse or death from any cause. Implant survival was defined as implant complication whether required revision or not. The OS, DFS and implant survival was analyzed with the Kaplan-Meier method. The log-rank test was used to compare the overall survival difference between the two groups. A p-value <0.05 was considered to indicate a statistically significant difference. Statistical analysis was performed with STATA 14.0 (StataCorp LLC., Texas, USA).

RESULTS

According to the Enneking and Dunham system (27), all patients were operated on a Type I/IV resection. Primary tumor origins and stage based on the Enneking staging system (28) were osteosarcomas in 12 patients (42.9%) with IIB, chondrosarcomas in 8 (25.8%) with IIB, Ewing sarcomas in 2 (7.1%) with IIB, giant cell tumor in 2 (7.1%) (malignant in one with IIB and benign in one with stage 3), and aneurysmal bone cyst in 1 (3.5%) with stage 3. Three patients diagnosed with metastatic cancers, which consist of pulmonary origin and renal cancer, were classified as stage III. The baseline data regarding age, gender, and adjuvant therapy in two groups showing no statistical significance. (p= 0.20, p=0.71 and p=0.68, respectively) (**Table 2**). The median follow-up in this study was 47 months (range, 10 to 128 months) for all patients and 28.5 months for the 3D-printed endoprosthesis group (range, 10 to 48 months) and 52 months for the PRSS group (range, 10 to 128 months). No patient lost follow-up by the time when data collected, or until the death of the patient. Adequate margins (wide margin) were biopsy-confirmed and were achieved in 9 (90.0%) patients in the

TABLE 2 | Comparison of baseline data, clinical outcomes, and complication between two groups.

	Pedicle rod-screw system	3D-printed endoprosthesis	*P*-value
Age	39.0 ± 14.0	32.70 ± 7.45	0.20
Gender			0.71[a]
Male	9	6	
Female	9	4	
Adjuvant therapy			
Chemotherapy	10	7	0.68[a]
Surgical margin			
Wide	10	9	0.09[a]
Wide-contaminated	2	1	
Marginal	2	0	
Intralesional	4	0	
MSTS-93[b]	19.83 ± 3.82	23.9 ± 3.76	0.012
Intraoperative hemorrhage	3,000 (1600, 7700)	2,000 (1600, 4000)	0.032[c]
Operation time	307.78 ± 70.0	251 ± 52.16	0.034
Limb discrepancy	2.5 (1, 4)	1.5 (1, 2)	0.03[c]
Recurrence			0.36
Yes	6	1	
No	12	9	
Complications[d]	12	2	0.046[a]
Deep infection	5	0	
Implant failures	6	0	
Wound-related	8	2	
Pulmonary embolism	1	0	

[a]$\chi 2$ test and Fisher exact probability method were used to compare the rate of wide resection and overall complication rate between two groups. [b]MSTS-93, the 1993 version of the Musculoskeletal Tumor Society score. [c]Mann-Whitney U test was used for the non-normal distribution of the data. The data was expressed as median and range. [d]Deep infections occurred in 3 patients with delayed wound union. Implant failures occurred in 2 patients with deep infection.

endoprosthesis group and 10 patients (55.56%) in the PRSS group, which presented no statistical significance (p=0.09). We didn't find significance regarding local recurrence rates between the endoprosthesis group (1/10, 10%) and PRSS group (6/18, 33.3%) (p=0.36). The cumulative OS was 96.4% (95% confidence interval, 77.2% to 99.5%), and 79.3% (95% confidence interval, 56.9% to 90.0%), 45.3% (95% confidence interval, 17.0% to 70.1%) at 1 year, 3 years, and 5 years, respectively for all patients. The DFS was 85.7% (95% confidence interval, 66.3% to 94.4%), and 69.5% (95% confidence interval, 47.9% to 83.6%), 43.3% (95% confidence interval, 18.7% to 66.0%) at 1 year, 3 years, and 5 years, respectively for all patients. Log-rank test for equality of overall survivor functions and disease-free survival showing no statistical significance (**Figures 5A, B**) (p = 0.68, p = 0.94, respectively).

We observed less intraoperative surgical trauma in patients who underwent 3D-printed endoprosthesis reconstruction evaluated by blood loss and operative time in this study. The median intraoperative hemorrhage was 3000 ml (range, 1600, 7700ml) in PRSS group, which was higher than 2000ml (range, 1600, 4000ml) in endoprosthesis group with statistical significance (p=0.032). The mean operation duration showing a statistically higher time cost of 307.78 ± 70.0 (range, 170, 430) minutes in PRSS reconstruction procedure compared with 251 ± 52.16 minutes (150, 350) in endoprosthesis group (p = 0.034).

The mean postoperative MSTS-93 score (%) at the last follow-up was 23.9 ± 3.76 (79.6%, range, 50% to 93.3%) in endoprosthesis group, compared with 19.83 ± 3.82 (66.1%, range, 33.3% to 86.7%) in PRSS group (p=0.012). Limb discrepancy was identified in four patients received endoprosthesis reconstruction and 12 in the PRSS group, which showed a significant difference of limb-length discrepancy between the endoprosthesis group (median=1.5 cm, range, 1 to 2 cm) and PRSS group (median=2.5 cm, range, 1 to 4 cm) (p=0.03). Seven of 18 patients in the PRSS group had more than 2 cm of discrepancy, while no patient with more than 2cm of discrepancy was observed in endoprosthesis group. The patient in 3DMMI group, with mildly abnormal gait, could walk and squat in a full range of motion freely without mobility assistive devices at the final follow-up (**Videos S2** and **S3**).

We observed 22 complications in 14 patients (50%), which presented as 20 complications in 12 patients in PRSS group compared with 2 patients in endoprosthesis group (p=0.046) (**Tables 1** and **2**). Wound-related problem (10/28, 35.7%) was the most frequent complication in this study. We treated these patients with dressing change, bacterial culture, and silver ion dressing (Atrauman Ag, Paul Hartmann Ag, German) and found no subsequent infection. One patient with pulmonary embolism was treated with anticoagulation therapy. Deep infection was found in 5 patients and was treated by debridement, intravenous antibiotics, and dressing change. The cumulative implant survival for PRSS group was 88.9% (95% confidence interval, 62.4% to 97.1%), and 82.1% (95% confidence interval, 53.7% to 93.9%), 67.1% (95% confidence interval, 37.5% to 85.1%) at 1 year, 3 years, and 5 years, respectively. Since no components related loosening, breakage, or implant-related revision was found in endoprosthesis group, we could not perform a log-rank test for comparison. The overall implant survival was shown in **Figure 5C**. Two patients (#14 and #27) with infection underwent curettage of the bony lesion in the debridement and were found subsequent implant-related complications, namely screw loosening and breakage. They presented chronic pain and walked with crutches and were treated with NSAIDs, and were closely followed without further surgical intervene. Another two patients (#2 and #8) were found screw breakages at the 24-month and 40-month follow-up. One (#2) of them was diagnosed with pulmonary metastasis with poor condition and refused further treatment. Another patient had screw breakage at residual ilium site with bursitis and received revision. Malposition of loosening rods occurred in Case 9 and Case 16 with restriction of activity and pain. They were all young patients and received revision surgery for functional demands.

DISCUSSION

Limb-sparing surgical procedure is much more challenging and demanding in the pelvis as compared with hindquarter amputation but has been proved to be associated with comparable life expectancies, relapse-free survival, and improved QOL (quality-of-life) (1, 7, 25). Due to the complex three-dimensional structures of the pelvis, especially when iliosacral regions involved, tumors are frequently related to the invasion of pelvic viscera and neurovascular structures and tend

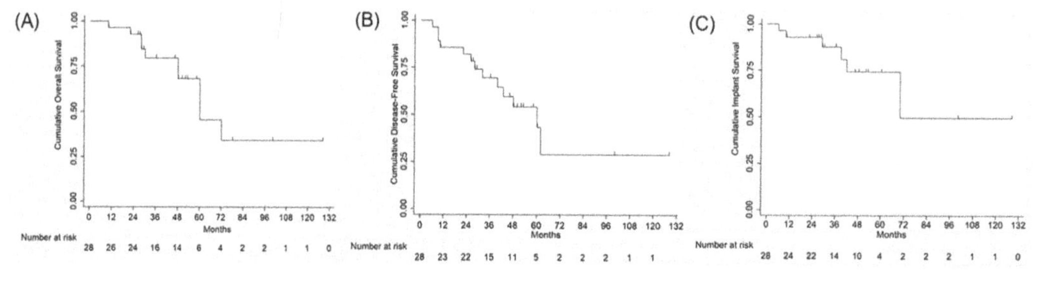

FIGURE 5 | **(A, B)** Survival analysis using Kaplan-Meier curve showing the cumulative overall survival **(A)**, and disease-free survival **(B)** and implant survival **(C)** for all patients.

to develop into considerable sizes before confirmed, which render Type I + IV resection more difficult to achieve (1, 4, 7, 26). When the supra-acetabular region and the partial sacrum are resected, the discontinuity of the posterior pelvic girdle contributed to considerable limb shortening and decreased lumbopelvic stability if without reconstruction (19, 25). Nevertheless, few studies have presented reasonable outcomes in selected participants with no reconstruction (11, 12, 29). Currently, rare studies have unequivocally provided preferable functional outcomes with the known reconstruction methods (1, 7, 10, 25). The major concern is that practicable reconstructive modalities have not been proved to remain preferable functional outcomes and are related to various complications regarding mechanical failures and deep infections (7, 25, 30). To address the current issues, we adopted 3DMMI techniques with Patient-Specific Instruments (PSI) and customized 3D printed endoprosthesis, which allows surgeons to precisely resect the involved pelvis, restore integrity between the sacrum and the ilium and retain the acceptable functional outcomes.

Since the massive musculoskeletal resections are frequently mandatory for iliosacral tumors, it is still under debate whether the unstable pelvic girdle defects should be reconstructed (11, 12, 29). Beadel et al. (12) reported a retrospective case-control study with 16 patients who underwent Type I + IV resections involved, of which 12 patients received no reconstruction. In their study, shorter operative duration, minor hemorrhage, and fewer complications were observed in patients without reconstruction with functional evaluation showing no statistical difference in the two groups. In their updated retrospective observational study (29), 32 patients who underwent Type I or Type I/IV resections without reconstruction were enrolled with a mean MSTS-93 score of 67.3% and a 3% local recurrence rate. However, the complications were observed in 17 patients with 40.6% (13 of 32 patients) wound-related complications. They have achieved favorable oncological outcomes with adequate margins, which may indicate that more structures must be removed as they stated 'aggressive resections'. If excessive resection without reconstruction, especially in the sacrum, the insufficient vascularized tissues with a large residual cavity may contribute to the infection (7). The main concept they prefer no reconstruction is that iliosacral defect induces the medialization of the hip joint center, accompanied with decreased body-weight moment exerting on a shorter abductor lever arm, which leads to an improved single-leg gait (12, 29). Nevertheless, the limb function is at the cost of the loss of lumbopelvic stability and integrity of pelvic ring. Besides, several studies have reported that sacroiliac arthrodesis contributes to progressive scoliosis and flail hips with considerable limb shortening (5, 7, 31). Wang et al. (32) reported a contrasting view that the functional outcomes of 12 patients with autograft and plate or pedicle screw fixation were superior to 12 cases without reconstruction, and the minor limb-length discrepancy was also defined in the reconstruction group. In the current study, we found no patient with more than 2cm limb discrepancy in endoprosthesis group, which leads us to believe that the lumbopelvic stability and pelvic girdle integrity should be restored with comparable results after Type I/IV resection.

The precision of resection with safe margins has a substantial impact on the oncological outcomes with regard to local relapse and patient survival. Peripheral regions of tumor are abundant with blood supply, which means resection process with positive margin is associated with a higher amount of hemorrhage and longer intraoperative duration. The results in our study have shown a minor surgical trauma in the prosthesis group with mean blood loss of 2270 ml (1600, 4000 ml) and mean operation time of 251 minutes (range, 150 to 350 minutes) which was comparable to the results of other studies ranging from 3153 to 5600ml and 256 minutes to 5.27 hours in similar resections regardless whether reconstruction performed or not (10–12, 26, 32, 33). Adequate surgical margins are particularly difficult to achieve when the sacroiliac joint is invaded (34) because substantial tumor size is frequently combined with extracompartmental feature, and occasionally responsible for distant tumor thrombi in the Baston plexus (31). Thus, 3D-printed endoprosthesis, characterized with individual design to fit the defects and improved accuracy of resection, is gaining growing popularities for precise resection purposes. However, most published literature presented their application of 3D-printed endoprosthesis based on one or two modalities of radiography with extremely limited structures merged into a 3D model (8, 13, 19, 35). Besides, the lack of PSI may lead to higher demands of surgical skills because inaccuracy resection wound make this technically difficult procedure even harder to perform (19). In this study, the cost for 3DMMI design was ¥3,000 to ¥5,000 and for PSI manufacture and 3D-printed endoprosthesis was ¥800 and ¥50,000, respectively, which is cost efficient when compared with the cost ranging from ¥50,000 to ¥60,000 in PRSS.

Although endoprosthesis group showed better outcomes than PRSS group regarding margin status, local relapse, we did not find a statistical difference between the two groups. The current study presenting an overall recurrence rate of 10% in the 3DMMI group with a wide margin rate of 90% is superior in resection of similar studies (**Table 3**). The reasons may be as follows. First, multiple modalities (CT, CTA, MRI, and MRWI) can be utilized and more details of the tumor can be presented, resulting in improved preoperative imaging assessments for the following resection and reconstruction. Unlike the most frequently used 3D printed endoprosthesis, designed and manufactured on the basis of a single modality of image mainly depends on bony structure (three-dimensional CT scan of the pelvis, design in Mimics), our 3DMMI technique implementing the algorithm in symmetric diffeomorphic and growcut manner, regionalization-adaptive registration, nD morphological contour interpolation, and Gaussian smoothing (18). Second, the application of PSI based on 3DMMI was precisely designed to be fixed in the tumor-free anatomic regions guarantees the reliability of the margin and accuracy. Due to the irregular shape of the pelvis and heterogeneity of the individuals, each PSI was unique and customized, which can only be fixed on the previously designated site. Third, the resection process was done in a straight-forward manner with time saved. PSI was firmly fixed on with K-wires and was designed with a groove. Osteotomy can easily be performed using a swing saw through the groove, which

TABLE 3 | A review of previous studies on sacroiliac resection and reconstruction, the margin, blood loss, proportion of patients with complications, and functional outcomes.

Study	Number of patients	Type of resection	Margin	Blood loss (mean, ml)	Reconstruction method	Follow-up (months)	Function (Mean)	Complications
Beadel et al. (12)	16 in total 12 (WR) 4 (R)	Type I for 16	Wide in 8 (50%) Microscopic or grossly positive in 8 (50%)	Mean 4325 for WR Mean 6250 for R	Four of 16 patients One (autograft + screw) Three (allograft + screw + cement)	Mean 45 for WR Mean 43 for R	Mean MSTS-93[c] 58% for WR (n = 12) 51% for R (n = 4)	Overall complication rate: NR intraoperative vascular injury in 1 (6.3%, n = 16) Allograft fractured in 1 (6.3%, n = 16) Allograft nonunion in 2 (12.5%, n = 16) Spinal deformity in 1 (8.3%, n = 12) Wound infection or necrosis in 7 (58.3%, n = 12)
Gupta et al. (29)	32	Type I in 8 Type I/IV in 24	R0 in 21 (65.6%) R1 in 8 (25%) R2 in 3 (9.4%)	NR	WR for all patients	159	Mean MSTS-93 67.3%	Overall 53.1% (17 of 32 patients) Wound- or infection-related complication in 13 (40.6%, n = 32) Postoperative fracture in 2 (6.3%, n = 32) Local recurrence in 1 (3%, n = 32)
Lin et al. (1)	30	Type I in 24 Type I/IV in 6	NR	NR	PRSS[4] ± bone cement ± bone graft	Mean 40.4(13.1 to 162.2)	Overall MSTS 81.0% (n=30)	Overall 40% (12 of 30 patients) Wound complications in 4 (13.3%, n = 30) Neurologic defects in 4 (13.3% n = 30) Bone nonunion in 1 (3.3% n = 30) mechanical failures in 5 (16.6% n = 30) (implant breakage in 1 and lessening in 4) Local recurrence in 10 (33.3%)
Jin et al. (11)	21	Type I/IV	Wide in 9 (42.9%) Marginal in 5 (23.8%) Intralesional in 7 (33.3%)	Mean 1988 for WR (n=18) Mean 3266 for R (n=3)	No reconstruction in 18 Autograft + screw in 3	Mean 67.3 (14 to 163)	Mean MSTS-93 93.3% for WR and R	Overall complication rate: NR Autograft absorption 1 (33.3%, n=3) Intraoperative sacral nerve damage in 1 (4.8%, n = 21) Dislocation in 1 (4.8%, n = 21) Wound necrosis in 2 (9.6%, n = 21) Screw loosening in 1 (4.8%, n = 21) Local recurrence 16.7%
Wang et al. (10)	25	Type I +II+IV	Wide in 12 (48%) Marginal in 6 (24%) Intralesinal in 7 (28%)	Mean 5600	Combined hemipelvic endoprosthesis (PRSS)	Median 48 (23 to 87)	Mean MSTS-93 48.0% (range, 30.0–66.7%)	Overall 56% (14 of 25 patients) Wound disturbances in 7 (28.0%, n = 25 patients) Deep infections in 4 patients (16.0%, n = 25) Prosthesis-related complication in 7

(Continued)

TABLE 3 | Continued

Study	Number of patients	Type of resection	Margin	Blood loss (mean, ml)	Reconstruction method	Follow-up (months)	Function (Mean)	Complications
								(24.0%, n = 25) Intraoperative sacral nerve damage in 2 (80%, n = 25) Local recurrence in 8 (32.0%, n = 25)
Court et al. (7)	40	Type I/IV in 33 Type I/II/IV in 4 Type I/II/III/IV in 3	Wide in 20 (52.6%) Marginal in 8 (21.1%) Wide-contaminated 4 (10.5%) Marginal-contaminated 2 of 38 (5.3%) Intralesional in 4 (10.5%)	NR	PRSS in 21 Various pseudarthrosis/ arthrodesis ± osteosynthesis in 19	Mean 70 (12-180)	Overall mean MSTS: NA 20% to 80% in different subgroups	Deep infection in 15 (37.5%, n = 40) Wound necrosis in 1 (2.5%, n = 40) Implant loosening in 5 (12.5%, n =40) Lumbosacral destabilization in 2 (5%, n = 40) Local recurrence in 9 (22.5%, n = 40)
Zang et al. (25)	17	Type I/II/IV in 16 Type I/II/III/IV in 1	Wide in 9 (52.9%) Intralesional in 4 ()	3153 (1700 to 6000)	Combined hemipelvic endoprosthesis (Combined with PRSS)	Mean 33 (15 to 59)	Mean MSTS 58% (33 to 77)	Overall 47.1% (8/17) Deep infection in 2 (11.8%, n = 17) wound healing in 5 (29.4%, n = 17) Dislocation in 1 (5.9%, n = 17) Local recurrence in 6 (35.3%, n = 17)
Zhang et al. (19)	20	Type I/II/IV in 9 Type I/II/III/IV in 6	Wide in 8 (40%) Marginal in 10 (50%) Intralesional in 2 (10%)	NR	Combined hemipelvic endoprosthesis (Combined with PRSS)	Median 36 (6 to 60)	Median MSTS 19 (5 to 26) for patients with 12 months survival or more (n = 16)	Overall in 12 (60%, n=20) Deep infection in 1 (5%, n=20) Dislocation in 2 (10%, n=20) Local recurrence in 3 (15%, n=20)
Ozaki et al. (30)	12	Type I/II/IV in 8 Type II/III in 4	Wide in 7 (58.3%) Marginal in 5 (41.7%)	NR	Custom-made hemipelvic endoprosthesis	Median 57 (26 to 77)	Overall mean MSTS 33.3% for patients that were recorded (n=8) Mean MSTS 37% for patients with prosthesis (n = NR)	Deep infection in 4 (33.3%, n = 12) Dislocation in 1 (8.3%, n = 12) Screw loosening/ breakage in 2 (12.6%, n = 12) Local recurrence in 5 (41.6%, n = 12)
Wang et al. (32)	26	Type I/IV	Wide in 19 Marginal in 7	Mean 1,300 (range, 600–3,600) The mean operative time was 280 (range, 230–380) min	Fibular grafts and plate and/or PRSS	Median 84.4 (32 to 165)	MSTS WR: 20.36 ± 2.56 R: 25.25 ± 2.93	Overall 26.9% (7/26) Delayed wound healing in 1 (3.8%, n = 26 Screw breakage in 1 (3.8%, n = 26
Nassif et al. (34)	6	Type I/IV	wide in 3 marginal in 3	median of 256 minutes (range, 212–339 minutes). The Median reported blood loss was1400 cc (range, 900–6000 cc)	Autogenous iliac graft with PRSS	median 33(6 to 53)	Mean MSTS '93 score was 72%	Overall 67.7% (4 of 6 patients) Delayed wound healing in 2 (33.3%, n = 6) Deep infection in 1 (16.7%, n = 6) Implant failure in 1 (16.7%, n = 6)
Sabourin et al. (26)	24	Type I in 13 Type I/IV	Marginal in 11 Wide in 12 Contaminated in 1	Average 5.27 hours (2.5—12).	Autogenous graft with pedicle s r	Mean 57.6 (4 to 240)	Mean MSTS-93 61.1%	Overall 75% (18/24) Deep infections in 8 (33.3%, n = 24) Hematomas in 6 (25%,

(Continued)

TABLE 3 | Continued

Study	Number of patients	Type of resection	Margin	Blood loss (mean, ml)	Reconstruction method	Follow-up (months)	Function (Mean)	Complications
		in 4 SI in 7						n = 24) Scar necroses in 8 (33.3%, n = 24) Graft nonunion in 42% (n = NR)
Gebert et al. (45)	35	Type I/IV	Wide in 32 Marginal in 3	NR	PRSS with bonce cement in 29 PRSS in 6	Mean 46 (1.9 to 139.5)	Mean MSTS 21.2 (10 to 27).	Delayed wound healing in 8 (22.9%, n = 35) Deep infections in 5 (14%, n = 35) Implant failure in 6 (17.1%, n = 35) Neurological defect in 12 (34%, n = 35) Local recurrence in 1 (2.9%, n = 35)

MSTS, Musculoskeletal Tumor Society score; WR, patients without reconstruction; R, patients with reconstruction; NR, not report, PRSS, pedicle rod-screw system.

can prevent insufficient or excessive resection. Fourth, the preoperative virtual operation was performed, on the 3D-printed pelvis model with a customized endoprosthesis. Thus, we can test modify the design and operation plan to minimize the possible error and risk before surgery.

Among the existing reconstruction methods, we prefer to adopt endoprosthesis reconstruction of pelvic girdle for its mechanical superiority of transferring weight-bearing force from the lumbar spine to hip and limb *via* sacroiliac joint. In this study, the conjunction between the prosthesis and residual sacrum was enhanced by enlarged implant-sacrum contact surface and more screw fixation compared with similar studies (8, 19, 25). The contact of implant-sacrum was anatomic match with three screws perpendicularly fixed and one extra rod-screw fixation perpendicular to sacroiliac joint, while the interface of implant-ilium was strengthened by an 'L' shaped design with crossed screws fixed. The polyaxial screw design can be either directly fixed or adjusted for a rod-screw fixation purpose. The advantage of this design lies in transferring the shear stress to compression stress in the stress conduction (35). Pedicle screw and rod systems were favored predominantly in many studies. In this type of reconstruction, stress mainly concentrated on both ends of the connecting rods in the supraacetabular region, and on the pedicle bodies of L4/L5 or residual sacrum, which is vulnerable to torsional force (36, 37). Hence, some studies recommended a compound rod and screw system with bone grafts for improved lumbopelvic stability (1, 19, 32, 37). However, problems remain for bone healing, graft fracture, and infections (1, 7, 26, 32). Allografts have been widely recognized with high infection risks (1, 30), whereas autografts are limited by donor site morbidities and extra operations (1, 33). Despite the superiorities of autograft, Sabourin et al. reported poor functional outcomes and a graft nonunion rate of 42% using polyaxial screws and titanium rods in 24 patients who underwent autogenous graft with pedicle screw-rod system fixation (26).

Endoprosthesis reconstructions presented various functional performance according to types of resection and reconstruction, which include allograft/prosthesis composite (38), modular hemipelvic endoprosthesis (39, 40), modular saddle prosthesis (41), and custom-made hemipelvic endoprosthesis (19, 25, 42) (**Table 3**). Combined pedicle-hemipelvic endoprosthesis, the most frequently applied method in treating pelvis tumors invading sacroiliac joint, of which the mean MSTS score ranging from 48% to 63% (8, 10, 19, 25). These prostheses were pedicle-hemipelvic design with connecting rods fixed on the acetabular components and L4/L5 vertebra (8, 10, 25). The similar problems confronting the connecting rods with peak prosthetic stress at the conjunction regions (10, 37), as Wang et al. highlighted in their continuous studies (8, 10). Zhang et al. reported high complications concerning pedicle screw-rod failures, and prosthetic dislocation in their previous study (25) and improve the prosthesis design with enhanced stabilization by extra fixation to the residual sacrum (19). These pedicle-hemipelvic prostheses emphasized the fixation should be embedded in bone cement, thus enhanced stabilization can be retained. However, bone cement is well compression-resistant but vulnerable to torsion, as proved by the high failure rates of screw-rod with bone cement enhancement (19). Since studies specifically focused on this anatomic region are rare, it is difficult to make between-approach comparisons with other endoprosthesis. However, our endoprosthesis showing a mean MSTS-93 score of 23.9 (79.7%) was favorable in the Type I + IV resections. Apart from the mechanical limitations of stress concentration of connecting rods and screws, the sacroiliac joint is characterized with physiological micromotion and hip movements induce rotation in the supraacetabular region (43). This type of enhancements may yield initial stability rather than long-term benefits. Our implant failure of 33.3% in PRSS group may also support the above statements. The fixation of rod-screw on L5 or L4/5 may be another potential risk for decreased implant stability. Lin et al. conducted a study with various types of pedicle rod-screw fixations and found that extrapelvic fixation in L4/5 was less stable than intrapelvic fixation in residual sacrum (1). The study recommends intrapelvic fixation if possible, because micromotions between intervertebral discs may contribute to increased stress level (8) and further fatigue broken or loosening of implant (1).

Other complications that are mainly focused on wound-related disturbances and deep infections were the most frequent complications in this study, as widely recognized (7, 25, 29, 35). We found two delayed unions (20%) and no deep infection in the endoprosthesis group, compared with 44.4% and 27.8% in PRSS group. Apart from inherent potential risks that sacrum adjacent to rectum, presacral venous hemorrhage, and undermined tissue regeneration caused by neoadjuvant therapy, the prolonged operative duration, increased blood loss and insufficient soft tissue coverage may also contribute to the infection and wound union (9, 44). Minor surgical trauma is difficult to achieve by conventional freehand surgical techniques that reported deep infection rate ranging from 11.8% to 37.5% (7, 10, 25, 26, 33, 34, 45). However, we minimized the chances of infection in a few aspects. On the one hand, the size and shape of endoprosthesis volume are not necessary to be the same as the bone defect. Decreased volume design of endoprosthesis that maintain the biomechanics contributes to better soft-tissue coverage. On the other hand, PSI based on 3DMMI allows the surgeon to perform planned resections, which diminish unnecessary surgical manipulations (9, 14, 46). Hence, we think patients may benefit from a well-designed implant with 3DMMI-based preoperative evaluation, which yields decreased infection in this study.

Though we presented encouraging clinical outcomes in patients with endoprosthesis reconstruction in Type I/IV resections, this study had a few limitations. First, the present study was retrospective in nature and was limited by its small sample enrolled. However, studies focused on Type I/IV resection are few (4) and mainly included Type I resection without a control group. Hence, the clinical outcomes may be comparable and able to justify the application of the novel prosthesis design. Second, the follow-up was not long enough to detect major complications, especially implant-related complications in the endoprosthesis group. Since the contact surface of endoprosthesis was highly porous surface design mimicking bone trabecula structure, we think a mean follow-up of 30.1 months (endoprosthesis group) in a group with a limited lifespan may be sufficient to report its early implant function, as the similar design has proved its long-term stability (19, 44). Third, tumor heterogeneity exists in this study. Despite we included benign tumors, the main purpose of this study was to evaluate the performance of resection and reconstruction adopting this novel design with 3DMMI and PSI. And the baseline data were comparable between groups. To date, this may be the first study reporting specific Type I/IV resections reconstructed with 3D-printed endoprosthesis assisted by 3DMMI and PSI.

In conclusion, the novel design of this 3D-printed endoprosthesis, together with 3DMMI and PSI assisted, are technically accessible with relatively minor trauma and better implant stability in facilitating Type I/IV resections compared with PRSS. It must be noted that long-term follow-up is essential to validate its capacity.

ETHICS STATEMENT

The studies involving human participants were reviewed and approved by Medical Ethics Committee of West China Hospital, Sichuan University. The patients/participants provided their written informed consent to participate in this study. Written informed consent was obtained from the individual(s) for the publication of any potentially identifiable images or data included in this article.

AUTHOR CONTRIBUTIONS

Study Design: HD. Data Collection: ZY and WZ. Methodology: ZY, XF, and CT. Written Work: ZY and WZ. Review and Revision: HD and WZ. Visualization: HD and WZ. Resource: HD and CT. Project Administration: HD and CT. All authors contributed to the article and approved the submitted version.

REFERENCES

1. Lin P, Shao Y, Lu H, Zhang Z, Lin H, Wang S, et al. Pelvic reconstruction with different rod-screw systems following Enneking type I/I + IV resection: a clinical study. *Oncotarget* (2017) 8:38978–89. doi: 10.18632/oncotarget.17164
2. Wei R, Guo W, Yang R, Tang X, Yang Y, Ji T, et al. Reconstruction of the pelvic ring after total en bloc sacrectomy using a 3D-printed sacral endoprosthesis with re-establishment of spinopelvic stability. *Bone Joint J* (2019) 101:9. doi: 10.1302/0301-620X.101B7.BJJ-2018-1010.R2
3. Li D, Guo W, Tang X, Yang R, Tang S, Qu H, et al. Preservation of the contralateral sacral nerves during hemisacrectomy for sacral malignancies. *Eur Spine J* (2014) 23:1933–9. doi: 10.1007/s00586-013-3136-3
4. Xu M, Zheng K, Zhao J, Bai W, Yu X. En Bloc Resection and Pelvic Ring Reconstruction for Primary Malignant Bone Tumors Involving Sacroiliac Joint. *Orthop Surg* (2019) 11:1120–6. doi: 10.1111/os.12563
5. Kollender Y, Shabat S, Bickels J, Flusser G, Isakov J, Neuman Y, et al. Internal hemipelvectomy for bone sarcomas in children and young adults: surgical considerations. *Eur J Surg Oncol* (2000) 26:398–404. doi: 10.1053/ejso.1999.0906
6. Sucato DJ, Rougraff B, Mcgrath BE, Sizinski J, Mindell ER. Ewing's sarcoma of the pelvis. Long-term survival and functional outcome. *Clin Orthop Relat Res* (2000) 373:193–201. doi: 10.1097/00003086-200004000-00023
7. Court C, Bosca L, Cesne AL, Nordin JY, Missenard G. Surgical Excision of Bone Sarcomas Involving the Sacroiliac Joint. *Clin Orthop Relat Res* (2006) 451:189–94. doi: 10.1097/01.blo.0000229279.58947.91
8. Wang B, Sun P, Xie X, Wu W, Tu J, Ouyang J, et al. A novel combined hemipelvic endoprosthesis for peri-acetabular tumours involving sacroiliac joint: a finite element study. *Int Orthop (SICOT)* (2015) 39:2253–9. doi: 10.1007/s00264-015-2891-7
9. Cartiaux O, Paul L, Francq BG, Banse X, Docquier P-L. Improved Accuracy with 3D Planning and Patient-Specific Instruments During Simulated Pelvic Bone Tumor Surgery. *Ann BioMed Eng* (2014) 42:205–13. doi: 10.1007/s10439-013-0890-7
10. Wang B, Zou C, Hu X, Tu J, Yao H, Yin J, et al. Reconstruction with a novel combined hemipelvic endoprosthesis after resection of periacetabular tumors involving the sacroiliac joint: a report of 25 consecutive cases. *BMC Cancer* (2019) 19:861. doi: 10.1186/s12885-019-6049-7

11. Jin T, Liu W, Xu H, Li Y, Hao L, Niu X. How does iliosacral bone tumor resection without reconstruction affect the ipsilateral hip joint? *BMC Musculoskelet Disord* (2018) 19:102. doi: 10.1186/s12891-018-2023-9
12. Beadel GP, McLaughlin CE, Aljassir F, Turcotte RE, Isler MH, Ferguson P, et al. Iliosacral Resection for Primary Bone Tumors: Is Pelvic Reconstruction Necessary? *Clin Orthop Relat Res* (2005) NA:22–9. doi: 10.1097/01.blo.0000180046.97466.bc
13. Ji T, Yang Y, Tang X, Liang H, Yan T, Yang R, et al. 3D-Printed Modular Hemipelvic Endoprosthetic Reconstruction Following Periacetabular Tumor Resection: Early Results of 80 Consecutive Cases. *J Bone Joint Surg* (2020) 1530–41. doi: 10.2106/JBJS.19.01437
14. Jentzsch T, Vlachopoulos L, Fürnstahl P, Müller DA, Fuchs B. Tumor resection at the pelvis using three-dimensional planning and patient-specific instruments: a case series. *World J Surg Onc* (2016) 14:249. doi: 10.1186/s12957-016-1006-2
15. Nomikos GC, Murphey MD, Kransdorf MJ, Bancroft LW, Peterson JJ. Primary bone tumors of the lower extremities. *Radiol Clin North Am* (2002) 40:971–90. doi: 10.1016/s0033-8389(02)00038-6
16. Murphy MA, O'Brien TJ, Morris K, Cook MJ. Multimodality image-guided surgery for the treatment of medically refractory epilepsy. *J Neurosurg* (2004) 100:452–62. doi: 10.3171/jns.2004.100.3.0452
17. Nowell M, Rodionov R, Zombori G, Sparks R, Winston G, Kinghorn J, et al. Utility of 3D multimodality imaging in the implantation of intracranial electrodes in epilepsy. *Epilepsia* (2015) 56:403–13. doi: 10.1111/epi.12924
18. Cao X, Yang J, Gao Y, Wang Q, Shen D. Region-adaptive Deformable Registration of CT/MRI Pelvic Images via Learning-based Image Synthesis. *IEEE Trans Image Process* (2018) 3500–12. doi: 10.1109/TIP.2018.2820424
19. Zhang Y, Tang X, Ji T, Yan T, Yang R, Yang Y, et al. Is a Modular Pedicle-hemipelvic Endoprosthesis Durable at Short Term in Patients Undergoing Enneking Type I + II Tumor Resections With or Without Sacroiliac Involvement? *Clin Orthop Relat Res* (2018) 476:1751–61. doi: 10.1007/s11999.0000000000000121
20. Yushkevich PA, Piven J, Hazlett HC, Smith RG, Ho S, Gee JC, et al. User-guided 3D active contour segmentation of anatomical structures: significantly improved efficiency and reliability. *Neuroimage* (2006) 31:1116–28. doi: 10.1016/j.neuroimage.2006.01.015
21. Wong KC, Kumta SM, Geel NV, Demol J. One-step reconstruction with a 3D-printed, biomechanically evaluated custom implant after complex pelvic tumor resection. *Comput Aided Surg* (2015) 20:14–23. doi: 10.3109/10929088.2015.1076039
22. Nandra R, Matharu G, Stevenson J, Parry M, Grimer R, Jeys L. Long-term outcomes after an initial experience of computer-navigated resection of primary pelvic and sacral bone tumours: soft-tissue margins must be adequate to reduce local recurrences. *Bone Joint J* (2019) 101-B:484–90. doi: 10.1302/0301-620X.101B4.BJJ-2018-0981.R1
23. Zhang Y, Guo W, Tang X, Yang R, Ji T, Yang Y, et al. En bloc resection of pelvic sarcomas with sacral invasion: a classification of surgical approaches and outcomes. *Bone Joint J* (2018) 100-B:798–805. doi: 10.1302/0301-620X.100B6.BJJ-2017-1212.R1
24. Kawaguchi N, Ahmed AR, Matsumoto S, Manabe J, Matsushita Y. The concept of curative margin in surgery for bone and soft tissue sarcoma. *Clin Orthop Relat Res* (2004) 419:165–72. doi: 10.1097/00003086-200402000-00027
25. Zang J, Guo W, Yang Y, Xie L. Reconstruction of the hemipelvis with a modular prosthesis after resection of a primary malignant peri-acetabular tumour involving the sacroiliac joint. *Bone Joint J* (2014) 96-B:399–405. doi: 10.1302/0301-620X.96B3.32387
26. Sabourin M, Biau D, Babinet A, Dumaine V, Tomeno B, Anract P. Surgical management of pelvic primary bone tumors involving the sacroiliac joint. *Orthop Traumatol: Surg Res* (2009) 95:284–92. doi: 10.1016/j.otsr.2009.04.008
27. Enneking WF, Dunham WK. Resection and reconstruction for primary neoplasms involving the innominate bone. *J Bone Joint Surg Am* (1978) 60:731–46. doi: 10.2106/00004623-197860060-00002
28. Enneking WF, Spanier SS, Goodman MA. A system for the surgical staging of musculoskeletal sarcoma. *Clin Orthop Relat Res* (1980) 153:106–20. doi: 10.1097/00003086-198011000-00013
29. Gupta S, Griffin AM, Gundle K, Kafchinski L, Zarnett O, Ferguson PC, et al. Long-term outcome of iliosacral resection without reconstruction for primary bone tumours. *Bone Joint J* (2020) 102-B:779–87. doi: 10.1302/0301-620X.102B6.BJJ-2020-0004
30. Ozaki T, Hoffmann C, Hillmann A, Gosheger G, Lindner N, Winkelmann W. Implantation of Hemipelvic Prosthesis After Resection of Sarcoma. *Clin Orthop Relat Res* (2002) 396:197–205. doi: 10.1097/00003086-200203000-00030
31. Wirbel RJ, Schulte M, Mutschler WE. Surgical treatment of pelvic sarcomas: oncologic and functional outcome. *Clin Orthop Relat Res* (2001) 390:190–205. doi: 10.1097/00003086-200109000-00022
32. Wang J, Tang Q, Xie X, Yin J, Zhao Z, Li Z, et al. Iliosacral Resections of Pelvic Malignant Tumors and Reconstruction with Nonvascular Bilateral Fibular Autografts. *Ann Surg Oncol* (2012) 19:4043–51. doi: 10.1245/s10434-012-2339-x
33. Nassif NA, Buchowski JM, Osterman K, McDonald DJ. Surgical Technique: Iliosacral Reconstruction With Minimal Spinal Instrumentation. *Clin Orthop Relat Res* (2013) 471:947–55. doi: 10.1007/s11999-012-2643-6
34. Ozaki T, Flege S, Kevric M, Lindner N, Maas R, Delling G, et al. Osteosarcoma of the pelvis: experience of the Cooperative Osteosarcoma Study Group. *J Clin Oncol* (2003) 21:334–41. doi: 10.1200/JCO.2003.01.142
35. Dai K-R, Yan M-N, Zhu Z-A, Sun Y-H. Computer-Aided Custom-Made Hemipelvic Prosthesis Used in Extensive Pelvic Lesions. *J Arthroplasty* (2007) 22:981–6. doi: 10.1016/j.arth.2007.05.002
36. Jia Y, Cheng L, Yu G, Du C, Yang Z, Yu Y, et al. A finite element analysis of the pelvic reconstruction using fibular transplantation fixed with four different rod-screw systems after type I resection. *Chin Med J (Engl)* (2008) 121:321–6. doi: 10.1097/00029330-200802020-00008
37. Wu T, Ren X, Cui Y, Cheng X, Peng S, Hou Z, et al. Biomechanical study of three kinds of internal fixation for the treatment of sacroiliac joint disruption using biomechanical test and finite element analysis. *J Orthop Surg Res* (2018) 13:152. doi: 10.1186/s13018-018-0858-2
38. Schwameis E, Dominkus M, Krepler P, Dorotka R, Lang S, Windhager R, et al. Reconstruction of the pelvis after tumor resection in children and adolescents. *Clin Orthop Relat Res* (2002) 402:220–35. doi: 10.1097/00003086-200209000-00022
39. Tang X, Guo W, Ji T. Reconstruction with modular hemipelvic prosthesis for the resection of solitary periacetabular metastasis. *Arch Orthop Trauma Surg* (2011) 131:1609–15. doi: 10.1007/s00402-011-1359-5
40. Zhou Y, Duan H, Liu Y, Min L, Kong Q, Tu C. Outcome after pelvic sarcoma resection and reconstruction with a modular hemipelvic prostheses. *Int Orthop (SICOT)* (2011) 35:1839–46. doi: 10.1007/s00264-011-1222-x
41. Aljassir F, Beadel GP, Turcotte RE, Griffin AM, Bell RS, Wunder JS, et al. Outcome after pelvic sarcoma resection reconstructed with saddle prosthesis. *Clin Orthop Relat Res* (2005) 438:36–41. doi: 10.1097/00003086-200509000-00009
42. Barrientos-Ruiz I, Ortiz-Cruz EJ, Peleteiro-Pensado M. Reconstruction After Hemipelvectomy With the Ice-Cream Cone Prosthesis: What Are the Short-term Clinical Results? *Clin Orthop Relat Res* (2017) 475:735–41. doi: 10.1007/s11999-016-4747-x
43. The sacroiliac joint: an overview of its anatomy, function and potential clinical implications. Available at: https://www.ncbi.nlm.nih.gov/pmc/articles/PMC3512279/ (Accessed September 2, 2020).
44. Wang J, Min L, Lu M, Zhang Y, Wang Y, Luo Y, et al. What are the Complications of Three-dimensionally Printed, Custom-made, Integrative Hemipelvic Endoprostheses in Patients with Primary Malignancies Involving the Acetabulum, and What is the Function of These Patients? *Clin Orthop Relat Res* (2020) 478:2487–501. doi: 10.1097/CORR.00000 00000001297
45. Gebert C, Wessling M, Gosheger G, Aach M, Streitbürger A, Henrichs MP, et al. Pelvic reconstruction with compound osteosynthesis following hemipelvectomy: A clinical study. *Bone Joint J* (2013) 95-B:1410– doi: 10.1302/0301-620X.95B10.31123
46. Wong K-C, Sze K-Y, Wong IO-L, Wong C-M, Kumta S-M. Patient-specific instrument can achieve same accuracy with less resection time than navigation assistance in periacetabular pelvic tumor surgery: a cadaveric study. *Int J CARS* (2016) 11:307–16. doi: 10.1007/s11548-015-1250-x

6

Current Trends for Improving Safety of Stereotactic Brain Biopsies: Advanced Optical Methods for Vessel Avoidance and Tumor Detection

Serik K. Akshulakov[1], *Talgat T. Kerimbayev*[1], *Michael Y. Biryuchkov*[2], *Yermek A. Urunbayev*[1], *Dara S. Farhadi*[3] *and Vadim A. Byvaltsev*[1,4*]

[1] Department of Neurosurgery, JSC "National Center for Neurosurgery", Nur-Sultan, Kazakhstan, [2] Department of Neurosurgery and Traumatology, West Kazakhstan Marat Ospanov State Medical University, Aktobe, Kazakhstan, [3] University of Arizona College of Medicine, Phoenix, AZ, United States, [4] Department of Neurosurgery and Innovative Medicine, Irkutsk State Medical University, Irkutsk, Russia

***Correspondence:**
Vadim A. Byvaltsev
email@uni.edu;
byval75vadim@yandex.ru

Stereotactic brain needle biopsies are indicated for deep-seated or multiple brain lesions and for patients with poor prognosis in whom the risks of resection outweigh the potential outcome benefits. The main goal of such procedures is not to improve the resection extent but to safely acquire viable tissue representative of the lesion for further comprehensive histological, immunohistochemical, and molecular analyses. Herein, we review advanced optical techniques for improvement of safety and efficacy of stereotactic needle biopsy procedures. These technologies are aimed at three main areas of improvement: (1) avoidance of vessel injury, (2) guidance for biopsy acquisition of the viable diagnostic tissue, and (3) methods for rapid intraoperative assessment of stereotactic biopsy specimens. The recent technological developments in stereotactic biopsy probe design include the incorporation of fluorescence imaging, spectroscopy, and label-free imaging techniques. The future advancements of stereotactic biopsy procedures in neuro-oncology include the incorporation of optical probes for real-time vessel detection along and around the biopsy needle trajectory and *in vivo* confirmation of the diagnostic tumor tissue prior to sample acquisition.

Keywords: fluorescence, 5-aminolevulinic acid, stereotactic, spectroscopy, optical, biopsy, fluorescein sodium

INTRODUCTION

Brain needle biopsies are indicated for deep-seated or multiple brain lesions and for patients with poor prognosis in whom the risks of resection outweigh the potential outcome benefits. A recent systematic review and evidence-based clinical practice guideline investigating the role of stereotactic brain biopsy for low-grade gliomas provided level III evidence in support of brain biopsies and recommended that surgeons consider using advanced imaging techniques to improve diagnostic accuracy (1). In suspected low-grade tumors that are not considered for resection, biopsy location should be planned based on molecular guidance techniques, such as positron emission tomography, magnetic resonance (MR) spectroscopy, or others in order to provide a reliable molecular diagnosis (2).

The current standard-of-care method for stereotactic brain needle biopsy involves a 1.6- to 2-mm-diameter needle cannula insertion through a cranial burr-hole aligned to a predetermined trajectory. The two cannulas have overlapping side windows. When the desired position is reached, these windows are aligned, and brain tissue is lodged into cannula using suction and cut by sliding the inner cannula.

Despite the minimally invasive nature of the needle brain biopsy, the limitations and risks are still present and include the following:

1. Non-diagnostic biopsy yield. The frequency of non-diagnostic biopsies ranges in various studies
    - Not-specified non-diagnostic biopsy rate−5.2% (3), 9% (4), 10.7% (5), 13% (6);
    - Biopsy performed without intraoperative frozen section−11%;
    - Biopsy performed with frozen section on demand−1% (7);
2. Technical failure rate is 2.4–3.7% (7)
3. Complications rate:
    - Overall complications rate−1.2% (3), 7.36% (4);
    - Perioperative−6.3–4.8% (7);
    - Postoperative−10.5–4.8% (7);
    - Hemorrhagic/vessel injury complications: 2.1% (6), 3% (7), 4.35% (4), overall 8.8%, including 1% symptomatic, or >1 cm (8). One study reported the overall rate of hemorrhages on postoperative computerized tomography (CT) as 59.8%, including 41.1% of bleeds <5 mm in diameter and 8.9% of bleeds 3–4 cm in diameter (9).
4. Mortality rate was 0.6% (3), 1.34% (4), and 0.6–3.7% (7) in various studies.

Vessel injury is one of the most feared complications during minimally invasive stereotactic procedures. The rounded tip design of the biopsy needle intends to push aside any vessel encountered along the biopsy needle trajectory. However, such a design does not completely eliminate the potential for vessel injury during the forward movement of the needle. Moreover, the risk of vessel injury is believed to be higher during the side-cutting movement during biopsy acquisition. Therefore, apart from techniques for navigation on the anatomical level, like MR spectroscopy (10, 11), perfusion (12), and metabolism (13), improvements of intraoperative tools for biopsy acquisition and rapid assessment would be beneficial.

This paper aims to provide a concise review of novel fluorescence-based and other optical techniques for improvement of safety and efficacy of minimally invasive stereotactic needle biopsy procedures in neuro-oncology. The main goal of such procedures is not to improve the resection extent but to safely acquire viable tissue representative of the lesion for further comprehensive histological, immunohistochemical, and molecular analyses. Here, we do omit discussion of MR, computed tomography, and ultrasound Doppler (14, 15)-based navigation techniques. Although the potential value of these techniques is undeniable, we focus this review on recently proposed optical methods. The basics of optical techniques are found in recently published reviews of this subject that describe the basics of fluorescence guidance in neuro-oncology (16–21).

METHODS

We performed a literature search in the PubMed database using the terms "biopsy," "stereotactic," "fluorescence," "Raman," "spectroscopy," "brain," "optical," and "optical probe" in various combinations. Our search included papers published up to November 2018. We did not set a lower bound for this search. The titles were scanned and relevant articles were selected for full-text review, resulting in relevant articles for analysis as presented in the **Supplementary Data 1**. Additional articles were added from reference lists if deemed relevant. After reviewing the articles, the three key areas for analysis and discussion were selected: (1) avoidance of vessel injury during stereotactic biopsies, (2) probe-based guidance methods for biopsy acquisition, and (3) methods for rapid intraoperative assessment of stereotactic biopsy specimens. The latter two areas were united in one section for discussion due to the similarity in the used optical principles toward the common goal for differentiation of tumor and normal tissues, which can be done *in vivo* (using the miniaturized probes) or *ex vivo* after the biopsy has been acquired (using either miniaturized or benchtop systems).

RESULTS AND DISCUSSION

Avoidance of Vessel Injury During Stereotactic Biopsy (Table 1)

Intravascular Contrast Detection

Göbel et al. described a small contact forward-viewing endoscopic probe that can fit into a standard biopsy needle and visualize fluorescence signals of protoporphyrin IX (PpIX) and indocyanine green (ICG) (**Figure 1A**) (22). PpIX is a fluorophore (excitation maximum wavelength is 405 nm; emission maximum, 630 nm) commonly used as the basis of fluorescent-guided neuro-oncology (31), while ICG is a near-infrared fluorophore (excitation maximum wavelength is 780–800 nm; emission maximum, 830 nm) commonly used for vascular flow visualization (32). The multifiber probe includes two excitation diode lasers (405 and 785 nm for PpIX autofluorescence and ICG, respectively) and a charge-coupled device camera for signal detection. This endoscope allowed ICG detection through the brain tissue (about 1 mm thickness) on a phantom model. It also showed reliable detection of a red PpIX fluorescence from the tumor in a mouse glioma model. Subsequently, in a pilot clinical trial ($n = 1$), this needle endoscope was used instead of the standard brain biopsy needle mandarin to visualize fluorescence during probe advancement. The actual biopsy acquisition was performed with a small forward biting biopsy forceps. Although bright

Abbreviations: PpIX, protoporphyrin IX; ICG, indocyanine green.

TABLE 1 | Techniques for vessel detection during stereotactic brain biopsies.

Author, year	Technique	Clinical data	Main findings	Limitations	Safety
FLUORESCENT CONTRAST DETECTION					
Göbel et al. (22)	1.5-mm-diameter multifiber forward-viewing needle endoscope for dual fluorescence (PpIX, ICG) and autofluorescence imaging. Results in multicolor images.	Pilot clinical trial ($n = 1$) showed feasibility of autofluorescence and PpIX visualization; however, safety, and vessel detection were not evaluated.	Established feasibility on phantom and characterized detection capability of the vessels, normal brain, and viable tumor tissue.	Forward-viewing probe.	Light power was 10 mW.
Rühm et al. (23)	Fiber-based ICG detection in the vessels for stereotactic procedures.	No. Only computer simulation model.	Established safety corridor for excitation light power to prevent normal brain destruction.	Simulation computer model experiment.	Established light intensity safety corridor for ICG.
STAIN-LESS REFLECTANCE IMAGING APPROACHES					
Pichette et al. (24) Goyette et al. (25)	24-fiber, 1.7-mm-diameter probe for interstitial sub-diffuse optical tomography. Technology is based on the spectroscopic detection of hemoglobin remittance and sub-diffused light spectra. Creates a 2D map visualizing potential locations of vessels and their proximity to the probe's tip.	No. Only preclinical study on phantom models.	Established feasibility and characterized detection capability of the vessels of various locations and sizes.	Extravascular blood could affect interpretation of the data. Complex probe design.	N/R.
Markwardt et al. (26)	Double fiber-based probe inserted in biopsy needle for hemoglobin remission spectrometry. Allows detection of proximity and size of blood vessels.	No. Only preclinical study on phantom models.	Established feasibility and characterized detection capability of the vessels of various locations and sizes.	Extravascular blood could affect interpretation of the data.	Light power intensity below MPE for the skin of 2 kW/m^2.
Ramakonar et al. (27)	Side-viewing fiber OCT probe fitting the standard brain biopsy needle with automatic vessel detection on B-imaging mode.	Pilot clinical trial ($n = 11$) demonstrated feasibility of automatic vessel detection.	Established feasibility and characterized detection capability of the vessels.	No forward viewing.	N/R, although considered safe based on the patient data.
LASER DOPPLER FLOWMETRY					
Haj-Hosseini et al. (28)	9-fiber, forward-viewing probe fitting the biopsy needle for simultaneous laser Doppler flowmetry and PpIX fluorescence spectral detection.	Similar probes for laser Doppler flowmetry imaging have been studied in stereotactic procedures under IRB approval in previous studies (29, 30).	Established feasibility and characterized brain perfusion along the biopsy needle trajectory.	No side viewing.	Light power 10 mW for PpIX excitation.

ICG, indocyanine green; N/R, not reported; PpIX, protoporphyrin IX; ICG, indocyanine green; OCT, optical coherence tomography; MPE, maximal permissible exposure.

PpIX fluorescence from the viable tumor core was visible, no fluorescence in the surrounding needle positions was evident. For vessel visualization, a 200 mg/kg dose of ICG was used in the mouse model. With this, near-infrared ICG fluorescence appeared inside the blood vessels at an excitation of 785 nm (**Figure 1A**, top panel). With autofluorescence at 405-nm excitation, the vessels appear clearer and darker (**Figure 1A**, middle panel). With a combination of autofluorescence and ICG visualization simultaneously, the vessels also display clear visualization (**Figure 1A**, bottom panel). Vessel visualization in a human tissue was not performed.

Ruhm et al. investigated forward-viewing microfiber probe for ICG detection using a computer simulation of ICG fluorescence excited and detected through the same fiber-optic system in homogeneous human brain tissue (23). Although detection of intravascular ICG is widely used in open vascular neurosurgery (33), its application for detection of deep vessels might not be optimal due to the fast redistribution and ICG fluorescence decay. Leakage of blood or trace amounts of blood containing ICG in the vicinity of the probe would result in false-positive measurements. Furthermore, the dosage and timing of ICG administration would need to be optimized, and the necessity for additional drug injection should be considered, especially when comparing to other methods for vessel detection.

Laser Doppler Flowmetry

Another recently reported tool is a 2.2-mm-diameter forward-viewing needle probe that combines fluorescence spectral detection and laser Doppler flowmetry (28). The probe was designed to fit the Leksell® Stereotactic System. By measuring the frequency shift in the 780-nm backscattered laser light caused by the cell movements in the capillaries, the device assesses brain perfusion and blood flow. The pilot study on three patients demonstrated reliable detection of PpIX spectra (405

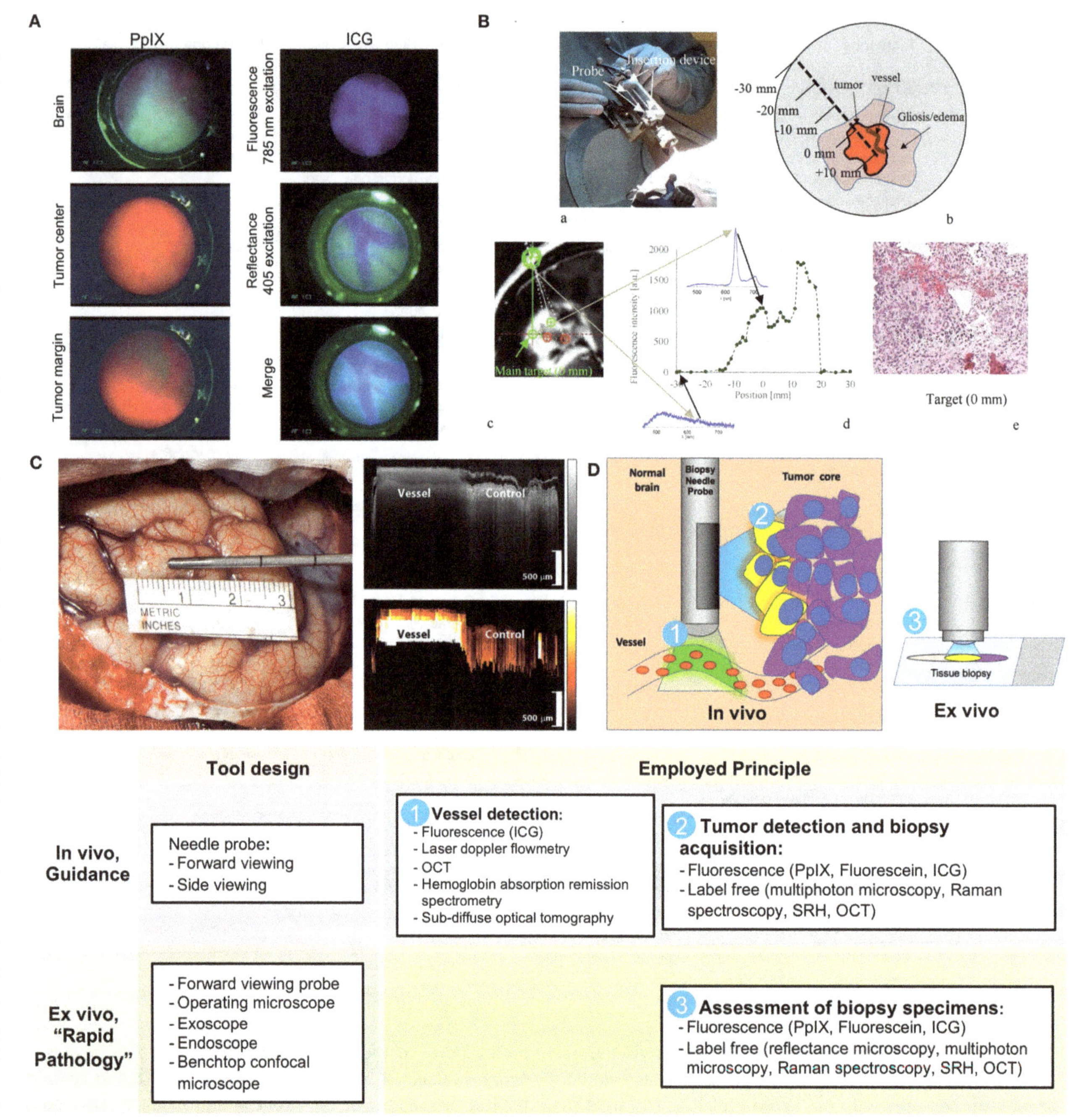

FIGURE 1 | Examples of the optical technologies for brain needle biopsies. **(A)** Images from the fluorescence optical needle endoscope described by Göbel et al. (22) for PpIX visualization in the tumor (left column) and vessel visualization using ICG (right column) in a mouse model. Adapted with permission from Göbel et al. (22)© The Optical Society. **(B)** Illustration of PpIX spectroscopy method for tumor detection during stereotactic biopsy described by Haj-Hosseini et al. (28). The top two panels show the probe positioned in the stereotactic frame and the concept of measurements along the trajectory. The bottom panels show an MR image with calculated targets, spectral data of PpIX along the injection trajectory, and the histopathology slide of the target. Adapted with permission from Haj-Hosseini et al. (28)© The Optical Society. **(C)** Stain-less reflectance imaging method from Ramakonar et al. (27). Left panel shows a photo of an imaging needle rolled over a vessel of 650 μm. The imaging window of the probe is not visible and is facing toward the tissue. The upper right panel displays OCT B-scan consisting of A-scans. The tissue surface corresponds to the top of the image. Depth increases going down the image. The bottom right panel displays a speckle decorrelation image calculated form the OCT scan with high decorrelation as white and low decorrelation as dark red. Adapted from Ramakonar et al. (27) under Creative Commons Attribution license. **(D)** Schematic summary of advanced optical methods and tool designs, for increasing safety of stereotactic brain biopsies. OCT, optical coherence tomography; PpIX, protoporphyrin IX; ICG, indocyanine green; SRH, Stimulated Raman Histology.

excitation laser) along the trajectory of the device (**Figure 1B**). Although increased perfusion was detected in two biopsy locations, no information regarding the changes in the surgical plan or needle trajectory was reported (28). A similar stand-alone forward-viewing laser Doppler flowmetry needle probe had been investigated by the same group during the electrode placement for deep brain stimulation in patients (29, 30). Although the main goal of these studies was to establish the link between the measured blood flow and anatomy along trajectories, the authors did encounter one bleeding episode evidenced by significantly increased blood flow measures, which was later confirmed by CT (29). Subsequently, the authors suggested that this method could detect small vessels and thus decrease the risk of bleeding complications in stereotactic procedures (30). Obtaining measurements every 0.5 mm along the injection trajectory was proposed; however, it would result in a significant increase of surgical time (20 s per measurement resulting in at least 33.3 min for 5-cm trajectory) (28). Additionally, this probe has not been integrated into a brain biopsy needle for side view assessment. Future studies are necessary to assess if vascular imaging is helpful to guide intraoperative adjustments of the surgical plan and prevent vessel injury and bleeding.

Stain-Less Reflectance Imaging Approaches

Ramakonar et al. reported the performance of a side-viewing probe that fit a standard side-cutting brain biopsy needle for optical coherence tomography (OCT) imaging and differentiation of solid tissue and vessels (**Figure 1C**) (27). This imaging method is based on the detection and reconstruction of backscattered light from the 1,300-nm near-infrared illumination light, allowing 1–1.5 mm penetration depth and 5–20 μm resolution. OCT imaging was presented in an earlier paper by Kut et al. that demonstrated the modality's efficacy as a label-free technique for differentiating cancer from non-cancer in human brain tissues at a 1- to 1.5-mm penetration depth (34). To overcome the challenge of OCT's shallow depth, Ramakonar et al. was able to develop an optically guided biopsy needle capable of OCT imaging in order to visualize blood vessels at greater tissue depths. The information is then displayed on a monitor as a B-scan acquired during needle movements. Initial analysis of surface cortical vessels in patients that underwent craniotomy showed that the device detected blood vessels with a diameter of >500 μm with a sensitivity of 91.2% and a specificity of 97.7% (27). Furthermore, the authors validated these findings by demonstrating deep brain vessel detection capability (vessels were preselected on MRI) during brain needle biopsies in three patients (27).

Markwardt et al. in a phantom model and in *ex vivo* porcine brains demonstrated that a side-viewing double fiber probe for remission spectrometry inserted in a side-cutting biopsy needle can determine the proximity of the vessel to the needle (26). The method is based on the illumination of the tissue with a light from a broad wavelength light emitting diode (LED) light source (400–700 nm) and spectroscopic analysis of the remitted light. The remitted light is assessed at wavelengths that are characteristic of hemoglobin absorption (578 and 650 nm for oxygenated and deoxygenated, respectively), allowing the estimation of the proximity of the vessels to the probe. The method results are displayed as ratio values that represent the proximity, size, and orientation of the hemoglobin-containing vessels to the probe. Although there is no visual information regarding the appearance of the tissue, the technique is relatively simple and inexpensive.

Pichette et al. in phantom experiments demonstrated that interstitial sub-diffuse optical tomography technology can detect vessels with diameters of more than 300 μm for up to 2 mm from the biopsy needle (24). The 1.7-mm-diameter probe consists of 24 side-viewing fibers that provide circumferential scanning and detection of the spectrally resolved remitted light from the tissue around the needle guide. The main advantage of this method is that the probe scans the whole volume of tissues surrounding the needle, creating a two-dimensional visual signal map across the depth and circumference position. An additional advantage is higher tissue penetration depth when compared to optical coherence tomography (2 vs. ~1 mm) (24). Remission spectrometry and sub-diffuse optical tomography both rely on the hemoglobin absorption spectra and do not require additional contrast agents (24, 26).

METHODS FOR BIOPSY ACQUISITION GUIDANCE AND FOR RAPID INTRAOPERATIVE ASSESSMENT OF OBTAINED SPECIMENS

Identification of Viable Diagnostic Tissue

Decreasing the number of stereotactic biopsies represents another strategy to minimize the risk of brain and vascular damage. Therefore, technologies that allow for the detection of viable tumor tissue along the biopsy needle trajectory are valuable. Such techniques allow not only to increase accuracy for diagnostic sample acquisition for proper histopathological diagnostics but also to avoid unnecessary repetitive needle biopsies.

Methods Based on the Detection of Molecular Labels in the Tumor Tissue

The presence of 5-aminolevulinic (5-ALA)-induced PpIX fluorescence is diagnostic for malignant tumors and can be used to assess stereotactic biopsy samples before submitting them to pathology, while the absence of fluorescence can filter out necrotic areas and inflammatory reactive tissue without malignant cells. This method was confirmed in multiple studies (35–40). Detection of PpIX fluorescence was highly diagnostic for viable tumor tissue in patients with intracranial lymphomas (41), high-grade gliomas, and anaplastic foci in patients with low-grade gliomas (42). Fluorescence positive samples might even not require intraoperative frozen section analysis and could be sent directly for a permanent section because of the high positive predictive value of PpIX fluorescence (39, 43, 44). In cases of low or negative fluorescence, the intraoperative frozen section analysis is recommended with subsequent biopsies upon the results of the intraoperative histopathological analysis (43).

Excitation of PpIX at 633 nm can further increase the diagnostic utility of such a method, as it allows for deeper imaging through a small layer of blood or tissue, which was previously impossible with 405-nm excitation (45, 46).

Similarly to 5-ALA, fluorescein sodium can be used to assess stereotactic biopsy specimens under the special fluorescence mode of the surgical microscope. High-grade glioma tissue shows strong yellow fluorescence when excited at about 488 nm (47). Being a relatively inexpensive drug, fluorescein sodium could also be visualized using a low-cost miniature device, Fluoropen, which is essentially a LED torch with a blue filter mounted at the light source for excitation and a yellow filter attached around the torch as a cone collar (48). The device is positioned close to the specimen and yellow fluorescence is observed through the yellow filter (48). Observation of fluorescein fluorescence from the specimens had a 100% positive predictive value and a 25% negative predictive value of a lesional tissue (49). Overall, the fluorescein-based method was shown to be as effective as frozen section analysis for the diagnostic biopsy screening (49).

ICG may also be used as a highlighter of the tumor tissue (50–54). Although there are few reports about the ICG use for tumor detection during stereotactic biopsies (16), open surgical visualization showed high sensitivity but low specificity of the second-window ICG (52). Other targeted molecular labels that can be used for open fluorescence-guided surgery, for example, BLZ-100, an ICG-conjugated tumor-targeting peptide chlorotoxin used for imaging, also hold potential for stereotactic needle biopsy procedures (55).

Apart from the macroscopic identification of the retained fluorescent drug, the obtained stereotactic biopsy specimens could be subjected to analysis with other methods alternative to a frozen section. Such methods might be less laborious and time-consuming. Stereotactic samples could be stained with rapid fluorophores *ex vivo* and scanned with a confocal microscope (56, 57). Miniaturized handheld confocal laser endomicroscopy with fluorescein sodium injected intraoperatively as a contrast can visualize the histological architecture of brain biopsies *ex vivo* and *in vivo* (58–62). However, this probe has not been assessed in stereotactic procedures.

A thin forward-viewing fiber-based confocal laser endomicroscope that can fit biopsy needles is available for 488-nm and 660-nm excitable fluorophores (fluorescein sodium and ICG, respectively) (63, 64). A pilot study has demonstrated that such an endomicroscope with fluorescein as a contrast can visualize brain tumor architecture during a stereotactic brain biopsy procedure in humans (65). A similar technique was tested by Lynagh et al. in a proof-of-concept study for the detection of fluorescein and blue-fluorescence protein labeled glioma cells in a rat model using a 0.65-mm fiber microendoscope coupled with a clinical stereotactic biopsy needle (66). Microendoscopy technology is similar to a needle-based contact endoscope (22) and other fiber probes for spectral measurements that were discussed above (28, 35, 44), but is able to provide fluorescence tissue image with higher resolution down to the cellular level.

Label-Free Methods

Various microscopy imaging methods that are not dependent on the drug-induced contrast and instead rely on intrinsic optical properties of the tissues recently received clinical attention. Such methods could be used for rapid intraoperative assessment of the acquired stereotactic brain biopsies to increase diagnostic yield and improve pathology workflow.

It has been shown that measurements of reflectance and fluorescence spectra of unstained brain tissues can differentiate radiation necrosis in brain tumor tissue (67). Reflectance confocal microscopy can differentiate viable brain tumor tissue from necrotic tissue and further characterize histological appearance with high diagnostic accuracy (68, 69). Label-free multiphoton microscopy methods were successfully used for the imaging of Alzheimer's disease brain samples (70). Raman microspectroscopic microscopy imaging has been studied for histological assessment of brain tumor biopsies (71). A notably successful variant of Raman microscopy is the Stimulated Raman Histology (SRH) technique, which has been used for *ex vivo* histological assessment of brain tumor biopsies. SRH provided high-resolution digital images that look similar to the standard hematoxylin and eosin staining (72, 73). SRH is a stand-alone imaging system that can be positioned in the operating room for rapid intraoperative pathological assessment (72, 73). Although most of the imaging studies were performed on benchtop microscopes, some multiphoton microscopy modes (CARS and TREF) will be available in endoscopes and needle-size probes in the near future (74).

Stevens et al. described a 1.8-mm-diameter forward-viewing 830-nm Raman-based spectroscopy probe without fibers that fit a standard brain biopsy needle (75, 76). The new design of the probe resulted in significant noise reduction compared to the silica-fiber-based Raman imaging and demonstrated discrimination of various porcine brain structures including white matter, gray matter, and blood vessels based on the Raman spectra (75).

SUMMARY

Current developments for increasing the safety and efficacy of stereotactic brain biopsy procedures are centered around the two main areas: avoidance of the vessels and detection of the viable diagnostic tissue, which could be achieved *in vivo* or *ex vivo* (**Figure 1D**).

Because vessel avoidance is a major component for the safety of any stereotactic needle-based procedure including needle brain biopsy, deep brain stimulation (77), or interstitial laser thermal therapy (78, 79), advancements in the surgical tools that allow for timely vessel detection is of utmost importance. Several technologies for vessel detection implemented into a biopsy needle included detection of fluorescent intravascular contrast, laser Doppler flowmetry, optical coherence and interstitial sub-diffuse tomography, and remission spectrometry. Non-fluorescence methods based on the blood flow and hemoglobin detection are thought to be the most promising as they avoid dealing with fluctuations in the intravascular contrast concentrations after injection. It should be noted that the current literature does not provide definitive evidence on the efficacy of such methods for vessel injury avoidance; therefore, more clinical studies are necessary.

Ex vivo confirmation of PpIX or fluorescein fluorescence from biopsy samples has been established to have a high positive predictive value of a diagnostic biopsy in multiple studies and can be recommended as a routine method for stereotactic biopsy at this current stage. However, the possibility for identification of the correct biopsy needle position *in vivo* prior to actual biopsy acquisition with a small optical tool is even more exciting. Most of such reports are based on the detection of the intra-tumoral fluorescent molecules (PpIX, fluorescein, and ICG); however, the development of reflectance and multiphoton microscopy techniques and militarization of microscopes would allow label-free tumor tissue identification through a biopsy needle in the future. There is a marked diversity in qualitative and quantitative optical methods for brain tumor tissue identification, and each of them requires a significant learning curve and dedication. So far, the most progress has been achieved with 5-ALA-induced PpIX, which is highly specific for malignant tissues and can be detected spectroscopically with a single optical fiber inserted in the biopsy needle.

Another limitation is that most of the discussed methods require timely interpretation and adjustments of multiple parameters during the procedure to ensure optimal performance, which is not always practical and may lead to information overload. For example, results of quantitative spectroscopy are usually displayed on the screen in a graph form. This information could be converted into an auditory format, which would be easy to understand and non-disruptive during the surgery (80). Finally, the possibility of light-induced tissue damage should be carefully considered when developing novel optical and fluorescent tools for *in vivo* diagnostics.

When considering the design of an ideal probe, it should incorporate vessel detection as well as tumor detection modules, most likely in forward and side views simultaneously for the safest possible probe insertion and biopsy acquisition. Machine learning, coupled with optical visualization technologies, would be a basis for computer-aided, real-time tissue image analysis for the selection of the best probe trajectory or location for biopsy acquisition. Besides these technologies that are used for vessel avoidance and tumor detection, future development of probes could also include augmented or virtual reality for clinicians to perform more accurate probe trajectory planning.

AUTHOR CONTRIBUTIONS

All authors listed have made a substantial, direct and intellectual contribution to the work, and approved it for publication.

REFERENCES

1. Ragel BT, Ryken TC, Kalkanis SN, Ziu M, Cahill D, Olson JJ. The role of biopsy in the management of patients with presumed diffuse low grade glioma. *J Neuro Oncol.* (2015) 125:481–501. doi: 10.1007/s11060-015-1866-2
2. Schwartz C, Kreth FW. Comment on: the role of biopsy in the management of patients with presumed diffuse low grade glioma: a systematic review and evidence-based clinical practice guideline. *J Neuro Oncol.* (2016) 128:173. doi: 10.1007/s11060-016-2086-0
3. Teixeira MJ, Fonoff ET, Mandel M, Alves HL, Rosemberg S. Stereotactic biopsies of brain lesions. *Arq Neuropsiquiatr.* (2009) 67:74–7. doi: 10.1590/S0004-282X2009000100018
4. Chen CC, Hsu PW, Erich Wu TW, Lee ST, Chang CN, Wei KC, et al. Stereotactic brain biopsy: Single center retrospective analysis of complications. *Clin Neurol Neurosurg.* (2009) 111:835–9. doi: 10.1016/j.clineuro.2009.08.013
5. Shastri-Hurst N, Tsegaye M, Robson DK, Lowe JS, Macarthur DC. Stereotactic brain biopsy: an audit of sampling reliability in a clinical case series. *Br J Neurosurg.* (2009) 20:222–6. doi: 10.1080/02688690600875507
6. Bander ED, Jones SH, Pisapia D, Magge R, Fine H, Schwartz TH, et al. Tubular brain tumor biopsy improves diagnostic yield for subcortical lesions. *J Neurooncol.* (2019) 141:121–9. doi: 10.1007/s11060-018-03014-w
7. Dammers R, Schouten JW, Haitsma IK, Vincent AJ, Kros JM, Dirven CM. Towards improving the safety and diagnostic yield of stereotactic biopsy in a single centre. *Acta Neurochir.* (2010) 152:1915–21. doi: 10.1007/s00701-010-0752-0
8. Frati A, Pichierri A, Bastianello S, Raco A, Santoro A, Esposito V, et al. Frameless stereotactic cerebral biopsy: our experience in 296 cases. *Stereotact Funct Neurosurg.* (2011) 89:234–45. doi: 10.1159/0003 25704
9. Kulkarni AV, Guha A, Lozano A, Bernstein M. Incidence of silent hemorrhage and delayed deterioration after stereotactic brain biopsy. *J Neurosurg.* (1998) 89:31–5. doi: 10.3171/jns.1998.89.1.0031
10. Preul MC, Caramanos Z, Collins DL, Villemure JG, Leblanc R, Olivier A, et al. Accurate, noninvasive diagnosis of human brain tumors by using proton magnetic resonance spectroscopy. *Nat Med.* (1996) 2:323–5. doi: 10.1038/nm0396-323
11. Chernov MF, Muragaki Y, Ochiai T, Taira T, Ono Y, Usukura M, et al. Spectroscopy-supported frame-based image-guided stereotactic biopsy of parenchymal brain lesions: comparative evaluation of diagnostic yield and diagnostic accuracy. *Clin Neurol Neurosurg.* (2009) 111:527–35. doi: 10.1016/j.clineuro.2009.03.006
12. Lefranc M, Monet P, Desenclos C, Peltier J, Fichten A, Toussaint P, et al. Perfusion MRI as a neurosurgical tool for improved targeting in stereotactic tumor biopsies. *Stereotact Funct Neurosurg.* (2012) 90:240–7. doi: 10.1159/000338092
13. Levivier M, Goldman S, Pirotte B, Brucher JM, Baleriaux D, Luxen A, et al. Diagnostic yield of stereotactic brain biopsy guided by positron emission tomography with [18F]fluorodeoxyglucose. *J Neurosurg.* (1995) 82:445–52. doi: 10.3171/jns.1995.82.3.0445
14. Gilsbach J, Mohadjer M, Mundinger F. A new safety device to prevent bleeding complications during stereotactic biopsy—The "stereotactic" Doppler sonography. *Acta Neurochir.* (1987) 89:77–9. doi: 10.1007/BF01406671
15. Virdyawan V, Y Baena FR. Vessel pose estimation for obstacle avoidance in needle steering surgery using multiple forward looking sensors. In: *2018 IEEE/RSJ International Conference on Intelligent Robots and Systems (IROS).* (2018). p. 3845–52. doi: 10.1109/IROS.2018.8594198
16. Cho SS, Salinas R, Lee JYK. Indocyanine-green for fluorescence-guided surgery of brain tumors: evidence, techniques, and practical experience. *Front Surg.* (2019) 6:11. doi: 10.3389/fsurg.2019.00011

17. Zhang DY, Singhal S, Lee JYK. Optical principles of fluorescence-guided brain tumor surgery: a practical primer for the neurosurgeon. *Neurosurgery.* (2019) 85:312–4. doi: 10.1093/neuros/nyy315
18. Wei L, Roberts DW, Sanai N, Liu JTC. Visualization technologies for 5-ALA-based fluorescence-guided surgeries. *J Neurooncol.* (2019) 141:495–505. doi: 10.1007/s11060-018-03077-9
19. Hadjipanayis CG, Stummer W. 5-ALA and FDA approval for glioma surgery. *J Neurooncol.* (2019) 141:479–86. doi: 10.1007/s11060-019-03098-y
20. Valdes PA, Juvekar P, Agar NYR, Gioux S, Golby AJ. Quantitative wide-field imaging techniques for fluorescence guided neurosurgery. *Front Surg.* (2019) 6:31. doi: 10.3389/fsurg.2019.00031
21. Lakomkin N, Hadjipanayis CG. The use of spectroscopy handheld tools in brain tumor surgery: current evidence and techniques. *Front Surg.* (2019) 6:30. doi: 10.3389/fsurg.2019.00030
22. Göbel W, Brucker D, Kienast Y, Johansson A, Kniebühler G, Rühm A, et al. Optical needle endoscope for safe and precise stereotactically guided biopsy sampling in neurosurgery. *Optics Exp.* (2012) 20:26117–26. doi: 10.1364/OE.20.026117
23. Ruhm A, Gobel W, Sroka R, Stepp H. ICG-assisted blood vessel detection during stereotactic neurosurgery: simulation study on excitation power limitations due to thermal effects in human brain tissue. *Photodiagnosis Photodyn Ther.* (2014) 11:307–18. doi: 10.1016/j.pdpdt.2014.03.007
24. Pichette J, Goyette A, Picot F, Tremblay M-A, Soulez G, Wilson BC, et al. Sensitivity analysis aimed at blood vessels detection using interstitial optical tomography during brain needle biopsy procedures. *Biomed Optics Exp.* (2015) 6:4238–54. doi: 10.1364/BOE.6.0 04238
25. Goyette A, Pichette J, Tremblay MA, Laurence A, Jermyn M, Mok K, et al. Sub-diffuse interstitial optical tomography to improve the safety of brain needle biopsies: a proof-of-concept study. *Optics Lett.* (2015) 40:170–3. doi: 10.1364/OL.40.000170
26. Markwardt NA, Stepp H, Franz G, Sroka R, Goetz M, Zelenkov P, et al. Remission spectrometry for blood vessel detection during stereotactic biopsy of brain tumors. *J Biophoton.* (2017) 10:1080–94. doi: 10.1002/jbio.201600193
27. Ramakonar H, Quirk BC, Kirk RW, Li J, Jacques A, Lind CRP, et al. Intraoperative detection of blood vessels with an imaging needle during neurosurgery in humans. *Sci Adv.* (2018) 4:eaav4992. doi: 10.1126/sciadv.aav4992
28. Haj-Hosseini N, Richter JCO, Milos P, Hallbeck M, Wårdell K. 5-ALA fluorescence and laser doppler flowmetry for guidance in a stereotactic brain tumor biopsy. *Biomed Optics Exp.* (2018) 9:2284–96. doi: 10.1364/BOE.9.002284
29. Wårdell K, Zsigmond P, Richter J, Hemm S. Relationship between laser doppler signals and anatomy during deep brain stimulation electrode implantation toward the ventral intermediate nucleus and subthalamic nucleus. *Oper Neurosurg.* (2013) 72:ons127–ons40. doi: 10.1227/NEU.0b013e31827e5821
30. Wårdell K, Hemm-Ode S, Rejmstad P, Zsigmond P. High-resolution laser Doppler measurements of microcirculation in the deep brain structures: a method for potential vessel tracking. *Stereotact Funct Neurosurg.* (2016) 94:1–9. doi: 10.1159/000442894
31. Stummer W, Pichlmeier U, Meinel T, Wiestler OD, Zanella F, Reulen HJ, et al. Fluorescence-guided surgery with 5-aminolevulinic acid for resection of malignant glioma: a randomised controlled multicentre phase III trial. *Lancet Oncol.* (2006) 7:392–401. doi: 10.1016/S1470-2045(06) 70665-9
32. Hanel RA, Nakaji P, Spetzler RF. Use of microscope-integrated near-infrared indocyanine green videoangiography in the surgical treatment of spinal dural arteriovenous fistulae. *Neurosurgery.* (2010) 66:978–84. discussion: 84–5. doi: 10.1227/01.NEU.0000368108.94233.22
33. Raabe A, Beck J, Gerlach R, Zimmermann M, Seifert V. Near-infrared Indocyanine green video angiography: a new method for intraoperative assessment of vascular flow. *Neurosurgery.* (2003) 32–9. discussion: 139. doi: 10.1097/00006123-200301000-00017
34. Kut C, Chaichana KL, Xi J, Raza SM, Ye X, McVeigh ER, et al. Detection of human brain cancer infiltration *ex vivo* and *in vivo* using quantitative optical coherence tomography. *Sci Transl Med.* (2015) 7:292ra100. doi: 10.1126/scitranslmed.3010611
35. Haj-Hosseini N, Richter JCO, Hallbeck M, Wårdell K. Low dose 5-aminolevulinic acid: Implications in spectroscopic measurements during brain tumor surgery. *Photodiagnosis Photodyn Ther.* (2015) 12:209–14. doi: 10.1016/j.pdpdt.2015.03.004
36. Piquer J, Llácer JL, Rovira V, Riesgo P, Rodriguez R, Cremades A. Fluorescence-guided surgery and biopsy in gliomas with an exoscope system. *BioMed Res Int.* (2014) 2014:1–6. doi: 10.1155/2014/207974
37. Hefti M, von Campe G, Moschopulos M, Siegner A, Looser H, Landolt H. 5-Aminolevulinic acid induced protoporphyrin IX fluorescence in high-grade glioma surgery: a one-year experience at a single institutuion. *Swiss Med Wkly.* (2008) 138:180–5. doi: 10.4414/smw.2008.12077
38. Moriuchi S, Yamada K, Dehara M, Teramoto Y, Soda T, Imakita M, et al. Use of 5-aminolevulinic acid for the confirmation of deep-seated brain tumors during stereotactic biopsy. Report of 2 cases. *J Neurosurg.* (2011) 115:278–80. doi: 10.3171/2011.4.JNS102137
39. von Campe G, Moschopulos M, Hefti M. 5-Aminolevulinic acid-induced protoporphyrin IX fluorescence as immediate intraoperative indicator to improve the safety of malignant or high-grade brain tumor diagnosis in frameless stereotactic biopsies. *Acta Neurochir.* (2012) 154:585–8. doi: 10.1007/s00701-012-1290-8
40. Yamaguchi F, Takahashi H, Teramoto A. Photodiagnosis for frameless stereotactic biopsy of brain tumor. *Photodiagnosis Photodyn Ther.* (2007) 4:71–5. doi: 10.1016/j.pdpdt.2006.09.005
41. Kiesel B, Millesi M, Woehrer A, Furtner J, Bavand A, Roetzer T, et al. 5-ALA–induced fluorescence as a marker for diagnostic tissue in stereotactic biopsies of intracranial lymphomas: experience in 41 patients. *Neurosurg Focus.* (2018) 44:E7. doi: 10.3171/2018.3.FOCUS1859
42. Arita H, Kinoshita M, Kagawa N, Fujimoto Y, Kishima H, Hashimoto N, et al. 11C-methionine uptake and intraoperative 5-aminolevulinic acid-induced fluorescence as separate index markers of cell density in glioma. *Cancer.* (2012) 118:1619–27. doi: 10.1002/cncr.26445
43. Widhalm G, Minchev G, Woehrer A, Preusser M, Kiesel B, Furtner J, et al. Strong 5-aminolevulinic acid-induced fluorescence is a novel intraoperative marker for representative tissue samples in stereotactic brain tumor biopsies. *Neurosurg Rev.* (2012) 35:381–91. doi: 10.1007/s10143-012-0374-5
44. Potapov AA, Goryaynov SA, Okhlopkov VA, Pitskhelauri DI, Kobyakov GL, Zhukov VY, et al. [Clinical guidelines for the use of intraoperative fluorescence diagnosis in brain tumor surgery]. *Zh Vopr Neirokhir Im N N Burdenko.* (2015) 79:91–101. doi: 10.17116/neiro201579591-101
45. Markwardt NA, Haj-Hosseini N, Hollnburger B, Stepp H, Zelenkov P, Rühm A. 405 nm versus 633 nm for protoporphyrin IX excitation in fluorescence-guided stereotactic biopsy of brain tumors. *J Biophoton.* (2016) 9:901–12. doi: 10.1002/jbio.201500195
46. Potapov AA, Goriainov SA, Loshchenov VB, Savel'eva TA, Gavrilov AG, Okhlopkov VA, et al. [Intraoperative combined spectroscopy (optical biopsy) of cerebral gliomas]. *Zh Vopr Neirokhir Im Burdenko.* (2013) 77:3–10.
47. Rey-Dios R, Hattab EM, Cohen-Gadol AA. Use of intraoperative fluorescein sodium fluorescence to improve the accuracy of tissue diagnosis during stereotactic needle biopsy of high-grade gliomas. *Acta Neurochir.* (2014) 156:1071–5. doi: 10.1007/s00701-014-2097-6
48. Thien A, Rao JP, Ng WH, King NKK. The fluoropen: a simple low-cost device to detect intraoperative fluorescein fluorescence in stereotactic needle biopsy of brain tumors. *Acta Neurochir.* (2016) 159:371–5. doi: 10.1007/s00701-016-3041-8
49. Thien A, Han JX, Kumar K, Ng YP, Rao JP, Ng WH, et al. Investigation of the usefulness of fluorescein sodium fluorescence in stereotactic brain biopsy. *Acta Neurochir.* (2017) 160:317–24. doi: 10.1007/s00701-017-3429-0
50. Catapano G, Sgulo F, Laleva L, Columbano L, Dallan I, de Notaris M. Multimodal use of indocyanine green endoscopy in neurosurgery: a single-center experience and review of the literature. *Neurosurg Rev.* (2018) 41:985–98. doi: 10.1007/s10143-017-0858-4
51. Hitti FL, Lee JYK. Endoscopic resection of an intraventricular tumor with second window indocyanine green: 2-dimensional operative video. *Oper Neurosurg.* (2018) 15:E53–E4. doi: 10.1093/ons/opy053
52. Lee JY, Thawani JP, Pierce J, Zeh R, Martinez-Lage M, Chanin M, et al. Intraoperative near-infrared optical imaging can localize gadolinium-enhancing gliomas during surgery. *Neurosurgery.* (2016) 79:856–71. doi: 10.1227/NEU.0000000000001450

53. Haglund MM, Hochman DW, Spence AM, Berger MS. Enhanced optical imaging of rat gliomas and tumor margins. *Neurosurgery.* (1994) 35:930–40. discussion: 40–1. doi: 10.1097/00006123-199411000-00019
54. Watson JR, Martirosyan N, Lemole GM, Trouard TP, Romanowski M. Intraoperative brain tumor resection with indocyanine green using augmented microscopy. *J Biomed Optics.* (2018) 23:1–4. doi: 10.1117/1.JBO.23.9.090501
55. Butte PV, Mamelak A, Parrish-Novak J, Drazin D, Shweikeh F, Gangalum PR, et al. Near-infrared imaging of brain tumors using the tumor paint BLZ-100 to achieve near-complete resection of brain tumors. *Neurosurg Focus.* (2014) 36:E1. doi: 10.3171/2013.11.FOCUS13497
56. Martirosyan NL, Georges J, Eschbacher JM, Belykh E, Carotenuto A, Spetzler RF, et al. Confocal scanning microscopy provides rapid, detailed intraoperative histological assessment of brain neoplasms: experience with 106 cases. *Clin Neurol Neurosurg.* (2018) 169:21–8. doi: 10.1016/j.clineuro.2018.03.015
57. Martirosyan NL, Georges J, Eschbacher JM, Cavalcanti DD, Elhadi AM, Abdelwahab MG, et al. Potential application of a handheld confocal endomicroscope imaging system using a variety of fluorophores in experimental gliomas and normal brain. *Neurosurg Focus.* (2014) 36:E16. doi: 10.3171/2013.11.FOCUS13486
58. Martirosyan NL, Eschbacher JM, Kalani MY, Turner JD, Belykh E, Spetzler RF, et al. Prospective evaluation of the utility of intraoperative confocal laser endomicroscopy in patients with brain neoplasms using fluorescein sodium: experience with 74 cases. *Neurosurg Focus.* (2016) 40:E11. doi: 10.3171/2016.1.FOCUS15559
59. Foersch S, Heimann A, Ayyad A, Spoden GA, Florin L, Mpoukouvalas K, et al. Confocal laser endomicroscopy for diagnosis and histomorphologic imaging of brain tumors *in vivo.* *PLoS ONE.* (2012) 7:e41760. doi: 10.1371/journal.pone.0041760
60. Breuskin D, Szczygielski J, Urbschat S, Kim YJ, Oertel J. Confocal laser endomicroscopy in neurosurgery—An alternative to instantaneous sections? *World Neurosurg.* (2017) 100:180–5. doi: 10.1016/j.wneu.2016.12.128
61. Sankar T, Delaney PM, Ryan RW, Eschbacher J, Abdelwahab M, Nakaji P, et al. Miniaturized handheld confocal microscopy for neurosurgery: results in an experimental glioblastoma model. *Neurosurgery.* (2010) 66:410–7. discussion: 7–8. doi: 10.1227/01.NEU.0000365772.66324.6F
62. Sanai N, Eschbacher J, Hattendorf G, Coons SW, Preul MC, Smith KA, et al. Intraoperative confocal microscopy for brain tumors: a feasibility analysis in humans. *Neurosurgery.* (2011) 68(2 Suppl Operative):282–90. discussion: 90. doi: 10.1227/NEU.0b013e318212464e
63. Giovannini M. Needle-based confocal laser endomicroscopy. *Endosc Ultrasound.* (2015) 4:284–8. doi: 10.4103/2303-9027.170405
64. Schneider C, Johnson SP, Gurusamy K, Cook RJ, Desjardins AE, Hawkes DJ, et al. Identification of liver metastases with probe-based confocal laser endomicroscopy at two excitation wavelengths. *Lasers Surg Med.* (2017) 49:280–92. doi: 10.1002/lsm.22617
65. Pavlov V, Meyronet D, Meyer-Bisch V, Armoiry X, Pikul B, Dumot C, et al. Intraoperative probe-based confocal laser endomicroscopy in surgery and stereotactic biopsy of low-grade and high-grade gliomas: a feasibility study in humans. *Neurosurgery.* (2016) 79:604–12. doi: 10.1227/NEU.0000000000001365
66. Lynagh R, Ishak M, Georges J, Lopez D, Osman H, Kakareka M, et al. Fluorescence-guided stereotactic biopsy: a proof-of-concept study. *J Neurosurg.* (2019) 22:1–7. doi: 10.3171/2018.11.JNS18629
67. Lin W-C, Mahadevan-Jansen A, Johnson MD, Weil RJ, Toms SA. *In vivo* optical spectroscopy detects radiation damage in brain tissue. *Neurosurgery.* (2005) 57:518–25. doi: 10.1227/01.NEU.0000170559.48166.AC
68. Eschbacher JM, Georges JF, Belykh E, Yazdanabadi MI, Martirosyan NL, Szeto E, et al. Immediate label-free *ex vivo* evaluation of human brain tumor biopsies with confocal reflectance microscopy. *J Neuropathol Exp Neurol.* (2017) 76:1008–22. doi: 10.1093/jnen/nlx089
69. Georges J, Zehri A, Carlson E, Nichols J, Mooney MA, Martirosyan NL, et al. Label-free microscopic assessment of glioblastoma biopsy specimens prior to biobanking [corrected]. *Neurosurg Focus.* (2014) 36:E8. doi: 10.3171/2013.11.FOCUS13478
70. Lee JH, Kim DH, Song WK, Oh M-K, Ko D-K. Label-free imaging and quantitative chemical analysis of Alzheimer's disease brain samples with multimodal multiphoton nonlinear optical microspectroscopy. *J Biomed Optics.* (2015) 20:056013. doi: 10.1117/1.JBO.20.5.056013
71. Krafft C, Belay B, Bergner N, Romeike BFM, Reichart R, Kalff R, et al. Advances in optical biopsy—Correlation of malignancy and cell density of primary brain tumors using Raman microspectroscopic imaging. *Analyst.* (2012) 137:5533–7. doi: 10.1039/c2an36083g
72. Hollon TC, Lewis S, Pandian B, Niknafs YS, Garrard MR, Garton H, et al. Rapid intraoperative diagnosis of pediatric brain tumors using stimulated Raman histology. *Cancer Res.* (2018) 78:278–89. doi: 10.1158/0008-5472.CAN-17-1974
73. Orringer DA, Pandian B, Niknafs YS, Hollon TC, Boyle J, Lewis S, et al. Rapid intraoperative histology of unprocessed surgical specimens via fibre-laser-based stimulated Raman scattering microscopy. *Nat Biomed Eng.* (2017) 1:0027. doi: 10.1038/s41551-016-0027
74. Romeike BFM, Meyer T, Reichart R, Kalff R, Petersen I, Dietzek B, et al. Coherent anti-stokes raman scattering and two photon excited fluorescence for neurosurgery. *Clin Neurol Neurosurg.* (2015) 131:42–6. doi: 10.1016/j.clineuro.2015.01.022
75. Mahadevan-Jansen A, Petrich W, Stevens OAC, Hutchings J, Gray W, Day JC. A low background Raman probe for optical biopsy of brain tissue. *Biomed Vibrational Spectrosc.* (2014). doi: 10.1117/12.2044139. [Epub ahead of print].
76. Stevens OAC, Hutchings J, Gray W, Vincent RL, Day JC. Miniature standoff Raman probe for neurosurgical applications. *J Biomed Optics.* (2016) 21:087002. doi: 10.1117/1.JBO.21.8.087002
77. Giller CA, Liu H, German DC, Kashyap D, Dewey RB. A stereotactic near-infrared probe for localization during functional neurosurgical procedures: further experience. *J Neurosurg.* 110:263–73. doi: 10.3171/2008.8.JNS08728
78. Lee I, Kalkanis S, Hadjipanayis CG. Stereotactic laser interstitial thermal therapy for recurrent high-grade gliomas. *Neurosurgery.* (2016) 79 (Suppl 1):S24–S34. doi: 10.1227/NEU.0000000000001443
79. Ashraf O, Patel NV, Hanft S, Danish SF. Laser-induced thermal therapy in neuro-oncology: a review. *World Neurosurg.* (2018) 112:166–77. doi: 10.1016/j.wneu.2018.01.123
80. Black D, Hahn HK, Kikinis R, Wårdell K, Haj-Hosseini N. Auditory display for fluorescence-guided open brain tumor surgery. *Int J Comput Assisted Radiol Surg.* (2017) 13:25–35. doi: 10.1007/s11548-017-1667-5

7

Confocal-Assisted Multispectral Fluorescent Microscopy for Brain Tumor Surgery

Patra Charalampaki [1*], Makoto Nakamura [1], Dimitrios Athanasopoulos [1] and Axel Heimann [2]

[1] Department of Neurosurgery, Cologne Medical Center, University Witten-Herdecke, Witten, Germany, [2] Institute of Neurosurgical Pathophysiology, Medical University Mainz, Mainz, Germany

Correspondence:
Patra Charalampaki
charalampaki@yahoo.de

Optimal surgical therapy for brain tumors is the combination of complete resection with minimal invasion and damage to the adjacent normal tissue. To achieve this goal, we need advanced imaging techniques on a scale from macro- to microscopic resolution. In the last decade, the development of fluorescence-guided surgery has been the most influential breakthrough, marginally improving outcomes in brain tumor surgery. Multispectral fluorescence microscopy (MFL) is a novel imaging technique that allows the overlapping of a fluorescent image and a white light image in real-time, with delivery of the merged image to the surgeon through the eyepieces of a surgical microscope. MFL permits the detection and characterization of brain tumors using fluorescent molecular markers such as 5-aminolevulinic acid (5-ALA) or indocyanine green (ICG), while simultaneously obtaining high definition white light images to create a pseudo-colored composite image in real-time. Limitations associated with the use of MFL include decreased light imaging intensity and decreased levels of magnification that may compromise maximal tumor resection on a cellular scale. Confocal laser endomicroscopy (CLE) is another novel advanced imaging technique that is based on miniaturization of the microscope imaging head in order to provide the possibility of *in vivo* microscopy at the cellular level. Clear visualization of the cellular cytoarchitecture can be achieved with 400-fold–1,000-fold magnification. CLE allows on the one hand the intra-operative detection and differentiation of single tumor cells (without the need for intra-operative histologic analysis of biopsy specimens) as well as the definition of borders between tumor and normal tissue at a cellular level, dramatically improving the accuracy of surgical resection. The application and implementation of CLE-assisted surgery in surgical oncology increases not only the number of options for real-time diagnostic imaging, but also the therapeutic options by extending the resection borders of cancer at a cellular level and, more importantly, by protecting the functionality of normal tissue in the adjacent areas of the human brain. In this article, we describe our experience using these new techniques of confocal-assisted fluorescent surgery including analysis on the technology, usability, indications, limitations, and further developments.

Keywords: fluorescent microscopy, brain tumor, surgery, confocal laser endomicroscopy (CLE), meningioma

INTRODUCTION

Microsurgery, the performing of surgical procedures with visualization of the surgical field under a surgical microscope, has nowadays become a standard in neurosurgery. The visualization of specific pathologic entities within the surgical field, such as vascular malformations, benign, and malignant lesions, as well as normal vasculature, can be further facilitated by using different fluorescent dyes, such as indocyanine green (ICG), 5-aminolevulinic acid (5-ALA), and fluorescein (FL). Intra-operative fluorescence uses a surgical microscope with integrated special filters for the visualization of the surgical field under a spectral band that corresponds to the peak spectral emission of a fluorescent agent such as ICG, 5-ALA, or fluorescein (1–3). Previously available fluorescent surgical microscopes have been limited by allowing only the visualization of either white light or the fluorescent signal, but not both. Without simultaneous visualization, the fluorescent image is usually delivered via a separate external monitor and not through the microscope's eyepiece, like the white light image. The surgeon must visualize and process the white light image and the fluorescent image separately, combining the information of both using their perception skills while performing surgery. Secondly, switching between white light imaging and fluorescent imaging is necessary several times during the procedure, since the surrounding anatomical structures (other than the highlighted ones) are not clearly visible under the fluorescent mode. This interchange continually interrupts the workflow of the surgeon.

In order to overcome the limitations and disadvantages associated with the currently available intra-operative fluorescence imaging techniques, we developed and investigated a novel intra-operative advanced imaging technique, multispectral fluorescence microscopy (MFL) (4). MFL uses the ARveo Glow800 surgical microscope (Leica Microsystems, Wetzlar, Germany), which enables the visualization of the surgical field under white light and fluorescence at the same time. This is achieved by the use of different filters integrated into the multispectral fluorescence microscope and a sophisticated software that overlaps the fluorescent image onto the white light image in real-time, creating a composite image. Furthermore, the overlaid image can be delivered to the surgeon directly through the eyepiece of the microscope and not only on an external monitor.

Despite the improvement of fluorescent surgical microscopes, complete surgical resection of central nervous system (CNS) tumors remains challenging. Fluorescence microscopy using markers such as 5-ALA allows for intraoperative macroscopic assessment of tumor tissue and is now routinely used as a marker for resection of high-grade gliomas in neurosurgery (5). Although this has been an important advancement, remaining significant challenges of tumor resection with 5-ALA include the quantitative assessment of the PpIX-fluorescence signal, tumor removal under microscopy "in the dark," and the limited magnification of surgical microscopes.

Therefore, the use of intra-operative histologic analysis of frozen biopsy specimens is the standard of care for the determination of complete surgical resection at the cellular level. This procedure is time-consuming and attended by several limitations, such as the occurrence of freezing artifacts, tissue sampling errors, and poor resolution of the final slide. In order to overcome these limitations, we have used confocal laser imaging for the intra-operative real-time high-resolution optical imaging of CNS tumors at the cellular level (6).

Confocal laser endomicroscopy (CLE) is a promising method that permits *in vivo* cellular and sub-cellular visualization in real-time and in high resolution without any need for special tissue preparation (7). However, CLE requires intra-venous or topical application of fluorescent dyes to achieve high-resolution images during examination (8). Ideal fluorophores should possess specific optical characteristics with a high quantum yield and they should be rapidly cleared from the blood stream and CNS tissue, while having an excellent safety profile for human application (7, 8). CLE works with miniaturized fiber-optic probes and has been successfully used in gastroenterology (7, 9), pulmonology (10, 11), gynecology (12), urology (13–15), otolaryngology (16, 17), and plastic surgery (18). Indeed, CLE has allowed rapid diagnosis of various diseases, such as inflammatory bowel disease (19), Barrett's esophagus (20), coeliac disease, and various types of neoplasias (21). In neurosurgery, CLE could improve the safe removal of tumors in CNS regions by providing real-time differentiation between malignant tissue and healthy tissue at a cellular level (6, 22–25). In addition to the use of CLE, in this article we also describe our experience with MFL using the Glow800 surgical microscope, demonstrating ICG fluorescence under high-definition white light imaging in combination with a confocal endomicroscope for the detection of ICG in the near infrared spectrum (NIR) at a cellular level. Our introduction and development of these innovative techniques, CLE and MFL for neurosurgery, are referred to as confocal-assisted fluorescent microsurgery. The focus of this work is the analysis of the procedural techniques, the combination of both in the same surgical performance, the description of the usability, indications, limitations, and further developments of these new concepts in advanced imaging for neurosurgery.

MATERIALS AND METHODS

Multispectral Fluorescent Surgical Microscope

The MFL microscope has the same basic structure and layout as a standard surgical microscope, capable of visualizing fluorescence, and white light in combination and in real-time. The Glow800 tool (ARveo Glow800, Leica microsystems, Wetzlar, Germany) that we used for our surgeries uses multispectral fluorescence for the excitation of fluorescent molecular markers in the NIR (around 800 nm). By means of custom-built software, it can combine the NIR signal with the white light visual signal (VL) and present an overlaid signal, and finally image, to the end user. Thus, the surgeon receives a combined image, in which both the anatomical orientation of the surgical field, similar to the simple VL image, as well as an artificially colored fluorescence signal are depicted simultaneously and in real-time. A pseudo-coloring algorithm is used to fuse the visible light video signal with the fluorescence values extracted from the NIR camera. The color choice of the fluorescent signal depends on the end user. In our surgeries we used a standardized bright green color, however surgeons who are red-green color-blind could choose other color options. This technique abolishes the previously usual black and white display of fluorescence images, although the visualization of fluorescence raw data (mere NIR spectrum) on a black background is also possible, depending on the mode the user selects to use for the device.

Confocal Laser Endomicroscope

The Cellvizio®-780 nm system (Mauna Kea Technologies, Paris, France) has a near-infrared scanning unit. The mini-optical probes of the Cellvizio® system are composed of 30,000 optical fibers and are available with various optical properties and lengths according to clinical needs. Confocal imaging was accomplished by the CystoFlex UHD C-R™ probe. The probe is 2 m long, has an internal diameter of 2.6 mm and has a lateral resolution of 1 μm. The maximum field of view is 240 μm with an imaging plane depth of 55–65 μm. To enable real-time imaging, a 4 kHz oscillating mirror has been incorporated for horizontal line scanning and a galvanometric mirror for frame scanning. The device has a frame rate of 12 images per second. A foot pedal allows starting and pausing of video image acquisition. These image files may subsequently be exported using the Cellvizio® software.

Fluorescent Agent Indocyanine Green (ICG)

ICG (Verdye, Germany; λ_{ex} 760–775 nm/λ_{em} 835 nm) was used off label to enhance tumor tissue contrast by highlighting tumor blood vessels. ICG is an approved fluorescent agent for use in everyday neurosurgical practice and has several other medical and diagnostic applications, such as in ophthalmology for the imaging of the retinal blood vessels. It is administered intravenously and tends to bind strongly to specific plasma proteins without being extravasated or binding to atherosclerotic plaques on the walls of blood vessels. This feature results in the fluorescent dye remaining within the vascular system and renders it a very useful tool for contrasting vascular structures and visualization of the blood flow. As it circulates in pathological tumor vessels, ICG extravasation as a tumor staining agent can be visualized. Furthermore, during tumor surgery ICG spreads locally in the tissue and binds to cytoplasmic proteins, which results in staining of the cell cytoplasm around the nucleus. In our study, ICG (50 mg) was administered intravenously 1 h before operative exposure of the tumor.

Confocal-Assisted Fluorescent Technique

All the confocal-assisted fluorescent procedures were performed after permission of the ethical committee of the medical association of Nordrhein-Westfalia, Germany and the ethical committee of the University Witten-Herdecke. The special consent obtained from the participants for participating in the study was both informed and written. Participants under the age of 18 were not included.

We intra-operatively applied the combined use of infrared multispectral fluorescence and CLE on different types of CNS pathologies, using ICG as the fluorescent agent. We first examined 22 rats in the lab with implanted C6 glioma using a combination of the above techniques and transferred our experience to the surgical theater, which is the subject of this study. We describe here our first experience on 13 patients. The pathologies included were gliomas ($n = 5$), meningiomas ($n = 3$), neurinomas ($n = 2$), and metastases ($n = 3$) in different locations within the CNS, such as brain parenchyma, skull base, and spinal cord.

After opening the dura, the tumor was exposed and visualized with the Glow800 microscope. Initial observation was performed for tumor localization and characterization of the lesion's extent within the surgical field, as well as the tumor blood supply and draining vessels in relation to the surrounding structures. Furthermore, we observed tumor vascularization with fluorescent contrast enhancement. During and after tumor resection, the pseudo-colored mode of multispectral fluorescence demonstrated the extent of tumor resection, the tumor margins, and the anatomical properties of the resection cavity, and its vasculature. In a similar fashion, after tumor exposure we used the CLE device to visualize the tumor cellular architecture and performed optical biopsies without the need of real tissue resection. At the end of the fluorescence-assisted removal of the tumor, we inserted the confocal scope again into the surgical field to search for remaining tumor. The endomicroscope was held by hand against the tissue if the tumors were located on the surface or in the parenchyma. Confocal image injection in the surgical microscope was easily possible. If the tumors were located in the skull base and we had to use the endoscope for deep, around the corner visualization, then the endomicroscope was inserted into the working channel of the endoscope (**Figure 1**). Post-operatively, the resected tumor biopsies were fixed with formalin and transported to the neuropathology department for histopathological and immunohistochemical analysis. The extra surgical time was 5–10 min in addition to the normal surgical time for getting the CLE images. The images were selected from three parts of the surgical field: (a) fluorescent part of the tumor, (b) tumor to normal brain transition zone, and (c) normal tissue.

SURGICAL TECHNIQUE ANALYSIS AND CASE DEMONSTRATIONS

The Glow800-mode was used after performing the approach and the initial exposure of the tumor. The VL mode provided an equal image to the standard surgical microscope throughout the entire procedure. Vascular anatomy of the tumors, especially the arterial blood supply of the tumors and their branches, the tumor blood vessels, capillaries, and neovascularization patterns, and the complex venous drainage of the tumors were clearly visible both with the pseudo-colored as well as with the classic NIR-mode. The pseudo-colored mode showed here a significant superiority to the NIR-mode, as it presented the exact localization and anatomical relation of each vascular structure to the tumor mass and the surrounding surgical field in a bright colored image. In cases of extravasation due to bleeding from a local tumor blood vessel, the pseudo-colored mode also assisted the visualization

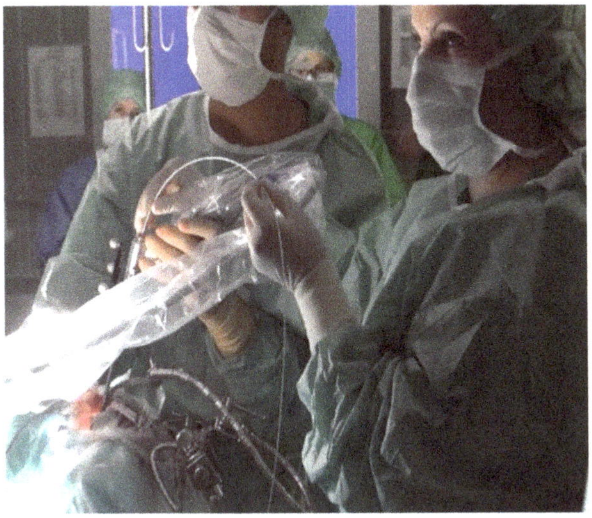

FIGURE 1 | On deep seated lesions, e.g., in the skull base, we inserted the confocal endomicroscope into the working channel of a classic endoscope performing a confocal-assisted endoscopic procedure.

of the bleeding spot and enabled instant hemostasis by the surgeon. After completion of tumor resection, the observation of the tumor margins under the pseudo-colored mode facilitated a better recognition of remaining pathologic tissue and neoplastic blood vessels, and therefore, their further removal. The image overlapping also allowed for quick and efficient recognition of these spots within and close to the resection hole without the need of several manipulations within the surgical field or switching to the VL or NIR-mode. As expected, these advantageous features of the pseudo-colored mode were more profound in more thickly vascularized tumors.

Due to bleeding during tumor removal, ICG was locally distributed in the surgical field and therefore, it could penetrate into the surrounding cells. The use of the CLE tool was important after dural opening and at the end for checking tumor margins at spots in the surgical field where fluorescence was not visible any more. When the probe was held directly with the hand, it was difficult to stabilize the imaging probe, which is a problematic issue. It was also difficult to control the uniform application of pressure of the probe against the tissue to provide artifact-free images. We obtained the best results for the multispectral infrared imaging of meningiomas, neurinomas, and metastatic tumors, while gliomas remained problematic on ICG uptake; high grade (WHO III, IV) gliomas were very marginal and not homogenously highlighted, while low grade gliomas were not highlighted at all. Therefore, we were surprised to see that confocal imaging, in contrast, was able to detect, at a cellular level, even those cells from tumors which were not highlighted at all with the fluorescent surgical microscope. However, the study's subject here is to show how the combination of both technologies together can affect intra-operative decision making on tumor resection and therefore, we present three cases out of 13 patients that demonstrate how we used both novel technologies as a confocal-assisted fluorescent technique.

Patient 1: Convexity Meningioma

This patient was scheduled for resection of a 6 × 5 × 4 cm convexity meningioma. The tumor was macroscopically well-defined. Once the dura was exposed, the Glow800 imaging system was used to demonstrate the accumulation of ICG in the tumor. With the CLE tool we also demonstrated the cytoarchitecture with cellular imaging of the tumor. Psammoma bodies, which are the typical characteristics of meningiomas, were clearly visible. Then, normal resection of the tumor, guided with the Glow800 module, was performed. When complete macroscopic removal was accomplished, CLE optical biopsies were performed to document complete resection with clear margins of normal tissue. *Ex vivo* CLE imaging was also performed on small pieces of the tumor infiltrating the dura matter and on the entire resection specimen by means of an interactive teleconference with the neuropathologists. The tissue areas imaged with CLE *in vivo* were the resection bed and the small parts of the normal brain surrounding the tumor that were exposed after dura opening (**Figure 2**). No residual tumor cells in the resection bed or the dura were seen.

Patient 2: Metastasis of a Ductal Carcinoma of the Breast

This patient was scheduled for the resection of a 5 × 5 × 4 cm metastasis of a ductal carcinoma of the breast located in the right parietal lobe. The tumor was macroscopically well-defined. Once the dura was opened, fluorescent imaging with the Glow800 demonstrated excellent accumulation of ICG onto the tumor surface. Then normal resection of the tumor with the Glow800 module was performed. During the resection, CLE optical biopsies were performed in order to check the histological type of the tumor and the margins between tumor and normal tissue. With the CLE tool we demonstrated the cytoarchitecture of the tumor. Typical cellular architecture of the carcinoma was well-identified with nests of cells featuring prominent nuclei with mitotic activities. *Ex vivo* CLE imaging was performed on the entire resection specimen and discussed in an interactive teleconference with the neuropathologist. The tissue areas visualized before dura closure with CLE *in vivo* were, as usual, the resection bed and the small parts of the normal brain surrounding the tumor on the brain surface exposed after initial dura opening (**Figure 3**).

Patient 3: Sphenoid Wing Meningioma With Compression of the Optic Nerve

This patient was scheduled for resection of a meningioma originating from the sphenoid wing with compression of the optic nerve. Using the fluorescent imaging system with the Glow800, we visualized during the 4 h tumor removal the different uptake steps of ICG into the tumor (**Figure 4**). After completing the tumor resection, CLE was performed on different structures on the skull base, especially on different parts of the exposed optic nerve and chiasm. In this case, the CLE probe was inserted in the operative channel of an endoscope for better stabilization and gentle manipulation of the CLE probe on the optic nerve. CLE video sequences of normal tissue, tumor, nerve,

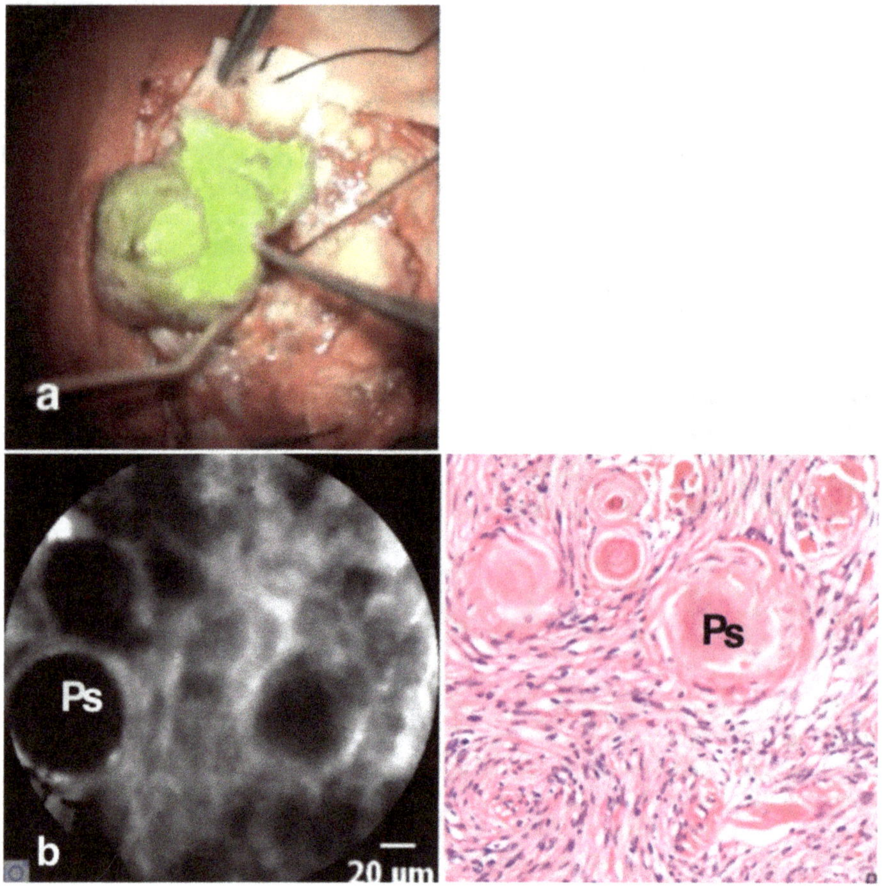

FIGURE 2 | The meningioma is visible as a "green" tumor **(a)** with very clear borders, while the normal brain around is without ICG uptake. *In vivo* confocal image **(b)** shows the cytoarchitecture of the meningioma with big psammoma bodies (Ps), while the H & E staining confirms the diagnosis.

and resection bed were acquired at the beginning, during, and after the resection. **Supplementary Video 1** shows the border between the tumor and nerve fibers (**Supplementary Video 1**). We performed CLE imaging *in vivo* from the resection bed and *ex vivo* directly from the tumor. In the same case, psammoma bodies, nerve, and normal brain tissue from the frontal lobe could be observed. The different cellular perspective pictures in longitudinally and transversely taken slices of the optic nerve were impressive. Within the nerve bundles, we observed insulated nerve fibers from their neighbors by neuroglia. Within the nerve fiber bundles, rows of supporting astrocytes, oligodendrocytes, and some microglial cells were also seen. A continuous glial membrane formed by the astrocytes separated the nerve fibers. ICG highlighted the cytoplasm of the surrounding glia and oligodendrocytes. Therefore, small white rings were visible on the transverse slices of the nerve. Histological sampling (H&E stain) of the optic nerve was not performed as we protected the optic nerve.

DISCUSSION

Over the previous years, the aim of optimizing microsurgery and maximizing its safety and efficiency has brought forward several intra-operative techniques for the visualization and contrast imaging of tumor and normal tissue. In tumor surgery, the visualization of the blood vessels of the tumor and the surrounding tissues has not yet been the major point of interest, with the most cutting edge feature being 5-ALA fluorescence, which uses the metabolic features of tumor cells to help identify neoplastic tissue within the surgical field (5). The currently existing infrared fluorescence surgical microscopes allow fluorescent image delivery through an external monitor and not through the eyepiece of the microscope, thus forcing interruption of the surgical workflow for assessment of the white light and fluorescent images.

The Glow800 tool is a surgical-microscope-integrated software and hardware system that enables the superimposition of an ICG fluorescent image onto a white light image, producing a merged image that delivers both the white light anatomical data as well as the dynamic information of ICG fluorescence in a real-time fashion. It shows the fluorescent signal of ICG in green (also visible in seven different other colors) onto a white light pseudo-colored anatomical background. After visualization of the tumor as a green-colored mass, the confocal endomicroscope was used to characterize the cellular cytoarchitecture of the tumor and scan the intra-operative field for remaining tumor tissue.

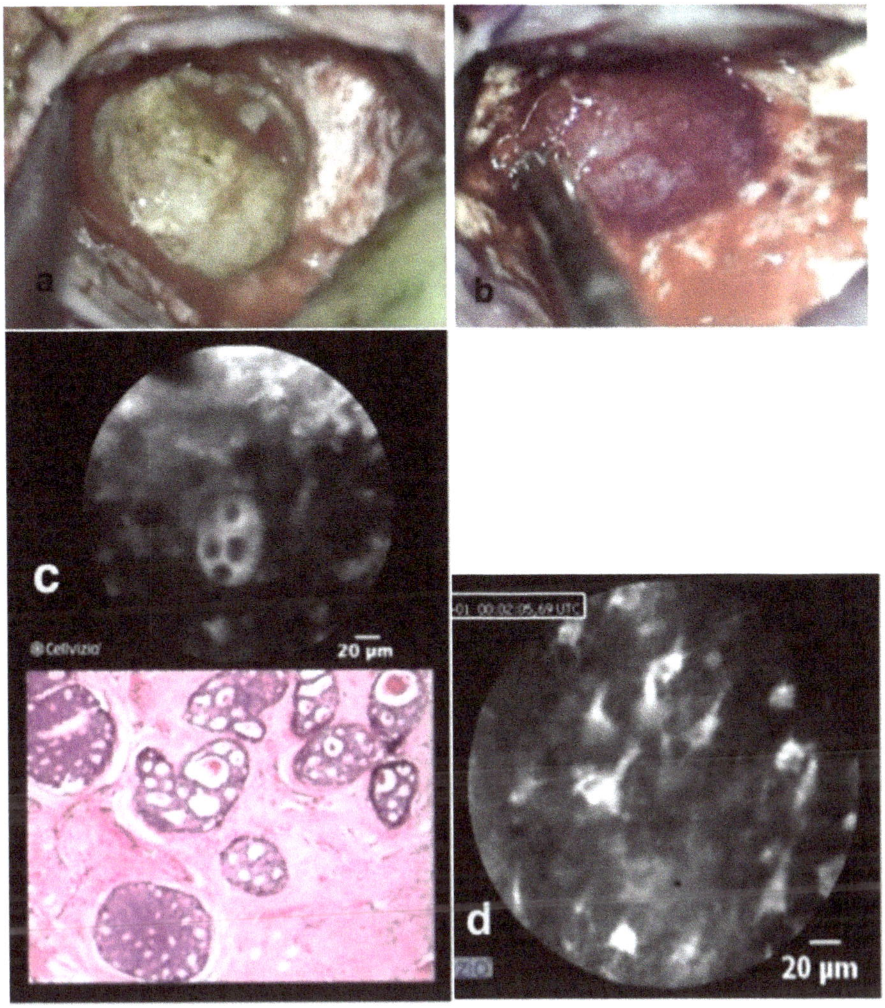

FIGURE 3 | Brain metastasis of ductal breast cancer in two different colors pictured **(a,b)**. *In vivo* confocal imaging **(c)** shows the cell nester with prominent nucleus with the analog H & E staining typical for breast metastasis. The confocal scanning with the scope on the remaining brain tissue shows normal brain structures **(d)** with astrocytes, pyramidal, and bipolar cells.

The current study tested the MFL technique with the Glow800 tool on a series of 13 patients in interaction with confocal endomicroscopy, trying to prove the feasibility and superiority of this so called confocal-assisted fluorescent technique over the existing standard in neurosurgical practice.

In tumor surgery, the presentation of the anatomical structures related to the tumor and the tumor vessels in the pseudo-colored mode provided a substantially larger and crucial amount of information regarding tumor appearance and borders while performing surgery. Although administration of high dose ICG with the second window detection has been reported previously (26–28), a high dose was not necessary in our study. The dose of ICG administered was 50 mg in all cases (two commercially available vials of 25 mg each) and the time of administration was only 1 h before the beginning of the surgical procedure (during introduction of anesthesia). The simultaneous use of CLE with the cellular analysis of tissue brings immediate answers during the surgical session about how far resection has to go.

A further technique, similar to the ICG fluorescence, which has been used by many groups for the visualization of tumor blood vessels, is fluorescein fluorescence (29–33). It also requires a surgical microscope that can detect fluorescent images and delivers the fluorescein highlighting blood vessels over an anatomical white light image of the surgical field. The disadvantages of fluorescein fluorescence, however, include the lack of FDA approval for this fluorescent agent in neurosurgery, the extensive extravasation of fluorescein when injected in high concentrations—and therefore, lack of a quick washout, preventing intravenous injections,—and its extensive binding to atherosclerotic plaques, leading to prolonged highlighting of atherosclerotic blood vessels and potentially generating a false impression of present blood flow. The use of fluorescein in confocal endomicroscopy also faces some limitations in

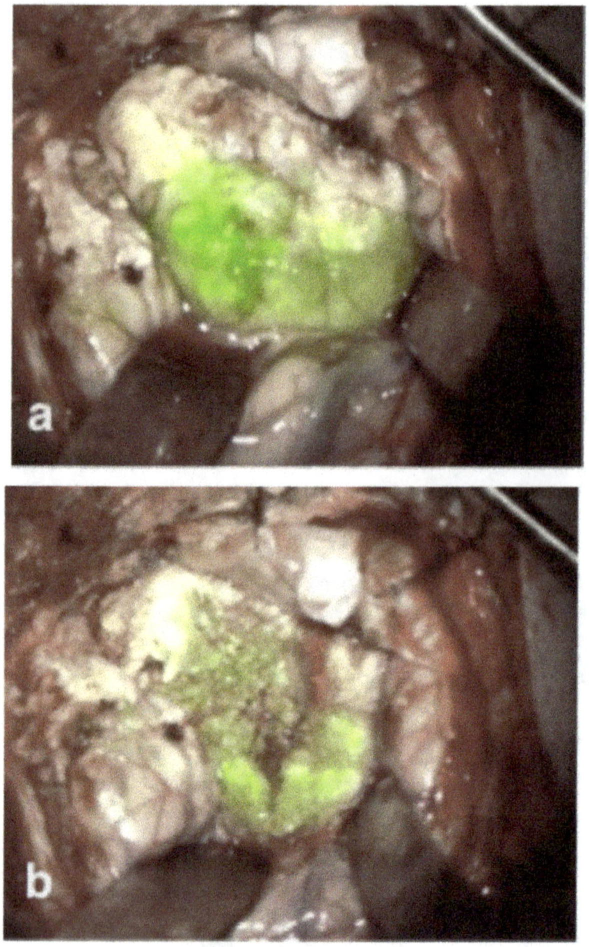

FIGURE 4 | The skull base meningioma shows strong ICG uptake at the beginning of tumor resection immediately after tumor exposure **(a)**. During the tumor resection ICG seemed to be still active in its accumulation into the tumor, as we observed an increased fluorescence signal into the tumor volume **(b)**.

comparison to ICG. Fluorescein remains extracellular and highlights the extracellular space (34). Therefore, cell architecture is not as clearly visible as it is with ICG, which binds intra-cellularly on cytoplasmic proteins and highlights the cell itself. Another disadvantage is that the detection spectrum of fluorescein interacts with the spectrum of hemoglobin on around 530–550 nm. This means that, working with fluorescein intra-operatively at the cellular level, the visualization of fluorescein fluorescence could be blocked due to overlying erythrocytes (hemoglobin), which would not be the case with ICG in infrared (780–800 nm) since confocal endomicroscopes that are able to detect in infrared are "blind" to light emission in lower spectra. In infrared, the view is open to see behind the "wall" of erythrocytes. Furthermore, infrared light (needed for detecting ICG) penetrates deeper in the tissue compared to light at a shorter spectral range (needed for FL). In tumor surgery, even if 5-ALA or ICG fluorescence is not visible, there could be tumor cells present in a depth of 1–2 mm spread behind the tumor bed. Therefore, for cellular imaging we need detection sources able to penetrate as deeply as possible inside the tissue. Those light ranges are found in infrared and beyond.

In oncologic surgery, the CLE-assisted fluorescent technique allows for intra-operative detection of green-colored tumor on a macroscale as well as differentiation and identification of individual tumor cells at a subcellular or subnuclear level. This technique provides immediate online diagnosis without the need for rapid biopsies and therefore, helps to define the borders between tumor and normal tissue at a cellular level. The application and implementation of CLE-assisted surgery in surgical oncology would increase the range of available diagnostic and therapeutic options by extending the resection borders of cancer at a cellular level and, more importantly, by automatically protecting the functionality of normal tissue in eloquent areas of the human brain. Confocal-assisted fluorescent surgery offers, in different regions of the neuronal axis, an excellent addition to the intra-operative navigation because of the cellular confocal-fluorescence guidance, which provides real-time images, so that brain shift is no longer a problem. The surgical CLE prototype device we used in our surgeries provides ~400-fold magnification of the observed tissue structures during surgery. Widely used microscopy and standard endoscopy offer only a very slight increase in the visualization of structures, about 10-fold and 2-fold, respectively. Therefore, we used the combination of the new fluorescent microscope and the confocal endomicroscope in interaction during surgery. Using the confocal-assisted fluorescent microscopic technique, we were able to clearly identify the tumor on a macroscale while operating with fluorescence-guidance and we were then able to magnify the surrounding environment on a microscale of 400-fold to check the tissue at a cellular level.

There are also limitations in our approach of *in vivo* histopathological imaging with CLE. Intravenous injection and local application of some fluorescent agents such as ICG or fluorescein in tumor surgery are off-label. With the Glow800, we were able to use ICG to detect tumor vascularization and to highlight the tumors while using a small dose of ICG and relatively simple protocol. Although we observed a good accumulation of ICG on benign and metastatic processes, visualization of ICG uptake in gliomas remained problematic. Although we observed the strongest fluorescence signal on the tissue surface, the limited infiltration depth and field of view of the confocal endomicroscope is a drawback if the instrument has to show borders between tumors and normal brain. However, this could be overcome with the next generation of confocal systems, which could be able to penetrate deeper into the tissue and provide larger field of view. In the future, confocal systems with multiple excitation wavelengths, such as in bench-top confocal imaging, may facilitate clinical use, and a combination of a surgical microscope with a confocal endomicroscope could also be of great advantage. Regarding the MFL technique, we are now in the process of extending the usability also to other fluorescent agents like 5-ALA and fluorescein. In the near future, the surgeon will be able to see and operate on the tumor under white light while simultaneously viewing the accumulation 5-ALA or/and fluorescein as colored overlay, therefore, overcoming the individual limitations of dark blue or dark yellow light.

In this study, we described the application of MFL together with confocal laser endomicroscopy as "CLE-assisted fluorescent microsurgical technique," its implementation in the operative theater, its advantages, limitations, and future perspectives with planned developments in oncological surgery. With CLE-assisted fluorescent surgery, we were able to achieve both an improved representation of the borders between tumor (multi-color highlight) and normal tissue as a significant improvement in the representation of immediate histological diagnosis compared with the time-consuming multiple-day hematoxylin and eosin staining.

AUTHOR CONTRIBUTIONS

PC: concept design, performance of the clinical testings, and drafted the manuscript. MN: clinical testings and corrected the manuscript. DA: performance of part of clinical testings and edited the manuscript text. AH: contribution on study design according to previous animal experiments.

REFERENCES

1. Martirosyan NL, Skoch J, Watson, Lemole GM Jr, Romanowski M, Anton R. Integration of indocyanine green videoangiography with operative microscope. *Neurosurgery.* (2015) 11:252–8 doi: 10.1227/NEU.0000000000000681
2. Raabe A, Nakaji P, Beck J, Kim LJ, Hsu FP, Kamerman JD, et al. Prospective evaluation of surgical microscope-integrated intraoperative near-infrared indocyanine green videoangiography during aneurysm surgery. *J Neurosurg.* (2005) 103:982–9. doi: 10.3171/jns.2005.103.6.0982
3. Raabe A, Beck J, Seifert V. Technique and image quality of intraoperative indocyanine green angiography during aneurysm surgery using surgical microscope integrated near-infrared video technology. *Zentralbl Neurochir.* (2005) 66:1–6. doi: 10.1055/s-2004-836223
4. Nickele C, Nguyen V, Fisher W, Couldwell W, Aboud E, David C, et al. A pilot comparison of multispectral fluorescence to indocyanine green videoangiography and other modalities for intraoperative assessment in vascular neurosurgery. *Oper Neurosurg (Hagerstown).* (2018) 17:103–9. doi: 10.1093/ons/opy237
5. Stummer W, Pichlmeier U, Meinel T, Wiestler OD, Zanella F, Reulen HJ, et al. Fluorescence-guided surgery with 5-aminolevulinic acid for resection of malignant glioma: a randomised controlled multicentre phase III trial. *Lancet Oncol.* (2006) 7:392–401. doi: 10.1016/S1470-2045(06)70665-9
6. Foersch S, Heimann A, Ayyad A, Spoden GA, Florin L, Mpoukouvalas K, et al. Confocal laser endomicroscopy for diagnosis and histomorphologic imaging of brain tumors *in vivo. PLoS ONE.* (2012) 7:e41760. doi: 10.1371/journal.pone.0041760
7. Kiesslich R, Burg J, Vieth M, Gnaendiger J, Enders M, Delaney P, et al. Confocal laser endoscopy for diagnosing intraepithelial neoplasias and colorectal cancer *in vivo. Gastroenterology.* (2004) 127:706–13. doi: 10.1053/j.gastro.2004.06.050
8. Zehri AH, Ramey W, Georges JF, Mooney MA, Martirosyan NL, Preul MC, et al. Neurosurgical confocal endomicroscopy: a review of contrast agents, confocal systems, and future imaging modalities. *Surg Neurol Int.* (2014) 5:60. doi: 10.4103/2152-7806.131638
9. Polglase AL, McLaren WJ, Skinner SA, Kiesslich R, Neurath MF, Delaney PM. A fluorescence confocal endomicroscope for *in vivo* microscopy of the upper- and the lower-GI tract. *Gastrointest Endosc.* (2005) 62:686–95. doi: 10.1016/j.gie.2005.05.021
10. Lane PM, Lam S, McWilliams A, Leriche JC, Anderson MW, Macaulay CE. Confocal fluorescence microendoscopy of bronchial epithelium. *J biomed optics.* (2009) 14:024008. doi: 10.1117/1.3103583
11. Thiberville L, Moreno-Swirc S, Vercauteren T, Peltier E, Cave C, Bourg Heckly G. *In vivo* imaging of the bronchial wall microstructure using fibered confocal fluorescence microscopy. *Am j resp crit care med.* (2007) 175:22–31. doi: 10.1164/rccm.200605-684OC
12. Tan J, Quinn MA, Pyman JM, Delaney PM, McLaren WJ. Detection of cervical intraepithelial neoplasia *in vivo* using confocal endomicroscopy. *Bjog.* (2009) 116:1663–70. doi: 10.1111/j.1471-0528.2009.02261.x
13. Sonn GA, Jones SN, Tarin TV, Du CB, Mach KE, Jensen KC, et al. Optical biopsy of human bladder neoplasia with *in vivo* confocal laser endomicroscopy. *J urol.* (2009) 182:1299–305. doi: 10.1016/j.juro.2009.06.039
14. Wiesner C, Jager W, Salzer A, Biesterfeld S, Kiesslich R, Hampel C, et al. Confocal laser endomicroscopy for the diagnosis of urothelial bladder neoplasia: a technology of the future? *BJU inter.* (2011) 107:399–403. doi: 10.1111/j.1464-410X.2010.09540.x
15. Bui D, Mach KE, Zlatev DV, Rouse RV, Leppert JT, Liao JC. A pilot study of *in vivo* confocal laser endomicroscopy of upper tract urothelial carcinoma. *J Endourol.* (2015) 29:1418–23. doi: 10.1089/end.2015.0523
16. Haxel BR, Goetz M, Kiesslich R, Gosepath J. Confocal endomicroscopy: a novel application for imaging of oral and oropharyngeal mucosa in human. *Eur Arch Otorhinolaryngol.* (2010) 267:443–8. doi: 10.1007/s00405-009-1035-3
17. Linxweiler M, Kadah BA, Bozzato A, Bozzato V, Hasenfus A, Kim YJ, et al. Noninvasive histological imaging of head and neck squamous cell carcinomas using confocal laser endomicroscopy. *Eur Arch Otorhinolaryngol.* (2016) 273:4473–83. doi: 10.1007/s00405-016-4145-8
18. Schulz A, Daali S, Javed M, Fuchs PC, Brockmann M, Igressa A, et al. Presurgical mapping of basal cell carcinoma or squamous cell carcinoma by confocal laser endomicroscopy compared to traditional micrographic surgery: a single-centre prospective feasibility study. *Eur J Dermatol.* (2016) 26:572–9. doi: 10.1684/ejd.2016.2874
19. Malmstrom ML, Karstensen JG, A SF, Riis LB, Gogenur I, Vilmann P. Confocal laser endomicroscopy is a new endoscopic technique for diagnosing colorectal neoplasia and inflammatory bowel disease. *Ugeskr Laeger.* (2014) 176:V05130311.
20. Trovato C, Sonzogni A, Ravizza D, Fiori G, Tamayo D, De Roberto G, et al. Confocal laser endomicroscopy for *in vivo* diagnosis of Barrett's oesophagus and associated neoplasia: a pilot study conducted in a single Italian centre. *Dig Liver Dis.* (2013) 45:396–402. doi: 10.1016/j.dld.2012.12.016
21. Buchner AM, Wallace MB. *In-vivo* microscopy in the diagnosis of intestinal neoplasia and inflammatory conditions. *Histopathology.* (2015) 66:137–46. doi: 10.1111/his.12597
22. Charalampaki P, Javed M, Daali S, Heiroth HJ, Igressa A, Weber F. Confocal laser endomicroscopy for real-time histomorphological diagnosis: our clinical experience with 150 brain and spinal tumor cases. *Neurosurgery.* (2015) 62(Suppl 1):171–6. doi: 10.1227/NEU.0000000000000805
23. Martirosyan NL, Georges J, Eschbacher JM, Cavalcanti DD, Elhadi AM, Abdelwahab MG, et al. Potential application of a handheld confocal endomicroscope imaging system using a variety of fluorophores in experimental gliomas and normal brain. *Neurosurg Focus.* (2014) 36:E16. doi: 10.3171/2013.11.FOCUS13486
24. Martirosyan NL, Cavalcanti DD, Eschbacher JM, Delaney PM, Scheck AC, Abdelwahab MG, et al. Use of *in vivo* near-infrared laser confocal endomicroscopy with indocyanine green to detect the boundary of infiltrative tumor. *J neurosurg.* (2011) 115:1131–8. doi: 10.3171/2011.8.JNS11559
25. Eschbacher J, Martirosyan NL, Nakaji P, Sanai N, Preul MC, Smith KA, et al. *In vivo* intraoperative confocal microscopy for real-time histopathological imaging of brain tumors. *J Neurosurg.* (2012) 116:854–60. doi: 10.3171/2011.12.JNS11696
26. Zeh R, Sheikh S, Xia L, Pierce J, Newton A, Predina J, et al. The second window ICG technique demonstrates a broad plateau period for near infrared fluorescence tumor contrast in glioblastoma. *PLoS ONE.* (2017) 12:e0182034. doi: 10.1371/journal.pone.0182034

27. Lee JYK, Pierce JT, Zeh R, Cho SS, Salinas R, Nie S, et al. Intraoperative near-infrared optical contrast can localize brain metastases. *World Neurosurg.* (2017) 106:120–30. doi: 10.1016/j.wneu.2017.06.128
28. Lee JYK, Pierce JT, Thawani JP, Zeh R, Nie S, Martinez-Lage M, et al. Near-infrared fluorescent image-guided surgery for intracranial meningioma. *J Neurosurg.* (2018) 128:380–90. doi: 10.3171/2016.10.JNS161636
29. Belykh E, Cavallo C, Gandhi S, Zhao X, Veljanoski D, Izady Yazdanabadi M, et al. Utilization of intraoperative confocal laser endomicroscopy in brain tumor surgery. *J Neurosurg Sci.* (2018) 62:704–17. doi: 10.23736/S0390-5616.18.04553-8
30. Belykh E, Martirosyan NL, Yagmurlu K, Miller EJ, Eschbacher JM, Izadyyazdanabadi M, et al. Intraoperative fluorescence imaging for personalized brain tumor resection: current state and future directions. *Front Surg.* (2016) 3:55. doi: 10.3389/fsurg.2016.00055
31. Li Y, Rey-Dios R, Roberts DW, Valdés PA, Cohen-Gadol AA. Intraoperative fluorescence-guided resection of high-grade gliomas: a comparison of the present techniques and evolution of future strategies. *World Neurosurg.* (2014) 82:175–85. doi: 10.1016/j.wneu.2013.06.014
32. Lane BC, Cohen-Gadol AA. Fluorescein fluorescence use in the management of intracranial neoplastic and vascular lesions: a review and report of a new technique. *Curr Drug Discov Technol.* (2013) 10:160–9. doi: 10.2174/1570163811310020009
33. Diaz RJ, Dios RR, Hattab EM, Burrell K, Rakopoulos P, Sabha N, et al. Study of the biodistribution of fluorescein in glioma-infiltrated mouse brain and histopathological correlation of intraoperative findings in high-grade gliomas resected under fluorescein fluorescence guidance. *J Neurosurg.* (2015) 122:1360–9. doi: 10.3171/2015.2.JNS 132507
34. Martirosyan NL, Georges J, Eschbacher JM, Belykh E, Carotenuto A, Spetzler RF, et al. Confocal scanning microscopy provides rapid, detailed intraoperative histological assessment of brain neoplasms: experience with 106 cases. *Clin Neurol Neurosurg.* (2018) 169:21–8. doi: 10.1016/j.clineuro.2018.03.015

8

Receptor-Targeted Fluorescence-Guided Surgery with Low Molecular Weight Agents

Servando Hernandez Vargas[1,2], Christie Lin[3], Hop S. Tran Cao[4], Naruhiko Ikoma[4], Solmaz AghaAmiri[1], Sukhen C. Ghosh[1], Adam J. Uselmann[3] and Ali Azhdarinia[1,2*]*

[1] The Brown Foundation Institute of Molecular Medicine, McGovern Medical School, The University of Texas Health Science Center at Houston, Houston, TX, United States, [2] Therapeutics & Pharmacology Program, The University of Texas MD Anderson UTHealth Graduate School of Biomedical Sciences, Houston, TX, United States, [3] OnLume, Inc., Madison, WI, United States, [4] Department of Surgical Oncology, Division of Surgery, The University of Texas MD Anderson Cancer Center, Houston, TX, United States

***Correspondence:**
Servando Hernandez Vargas
Servando.HernandezVargas@uth.tmc.edu
Ali Azhdarinia
ali.azhdarinia@uth.tmc.edu

Cancer surgery remains the primary treatment option for most solid tumors and can be curative if all malignant cells are removed. Surgeons have historically relied on visual and tactile cues to maximize tumor resection, but clinical data suggest that relapse occurs partially due to incomplete cancer removal. As a result, the introduction of technologies that enhance the ability to visualize tumors in the operating room represents a pressing need. Such technologies have the potential to revolutionize the surgical standard-of-care by enabling real-time detection of surgical margins, subclinical residual disease, lymph node metastases and synchronous/metachronous tumors. Fluorescence-guided surgery (FGS) in the near-infrared (NIRF) spectrum has shown tremendous promise as an intraoperative imaging modality. An increasing number of clinical studies have demonstrated that tumor-selective FGS agents can improve the predictive value of fluorescence over non-targeted dyes. Whereas NIRF-labeled macromolecules (i.e., antibodies) spearheaded the widespread clinical translation of tumor-selective FGS drugs, peptides and small-molecules are emerging as valuable alternatives. Here, we first review the state-of-the-art of promising low molecular weight agents that are in clinical development for FGS; we then discuss the significance, application and constraints of emerging tumor-selective FGS technologies.

Keywords: surgical oncology, fluorescence-guided surgery, contrast agents, low molecular weight agents, cancer-targeted agents, receptor targeted imaging

INTRODUCTION

Fluorescence-guided surgery (FGS) is an imaging technique that is uniquely suited to bridge the gap between pre-operative radiologic imaging and post-operative histopathological assessment of cancer. The administration of a fluorescent contrast agent, its localization to sites of interest, and detection by an optical imaging device are the fundamental steps for generating an intraoperative fluorescent image. If effective, a fluorescent agent augments visual feedback to complement tactile guidance in open surgery or overcome the lack of tactile feedback in minimally invasive surgery (MIS), thereby potentially increasing complete tumor resection rates. Indeed, clinical FGS studies have reported improved surgical outcomes and patient benefit with a variety of contrast agents (1–4). The most widely used FGS agent is indocyanine green (ICG; molecular weight [MW] = 776 g/mol; $\lambda_{Excitation}/\lambda_{Emission}$ [Ex/Em] = 780/820 nm), a non-targeted, water-soluble tricarbocyanine dye and the only FDA-approved near-infrared fluorescence (NIRF) fluorophore. The excellent safety profile and favorable spectral properties of ICG have led to its use in numerous clinical applications such as angiography, tissue perfusion, sentinel lymph node mapping, and tumor imaging (5, 6). Moreover, its hepatic clearance and biliary excretion makes ICG an ideal agent for fluorescence cholangiography, and is increasingly used for safe cholecystectomy (7). Although ICG has been instrumental in demonstrating the utility of FGS (8, 9), there is a critical need to expand FGS applications with agents that possess improved tumor specificity.

Monoclonal antibodies (mAbs) were among the earliest targeted FGS agents to be translated into patients based largely on the repurposing of therapeutic mAbs for imaging (10). Standard bioconjugation techniques, such as N-hydroxysuccinimide (NHS) ester-activated crosslinkers, allowed fluorescent dyes to be reacted with primary amines on lysine residues of mAbs, producing, for example, fluorescent analogs of cetuximab and panitumumab (epidermal growth factor receptor [EGFR] targeting), or bevacizumab (vascular endothelial growth factor receptor [VEGFR] targeting). Clinical studies with these immunoconjugates demonstrated selective receptor binding and feasibility of tumor-specific FGS in several cancers (11–13). However, their large molecular weight produces prolonged serum half-life and slow clearance from non-target tissues. As a result, the time interval between injection and intraoperative imaging with fluorescent mAbs can be as long as one week to generate sufficient tumor contrast. Furthermore, interactions between the Fc region of mAbs and cognate receptors on immune effector cells produce additional background fluorescence that can confound tumor imaging. Low molecular weight (LMW) agents, such as peptides and small molecules, also possess high binding affinity to cancer biomarkers but have more favorable pharmacokinetic (PK) properties than mAb-based agents; for instance, a circulating half-life of a few hours and predominant renal excretion (14). Collectively, these properties have the potential to provide high tumor contrast within a few hours after injection (15, 16). Other key advantages of FGS with LMW agents include tumor visualization at microdose levels, amenability to chemical modification and the absence of immunogenic effects (17, 18).

To further illustrate the clinical potential of LMW agents for FGS, a recent review by Barth and Gibbs listed 39 novel fluorescent agents that are under investigation in clinical trials, 25 of which were classified as peptides or small molecules (19). Several recent review articles have highlighted the clinical development of promising FGS agents (19–22). Here, we focus on LMW agents and their potential to improve intraoperative visualization in surgical oncology. Furthermore, we discuss the significance, application and constraints of emerging tumor-selective FGS technologies.

TRANSLATING LMW AGENTS INTO THE OPERATING ROOM

The pressing need for improved tumor visualization in the operating room is reflected by the rapidly increasing number of studies under clinical investigation. Although the overarching goals of such studies are clear (i.e., determining safety and efficacy), clinical trial design and endpoint selection are driven by complex factors related to the semi-quantitative and combinatorial nature of FGS (22–24). The lack of standard methods and objective measures of efficacy (25) further complicate the assessment of trial results and trial comparison (26), even when the same drug is used (e.g., in combination with a different imaging device). However, several converging and diverging points during clinical development of LMW agents can be identified. Similarities in early phase trials include determination of an optimal dose and imaging time point along with safety and tolerability, thereby establishing feasibility of the approach. Diverging points are plenty and may be attributed to unique requirements of each clinical application; for instance, anatomical location, spectral properties of the tissue, the identification of margins *vs.* multifocal lesions, etc. (27, 28).

FGS seeks to increase the surgical sensitivity. To date, LMW agents have clinically demonstrated a promising avenue to do so. In this section, we first describe the development of LMW agents that have progressed to clinical studies and meet the specifications outlined in "*Selection Criteria, Search Strategy and Results.*" To contextualize the feasibility of the approach, we then aim to provide a brief description of study design per agent (classified by cancer type), associated endpoints, and emerging applications of FGS that complement current clinical workflows, where appropriate. Finally, in **Tables 1** and **2** we summarize key parameters for discussed studies such as dose, imaging time, device, tumor-to-background ratios (TBRs) and diagnostic accuracy, if available.

Selection Criteria, Search Strategy and Results

For reviewed agents, we applied the inclusion criteria listed below to the best of our ability:

- Tumor selectivity must be afforded by receptor-mediated uptake
- The conjugate must be <10,000 g/mol
- Must not be a nanoparticle
- Contrast must be provided in the NIRF spectrum (emission range: 750-900 nm)
- Must have advanced to clinical trials
- Must be intravenously administered
- References published on or before November 6th, 2020 were considered
- Only papers published in the English language were reviewed
- Final list of agents discussed was produced based on relevance to the present work

Methodology and Search Engines

On November, 6th, 2020, we used the clinical trial registry ran by the United States National Institute of Health (NIH), https://clinicaltrials.gov/, to search the following keywords: "cancer, fluorescence, surgery" and found a total of 251 studies.

We then manually checked each study to catalog fluorescent agents used. Applying the aforementioned selection criteria, we identified a total of 6 agents: OTL38, BLZ-100, ABY-029, LS301, cRGD-ZW800-1 and BBN-IRdye800CW. We then searched the name identifier of each agent in https://clinicaltrials.gov/ and https://pubmed.ncbi.nlm.nih.gov/ to retrieve published content. We also searched the keyword "cRGD-ZW800-1" in https://www.trialregister.nl/, a Netherlands trial register for clinical studies being conducted in the Netherlands.

OTL38 (SMALL MOLECULE)

The first clinical report demonstrating that tumor-specific FGS can increase intraoperative detection of cancer used a folate motif linked to fluorescein-isothiocyanate (folate-FITC, EC17; Ex/Em = 494/521 nm) to target the folate receptor α (FRα) in ovarian cancer (29). Unfortunately, the benefits of EC17 are hindered by its emission in the visible wavelength and thus, restricts detection of occult lesions. To overcome detection-depth limits, the folate motif was modified to enable conjugation of the NIRF dye, S0456 (indole cyanine-like green), producing OTL38 (MW = 1,414 g/mol; Ex/Em = 776/793 nm; **Figure 1**) (31). *In vivo* studies using mouse models and canine patients demonstrated the advantages of imaging in the NIRF range and supported the continued development of OTL38 (32, 33). To date, at least 9 clinical trials have begun (Phase I-III) using OTL38 and initial results (**Table 1**) are encouraging as described below.

Ovarian cancer: The main role of surgery in ovarian cancer is cytoreduction and thus, the major value of tumor-specific FGS in this setting is to increase debulking rates. Using OTL38, Hoogstins et al. demonstrated an increase of 29% more lesions resected compared to direct visual inspection and palpation (30). To select the optimal dose and time window for imaging, the authors first performed a randomized, placebo-controlled dose-escalation study in healthy volunteers to assess PK in skin and plasma. In patient studies, tolerability, PK, and efficacy were investigated. Efficacy in the intraoperative setting was assessed by measuring (i) TBRs, (ii) congruence between pathology and fluorescence, (iii) number and location of FRα+ lesions identified using standard-of-care and imaging, and (iv) the surgeon's evaluation of the practicality of the approach. In addition to standard-of-care, study design permitted tumor tissues identified by imaging to be eligible for resection if deemed clinically beneficial and surgically feasible. In another study, which supported progression to Phase III, Randall et al. further investigated safety along with the diagnostic accuracy of OTL38 in 44 patients (34). Results showed the approach to be safe with sensitivity and positive predictive values (PPVs) of over

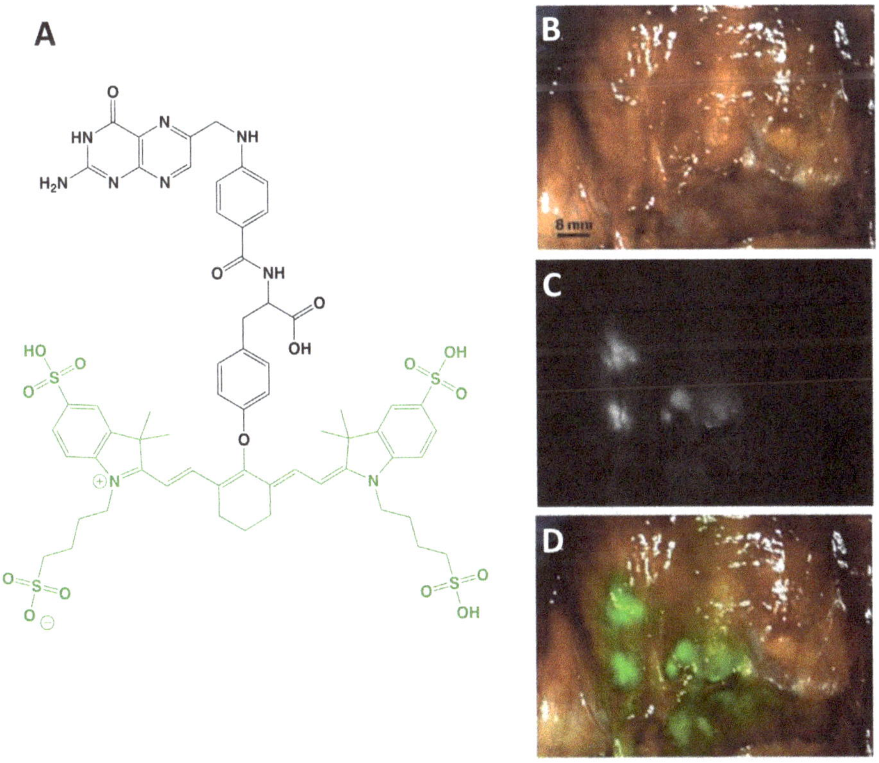

FIGURE 1 | OTL38. Chemical structure; folate motif (ligand) and linker in black, S0456 (dye) in green **(A)**. Intraoperative detection of ovarian cancer metastases with OTL38 administered 2-3 h prior to surgery: white-light only **(B)**, NIRF only **(C)** and white-light with NIRF overlay **(D)**. Panels **(B–D)** are adapted from (30) with permission.

TABLE 1 | Summary of key parameters in clinical studies with LMW contrast agents.

Agent	Type	Phase	Target	Cancer type	Dose (mg/kg)	Imaging time (h)	Image contrast*	Imaging device	Reference
OTL38	Small molecule	I-III	FRα	Ovarian	0.0125 to 0.2	2-3	3.5-5.4	Artemis (Quest medical imaging); PINPOINT (Novadaq); Iridium (Visionsense)	(30, 34)
				Lung	0.025 (1.48-3.29 mg total)	3-6	1.0-6.2	Iridium (Visionsense)	(35–40)
				Renal	0.025	2	N/A	da Vinci Fluorescence Imaging Vision System (Intuitive Surgical)	(41, 42)
				Gastric adenocarcinoma	0.025	1.5-6	2.6-7.4	VS3 Iridium system (Medtronic)	(43)
				Endometrial carcinoma	0.0125	2-3	2.9-13.0	Artemis (Quest medical imaging)	(44)
				Osteosarcoma	0.025	4	2.9-3.0	Iridium (Visionsense)	(45)
				Pituitary adenoma	0.025	2-4	1.6-3.2	Iridium (Visionsense)	(46, 47)
BLZ-100 (Tozuleristide, Tumor Paint™)	Peptide	I-III	Multiple	Gliomas (adult and pediatric)	3-30 mg	3-29	N/A (reported as -, weak or +)	FLUOBEAM 800 (Fluoptics); SIRIS (Teal Light Surgical)	(48, 49)
				Breast carcinoma	6-12 mg	1-26	N/A	SIRIS (Teal Light Surgical)	(50)
ABY-029	Affibody	0-I	EGFR	Soft tissue sarcoma	237 µg (30 nanomoles)	1-3	2.0 (n = 1)	Solaris (PerkinElmer)	(51)
BBN-IRdye800CW	Peptide	I	GRPR	Glioblastoma	1 mg	2-16	3.2-4.9	DPM-III-01 (Zhuhai Dipu Medical Technology)	(52, 53)
cRGD-ZW800-1	Small molecule	I-II	Integrins	Colorectal carcinoma	0.005-0.05	2-18	*In vivo*, 1.1-1.6; *ex vivo*, 1.4-6.2	Olympus Visera Elite II (CLV-S200-IR); Quest Spectrum Platform (Quest Medical Imaging)	(54)
LS301	Peptide	I-II	Annexin A2, others	Breast, liver, pancreas, gastric	-	-	-	-	-

*Rows are color coded to facilitate differentiation among agents. *In the image contrast column, we report the average lower and upper limit contrast (e.g., TBR) among all studies in the reference column and may include in situ, ex vivo values.*

94.9% when lesions were FRα+ and the statistical model used patients as random effect (**Table 2**).

Lung cancer: The major value of tumor-specific FGS in lung cancer is to facilitate tumor localization and afford margin assessment. Several feasibility studies (35–38) using OTL38 in lung cancer have demonstrated accurate identification of known lesions as determined by standard-of-care methods and importantly, enabled detection of otherwise undetectable synchronous subcentimeter processes. Using multivariate analysis, Predina et al. (39) investigated the variables impacting *in situ* tumor fluorescence and found that only nodule depth, but not nodule size, dose administered, imaging time, nor standardized uptake value by positron emission tomography (PET) with fluorodeoxyglucose (^{18}F-FDG), predicted *in situ* fluorescence. In another study, Predina and colleagues (40) demonstrated how FGS can synergize with preoperative imaging to translate diagnostic findings into the operating room. Patients who had undergone PET with ^{18}F-FDG were eligible for FGS with OTL38. Results showed that 56 of 59 nodules (94.9%) identified preoperatively were targeted by OTL38; remarkably, OTL38 detected 9 additional unknown lesions, which resulted in upstaging and improved management in 12% and 30% of patients, respectively. The authors concluded that the combination of PET (73% sensitivity, 89.3% PPV) with FGS (95.6% sensitivity, 94.2% PPV; **Table 2**) provided superior oncologic outcomes.

Renal cancer: Maximal tumor resection without excessive removal of normal parenchyma is the primary role of surgery in renal cancer and FGS could improve outcomes. Folate receptors are highly abundant in normal kidneys, but physiological expression is downregulated upon malignant transformation. Shum et al. (41) and Bahler et al. (42) exploited this phenomenon by applying "reverse-FGS" using OTL38 during surgical resection of kidney tumors. The investigators hypothesized that the lack of FR-mediated fluorescence demarcates renal tumors. Preliminary results in 3 patients supported the hypothesis: "dark" tumors were surrounded by fluorescent parenchyma prior to resection and a uniformly fluorescent parenchyma post-resection indicated intact margins. These observations were confirmed by immunohistochemistry (IHC) analysis.

Gastric adenocarcinomas, endometrial carcinoma, osteosarcomas, pituitary adenomas: The clinical evaluation of OTL38 has been expanded to other cancers and yielded favorable results. Accurate staging of gastric adenocarcinomas is challenging and existing techniques are limited. In a pilot clinical trial, Newton et al. (43) demonstrated the ability of OTL38 to color code tumors with a high TBR (4.1 ± 2.9) in 3/5 patients and concluded that the approach is feasible. In 4 high-risk endometrial cancer patients, Boogerd and

TABLE 2 | Diagnostic accuracy of LMW contrast agents in clinical studies.

Agent	Cancer type	Test description	Sensitivity (95% CI)	Specificity (95% CI)	PPV (95% CI)	NPV (95% CI)	Reference
OTL38	Ovarian	Any lesion (FRα + or -)	83.9%-96.8% *	-	85.3%-92.6% *	-	(34)
		FRα + only	85.9%-97.9% *	-	88.1%-94.9% *	-	
	Lung	>1 cm nodules	95.6% (87.6%–99.1%)	42.9% (9.9%–81.6%)	94.2% (85.8%–98.4%)	50% (11.8%–88.2%)	(40)
		<1 cm nodules	100% (78.2%–100%)	50.0% (1.2%–98.7%)	93.8% (69.8%–99.8%)	100% (2.5%–100%)	
	Pituitary adenoma	Nonfunctioning adenoma	75% (51–90%)	100% (60–100%)	100% (75–100%)	62% (43–77%)	(47)
		FRα-overexpressing adenoma	100% (75–100%)	100% (31–100%)	100% (75–100%)	100% (31–100%)	
		Margin detection with high FRα-expression	100%	100%	100%	100%	(46)
		Margin samples	100% (54–100%)	100% (63–100%)	100% (54–100%)	100% (63–100%)	(55)
BBN-IRdye800CW	Glioblastoma	From 42 foci of fluorescent-guided sampling	93.9% (79.8%–99.3%)	100% (66.4%–100%)	100% (88.8%–100%)	81.8% (48.2%–97.7%)	(52)
		From 89 harvested samples	94.4% (85.6%–98.2%)	88.2% (62.2%–97.9%)	–	–	(53)
cRGD-ZW800-1	Colorectal carcinoma; *ex vivo* lymph node detection	0.005 mg/kg, 2-4 h	74%	79%	71%	82%	(54)
		0.015 mg/kg, 2-4 h	100%	69%	6%	100%	
		0.05 mg/kg, 2-4 h	100%	73%	70%	100%	
		0.05 mg/kg, 18 h	100%	87%	33%	100%	

*All rows except white are color coded to indicate diagnostic accuracy within the same reference but as classified by the test description column. *Range with or without patient as random effect. PPV, positive predictive value. NPV, negative predictive value. CI, confidence interval.*

colleagues (44) showed the utility of OTL38 to paint tumors *in situ* (3/4 patients) and lymph node metastases (n = 16), including one otherwise undetectable malignant deposit. The authors also noted 17 false-positives in 50 non-metastatic lymph nodes, which was caused by targeting of the FR variant, FRβ, expressed in tumor-associated macrophages. Further utility of OTL38 was described for improving pulmonary metastasectomy in osteosarcoma, which could possibly extend survival or provide cure. During minimally invasive pulmonary resection, Predina et al. (45) reported the first successful use of molecular imaging for osteosarcomas in a patient, which was deemed safe, feasible and useful. Resection of pituitary adenomas is an essential treatment, but 20% of patients relapse. In one study, Lee et al. (46) reported that OTL38 afforded tumor visualization in 15/15 patients with an average TBR of 1.9 ± 0.70 (high FRα, 3.0 ± 0.29; low FRα, 1.6 ± 0.43) and 100% sensitivity/specificity (**Table 2**). In another study, Cho et al. (47) evaluated the benefits of non-specific (ICG) *vs.* tumor-specific (OTL38) FGS compared to standard-of-care in pituitary adenomas. Results showed that standard-of-care MIS of pituitary adenomas had 88% sensitivity and 90% specificity; ICG increased sensitivity to 100%, but had a specificity of 29% for both functioning and non-functioning adenomas. By contrast, tumor-specific FGS was 75% sensitive and 100% specific, but when the analysis was limited to FRα+ adenomas, sensitivity and specificity were both 100% (**Table 2**).

BLZ-100 (TOZULERISTIDE, TUMOR PAINT™; PEPTIDE)

BLZ-100 (MW = 5,124 g/mol; **Figure 2**) is the first receptor-selective NIRF agent for fluorescence-guided neurosurgery that advanced to clinical studies. It is composed of a chlorotoxin (CTX) peptide coupled *via* standard NHS chemistry to the NIRF dye, Cy5.5 (Ex/Em = 675/700-750 nm; ICG derivative). The CTX targeting motif, a 36 amino acid peptide with four disulfide bridges derived from scorpion venom, has been postulated to bind to a number of targets overexpressed in tumors including matrix metalloproteinases, Annexin A2, chloride ion channels, and others (56). The rationale for selecting CTX for FGS drug development came from several studies showing selective targeting of glioma cells compared with non-neoplastic cells or normal brain (57). Furthermore, a radiopharmaceutical analog of CTX, ^{131}I-TM-601, demonstrated negligible toxicity in phase I/II clinical trials for human brain cancer therapy (58). In addition to characterization in mouse xenograft models using commercial instrumentation, BLZ-100 has been investigated in combination with a customized device in a drug-device development fashion. Butte and colleagues (59) rationalized their approach on the fact that many commercially available imaging systems are not designed for detection of low ICG concentrations, emphasizing that non-optimal excitation, acquisition and sensitivity settings for imaging a tumor-selective agent may lead to underperformance. From this study, the authors demonstrated an approach to reduce the size and cost of the imaging system, while optimizing sensitivity with low noise. To facilitate clinical translation, the utility of BLZ-100 was evaluated in canine patients using a dose-escalation strategy in combination with commercial and custom imaging devices (60). Additionally, the toxicology and PK profile of BLZ-100 was evaluated in mice, rats, canines, and nonhuman primates, with results supporting first-in-human clinical trials. To date, at least 5 clinical trials have begun (Phase I-III) using BLZ-100 (**Table 1**) and initial results are encouraging:

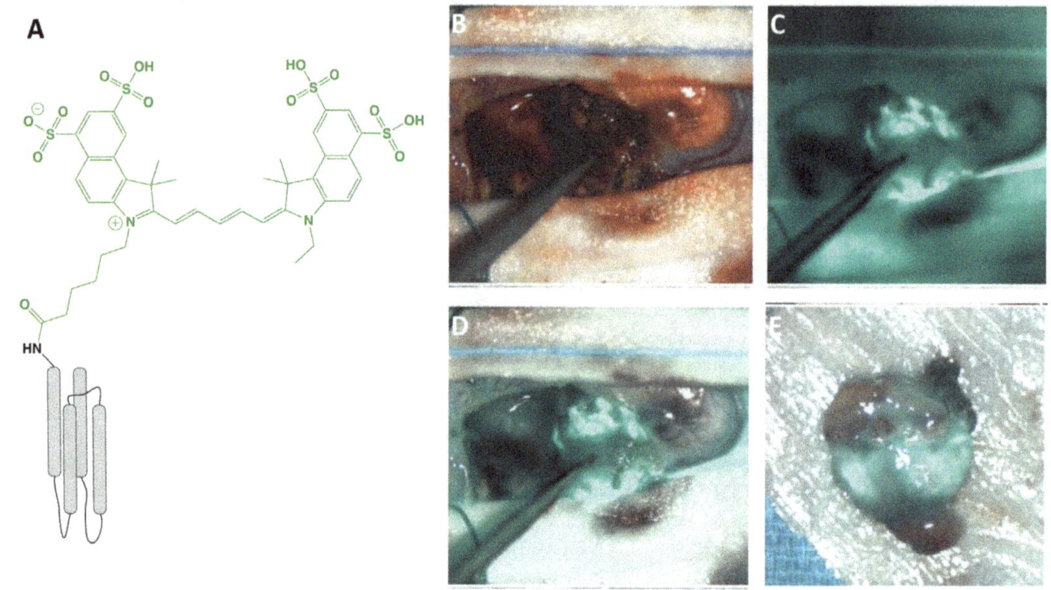

FIGURE 2 | BLZ-100 (Tozuleristide, Tumor Paint™). Schematic* of the peptide CTX (targeting motif; gray) labeled with Cy5.5 (dye; green) **(A)**. Intraoperative glioblastoma imaging with 18 mg total BLZ-100 administered 4 h prior to surgery: white-light only **(B)**, NIRF only **(C)** and white-light with NIRF overlay **(D)**. *Ex vivo* imaging, white-light with NIRF overlay **(E)**. Panels **(B–E)** are adapted from (48) with permission. *Not to scale.

Adult and pediatric gliomas: Patil et al. (48) performed a phase I clinical trial to characterize the safety and utility of BLZ-100 in 17 adults with glioma undergoing surgery. The primary objective was to establish the maximum tolerated dose by conducting a nonrandomized, single-dose, open label, 3 + 3 dose-escalation study (3-30 mg administered 3-29 h before surgery). Secondary objectives included evaluation of PK and fluorescence quantitation of *ex vivo* specimens, whereas exploratory objectives related to the assessment of fluorescence *in situ*. Study design provided standard-of-care to patients, and additionally allowed the surgeon to image the surgical cavity at any point and biopsy fluorescent regions at their discretion. No dose-limiting toxicity was observed and adverse events were not associated with agent administration. Although fluorescence was observed in both low- and high-grade gliomas, signal intensity was dose-dependent and time-independent only for high-grade gliomas. Image analysis was performed by independent reviewers who scored the observed fluorescence as negative, weak (contrast apparent but not well-defined) or strong (well-defined contrast). *Ex vivo* scores yielded 5 negative, 7 weak and 5 strong specimens; *in situ* scores yielded 11 negatives, 4 weak and 2 strong specimens. The investigators attributed the low fluorescence to the unoptimized commercial devices used in the study and intend to couple BLZ-100 with an adequately sensitive imager in the future. The authors concluded that further clinical trials are justified. Lee and colleagues (49) are investigating the safety and utility of BLZ-100 in a phase I study in pediatric brain tumor patients; preliminary results have shown the agent to be safe and yielded fluorescence in 13/15 tumors, including 5/7 low-grade gliomas.

Breast carcinoma: BLZ-100 has also been evaluated in breast cancer for fluorescence-guided pathology (50). The objective of this study was to investigate the feasibility of using BLZ-100 to (i) target breast carcinoma and (ii) enable demarcation of surgical margins. 23 patients undergoing surgery received either 6 or 12 mg of agent at least 1 h before the procedure. Resected specimens were imaged using an investigational device and fluorescent patterns were correlated with corresponding hematoxylin & eosin (H&E) stained sections. Furthermore, fluorescent intensity was correlated to clinical pathology, namely grade, histotype, prognostic biomarkers and margin measurements. Results showed that BLZ-100 afforded demarcation of pathologically-confirmed breast carcinoma (low- and high-grade) from normal tissue, independent of molecular marker/hormone receptor status.

ABY-029 (AFFIBODY)

The affibody conjugate ABY-029 (MW = 7,915 g/mol; **Figure 3**) has emerged as an innovative agent to expand the surgical armamentarium targeting EGFR. It is composed of the 58-amino acid synthetic peptide, Z03115-Cys, labeled with IRDye 800CW maleimide (Ex/Em = 774/789 nm). Rigorous evaluation of *in vitro* and *in vivo* performance showed excellent PK, specificity and utility for imaging (28, 61–63). Furthermore, toxicological characterization in Sprague Dawley rats found no pathological evidence of toxicity (64). Elliott et al. (65) demonstrated that ABY-029 is a promising candidate for image guidance of brain tumors, which overexpress EGFR in 50-70% of cases. In orthotopic mouse models of glioma, Elliott and colleagues investigated and

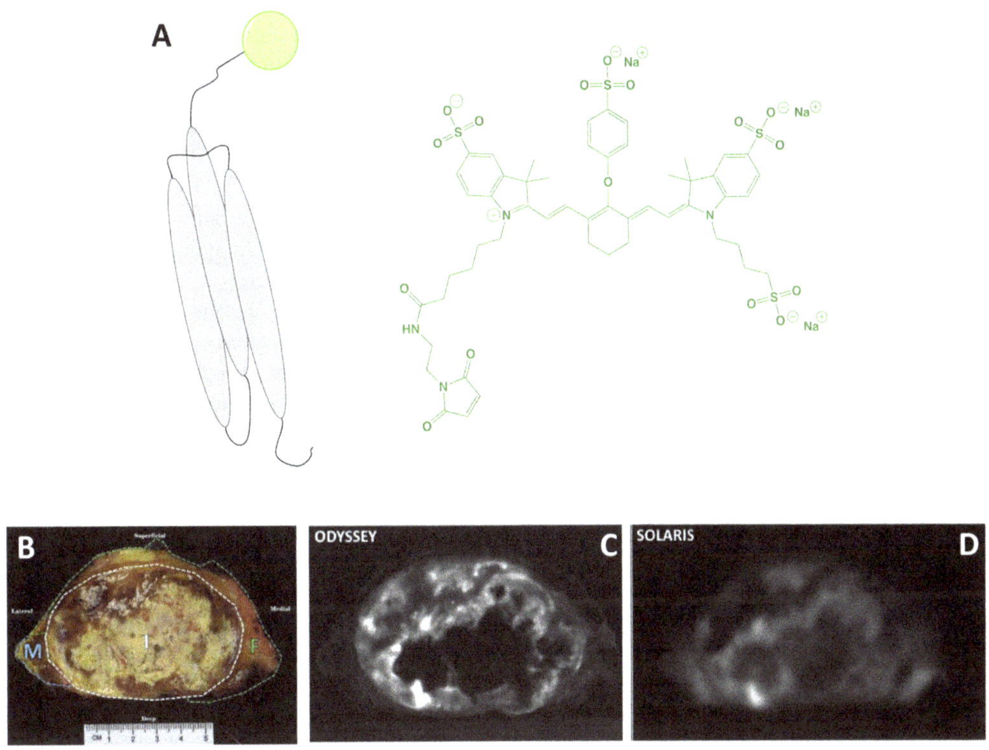

FIGURE 3 | ABY-029. Schematic* of the affibody Z03115-Cys (targeting motif; gray) labeled with IRDye800 (dye, represented as a green circle). The chemical structure of IRDye800 maleimide is also shown **(A)**. *Ex vivo* sarcoma imaging with 237 μg (30 nanomoles) ABY-029 administered 1-3 h prior to surgery: white-light of resected primary (breadloaf) **(B)**, NIRF using a flatbed, closed-box device **(C)** and NIRF using a wide-field device **(D)**. Panels **(B–D)** are adapted from (51) with permission. *Not to scale.

compared the image contrast provided by (i) receptor targeting (ABY-029), (ii) metabolic targeting (5-aminolevulinic acid [5-ALA]-induced Protoporphyrin IX [PpIX]; emerging clinical standard for FGS in glioma) and (iii) a permeability tracer (IRDye 680RD). Results showed that receptor targeting outperformed metabolic targeting by increasing TBRs at tumor margins and core by 50% and 60%, respectively. Given that commercial devices may be too insensitive, Elliott et al. (66) investigated the detection limits and *in vivo* efficacy of ABY-029 microdoses in combination with a custom-built imaging module, which enabled superior image contrast at all doses compared to a commercial counterpart. ABY-029 could also provide benefits during resection of soft tissue sarcomas, which overexpress EGFR in 43-78% of cases. To simulate the spectral properties of tissue surrounding sarcoma during wide local excision, Samkoe et al. (67) developed a phantom model to investigate how observed fluorescence signals change in relation to tumor size, tumor depth, bulk tissue type, and imaging system. Results validated the use of subsurface fluorescence to direct the resection of a tumor-mimicking inclusion to a desired margin thickness. ABY-029 has also been investigated for paired-agent imaging. This approach uses a tumor-specific agent in combination with a non-targeted or perfusion agent to subtract nonspecific signals, thereby improving contrast and/or measuring extracellular EGFR regions. Using ABY-029 along with IRDye 680RD conjugated to an affibody control or IRDye 700DX carboxylate, Samkoe et al. (68) and Sardar et al. (69) have demonstrated the feasibility of the approach in preclinical models of soft tissue sarcoma and head and neck cancer.

Notably, the clinical introduction of ABY-029 has followed a Phase 0 approach through submission of an exploratory investigational new drug (IND) to the FDA (70). This trial modality uses the concept of microdosing, namely sub-pharmacologic exposure, which is defined by the FDA as administration of ≤30 nmol of a protein product. It permits analytical toxicology in a single mammalian species and intends to expedite the estimation of key PK parameters of new drugs in a more economically viable pipeline (71). In practice, it is possible to request a modified Phase 0 study to the FDA with doses slightly above a microdose as long as the dose is 100x lower than the no observed adverse effect level in preclinical toxicity studies (72). Understanding that the clinical study of FGS drugs must be designed to maximize tumor contrast, Ribeiro de Souza et al. identified the optimal dose for imaging within a microdose framework in an orthotopic tumor model in rats (72). Results showed that increasing the microdose dose 5-fold, increased signal by 10-fold, which provided a rationale for performing a modified Phase 0 trial. Interestingly, the authors also found that whereas unlabeled cetuximab (anti-EGFR mAb) inhibited ABY-029 binding *in vitro*, it had no effect on *in vivo* tumor contrast when injected 1 or 24 h before ABY-029. To date, at least 3 clinical trials have begun (Phase 0-I) using ABY-029 and preliminary results are encouraging (**Table 1**):

Soft tissue sarcoma: Surgery can be curative if complete sarcoma resection is achieved, but positive margin rates of 22-34% have been reported and associated with recurrence. In a proof-of-concept study, Samkoe et al. (51) evaluated the ability of ABY-029 to selectively target EGFR and by extension, provide tumor-specific contrast. A resected specimen from a patient who had been administered a microdose (30 nmol, 237 μg) ~4 h prior to wide local excision was imaged *ex vivo* using flatbed, closed-box and open air, wide-field devices to investigate the observed fluorescence and contrast. Qualitative assessment showed clear fluorescence regardless of device and image analysis indicated comparable signal intensity in the tumor region. Interestingly, the closed-box system had increased image noise, which translated to a reduced contrast-to-noise ratio (CNR), despite having a higher TBR. Analysis of tumor samples for correlation of fluorescence with EGFR IHC was found to be moderately associated (r = 0.48), but could be improved by weighting the intensities by the area fraction of EGFR expression. Overall, the authors concluded that these results demonstrate the utility of ABY-029 for selective *ex vivo* imaging of sarcoma.

BBN-IRDYE800CW (PEPTIDE)

BBN-IRdye800CW (MW = 2,450 g/mol; Ex/Em = 778/795 nm; **Figure 4**) is the first LMW agent derived from a PET radiotracer to advance to clinical studies. It is composed of a gastrin-releasing peptide receptor (GRPR) targeting moiety, BBN(7-14) (amino acid sequence: Gln-Trp-Ala-Val-Gly-His-Leu-Met-NH_2), linked to the radiometal chelator, NOTA, and NIRF dye, IRdye 800CW NHS ester. The rationale for selecting a clinical radiotracer for FGS drug development is significant since the approach expands the imaging utility of a clinically-validated tumor-selective agent, thereby reducing concerns associated with toxicity and diagnostic efficacy (73). The safety and biodistribution of the parent compound, ^{68}Ga-NOTA-Aca-BBN(7–14), was shown to be well tolerated and have favorable PK (74). Preclinical *in vivo* evaluation was performed in an orthotopic model of glioblastoma in mice with a customized imaging device for real time visualization (52). To date, at least 2 clinical trials have begun (Phase I) using BBN-IRdye800CW and initial results are encouraging (**Table 1**):

Glioblastoma: Maximum safe resection during glioblastoma surgery remains a challenge despite FGS with non-targeted dyes (e.g., fluorescein sodium) and metabolic markers (e.g., 5-ALA). As an alternative, Li et al. (52) evaluated the utility of ^{68}Ga-BBN-IRdye800CW to provide receptor-mediated glioblastoma contrast for increased resection and margin assessment in 14 patients. The aim of the trial was to establish the safety and feasibility of PET and NIRF imaging with the same targeting vector (i.e., theranostics). To investigate the potential to translate pre-operative findings into the operating room, the authors performed PET scans in all patients with the parent radiotracer (n = 7), dual labeled counterpart (n = 4) or both (n = 3). Results showed similar tumor uptake and no significant biodistribution differences between radiotracers. For intraoperative imaging, 1 mg of unlabeled BBN-IRdye800CW was injected to patients 2 h before surgery. The fluorescent signal was well-visualized and provided superior ability to differentiate residual tumor from normal brain when compared to intraoperative white-light microscope imaging. Of note, the authors reported that the approach was not optimal for deep-seated tumors as signal-to-background ratios were not adequate during surgery in some instances. In another study, He et al. (53) investigated the extent of resection and survivability using BBN-IRdye800CW in 29 patients. To avoid confounding variability due to inter-surgeon differences, all procedures were performed by the same surgeon. Results showed that complete resection was achieved in ~83% of cases as determined by post-operative magnetic resonance imaging (MRI) scans. Median overall survival (OS) and progression-free survival (PFS) were 23.1 and 14.1 months, respectively, which is higher than values reported with standard-of-care techniques. Diagnostic accuracy for both studies is shown in **Table 2**.

cRGD-ZW800-1 (SMALL MOLECULE)

Zwitterionic (i.e., net-neutral) NIRF dyes have demonstrated reduced off-target interactions compared to commonly used NIRF dyes and position as valuable options to increase tumor contrast (75, 76). cRGD-ZW800-1 (MW = 1,729 g/mol; **Figure 5**) is the first tumor-selective agent to incorporate the zwitterionic-dye strategy to advance to clinical studies. It is composed of a cyclic Arg-Gly-Asp peptide, cRGDyK, conjugated to ZW800-1 NHS ester (Ex/Em = 772/788 nm). The cRGD motif targets integrins, which are transmembrane proteins that include $\alpha_5\beta_1$, $\alpha_8\beta_1$, $\alpha_v\beta_1$, $\alpha_v\beta_3$, $\alpha_v\beta_5$, $\alpha_v\beta_6$, $\alpha_v\beta_8$ and $\alpha_{II}\beta_3$. These cell-surface biomarkers have been associated with tumor angiogenesis and migration in a wide range of cancers, making them attractive candidates for tumor-selective FGS drug development. *In vivo* preclinical characterization using a clinical imager showed imaging utility in liver, lung, colorectal, breast, pancreatic and oral orthotopic mouse models, even at microdoses (77–79). In head-to-head comparison with IRDye 800CW and Cy5.5 analogs, cRGD-ZW800-1 demonstrated similar tumor uptake, but superior tumor contrast due to reduced background signal (TBR of 17.2 *vs.* 2.7-5.1) (77). The authors also found that the best scaling factor to extrapolate the dose of a targeted FGS drug from animal models to humans was to adjust by body surface area. Interestingly, a cRGD-ZW800-1 derivative has also been investigated in a dual labeled format, namely cRGD-ZW800-1-Forte-[^{89}Zr]Zr-DFO, to potentially develop a companion diagnostic for improved patient selection and surgical planning (80). Nonclinical toxicity studies of cRGD-ZW800-1 in rats were conducted according to ICH M3 (R2), FDA, EMEA, and GLP regulations, and showed no significant clinical signs or pathological changes. To date, at least 2 clinical trials have begun (Phase I-II) using cRGD-ZW800-1 and initial results are promising (**Table 1**):

Colon carcinoma: Partial or excessive resection in colon cancer is associated with increased morbidity and mortality. The establishment of neoadjuvant chemoradiotherapy as the standard for locally advanced rectal cancer further complicates

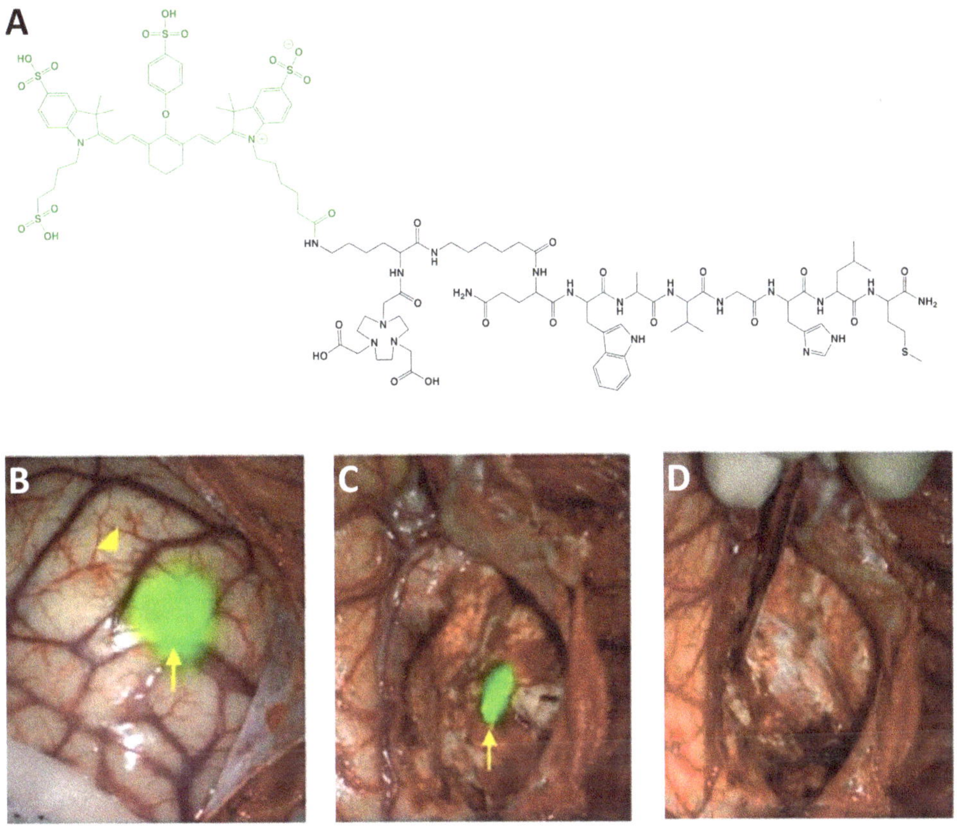

FIGURE 4 | BBN-IRdye800CW. Chemical structure; BBN(7-14) (ligand) and NOTA (Chelator) in black, IRdye800CW (dye) in green **(A)**. Intraoperative glioblastoma multiforme imaging with 1 mg total BBN-IRdye800CW administered 16 h prior to surgery: NIRF prior to resection **(B)**, residual fluorescence after initial tumor removal **(C)** and tumor-cavity after complete resection **(D)**. Panels **(B–D)** are adapted from (53) with permission.

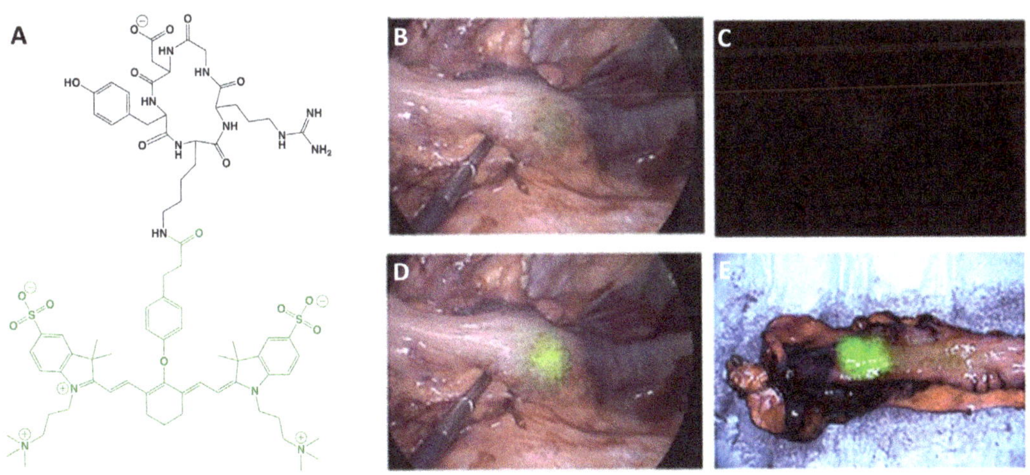

FIGURE 5 | cRGD-ZW800-1. Chemical structure; cRGDyK (ligand) in black, ZW800-1 (dye) in green **(A)**. Intraoperative colon cancer imaging with 0.05 mg/kg cRGD-ZW800-1 administered 18 h prior to surgery: white-light only **(B)**, NIRF only **(C)** and white-light with NIRF overlay **(D)**. *Ex vivo* imaging, white-light with NIRF overlay **(E)**. Panels **(B–E)** are adapted from (54) with permission.

eventual surgical resection with MIS due to obscuring of critical visual information. To overcome these challenges, de Valk et al. (54) evaluated the utility of cRGD-ZW800-1 to provide real time discrimination between tumor and normal tissues. The Phase I trial was a randomized, placebo-controlled, double-blinded, microdosing study to evaluate safety, tolerability and PK. Results showed no acute or toxic effects at all doses and measurable blood concentrations of drug up to 8 h after injection. The objective of the Phase II study was to demonstrate the feasibility of the approach and to determine optimal dose and imaging time point. Study design was an open-label ascending dose study in 12 patients and allowed MIS (n = 11) or open surgery (n = 1) 2-18 h after agent administration. Although $\alpha_v\beta_6$ was selected as the biomarker for IHC staining, selective targeting was solely based by correlating fluorescence and H&E. de Valk and colleagues measured intraoperative TBRs of 1.1-1.6 with fluorescence visualization through the bowel wall being only possible with the highest dose. *Ex vivo* fluorescence intensity in tumor and normal tissues increased in a dose-dependent manner in the 2-4 h post-injection cohort, with comparable TBRs for the median (4.0) and highest (4.1) doses. 18 h post-injection fluorescence intensity at the highest dose decreased in tumor and normal tissue but the TBR (6.2) did not change significantly. Negative predictive value (NPV) and PPV ranges for lymph node detection were 82-100% and 6-71%, respectively, depending on dose and time (**Table 2**). The authors concluded that (i) the approach is feasible but requires further dose and time optimization and (ii) widespread investigation of cRGD-ZW800-1 in cancer surgery is warranted.

LS301 (PEPTIDE)

Iterative pharmacophore optimization for improved performance is a hallmark facilitated by LMW agents. Such strategy was applied during the development of LS301 (MW = 1,469 g/mol; **Figure 6**) — a tumor-selective FGS agent consisting of the cyclic octapeptide, cyclic (d-Cys-Gly-Arg-Asp-Ser-Pro-Cys)-Lys-OH [c(CGRDSPC) K-OH], conjugated *via* standard methods to the ICG derivative, cypate (Ex/Em = 780/830 nm) (81). The pharmacophore c (CGRDSPC)K-OH was derived from the linear hexapeptide, Gly-Arg-Asp-Ser-Pro-Lys (GRDSPK), to enhance the stability of the first-generation agent, cypate-GRDSPK, *via* intramolecular disulfide cyclization (82). Recently, LS301 has been shown to target the phosphorylated phospholipid-binding protein Annexin A2, which is an abundant post-translational modification of the Annexin A2 preferentially found in tumor microenvironments (82). LS301 is also thought to bind to integrins (e.g., β_3), but their identities remain unknown (83). Overall, LS301 could be a versatile approach for targeting a wide range of solid tumors. In preclinical *in vivo* studies, LS301 has been shown to selectively accumulate in tumors and metastases of the breast, fibrosarcoma, pancreas and glioblastoma (82). Interestingly, the utility of LS301 for real-time intraoperative imaging has been investigated in combination with "cancer vision goggles" (84), an emerging interface for fluorescence visualization. To date, at least 2 clinical trials have been registered (Phase I-II) using LS301 (**Table 1**).

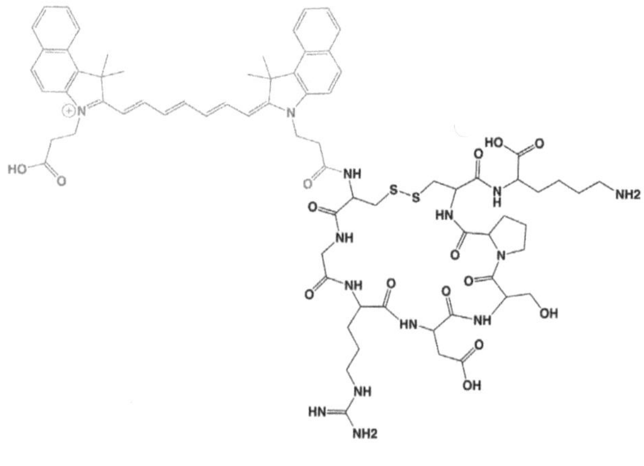

FIGURE 6 | LS301. Chemical structure; c(CGRDSPC)K-OH (ligand) in black, cypate (dye) in green.

PERSPECTIVE ON EMERGING TUMOR-SELECTIVE FGS TECHNOLOGIES

Significance and Application

FGS holds the promise of color-labeling the surgical field and enhancing surgical outcomes in several ways. Tumor-specific probes that delineate the location and extent of malignant tissues can improve staging accuracy and margin-negative resection; furthermore, they can potentially shorten operative time and avoid excessive removal of normal tissues. Indeed, the anatomy of normal tissues can be distorted by malignant processes, and safeguarding key structures during oncologic surgery can be as important a goal as complete resection of cancer (85). This point is especially important in neurosurgery, where destruction of non-cancerous brain tissue can lead to functional impairments. For gynecologic malignancies, fluorescence is used to evaluate and address disease burden during cytoreductive surgery. Conversely, improved detection of peritoneal dissemination in gastrointestinal cancers, such as cholangiocarcinomas, gastric and pancreatic cancers is critical as accurate tumor detection may spare patients a morbid and futile radical operation. The rapid evolution of MIS, particularly with robotic surgery platforms, has resulted in its widespread application for various cancer types (86–88). FGS technologies can also supplement these emerging surgical techniques with built-in fluorescent imaging systems to overcome the lack of tactile guidance. Maximal benefit, however, can only be realized if the fluorescent signal can accurately define tumor extent.

Development, Constraints and Outlook

FGS shares many similarities with nuclear medicine (e.g., PET) as a functional imaging modality; however, constraints in the translation of drugs for FGS are unique. For instance, nuclear medicine is inherently quantitative, with well-established methods for determining *in vivo* drug distribution and concentration based on collected images or signals (89). By contrast, the underlying physics of fluorescence imaging in bulk tissue (90), compounded with the myriad of FGS devices (91), leads to uncertainty in the quantitative evaluation of drug performance (92). Particularly, tumor-specific FGS relies on fluorescent drugs that accumulate preferentially in tumors and a device to detect their distribution and concentration to reveal measurable outputs such as tumor contrast (93, 94). For FGS imaging devices, confounding imaging factors include differences in spectral sensitivity, excitation and emission regimes, operating distance, ambient illumination, and efficiency of collection optics (25). Whereas many of these factors could be modeled and accounted for to directly compare commercial devices, this is unlikely to be achieved due to competitive concerns in sharing detailed specifications and optical schematics. Currently, most commercial FGS devices are designed to image ICG, matching its spectral and sensitivity requirements, which may differ from cancer-targeted probes. This is significant because non-optimal excitation and emission collection could lead to underperformance. Imaging efficiency may also be compromised by the tumoral concentration of a targeted dye, as was reported for the BLZ-100 clinical trials. Indeed, the concentration of a targeted dye is expected to be in the nanomolar range, as opposed to the micromolar levels of ICG, and may be a limiting factor (95). Regardless, as seen in **Table 1**, several commercial and experimental NIRF devices are compatible with LMW agents and demonstrate the feasibility of the approach. Optimal image quality [e.g., high signal-to-noise ratio (93)], however, will require instrumentation designed for imaging non-ICG NIRF dyes (e.g., with differing spectra) and with superior sensitivity (e.g., robust low nanomolar detection with low noise); such imaging devices are currently commercially limited or in experimental phases. In response to the growing need for second-generation imagers, specifications of ICG imagers and required capabilities to build upon them were outlined in the seminal work by DSouza et al. (91).

Tumor contrast also depends largely on the differential drug uptake between tumor and normal tissue. This suggests that superior contrast may be achieved by (i) increasing tumor uptake, (ii) decreasing background uptake, or (iii) a combination of (i) and (ii) (92). Points (i-iii) are clinically significant because they could enable contrast detectability with higher certainty, which may directly increase the positive and negative predictive value (96) of tumor-specific FGS for real-time decision making (97). From a chemical structure perspective, a strategy that could advance the specificity of targeted FGS agents involves modulating the physicochemical properties of dyes. Indeed, dye conjugation to tumor-specific vectors can impact the biodistribution of the native ligand, a phenomenon exacerbated for LMW motifs (98). This understanding has, for example, driven the emergence of NIRF dyes with a net-neutral charge (i.e., zwitterionic) that possess reduced nonspecific interactions and faster elimination from normal tissues (75, 76). In combination with high affinity targeting motifs, these attributes could enhance tumor selectivity along contrast in the operating room. Encouragingly, the first clinical application of this technology was with the LMW agent, cRGD-ZW800-1, as previously detailed.

This review focuses on six clinical-stage receptor-targeting LMW FGS agents to not only illustrate the safety and efficacy of the approach, but to also serve as roadmaps. In this sense, knowledge gained from these clinical-stage agents could be applied toward the development of FGS agents that are based on high-value cancer targets across different tumor types (99). For instance, radiolabeled peptides and small molecules have convincingly demonstrated the ability to target the somatostatin receptor subtype-2 (SSTR2) (100) and prostate-specific membrane antigen (PSMA) (101), which are hallmarks of neuroendocrine tumors and prostate cancer, respectively. Surgery is an essential treatment for both diseases and clinical data suggests that incomplete tumor resection can predict recurrence (102, 103). Thus, LMW fluorescent analogs that target SSTR2 (89) and PSMA (104–106) are promising candidates for translation.

Several factors ultimately define the translational route of a FGS agent and include mechanism of targeting, and importantly, whether the dye or ligand has been previously shown to be safe in humans (107). Generally, traditional or exploratory IND enabling studies are conducted first. The drug then undergoes Phase I, II, and III clinical trials to demonstrate safety and efficacy (108), likely resulting in FDA approval of the drug to be device agnostic. There is also the possibility for drug-device combination products to receive FDA approval following a pivotal Phase II clinical trial, which streamlines the regulatory process but requires the drug to be used with the device with which it was paired. Key organizational barriers that may affect the adoption of FGS agents in clinical practice [e.g., evidence-based care, clinical trial design (109)] must also be considered, and could be mitigated through consistent reporting methods and regulatory approaches that allow objective evaluation of these promising technologies [discussed in (94, 107, 108, 110)]. Regardless, the rapid growth of FGS in terms of new drugs, devices, and clinical applications is a testament to the multidisciplinary aspects of the field and its distinct stakeholders.

CONCLUSION

Several drug design approaches for tumor-selective FGS have been translated into the clinic with the overarching goal of improving diagnostic accuracy. The physicochemical properties of these drugs play an important role in their *in vivo* performance and can define clinical parameters such as dose and imaging time. FGS mediated by low molecular weight drugs is a safe and potentially efficacious approach to advance the precision of surgical oncology.

AUTHOR CONTRIBUTIONS

Conception and design: SHV, CL, AA. Development of methodology: SHV, CL. Acquisition of data: SHV. Analysis and interpretation of data: SHV, CL, HTC, NI, SA, SG, AU, AA. Writing, review, and/or revision of the manuscript: SHV, CL, HTC, NI, SA, SG, AU, AA. Administrative, technical, or material support (i.e., reporting or organizing data, constructing databases): SHV. Study supervision: SHV, CL, AA. All authors contributed to the article and approved the submitted version.

ACKNOWLEDGMENTS

This work was supported by the Cancer Prevention and Research Institute of Texas (RP180812), John S. Dunn Research Scholar Fund, Welch Foundation Endowment, and National Cancer Institute of the National Institutes of Health (R44CA206754, OnLume Inc.). The authors thank Lea Stitzlein for assistance with figure preparation.

REFERENCES

1. Moore GE, Peyton WT. The Clinical Use of Fluorescein in Neurosurgery; the Localization of Brain Tumors. *J Neurosurg* (1948) 5(4):392–8. doi: 10.3171/jns.1948.5.4.0392
2. Stummer W, Pichlmeier U, Meinel T, Wiestler OD, Zanella F, Reulen HJ, et al. Fluorescence-Guided Surgery With 5-Aminolevulinic Acid for Resection of Malignant Glioma: A Randomised Controlled Multicentre Phase III Trial. *Lancet Oncol* (2006) 7(5):392–401. doi: 10.1016/S1470-2045(06)70665-9
3. van der Vorst JR, Schaafsma BE, Hutteman M, Verbeek FP, Liefers GJ, Hartgrink HH, et al. Near-Infrared Fluorescence-Guided Resection of Colorectal Liver Metastases. *Cancer* (2013) 119(18):3411–8. doi: 10.1002/cncr.28203
4. van der Vorst JR, Schaafsma BE, Verbeek FP, Swijnenburg RJ, Tummers QR, Hutteman M, et al. Intraoperative Near-Infrared Fluorescence Imaging of Parathyroid Adenomas With Use of Low-Dose Methylene Blue. *Head Neck* (2014) 36(6):853–8. doi: 10.1002/hed.23384
5. Nagaya T, Nakamura YA, Choyke PL, Kobayashi H. Fluorescence-Guided Surgery. *Front Oncol* (2017) 7:314. doi: 10.3389/fonc.2017.00314
6. Alander JT, Kaartinen I, Laakso A, Patila T, Spillmann T, Tuchin VV, et al. A Review of Indocyanine Green Fluorescent Imaging in Surgery. *Int J BioMed Imaging* (2012) 2012:940585. doi: 10.1155/2012/940585
7. Daskalaki D, Fernandes E, Wang X, Bianco FM, Elli EF, Ayloo S, et al. Indocyanine Green (ICG) Fluorescent Cholangiography During Robotic Cholecystectomy: Results of 184 Consecutive Cases in a Single Institution. *Surg Innov* (2014) 21(6):615–21. doi: 10.1177/1553350614524839
8. Reinhart MB, Huntington CR, Blair LJ, Heniford BT, Augenstein VA. Indocyanine Green: Historical Context, Current Applications, and Future Considerations. *Surg Innov* (2016) 23(2):166–75. doi: 10.1177/1553350615604053
9. Dip F, Boni L, Bouvet M, Carus T, Diana M, Falco J, et al. Consensus Conference Statement on the General Use of Near-Infrared Fluorescence Imaging and Indocyanine Green Guided Surgery: Results of a Modified Delphi Study. *Ann Surg* (2020). doi: 10.1097/SLA.0000000000004412
10. Scheuer W, van Dam GM, Dobosz M, Schwaiger M, Ntziachristos V. Drug-based Optical Agents: Infiltrating Clinics At Lower Risk. *Sci Transl Med* (2012) 4(134):134ps11. doi: 10.1126/scitranslmed.3003572
11. Koller M, Qiu SQ, Linssen MD, Jansen L, Kelder W, de Vries J, et al. Implementation and Benchmarking of a Novel Analytical Framework to Clinically Evaluate Tumor-Specific Fluorescent Tracers. *Nat Commun* (2018) 9(1):3739. doi: 10.1038/s41467-018-05727-y
12. Rosenthal EL, Warram JM, de Boer E, Chung TK, Korb ML, Brandwein-Gensler M, et al. Safety and Tumor Specificity of Cetuximab-IRDye800 for Surgical Navigation in Head and Neck Cancer. *Clin Cancer Res* (2015) 21 (16):3658–66. doi: 10.1158/1078-0432.CCR-14-3284
13. Gao RW, Teraphongphom NT, van den Berg NS, Martin BA, Oberhelman NJ, Divi V, et al. Determination of Tumor Margins With Surgical Specimen Mapping Using Near-Infrared Fluorescence. *Cancer Res* (2018) 78 (17):5144–54. doi: 10.1158/0008-5472.CAN-18-0878
14. Schmidt MM, Wittrup KD. A Modeling Analysis of the Effects of Molecular Size and Binding Affinity on Tumor Targeting. *Mol Cancer Ther* (2009) 8 (10):2861–71. doi: 10.1158/1535-7163.MCT-09-0195
15. Krasniqi A, D'Huyvetter M, Devoogdt N, Frejd FY, Sorensen J, Orlova A, et al. Same-Day Imaging Using Small Proteins: Clinical Experience and Translational Prospects in Oncology. *J Nucl Med* (2018) 59(6):885–91. doi: 10.2967/jnumed.117.199901
16. Sadeghipour N, Rangnekar A, Folaron M, Strawbridge R, Samkoe K, Davis S, et al. Prediction of Optimal Contrast Times Post-Imaging Agent Administration to Inform Personalized Fluorescence-Guided Surgery. *J BioMed Opt* (2020) 25(11). doi: 10.1117/1.JBO.25.11.116005
17. Srinivasarao M, Galliford CV, Low PS. Principles in the Design of Ligand-Targeted Cancer Therapeutics and Imaging Agents. *Nat Rev Drug Discovery* (2015) 14(3):203–19. doi: 10.1038/nrd4519
18. Moss JA, Vavere AL, Azhdarinia A. Design of Peptide Imaging Agents for Whole-Body and Intraoperative Molecular Imaging. *Curr Med Chem* (2012) 19(20):3255–65. doi: 10.2174/092986712801215856
19. Barth CW, Gibbs SL. Fluorescence Image-Guided Surgery - A Perspective on Contrast Agent Development. *Proc SPIE Int Soc Opt Eng* (2020) 11222. doi: 10.1117/12.2545292
20. Zhang RR, Schroeder AB, Grudzinski JJ, Rosenthal EL, Warram JM, Pinchuk AN, et al. Beyond the Margins: Real-Time Detection of Cancer Using Targeted Fluorophores. *Nat Rev Clin Oncol* (2017) 14(6):347–64. doi: 10.1038/nrclinonc.2016.212
21. Hernot S, van Manen L, Debie P, Mieog JSD, Vahrmeijer AL. Latest Developments in Molecular Tracers for Fluorescence Image-Guided Cancer Surgery. *Lancet Oncol* (2019) 20(7):e354–67. doi: 10.1016/S1470-2045(19)30317-1
22. Lee JYK, Cho SS, Stummer W, Tanyi JL, Vahrmeijer AL, Rosenthal E, et al. Review of Clinical Trials in Intraoperative Molecular Imaging During Cancer Surgery. *J BioMed Opt* (2019) 24(12):1–8. doi: 10.1117/1.JBO.24.12.120901
23. Tipirneni KE, Warram JM, Moore LS, Prince AC, de Boer E, Jani AH, et al. Oncologic Procedures Amenable to Fluorescence-Guided Surgery. *Ann Surg* (2017) 266(1):36–47. doi: 10.1097/SLA.0000000000002127
24. Keereweer S, Van Driel PB, Snoeks TJ, Kerrebijn JD, Baatenburg de Jong RJ, Vahrmeijer AL, et al. Optical Image-Guided Cancer Surgery: Challenges and Limitations. *Clin Cancer Res* (2013) 19(14):3745–54. doi: 10.1158/1078-0432.CCR-12-3598
25. Koch M, Symvoulidis P, Ntziachristos V. Tackling Standardization in Fluorescence Molecular Imaging. *Nat Photonics* (2018) 12(9):505–15. doi: 10.1038/s41566-018-0221-5
26. Tummers WS, Warram JM, van den Berg NS, Miller SE, Swijnenburg RJ, Vahrmeijer AL, et al. Recommendations for Reporting on Emerging Optical Imaging Agents to Promote Clinical Approval. *Theranostics* (2018) 8 (19):5336–47. doi: 10.7150/thno.27384
27. Elliott JT, Dsouza AV, Davis SC, Olson JD, Paulsen KD, Roberts DW, et al. Review of Fluorescence Guided Surgery Visualization and Overlay Techniques. *BioMed Opt Express* (2015) 6(10):3765–82. doi: 10.1364/BOE.6.003765
28. Samkoe KS, Bates BD, Elliott JT, LaRochelle E, Gunn JR, Marra K, et al. Application of Fluorescence-Guided Surgery to Subsurface Cancers Requiring Wide Local Excision: Literature Review and Novel Developments Toward Indirect Visualization. *Cancer Control* (2018) 25 (1):1073274817752332. doi: 10.1177/1073274817752332
29. van Dam GM, Themelis G, Crane LM, Harlaar NJ, Pleijhuis RG, Kelder W, et al. Intraoperative Tumor-Specific Fluorescence Imaging in Ovarian Cancer by Folate Receptor-Alpha Targeting: First In-Human Results. *Nat Med* (2011) 17(10):1315–9. doi: 10.1038/nm.2472
30. Hoogstins CE, Tummers QR, Gaarenstroom KN, de Kroon CD, Trimbos JB, Bosse T, et al. A Novel Tumor-Specific Agent for Intraoperative Near-Infrared Fluorescence Imaging: A Translational Study in Healthy Volunteers and Patients With Ovarian Cancer. *Clin Cancer Res* (2016) 22(12):2929–38. doi: 10.1158/1078-0432.CCR-15-2640
31. Mahalingam SM, Kularatne SA, Myers CH, Gagare P, Norshi M, Liu X, et al. Evaluation of Novel Tumor-Targeted Near-Infrared Probe for Fluorescence-Guided Surgery of Cancer. *J Med Chem* (2018) 61(21):9637–46. doi: 10.1021/acs.jmedchem.8b01115
32. De Jesus E, Keating JJ, Kularatne SA, Jiang J, Judy R, Predina J, et al. Comparison of Folate Receptor Targeted Optical Contrast Agents for Intraoperative Molecular Imaging. *Int J Mol Imaging* (2015) 2015:469047. doi: 10.1155/2015/469047
33. Keating JJ, Runge JJ, Singhal S, Nims S, Venegas O, Durham AC, et al. Intraoperative Near-Infrared Fluorescence Imaging Targeting Folate Receptors Identifies Lung Cancer in A Large-Animal Model. *Cancer* (2017) 123(6):1051–60. doi: 10.1002/cncr.30419
34. Randall LM, Wenham RM, Low PS, Dowdy SC, Tanyi JL. A Phase II, Multicenter, Open-Label Trial of OTL38 Injection for the Intra-Operative Imaging of Folate Receptor-Alpha Positive Ovarian Cancer. *Gynecol Oncol* (2019) 155(1):63–8. doi: 10.1016/j.ygyno.2019.07.010
35. Predina JD, Newton AD, Connolly C, Dunbar A, Baldassari M, Deshpande C, et al. Identification of a Folate Receptor-Targeted Near-Infrared Molecular Contrast Agent to Localize Pulmonary Adenocarcinomas. *Mol Ther* (2018) 26(2):390–403. doi: 10.1016/j.ymthe.2017.10.016
36. Predina JD, Newton A, Connolly C, Singhal S. Folate Receptor-Targeted Molecular Imaging Improves Identification of Malignancy During Pulmonary Resection: A Case Report. *J Cardiothorac Surg* (2017) 12 (1):110. doi: 10.1186/s13019-017-0664-7

37. Predina JD, Newton A, Corbett C, Xia L, Sulyok LF, Shin M, et al. Localization of Pulmonary Ground-Glass Opacities With Folate Receptor-Targeted Intraoperative Molecular Imaging. *J Thorac Oncol* (2018) 13 (7):1028–36. doi: 10.1016/j.jtho.2018.03.023
38. Predina JD, Newton AD, Xia L, Corbett C, Connolly C, Shin M, et al. An Open Label Trial of Folate Receptor-Targeted Intraoperative Molecular Imaging to Localize Pulmonary Squamous Cell Carcinomas. *Oncotarget* (2018) 9(17):13517–29. doi: 10.18632/oncotarget.24399
39. Predina JD, Newton AD, Keating J, Dunbar A, Connolly C, Baldassari M, et al. A Phase I Clinical Trial of Targeted Intraoperative Molecular Imaging for Pulmonary Adenocarcinomas. *Ann Thorac Surg* (2018) 105(3):901–8. doi: 10.1016/j.athoracsur.2017.08.062
40. Predina JD, Newton AD, Keating J, Barbosa EM Jr., Okusanya O, Xia L, et al. Intraoperative Molecular Imaging Combined With Positron Emission Tomography Improves Surgical Management of Peripheral Malignant Pulmonary Nodules. *Ann Surg* (2017) 266(3):479–88. doi: 10.1097/SLA.0000000000002382
41. Shum CF, Bahler CD, Low PS, Ratliff TL, Kheyfets SV, Natarajan JP, et al. Novel Use of Folate-Targeted Intraoperative Fluorescence, OTL38, in Robot-Assisted Laparoscopic Partial Nephrectomy: Report of the First Three Cases. *J Endourol Case Rep* (2016) 2(1):189–97. doi: 10.1089/cren.2016.0104
42. Bahler CD, Maniar V, Marley KN, Kheyfets SV, Shum CF, Sundaram CP. Otl-38-Guided Fluorescent Imaging in Renal Cell Cancer Robotic Partial Nephrectomy. *J Endourol B Videourol* (2017) 31(3). doi: 10.1089/vid.2016.0068
43. Newton AD, Predina JD, Frenzel-Sulyok LG, Low PS, Singhal S, Roses RE. Intraoperative Molecular Imaging Utilizing a Folate Receptor-Targeted Near-Infrared Probe Can Identify Macroscopic Gastric Adenocarcinomas. *Mol Imaging Biol* (2021) 23(1):11–7. doi: 10.1007/s11307-020-01549-x
44. Boogerd LSF, Hoogstins CES, Gaarenstroom KN, de Kroon CD, Beltman JJ, Bosse T, et al. Folate Receptor-Alpha Targeted Near-Infrared Fluorescence Imaging in High-Risk Endometrial Cancer Patients: A Tissue Microarray and Clinical Feasibility Study. *Oncotarget* (2018) 9(1):791–801. doi: 10.18632/oncotarget.23155
45. Predina JD, Newton A, Deshpande C, Low P, Singhal S. Utilization of Targeted Near-Infrared Molecular Imaging to Improve Pulmonary Metastasectomy of Osteosarcomas. *J BioMed Opt* (2018) 23(1):1–4. doi: 10.1117/1.JBO.23.1.016005
46. Lee JYK, Cho SS, Zeh R, Pierce JT, Martinez-Lage M, Adappa ND, et al. Folate Receptor Overexpression Can Be Visualized in Real Time During Pituitary Adenoma Endoscopic Transsphenoidal Surgery With Near-Infrared Imaging. *J Neurosurg* (2018) 129(2):390–403. doi: 10.3171/2017.2.JNS163191
47. Cho SS, Jeon J, Buch L, Nag S, Nasrallah M, Low PS, et al. Intraoperative Near-Infrared Imaging With Receptor-Specific Versus Passive Delivery of Fluorescent Agents in Pituitary Adenomas. *J Neurosurg* (2018) 131(6):1974–84. doi: 10.3171/2018.7.JNS181642
48. Patil CG, Walker DG, Miller DM, Butte P, Morrison B, Kittle DS, et al. Phase 1 Safety, Pharmacokinetics, and Fluorescence Imaging Study of Tozuleristide (Blz-100) in Adults With Newly Diagnosed or Recurrent Gliomas. *Neurosurgery* (2019) 85(4):E641–9. doi: 10.1093/neuros/nyz125
49. Lee A, Cole B, Poliachik S, Ojemann J, Miller D, Novak J, et al. Trth-12. Phase 1 Safety, Pharmacokinetic and Imaging Study of BLZ-100 Tumor Paint in Pediatric Brain Tumor Patients. *Neuro-Oncology* (2017) 19 (suppl_4):iv54–4. doi: 10.1093/neuonc/nox083.224
50. Dintzis SM, Hansen S, Harrington KM, Tan LC, Miller DM, Ishak L, et al. Real-Time Visualization of Breast Carcinoma in Pathology Specimens From Patients Receiving Fluorescent Tumor-Marking Agent Tozuleristide. *Arch Pathol Lab Med* (2019) 143(9):1076–83. doi: 10.5858/arpa.2018-0197-OA
51. Samkoe KS, Sardar HS, Gunn J, Feldwisch J, Linos K, Henderson E, et al. Measuring Microdose ABY-029 Fluorescence Signal in a Primary Human Soft-Tissue Sarcoma Resection. *Proc SPIE Int Soc Opt Eng* (2019) 10862. doi: 10.1117/12.2510935
52. Li D, Zhang J, Chi C, Xiao X, Wang J, Lang L, et al. First-in-Human Study of PET and Optical Dual-Modality Image-Guided Surgery in Glioblastoma Using (68)Ga-Irdye800cw-BBN. *Theranostics* (2018) 8(9):2508–20. doi: 10.7150/thno.25599
53. He K, Chi C, Li D, Zhang J, Niu G, Lv F, et al. Resection and Survival Data From a Clinical Trial of Glioblastoma Multiforme-Specific IRDye800-BBN Fluorescence-Guided Surgery. *Bioeng Transl Med* (2021) 6(1):e10182. doi: 10.1002/btm2.10182
54. de Valk KS, Deken MM, Handgraaf HJM, Bhairosingh SS, Bijlstra OD, van Esdonk MJ, et al. First-In-Human Assessment of cRGD-ZW800-1, A Zwitterionic, Integrin-Targeted, Near-Infrared Fluorescent Peptide in Colon Carcinoma. *Clin Cancer Res* (2020) 26(15):3990–8. doi: 10.1158/1078-0432.CCR-19-4156
55. Cho SS, Zeh R, Pierce JT, Jeon J, Nasrallah M, Adappa ND, et al. Folate Receptor Near-Infrared Optical Imaging Provides Sensitive and Specific Intraoperative Visualization of Nonfunctional Pituitary Adenomas. *Oper Neurosurg (Hagerstown)* (2019) 16(1):59–70. doi: 10.1093/ons/opy034
56. McGonigle S, Majumder U, Kolber-Simonds D, Wu J, Hart A, Noland T, et al. Neuropilin-1 Drives Tumor-Specific Uptake of Chlorotoxin. *Cell Commun Signal* (2019) 17(1):67. doi: 10.1186/s12964-019-0368-9
57. Veiseh M, Gabikian P, Bahrami SB, Veiseh O, Zhang M, Hackman RC, et al. Tumor Paint: A Chlorotoxin:Cy5.5 Bioconjugate for Intraoperative Visualization of Cancer Foci. *Cancer Res* (2007) 67(14):6882–8. doi: 10.1158/0008-5472.CAN-06-3948
58. Hockaday DC, Shen S, Fiveash J, Raubitschek A, Colcher D, Liu A, et al. Imaging Glioma Extent With 131I-TM-601. *J Nucl Med* (2005) 46(4):580–6.
59. Butte PV, Mamelak A, Parrish-Novak J, Drazin D, Shweikeh F, Gangalum PR, et al. Near-Infrared Imaging of Brain Tumors Using the Tumor Paint BLZ-100 to Achieve Near-Complete Resection of Brain Tumors. *Neurosurg Focus* (2014) 36(2):E1. doi: 10.3171/2013.11.FOCUS13497
60. Fidel J, Kennedy KC, Dernell WS, Hansen S, Wiss V, Stroud MR, et al. Preclinical Validation of the Utility of BLZ-100 in Providing Fluorescence Contrast for Imaging Spontaneous Solid Tumors. *Cancer Res* (2015) 75 (20):4283–91. doi: 10.1158/0008-5472.CAN-15-0471
61. de Souza AL, Marra K, Gunn J, Samkoe KS, Hoopes PJ, Feldwisch J, et al. Fluorescent Affibody Molecule Administered *In Vivo* At a Microdose Level Labels EGFR Expressing Glioma Tumor Regions. *Mol Imaging Biol* (2017) 19(1):41–8. doi: 10.1007/s11307-016-0980-7
62. Xu X, Samkoe KS, Henderson ER. Effect of Preoperative Cancer Treatment on Epidermal Growth Factor Receptor (EGFR) Receptor Expression Level in ABY-029 Guided Sarcoma Surgery. *Proc SPIE Int Soc Opt Eng* (2020) 11222. doi: 10.1117/12.2546963
63. Samkoe KS, Schultz E, Solanki A, Wang L, Korber J, Tichauer KM, et al. Simultaneous Extracellular and Intracellular Quantification of EGFR Using Paired-Agent Imaging in an in Ovo Tumor Model. *Proc SPIE Int Soc Opt Eng* (2019) 10859. doi: 10.1117/12.2510778
64. Samkoe KS, Gunn JR, Marra K, Hull SM, Moodie KL, Feldwisch J, et al. Toxicity and Pharmacokinetic Profile for Single-Dose Injection of ABY-029: A Fluorescent Anti-EGFR Synthetic Affibody Molecule for Human Use. *Mol Imaging Biol* (2017) 19(4):512–21. doi: 10.1007/s11307-016-1033-y
65. Elliott JT, Marra K, Evans LT, Davis SC, Samkoe KS, Feldwisch J, et al. Simultaneous *In Vivo* Fluorescent Markers for Perfusion, Protoporphyrin Metabolism, and EGFR Expression for Optically Guided Identification of Orthotopic Glioma. *Clin Cancer Res* (2017) 23(9):2203–12. doi: 10.1158/1078-0432.CCR-16-1400
66. Elliott JT, Dsouza AV, Marra K, Pogue BW, Roberts DW, Paulsen KD. Microdose Fluorescence Imaging of ABY-029 on an Operating Microscope Adapted by Custom Illumination and Imaging Modules. *BioMed Opt Express* (2016) 7(9):3280–8. doi: 10.1364/BOE.7.003280
67. Samkoe KS, Bates BD, Tselepidakis NN, AV DS, Gunn JR, Ramkumar DB, et al. Development and Evaluation of a Connective Tissue Phantom Model for Subsurface Visualization of Cancers Requiring Wide Local Excision. *J BioMed Opt* (2017) 22(12):1–12. doi: 10.1117/1.JBO.22.12.121613
68. Samkoe KS, Park Y, Marra K, Chen EY, Tichauer KM. Paired-Agent Imaging for Detection of Head and Neck Cancers. *Proc SPIE Int Soc Opt Eng* (2019) 10853. doi: 10.1117/12.2510897
69. Sardar HS, Zai Q, Xu X, Gunn JR, Pogue BW, Paulsen KD, et al. Dual-Agent Fluorescent Labeling of Soft-Tissue Sarcomas Improves the Contrast Based Upon Targeting Both Interstitial and Cellular Components of the Tumor Milieu. *J Surg Oncol* (2020) 122(8):1711–20. doi: 10.1002/jso.26190
70. Pogue BW, Paulsen KD, Hull SM, Samkoe KS, Gunn J, Hoopes J, et al. Advancing Molecular-Guided Surgery Through Probe Development and

Testing in a Moderate Cost Evaluation Pipeline. *Proc SPIE Int Soc Opt Eng* (2015) 9311. doi: 10.1117/12.2083224

71. Burt T, Yoshida K, Lappin G, Vuong L, John C, de Wildt SN, et al. Microdosing and Other Phase 0 Clinical Trials: Facilitating Translation in Drug Development. *Clin Transl Sci* (2016) 9(2):74–88. doi: 10.1111/cts.12390
72. Ribeiro de Souza AL, Marra K, Gunn J, Samkoe KS, Hull S, Paulsen KD, et al. Optimizing Glioma Detection Using An EGFR-Targeted Fluorescent Affibody. *Photochem Photobiol* (2018) 94(6):1167–71. doi: 10.1111/php.13003
73. Hernandez Vargas S, Ghosh SC, Azhdarinia A. New Developments in Dual-Labeled Molecular Imaging Agents. *J Nucl Med* (2019) 60(4):459–65. doi: 10.2967/jnumed.118.213488
74. Zhang J, Li D, Lang L, Zhu Z, Wang L, Wu P, et al. 68ga-Nota-Aca-Bbn(7-14) PET/CT in Healthy Volunteers and Glioma Patients. *J Nucl Med* (2016) 57(1):9–14. doi: 10.2967/jnumed.115.165316
75. Choi HS, Nasr K, Alyabyev S, Feith D, Lee JH, Kim SH, et al. Synthesis and In Vivo Fate of Zwitterionic Near-Infrared Fluorophores. *Angew Chem Int Ed Engl* (2011) 50(28):6258–63. doi: 10.1002/anie.201102459
76. Luciano MP, Crooke SN, Nourian S, Dingle I, Nani RR, Kline G, et al. A Nonaggregating Heptamethine Cyanine for Building Brighter Labeled Biomolecules. *ACS Chem Biol* (2019) 14(5):934–40. doi: 10.1021/acschembio.9b00122
77. Choi HS, Gibbs SL, Lee JH, Kim SH, Ashitate Y, Liu F, et al. Targeted Zwitterionic Near-Infrared Fluorophores for Improved Optical Imaging. *Nat Biotechnol* (2013) 31(2):148–53. doi: 10.1038/nbt.2468
78. Handgraaf HJM, Boonstra MC, Prevoo H, Kuil J, Bordo MW, Boogerd LSF, et al. Real-Time Near-Infrared Fluorescence Imaging Using cRGD-ZW800-1 for Intraoperative Visualization of Multiple Cancer Types. *Oncotarget* (2017) 8(13):21054–66. doi: 10.18632/oncotarget.15486
79. Verbeek FP, van der Vorst JR, Tummers QR, Boonstra MC, de Rooij KE, Lowik CW, et al. Near-Infrared Fluorescence Imaging of Both Colorectal Cancer and Ureters Using a Low-Dose Integrin Targeted Probe. *Ann Surg Oncol* (2014) 21(Suppl 4):S528–37. doi: 10.1245/s10434-014-3524-x
80. Sibinga Mulder BG, Handgraaf HJ, Vugts DJ, Sewing C, Windhorst AD, Stammes M, et al. A Dual-Labeled Crgd-Based PET/optical Tracer for Pre-Operative Staging and Intraoperative Treatment of Colorectal Cancer. *Am J Nucl Med Mol Imaging* (2018) 8(5):282–91.
81. Liu Y, Bauer AQ, Akers WJ, Sudlow G, Liang K, Shen D, et al. Hands-Free, Wireless Goggles for Near-Infrared Fluorescence and Real-Time Image-Guided Surgery. *Surgery* (2011) 149(5):689–98. doi: 10.1016/j.surg.2011.02.007
82. Shen D, Xu B, Liang K, Tang R, Sudlow GP, Egbulefu C, et al. Selective Imaging of Solid Tumours Via the Calcium-Dependent High-Affinity Binding of A Cyclic Octapeptide to Phosphorylated Annexin A2. *Nat BioMed Eng* (2020) 4(3):298–313. doi: 10.1038/s41551-020-0528-7
83. Jones JE, Busi SB, Mitchem JB, Amos-Landgraf JM, Lewis MR. Evaluation of A Tumor-Targeting, Near-Infrared Fluorescent Peptide for Early Detection and Endoscopic Resection of Polyps in A Rat Model of Colorectal Cancer. *Mol Imaging* (2018) 17:1536012118790065. doi: 10.1177/1536012118790065
84. Liu Y, Njuguna R, Matthews T, Akers WJ, Sudlow GP, Mondal S, et al. Near-Infrared Fluorescence Goggle System With Complementary Metal-Oxide-Semiconductor Imaging Sensor and See-Through Display. *J BioMed Opt* (2013) 18(10):101303. doi: 10.1117/1.JBO.18.10.101303
85. Wyld L, Audisio RA, Poston GJ. The Evolution of Cancer Surgery and Future Perspectives. *Nat Rev Clin Oncol* (2015) 12(2):115–24. doi: 10.1038/nrclinonc.2014.191
86. Albright BB, Witte T, Tofte AN, Chou J, Black JD, Desai VB, et al. Robotic Versus Laparoscopic Hysterectomy for Benign Disease: A Systematic Review and Meta-Analysis of Randomized Trials. *J Minim Invasive Gynecol* (2016) 23(1):18–27. doi: 10.1016/j.jmig.2015.08.003
87. Zhou JY, Xin C, Mou YP, Xu XW, Zhang MZ, Zhou YC, et al. Robotic Versus Laparoscopic Distal Pancreatectomy: A Meta-Analysis of Short-Term Outcomes. *PloS One* (2016) 11(3):e0151189. doi: 10.1371/journal.pone.0151189
88. Kim HH, Han SU, Kim MC, Kim W, Lee HJ, Ryu SW, et al. Effect of Laparoscopic Distal Gastrectomy vs Open Distal Gastrectomy on Long-Term Survival Among Patients With Stage I Gastric Cancer: The KLASS-01 Randomized Clinical Trial. *JAMA Oncol* (2019) 5(4):506–13. doi: 10.1001/jamaoncol.2018.6727
89. Hernandez Vargas S, Kossatz S, Voss J, Ghosh SC, Tran Cao HS, Simien J, et al. Specific Targeting of Somatostatin Receptor Subtype-2 for Fluorescence-Guided Surgery. *Clin Cancer Res* (2019) 25(14):4332–42. doi: 10.1158/1078-0432.CCR-18-3312
90. Ntziachristos V, Ripoll J, Weissleder R. Would Near-Infrared Fluorescence Signals Propagate Through Large Human Organs for Clinical Studies? *Errata Opt Lett* (2002) 27(18):1652. doi: 10.1364/ol.27.001652
91. DSouza AV, Lin H, Henderson ER, Samkoe KS, Pogue BW. Review of Fluorescence Guided Surgery Systems: Identification of Key Performance Capabilities Beyond Indocyanine Green Imaging. *J BioMed Opt* (2016) 21 (8):80901. doi: 10.1117/1.JBO.21.8.080901
92. Hernandez Vargas S, Lin C, Voss J, Ghosh SC, Halperin DM, AghaAmiri S, et al. Development of a Drug-Device Combination for Fluorescence-Guided Surgery in Neuroendocrine Tumors. *J BioMed Opt* (2020) 25(12). doi: 10.1117/1.JBO.25.12.126002
93. Gharia A, Papageorgiou EP, Giverts S, Park C, Anwar M. Signal to Noise Ratio as a Cross-Platform Metric for Intraoperative Fluorescence Imaging. *Mol Imaging* (2020) 19:1536012120913693. doi: 10.1177/1536012120913693
94. Pogue BW, Rosenthal EL, Achilefu S, van Dam GM. Perspective Review of What Is Needed for Molecular-Specific Fluorescence-Guided Surgery. *J BioMed Opt* (2018) 23(10):1–9. doi: 10.1117/1.JBO.23.10.100601
95. Pogue BW, Paulsen KD, Samkoe KS, Elliott JT, Hasan T, Strong TV, et al. Vision 20/20: Molecular-guided Surgical Oncology Based Upon Tumor Metabolism or Immunologic Phenotype: Technological Pathways for Point of Care Imaging and Intervention. *Med Phys* (2016) 43(6):3143–56. doi: 10.1118/1.4951732
96. Mallett S, Halligan S, Thompson M, Collins GS, Altman DG. Interpreting Diagnostic Accuracy Studies for Patient Care. *BMJ* (2012) 345:e3999. doi: 10.1136/bmj.e3999
97. Lauwerends LJ, van Driel P, Baatenburg de Jong RJ, Hardillo JAU, Koljenovic S, Puppels G, et al. Real-Time Fluorescence Imaging in Intraoperative Decision Making for Cancer Surgery. *Lancet Oncol* (2021) 22(5):e186–e195. doi: 10.1016/S1470-2045(20)30600-8
98. Usama SM, Thapaliya ER, Luciano MP, Schnermann MJ. Not So Innocent: Impact of Fluorophore Chemistry on the *In Vivo* Properties of Bioconjugates. *Curr Opin Chem Biol* (2021) 63:38–45. doi: 10.1016/j.cbpa.2021.01.009
99. O'Connor JP, Aboagye EO, Adams JE, Aerts HJ, Barrington SF, Beer AJ, et al. Imaging Biomarker Roadmap for Cancer Studies. *Nat Rev Clin Oncol* (2017) 14(3):169–86. doi: 10.1038/nrclinonc.2016.162
100. Smit Duijzentkunst DA, Kwekkeboom DJ, Bodei L. Somatostatin Receptor 2-Targeting Compounds. *J Nucl Med* (2017) 58(Suppl 2):54S–60S. doi: 10.2967/jnumed.117.191015
101. Masters SC, Hofling AA, Gorovets A, Marzella L. Fda Approves Ga 68 PSMA-11 for Prostate Cancer Imaging. *Int J Radiat Oncol Biol Phys* (2021). doi: 10.1016/j.ijrobp.2021.03.055
102. Swanson GP, Basler JW. Prognostic Factors for Failure After Prostatectomy. *J Cancer* (2010) 2:1–19. doi: 10.7150/jca.2.1
103. Ramage JK, Ahmed A, Ardill J, Bax N, Breen DJ, Caplin ME, et al. Guidelines for the Management of Gastroenteropancreatic Neuroendocrine (Including Carcinoid) Tumours (Nets). *Gut* (2012) 61(1):6–32. doi: 10.1136/gutjnl-2011-300831
104. Baranski AC, Schafer M, Bauder-Wust U, Roscher M, Schmidt J, Stenau E, et al. Psma-11-Derived Dual-Labeled Psma Inhibitors for Preoperative Pet Imaging and Precise Fluorescence-Guided Surgery of Prostate Cancer. *J Nucl Med* (2018) 59(4):639–45. doi: 10.2967/jnumed.117.201293
105. Kularatne SA, Thomas M, Myers CH, Gagare P, Kanduluru AK, Crian CJ, et al. Evaluation of Novel Prostate-Specific Membrane Antigen-Targeted Near-Infrared Imaging Agent for Fluorescence-Guided Surgery of Prostate Cancer. *Clin Cancer Res* (2019) 25(1):177–87. doi: 10.1158/1078-0432.CCR-18-0803
106. Schottelius M, Wurzer A, Wissmiller K, Beck R, Koch M, Gorpas D, et al. Synthesis and Preclinical Characterization of the PSMA-Targeted Hybrid Tracer Psma-I&F for Nuclear and Fluorescence Imaging of Prostate Cancer. *J Nucl Med* (2019) 60(1):71–8. doi: 10.2967/jnumed.118.212720

107. Tummers WS, Warram JM, Tipirneni KE, Fengler J, Jacobs P, Shankar L, et al. Regulatory Aspects of Optical Methods and Exogenous Targets for Cancer Detection. *Cancer Res* (2017) 77(9):2197–206. doi: 10.1158/0008-5472.CAN-16-3217
108. Rosenthal EL, Warram JM, de Boer E, Basilion JP, Biel MA, Bogyo M, et al. Successful Translation of Fluorescence Navigation During Oncologic Surgery: A Consensus Report. *J Nucl Med* (2016) 57(1):144–50. doi: 10.2967/jnumed.115.158915
109. Achterberg FB, Deken MM, Meijer RPJ, Mieog JSD, Burggraaf J, van de Velde CJH, et al. Clinical Translation and Implementation of Optical Imaging Agents for Precision Image-Guided Cancer Surgery. *Eur J Nucl Med Mol Imaging* (2021) 48(2):332–9. doi: 10.1007/s00259-020-04970-0
110. Pogue BW, Zhu TC, Ntziachristos V, Paulsen KD, Wilson BC, Pfefer J, et al. Fluorescence-Guided Surgery and Intervention - An AAPM Emerging Technology Blue Paper. *Med Phys* (2018) 45(6):2681–8. doi: 10.1002/mp.12909

9

Blood-Brain Barrier, Blood-Brain Tumor Barrier and Fluorescence-Guided Neurosurgical Oncology: Delivering Optical Labels to Brain Tumors

Evgenii Belykh[1], *Kurt V. Shaffer*[1], *Chaoqun Lin*[2], *Vadim A. Byvaltsev*[3], *Mark C. Preul*[1*†] *and Lukui Chen*[4*†]

[1] Department of Neurosurgery, Barrow Neurological Institute, St. Joseph's Hospital and Medical Center, Phoenix, AZ, United States, [2] Department of Neurosurgery, School of Medicine, Southeast University, Nanjing, China, [3] Department of Neurosurgery, Irkutsk State Medical University, Irkutsk, Russia, [4] Department of Neurosurgery, Neuroscience Center, Cancer Center, Integrated Hospital of Traditional Chinese Medicine, Southern Medical University, Guangzhou, China

Correspondence:
Lukui Chen
neuro_clk@hotmail.com
Mark C. Preul
neuropub@barrowneuro.org

† These authors share senior authorship

Recent advances in maximum safe glioma resection have included the introduction of a host of visualization techniques to complement intraoperative white-light imaging of tumors. However, barriers to the effective use of these techniques within the central nervous system remain. In the healthy brain, the blood-brain barrier ensures the stability of the sensitive internal environment of the brain by protecting the active functions of the central nervous system and preventing the invasion of microorganisms and toxins. Brain tumors, however, often cause degradation and dysfunction of this barrier, resulting in a heterogeneous increase in vascular permeability throughout the tumor mass and outside it. Thus, the characteristics of both the blood-brain and blood-brain tumor barriers hinder the vascular delivery of a variety of therapeutic substances to brain tumors. Recent developments in fluorescent visualization of brain tumors offer improvements in the extent of maximal safe resection, but many of these fluorescent agents must reach the tumor via the vasculature. As a result, these fluorescence-guided resection techniques are often limited by the extent of vascular permeability in tumor regions and by the failure to stain the full volume of tumor tissue. In this review, we describe the structure and function of both the blood-brain and blood-brain tumor barriers in the context of the current state of fluorescence-guided imaging of brain tumors. We discuss features of currently used techniques for fluorescence-guided brain tumor resection, with an emphasis on their interactions with the blood-brain and blood-tumor barriers. Finally, we discuss a selection of novel preclinical techniques that have the potential to enhance the delivery of therapeutics to brain tumors in spite of the barrier properties of the brain.

Keywords: fluorescence-guided surgery, blood-brain barrier, blood-tumor barrier, 5-aminolevulinic acid, fluorescein sodium, indocyanine green, enhanced permeability and retention, drug delivery

INTRODUCTION

Gliomas account for nearly 80% of primary malignant tumors in the central nervous system (CNS) (1). Current recommended treatment for glioblastoma includes maximal safe resection, radiotherapy, temozolomide, and alternating electric field therapy (2). Despite all treatment efforts, glioma recurrence is inevitable due to the invasive nature of the tumor hampering complete tumor resection (3). Although it is practically impossible to eradicate every glioma cell surgically, increasing the precision of glioma removal with more accurate margin delineation predicts better treatment outcomes and preservation of quality of life (4–7). Because of the infiltrative growth pattern of gliomas, the tumor boundary is a mixture of tumor cells, reactive glial and immune cells, as well as normal brain cells. Such architecture complicates delivery of drugs to the invasive border region and restricts complete tumor resection. Margin delineation during resection is difficult and is inherently biased by both the subjective experience of the surgeon and the technical limitations of the operating microscope. Because of these factors, the goal of maximal safe resection of gliomas remains difficult to achieve, if not elusive.

In recent years, a number of intraoperative optical techniques, including fluorescence-guided surgery, have been developed to improve intraoperative visualization of cancers. These techniques can specifically label tumor cells, helping neurosurgeons to more objectively determine the boundary between the abnormal and surrounding normal tissues and to achieve more informed, maximum, and safe tumor resection. The impact of fluorescence techniques on extending progression-free and overall survival in high-grade gliomas is yet to be fully realized (8, 9). The most common drugs used for fluorescence-guided resection of high-grade gliomas are 5-aminolevulinic acid (5-ALA), fluorescein sodium (FLS), and indocyanine green (ICG), while multiple other fluorescent probes are currently in Phase I-II stages of investigation. Despite their mitigated success in clinical application for high-grade gliomas, current fluorescent labels often do not stain the overall area of the tumor, especially near the tumor margin, and do not delineate tumor margins in low-grade brain tumors. These difficulties are likely due to the effects of the blood-brain barrier (BBB), which maintains the sensitive environment of the brain by preventing the passage of blood-borne proteins, drugs, inflammatory cells, and other solutes. Consequently, delivery of fluorescent markers into the brain is also prevented, limiting the effectiveness of optical imaging techniques. Breakdown of the BBB is common in high-grade gliomas and brain metastases, producing what is known as the blood-brain tumor barrier (BBTB). It is this dysfunctional barrier that enables the extravasation of fluorescent markers into tumor tissue. However, the BBTB is more competent in low-grade gliomas and at the invasive border of high-grade gliomas (10, 11), complicating tumor staining (12, 13). Clearly, it would be advantageous to understand and manipulate the BBB and BBTB to overcome regional barriers to drug delivery and to target tumor cells where the BBTB is less disrupted.

In this review, we summarize the structure and function of the BBB and BBTB and their interactions with fluorescence visualization techniques for the optical guidance of invasive brain tumor resection. We review novel techniques that show potential for trans-BBB delivery of labels and therapeutics to elucidate the extent of brain tumors and to guide brain tumor surgery.

THE BLOOD-BRAIN BARRIER

The BBB is primarily composed of a continuous layer of non-fenestrated capillary endothelial cells covered by the glycocalyx and securely connected by a net of intercellular tight junctions (TJs) and adherens junctions, a basement membrane, pericytes, and perivascular astrocyte end-foot processes. Conceptually, the BBB contains three barriers arranged sequentially from the blood to the brain: the glycocalyx, endothelium, and extravascular compartment (14). A scaled schematic of these barriers is shown in **Figure 1**. Knowledge of the structure and function of these barriers is important not only for understanding the pharmacology of optical tracers in brain tumors and surrounding normal brain, but also for informing the design of novel drugs that can efficiently target invading tumor cells hidden behind regions of relatively intact BBTB.

Glycocalyx

The glycocalyx is an ~300-nm thick (15), gel-like structure on the luminal membrane of the endothelium consisting of negatively charged proteoglycans, glycosaminoglycans, and glycoproteins anchored in the luminal membrane by transmembrane proteins (16). A functional glycocalyx prevents the adhesion of circulating cells to the endothelium and serves as an initial malleable, sieve-like barrier to large molecules. For example, the concentration of intravascularly administered 150-kDa dextrans decreases by almost 50% within the glycocalyx layer, while the concentration of FLS (376 Da) remains above 90%, when compared to the center of the vessel (14, 17).

Endothelium

Endothelial cells create an ~200-nm thick, highly functionalized wall with luminal and abluminal membranes. These cells are tightly interconnected by TJs, lack fenestrations, and have a diminished number of pinocytic vesicles, limiting the transport of solutes across the BBB (18). Given these barrier properties, there are two main ways molecules pass the endothelial layer: via paracellular diffusion or using transcellular mechanisms.

Paracellular diffusion is significantly limited by the fence created by the continuous network of TJ complexes. TJs seal interendothelial clefts and anchor to the cytoskeleton, providing structural support. Brain endothelium differs from peripheral endothelium and epithelium in its expression of TJ proteins (high expression of occludin and claudin-5), which creates a tighter TJ network (19). Furthermore, alteration in the expression of the transmembrane proteins composing the TJs and their interactions modulate the gating of paracellular diffusion, allowing for dynamic control of paracellular diffusion (**Figure 2A**).

Transcellular diffusion is limited to those molecules that are relatively small, uncharged, and lipophilic (**Figure 2B**). More specifically, the intact BBB allows diffusion of hydrophobic

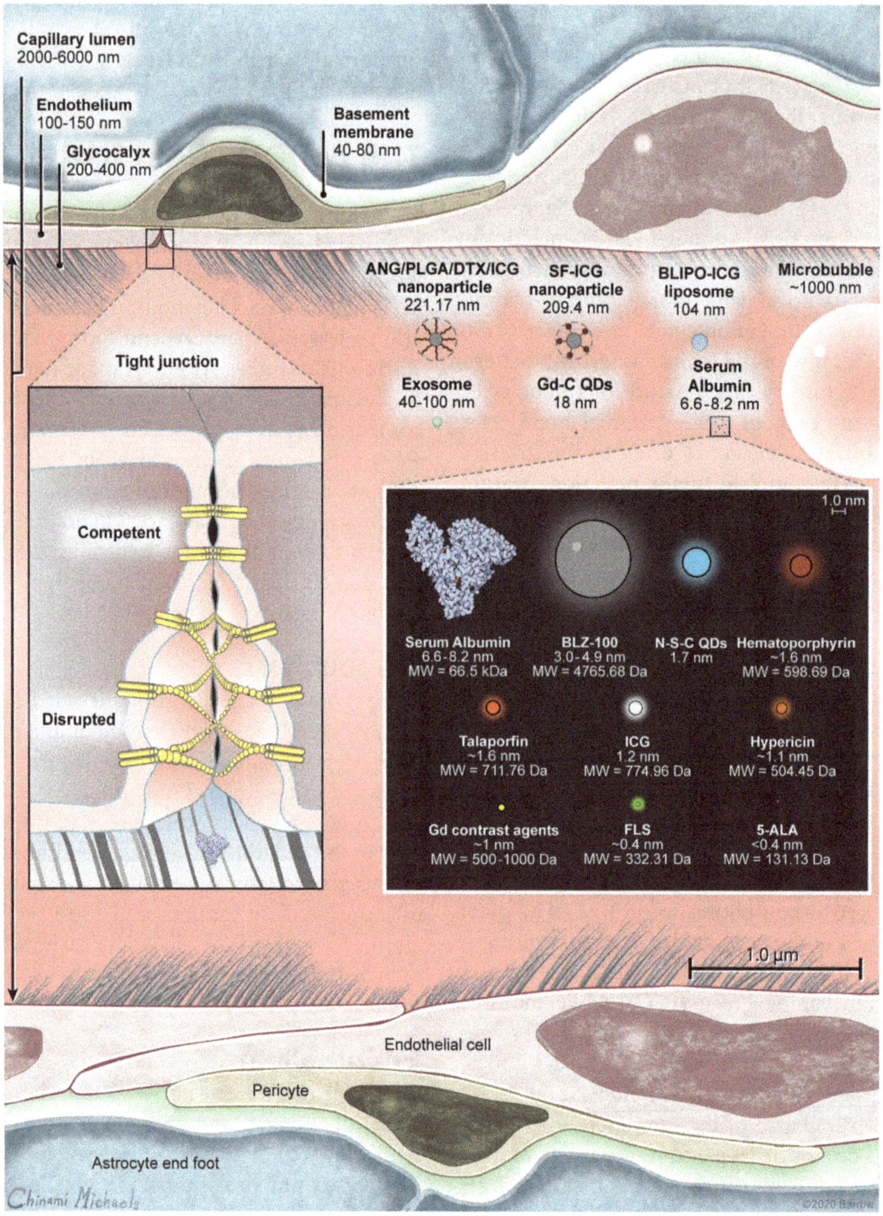

FIGURE 1 | A scale illustration of blood-brain barrier (BBB) structure with a selection of drugs and fluorescent markers discussed in this paper. Left inset shows the structure of the BBB including luminal glycocalyx, tight junctions (TJs), and the membranes of the neighboring endotheliocytes. In intact BBB, TJs secure the paracellular transport, while in disrupted BBB or in BBTB, TJs are deficient and allow for paracellular transport of large molecules through the interendothelial slits and pores. Human serum albumin is included because many small-molecule drugs (including ICG and FLS) bind extensively to serum proteins upon intravascular administration, thus changing their ability to cross the BBB. Right inset is scaled relative to the molecules within. Listed in nanometers are hydrodynamic diameters of molecules, when available, or molecular chain length estimated using PyMOL (The PyMOL Molecular Graphics System, Version 2.3 Schrödinger, LLC). 5-ALA, 5-aminolevulinic acid; ANG/PLGA/DTX/ICG, angiopep2/poly(lactic-co-glycolic acid)/docetaxel/indocyanine green; BLIPO-ICG, biomimetic liposome conjugated to indocyanine green; FLS, fluorescein sodium; Gd, gadolinium; Gd-C QD; gadolinium-carbon quantum dot; ICG, indocyanine green; N-S-C QD, nitrogen and sulfur co-doped carbon quantum dot; SF-ICG, silk fibroin indocyanine green conjugated. *Used with permission from Barrow Neurological Institute, Phoenix, Arizona.*

molecules that are less than 400–500 Da in size and form fewer than 8 to 10 hydrogen bonds with water (20). For ideal delivery, a drug should have an octanol:water partition coefficient (P_{ow}) of between 10:1 and 100:1 (21) or a total polar surface area less than 90 Å^2 (22). Coupled with endothelial TJs, this barrier to diffusion allows the endothelial expression and modulation of select transporters and receptors to dictate the flow of large molecules across the BBB (**Figures 2C–G**). Transporters at the endothelial cell membrane are primarily members of the solute carrier (SLC) family of passive membrane transporters (23–25) or of the adenosine triphosphate-binding cassette (ABC) family of active transporters (26–28). In contrast, the receptors

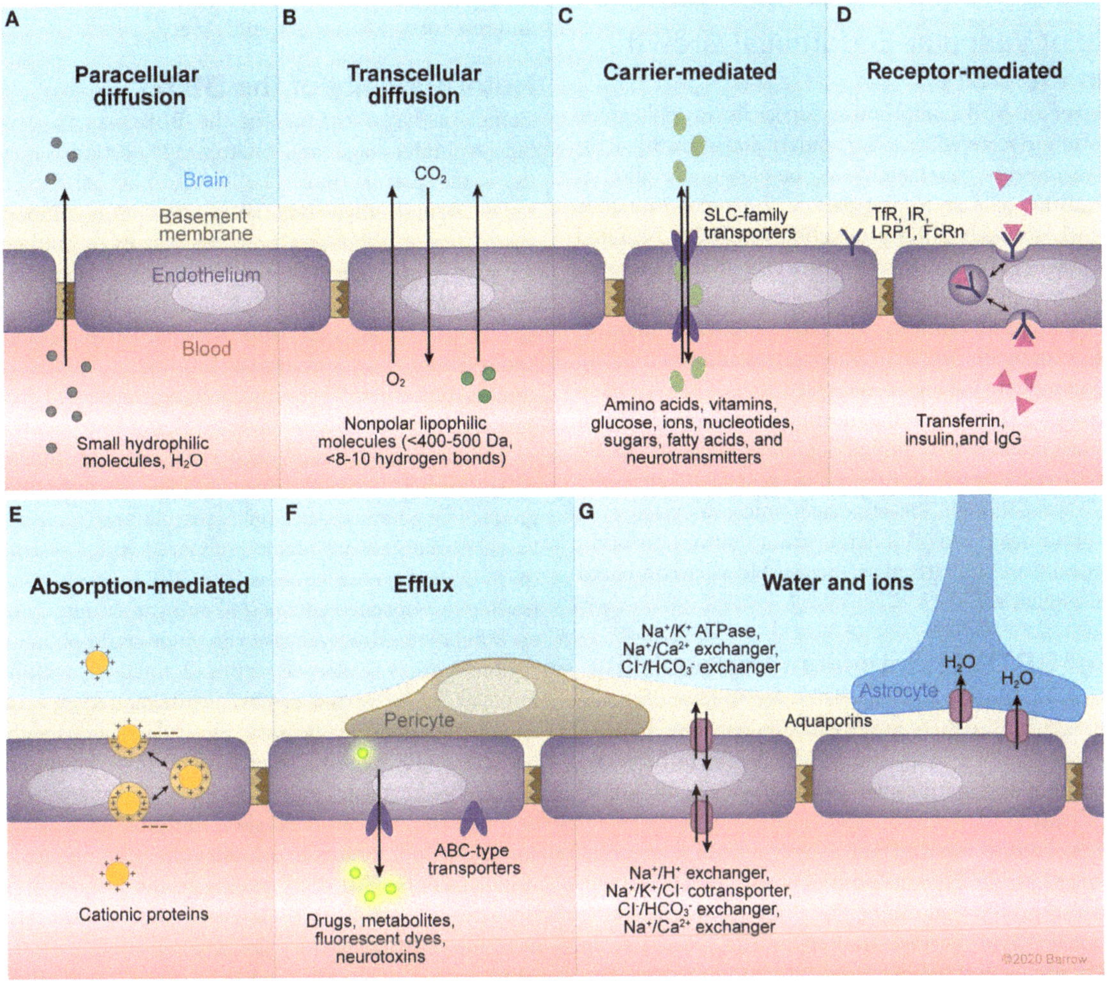

FIGURE 2 | Transport mechanisms of the blood-brain barrier (BBB). **(A)** Paracellular diffusion through intact tight junctions is possible for small, hydrophilic molecules and water. **(B)** Transcellular diffusion of small non-polar lipophilic molecules. **(C)** The facilitated diffusion of small molecules across the endothelium is mediated primarily by members of the solute carrier family of transporters, which transport a range of molecules including amino acids, vitamins, glucose, ions, nucleotides, sugars, fatty acids, and neurotransmitters. **(D)** Receptor-mediated transport allows for the transcellular passage of larger molecules across the endothelium via their binding to specific receptors. These receptors trigger endocytosis by conformational changes in cytoplasmic domains, allowing for the transcytosis or endocytosis of bound molecules. Examples of receptors expressed at the BBB include the transferrin receptor, insulin receptor, low-density lipoprotein related receptor 1, and the neonatal Fc receptor. **(E)** Cationic proteins can traverse the BBB via binding to negatively charged cell-surface molecules expressed in the capillary lumen, allowing for their transcytosis across the endothelium. **(F)** Members of the adenosine triphosphate (ATP) binding cassette family of transporters are expressed at the central nervous system endothelium, mediating the active efflux of a large selection of drugs, metabolites, neurotoxins, and fluorescent markers. **(G)** Proper osmolarity of the endothelial basement membrane and the adjacent brain interstitium is mediated by the selective expression of ion pumps and channels. Namely, the Na^+/K^+ ATPase, Na^+/Ca^{2+} exchanger, and Cl^-/HCO_3^- exchanger regulate abluminal ion equilibrium, while the Na^+/H^+ exchanger, $Na^+/K^+/Cl^-$ cotransporter, Cl^-/HCO_3^- exchanger, and Na^+/Ca^{2+} control ionic equilibrium with the blood. Additionally, expression of aquaporins 1 and 4 mediate the passive flow of water across endothelial cell and astrocyte membranes, respectively. ABC, adenosine triphosphate–binding cassette; FcRn, neonatal Fc receptor; IgG, immunoglobulin G; IR, insulin receptor; LRP1, low-density lipoprotein related receptor; SLC, solute carrier; TfR, transferrin receptor. *Used with permission from Barrow Neurological Institute, Phoenix, Arizona.*

expressed at the BBB are diverse, including the transferrin receptor (29), neonatal Fc receptor (30, 31), and low-density lipoprotein receptor 1 (LRP1) (25).

Extravascular Compartment

Other components of the BBB are pericytes, which cover 22–32% of the surface of the capillaries (32), the foot processes of neighboring astrocytes that completely encase the brain microvasculature (33), microglia, and neurons. These surrounding cells secrete signals that contribute to BBB development, provide physical and metabolic support, and are necessary to maintain dynamic integrity of the BBB (34–40). Altogether, these elements form a so-called neurovascular unit, capable of responding dynamically to local changes in physiology and environment (38, 41, 42). The composition, development, and regulation of the BBB have been previously reviewed in greater detail (21, 25, 38, 41–44), including a recent review of BBTB (45).

THE BLOOD-BRAIN TUMOR BARRIER

The Role of Vascular Endothelial Growth Factor in the BBTB

A major driver of BBB compromise, especially in high-grade gliomas, is tumor-secreted vascular endothelial growth factor (VEGF). The increased metabolic rate of high-grade gliomas results in local hypoxia and upregulation of hypoxia inducible factor-1, which stimulates the production of VEGF. Secreted VEGF then induces breakdown of existing BBB architecture and growth of structurally altered capillaries from the existing vessels (46, 47). This induced tumoral vascular endothelium displays an abnormal expression profile of transporters and receptors in order to accommodate the high metabolic demands of associated tumor cells (48–52). Unlike the normal brain vessels from which they originate, newly formed capillaries are structurally altered and are more permeable than even non-BBB peripheral capillaries (53). Although the abnormal microvasculature of high-grade brain neoplasms is different from that of non-brain solid tumors, both are similarly hyper-permeable when compared with normal capillaries.

Degree of BBTB Endothelium Permeability

The large size of interendothelial clefts and transendothelial fenestrations as well as their increased number contribute to the high degree of BBTB permeability. The degree of BBB and BBTB permeability is traditionally measured by using different-sized fluorescently labeled dextrans (54–58). The customizability of uniformly sized dextrans and their reactivity with fluorescent molecules such as fluorescein isothiocyanate (FITC) create easily assembled probes that can be visualized for interrogating BBB permeability. The average transendothelial pore size in intracranially implanted tumors is significantly smaller than that of extracranially implanted tumors (210–550 nm compared to 380–2,000 nm) (53). However, the hyperpermeability of the tumor capillaries to fluorescently labeled albumin (≈7 nm, 66 kDa) was associated with the number of pores, rather than their size (53). In average-size tumor vessels, about 30% had fenestrations and about 10% had open junctions (53). In a series of experiments with nine various-sized nanoparticles that tried to identify the maximal fenestration size in RG-2 glioma BBTB, 597 kDa molecules did not transgress the BBTB, while 330 kDa and smaller nanoparticles passed the BBTB (59).

To better portray the degree of BBTB hyperpermeability, tumor endothelium could be compared to non-brain endothelium, which is categorized into three groups based on permeability. (1) *Continuous non-fenestrated endothelium* is found in skin, heart, and lungs and is usually impermeable to molecules larger than 4–6 nm in diameter, but it may have intermittent discontinuities in TJs that create intercellular slits of up to 20 nm (60). (2) F*enestrated endothelium* of the intestines, kidneys, and choroid plexus has transcellular pores 25–60 nm in diameter, which are sealed by 5–6 nm thick diaphragms (61). (3) *Discontinuous endothelium* of the liver, spleen and bone marrow has large, 100–200 nm fenestrations without an underlying basement membrane (61). Consideration of the permeability of the various capillary types is important for the development of drugs, especially those that rely on the enhanced permeability and retention (EPR) effect for delivery.

Heterogeneity of the BBTB

Tumor-mediated changes in the BBB may vary with tumor type, volume, stage, and anatomical location, or even within the same tumor (62). The severity of barrier compromise ranges significantly, from critical disruption comparable to the vasculature in solid, non-brain neoplasms to mild compromise found in neurodegenerative disease, stroke, diabetes, and obesity, among other pathologies (18, 21, 43). Indeed, studies have shown that brain tumors possess all three distinct types of endothelium: non-fenestrated continuous, similar to normal cerebral blood vessels; continuous fenestrated; and discontinuous endothelium (63–65).

In low-grade gliomas, the structure and function of the BBTB largely resembles that of the normal BBB (66). In grade III gliomas, the microvasculature surface area and vascular diameter are higher compared with low-grade gliomas (67). In high-grade gliomas, the BBB is significantly altered, leading to associated edema (68) and gadolinium-based contrast accumulation. However, even in high-grade gliomas there are regions with vascular density and integrity within the same range as that of normal cerebral white matter, especially in non-enhancing regions or necrotic, avascular regions with decreased perfusion (10, 69, 70). Interestingly, this disruption does not necessarily correlate with the degree of infiltration of normal brain by tumor cells. A single infiltrating glioblastoma cell can cause the foot processes of astrocytes to migrate away from vascular endothelial cells, leading to the formation of localized fractures in the BBB (71). Alternatively, infiltrating glioma cells may be shielded by an intact BBB from intravascularly administered diagnostic and therapeutic agents (72, 73). This spectrum of BBB disruption seen in glioma is shown in **Figure 3**. An additional layer of complexity is added by the regional heterogeneity of immune cell populations that influence the BBTB in gliomas (74–76).

Glucocorticoids that are frequently used to manage peritumoral edema also influence the BBTB, reducing transendothelial flow by shrinking interendothelial gaps and increasing formation of intercellular junctions (77). However, preoperative steroid use was not associated with the efficacy of FLS staining of high-grade glioma tissue for wide-field fluorescence guidance and thus is unlikely to affect delivery of optical agents to the core of the tumor (78).

These characteristics depict the BBTB as a heterogeneous combination of preexisting and newly formed blood vessels, which provide nutrients and oxygen to the tumor. Although the BBTB is disrupted in the tumor core, it may retain characteristics of an intact BBB in certain areas, thus creating a barrier that, while compromised, still hinders delivery of diagnostic agents to the tumor, diminishing the diagnostic accuracy of intraoperative optical guidance techniques (52, 79). The fact that the BBTB is so disrupted in the core of high-grade gliomas leads some scientists to question the BBB as the major factor that limits the effectiveness of chemotherapy in these tumors (11). Therefore, in order to improve these techniques for brain tumor surgery, we

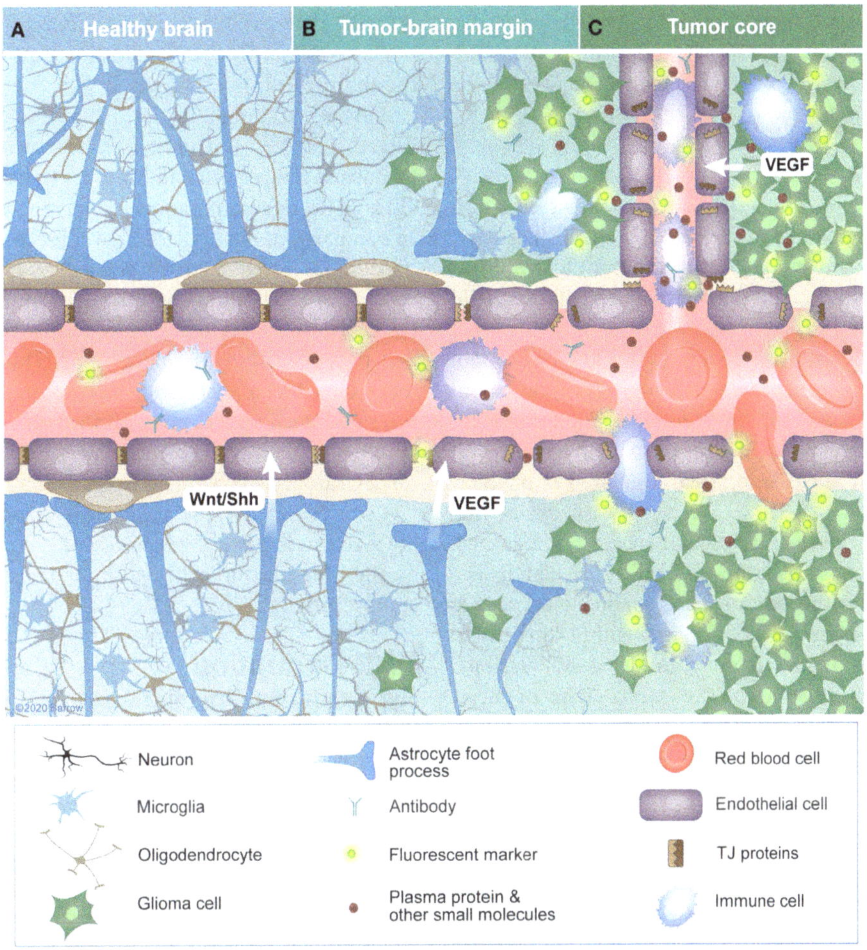

FIGURE 3 | Characteristics of the blood-brain (BBB) and blood-brain tumor barriers (BBTB) in glioma. **(A)** The healthy BBB selectively impedes the diffusion of blood contents across the central nervous system (CNS) endothelium. Controlled expression of tight-junction proteins and the endothelial cells themselves provide a physical barrier to the passage of these solutes into the brain parenchyma. Additionally, intimate associations among endothelial cells, pericytes, astrocytes, and neurons (the neurovascular unit) promote the continued integrity of the BBB. Sonic hedgehog and Wnt-family proteins secreted by astrocytes and pericytes are crucial for BBB maintenance. **(B)** In tumor margin zones, glioma cells may infiltrate into otherwise healthy parenchyma, causing disruption of local neural structures, including the BBB. This infiltration disrupts the connections between members of the neuro vascular unit, leading to the downregulation of tight-junction proteins and degradation of the BBB through tumor-secreted vascular endothelial growth factor. The resulting vascular permeability leads to the extravasation of blood contents, including solutes, antibodies, fluorescent markers, and immune cells. Alternatively, glioma cells may infiltrate in such a way that they do not disrupt the BBB, effectively shielding themselves with an intact BBB. **(C)** Within the tumor core, BBB disruption is often the greatest, especially in high-grade gliomas. The increased density of highly metabolically active cells in this area promotes hypoxia-driven expression of VEGF that promotes angiogenesis. These new vessels are often immature, lacking typical CNS barrier properties, leading to characteristics such as aberrant transporter expression, increased interstitial pressure, and edema. TJ, tight junctions; VEGF, vascular endothelial growth factor; Wnt/Shh, Wnt and sonic hedgehog family proteins. *Used with permission from Barrow Neurological Institute, Phoenix, Arizona.*

first need to understand the mechanisms that govern delivery of various optical labels across the heterogeneous BBTB in various tumor types. We also discuss approaches to circumvent the intact portions of the BBTB for more effective delivery of optical agents.

CURRENT STRATEGIES FOR DELIVERY OF TUMOR MARKERS ACROSS THE BBB AND BBTB

Efficacious drug delivery to the CNS has been difficult. The disrupted nature of the BBTB in high-grade gliomas permits increased delivery of drugs to the tumor core compared to surrounding normal brain, where the BBB is generally intact. Still, the invasive nature of high-grade gliomas and other non-enhancing brain tumors (80), in which cells migrate beyond the visible borders of gadolinium enhancement (81), presents a challenge for accurate delineation of the extent of tumor growth, for accurate diagnosis, and for intraoperative guidance.

Although many methods have been explored for drug delivery across the heterogeneous BBB and BBTB, these barriers remain a major obstacle (20, 21, 24, 52, 64, 82–92). In general, such methods can be classified into five broad categories: (1) passive delivery, (2) EPR of the BBTB, (3) BBTB disruption, (4) BBTB bypass, (5) BBTB targeting. We briefly discuss these categories of drug delivery and relate them to the current clinical tools and novel advancements for intraoperative optical guidance in neuro-oncology. Tumor markers reviewed in this manuscript are summarized in the **Table 1**.

Passive Delivery

Passive delivery through the intact BBTB is challenging, as most small lipophilic drugs that could diffuse through the BBB are not targeted and exhibit toxicity in high doses, and most hydrophilic molecules do not pass through the narrow TJs of the BBB (140, 141).

Passive delivery of small molecules (<40 kDa) through the disrupted BBTB proceeds down a blood-tumor diffusion gradient, similarly to drug delivery to non-brain tumors. Interestingly, low-molecular-weight drugs usually have a lower "tumor-to-normal brain" distribution ratio compared with larger molecules. This difference is due to the rapid wash out of the small-molecule drugs from the extracellular space and clearance from the blood (142). Accumulation of small molecular labels in tumor tissues peaks within minutes and gradually decreases within 4–6 h. Fluorescence-guided surgery within this time window of first-pass accumulation and clearance is still feasible, mainly because a healthy BBB limits the extravasation of these labels (for example FLS, ICG, and others) to areas of tumoral BBB degradation.

Enhanced Permeability and Retention

The EPR mechanism was initially described for non-brain solid tumors in 1986 (142, 143). This mechanism is based on four main components: (1) hypervascularization of the tumor, (2) enhanced permeability of tumor vasculature, (3) hampered absorption of macromolecules back into the vasculature, and (4) reduced drainage of molecules through the lymphatic system. Because the BBTB in high-grade gliomas is even more permeable than fenestrated non-brain capillaries, many optical guidance drugs reach the tumor via this mechanism. Furthermore, the lack of a lymphatic system in tumors prevents the clearance of large molecules and lipids from the interstitial space, greatly contributing to drug retention (142, 143). It is worth noting that some tumors do not have increased vascularity, and therefore the EPR effect is not observed in them. For example, metastatic prostate and liver cancers have low vascular densities (144, 145). This low vascular density potentially explains the lack of FLS-, ICG-, and 5-ALA-labeling of some brain metastases.

In order for the EPR effect to occur, the injected molecule should be biocompatible, have no clearance by the reticuloendothelial system, and be non-reactive to blood cells or the endothelium (142). The molecule should be large enough (>40 kDa) to avoid renal clearance through the pores in glomerular endothelium and have a weakly negative or neutral surface charge (142, 146). With respect to the upper limit of size of a molecule for EPR, researchers have demonstrated that 1-μm diameter *Lactobacilli* can be selectively delivered into the tumor with additional dilation of the tumor endothelial cell junctions by an angiotensin-converting enzyme inhibitor (147). Many drugs, including polymer conjugates, bind to albumin (60 kDa), increasing their molecular weight, thus satisfying the criteria for EPR delivery. For example, immunoglobulin G (160 kDa), polymer-drug conjugates, and liposome-encapsulated drugs fit the above-mentioned criteria.

Distinct accumulation of a high-molecular-weight drug via EPR can be seen within half an hour, with a maximum tumor-to-normal tissue ratio within hours to days after administration (142). The retention time usually ranges from hours to days. In comparison, low-molecular-weight contrast agents, including gadolinium-based contrast agents (500–1,000 Da in size) are capable of freely diffusing through the peripheral endothelium (148). These agents accumulate within the tumor because of a first-pass effect, but are not retained. Thus, compared to smaller molecules, the model EPR macromolecule is small enough to enter endothelial pores of the abnormal tumor vasculature, where it more preferentially accumulates, but large enough to avoid renal clearance, allowing prolonged circulation (142, 143).

Of note, all current clinically employed optical tracers for brain tumor imaging (FLS, ICG, and 5-ALA) rely to some degree on the EPR effect to exit the tumor microvasculature through a compromised BBTB.

BBB Disruption

Hyperosmolar Opening

Focus on drug delivery via disruption of the BBB began in the 1970s by Rapoport (149) and Rapoport et al. (150), establishing the effectiveness of temporary TJ opening with intraarterial infusion of a bolus of hyperosmolar mannitol (**Figure 4A**) (151). This method was subsequently adapted to increase the delivery of chemotherapeutics to brain tumors (152, 153). Although there are reports on the safety and efficacy of the selective endovascular hyperosmolar opening of the BBB for chemotherapeutics in cases of CNS lymphoma, anaplastic oligodendroglioma, and other brain malignancies (154, 155), overall effectiveness of this method is still debatable (91). The non-selective opening of the BBB allows for indiscriminate influx of blood-borne molecules, causing neurotoxicity, vasculopathy, seizure, and chronic neurologic defects, which limit its widespread clinical use (20, 91, 156). However, since the inception of this idea, there has been considerable advancement in other techniques to disrupt the BBB for theranostic applications.

Microbubble-Enhanced Focused Ultrasound

Microbubble-enhanced focused ultrasound (MEUS) techniques rely on the application of low-power ultrasound to a specific brain region in combination with intravenous (IV) administration of preformed, lipid-coated, echogenic microbubbles (**Figure 4A**) (160). The focused ultrasound induces stable cavitation in the bubbles as they pass through the ultrasound field, mediating precise and transient disruption of the BBB via the downregulation of TJ proteins (82), suppression of P-glycoprotein expression (161), and facilitation of pinocytosis (162). MEUS has been used recently in animal models to enhance BBB permeability to an array of therapeutics (160). Furthermore, this technique can be used under magnetic resonance imaging (MRI) guidance to evaluate the effectiveness of BBB opening. Such a combination has been explored clinically for targeted

TABLE 1 | Preclinical and early clinical agents for delivery of optical labels to brain tumors discussed in this review.

Agent	Interaction with BBB/BBTB	Stage of development	References
UNTARGETED AGENTS			
[^{18}F]-1; an [^{18}F]-labeled dasatinib derivative for ^{18}F-PET and fluorescence visualization *in vivo*	None; investigated using CED to bypass the BBB in mouse models	Preclinical	(93)
Collagen-based, ^{131}Cs-laden wafer for intracranial brachytherapy	None; intracranial implant to bypass the BBB	Clinical	(94)
PEGylated FLS	None; improved passive accumulation within tumor tissues via the EPR effect in U251 orthotopic mouse glioma	Preclinical	(95)
Albumin-bound 5-aminoFLS	None; improved passive accumulation within tumor tissues via the EPR effect intraoperatively	Clinical	(96, 97)
Second-window ICG	None; passive accumulation within tumor tissues via a delayed EPR effect	Clinical	(98–102)
Aptamer-conjugated PEGylated quantum dots	None; passive accumulation via the EPR effect and targeting via EGFRvIII-targeted aptamers in orthotopic mouse gliomas	Preclinical	(103)
Silk fibroin-ICG nanoparticles	None; improved passive accumulation within orthotopic C6 mouse glioma cells via the EPR effect	Preclinical	(104)
EPR Enhancers			
PGI2 agonists	Dilation of tumor vasculature to increase extravasation and accumulation via the EPR effect	Preclinical	(105)
TNF-a		Preclinical	(106)
Intraarterial angiotensin II		Clinical	(107)
ANTIBODY/AFFIBODY-BASED AGENTS			
ABY-029, an anti-EGFR affibody conjugated to the near infrared probe IRDye 800CW	Targeting to EGFR receptors overexpressed on glioma cells	Clinical	(108), NCT02901925
FITC-conjugated anti-EGFR antibody		Preclinical	(109)
IRDye 800CW-conjugated anti-EGFR antibody		Preclinical	(110)
OTHER TARGETED AGENTS			
ANG2, a synthetic peptide shown to target the BBB	RMT via low-density lipoprotein receptor 1 targets both BBB and BBTB	Clinical	(111, 112), NCT01967810, NCT02048059
ANG2/PLGA/DTX/ICG probe, an ANG2-coated, ICG- and docetaxel-laden PLGA nanoparticle	RMT via low-density lipoprotein receptor 1 targets both BBB and BBTB	Preclinical	(113)
ANG2/PEG-UCNP, an ANG2-conjugated, gadolinium-laden fluorescent upconversion nanoparticle	RMT via low-density lipoprotein receptor 1 targets both BBB and BBTB	Preclinical	(114)
AsT, a TGN- and AS1411-conjugated Cy3 fluorescent probe	Endothelial cell uptake and transcytosis into the brain via TGN-conjugation by an unknown mechanism and AS1411 aptamer-mediated glioma cell targeting	Preclinical	(115)
Lysine-methotrexate prodrug	CMT via L-type amino acid transporter 1 targets the BBB in a mouse model	Preclinical	(116)
Aspartate-, 2-amino-apidic acid-, and phenylalanine-conjugated dopamine prodrugs	CMT via large neutral amino acid transporter 1 targets BBB	Preclinical	(117)
ApoE3-labeled porphyrin-lipid nanoparticles	RMT via low-density lipoprotein receptor 1 targets both BBB and BBTB in a mouse model	Preclinical	(118)
Transferrin-functionalized lipid nanoparticles laden with temozolomide and bromodomain inhibitor JQ1	RMT via transferrin receptor in a mouse model	Preclinical	(119)
BLZ-100 (tozuleristide), ICG-conjugated chlorotoxin	RMT via binding to chloride channels to trigger endocytosis at the BBB or BBTB and MMP-2 binding for targeting of glioma cells	Clinical	(120–123), NCT03579602
IRDye 800CW-cyclic-RGD peptide	Targeting to integrin receptor overexpression on tumor vasculature and on tumor cells in a mouse glioma model	Preclinical	(124)
BLIPO-ICG, ICG-laden biomimetic proteolipid liposomes	Passive accumulation via the EPR effect and targeting to glioma cells via functionalization with glioma-derived surface markers in a mouse glioma model	Preclinical	(125)
5-ALA-COUPLED AGENTS			
5-ALA + MEK inhibitor selumetinib	Inhibition of ABCB1-mediated PpIX efflux and ferrochelatase-mediated PpIX metabolism at the BBB or BBTB in a mouse model	Preclinical	(126)

(Continued)

TABLE 1 | Continued

Agent	Interaction with BBB/BBTB	Stage of development	References
5-ALA + efflux pump inhibitors			
Ko143	Inhibition of ABCG2-mediated PpIX efflux at the BBB or BBTB	Preclinical	(127, 128)
Gefitinib		Preclinical	(129)
Imatinib mesylate		Preclinical	(130)
5-ALA + iron chelators	None; inhibition of PpIX metabolism to heme via ferrochelatase in tumor cells	Preclinical	(131–134)
5-ALA + differentiation agents			
Calcitriol	None; enhanced PpIX accumulation via upregulation of coproporphyrinogen oxidase in epithelial cancer and glioma cell cultures	Preclinical	(135, 136)
Vitamin E	None; enhanced PpIX accumulation via upregulation of coproporphyrinogen oxidase in epithelial cancer cell culture	Preclinical	(137)
5-ALA + heme oxygenase inhibitors	None; accumulation of PpIX via inhibition of downstream metabolism of heme by heme oxidase	Preclinical	(138, 139)

^{18}F, Fluorine-18; ^{131}Cs, Cesium-131; 5-ALA, 5-aminolevulinic acid; ABCB1, ATP-binding cassette subfamily B member 1; ABCG2, ATP-binding cassette subfamily G member 2; ANG2, angiopep-2; ApoE3; apolipoprotein E3; BBB, blood-brain barrier; BBTB, blood-brain tumor barrier; CMT, carrier-mediated transport; DCT, docetaxel; EPR, enhanced permeability and retention; FLS, fluorescein sodium; ICG, indocyanine green; MEK, mitogen-activated protein kinase kinase; MMP-2, matrix metalloproteinase 2; PEG, polyethylene glycol; PET, proton emission tomography; PLGA, poly(lactic-co-glycolic acid); PpIX, protoporphyrin IX; RMT, receptor-mediated transport; UCNP, up-conversion nanoparticle.

neuromodulation (163) and drug delivery in Alzheimer's disease (164). MEUS is designed for a non-invasive and highly targeted approach, mitigating the risks of non-specific hyperosmolar BBB disruption and surgical methods of drug delivery (165, 166).

Neurogenic Methods

Transcranial magnetic stimulation and sphenopalatine ganglion stimulation (**Figure 4D**) are novel methods that can affect neurovascular unit function and BBB permeability by acting on its neuronal component. Transcranial magnetic stimulation effects are based on neuronal activity and are mediated by an N-methyl-D-aspartate-receptor-dependent mechanism (167, 168). Transcranial magnetic stimulation has been used for the treatment of neurological disorders, including depression, but its potential for improving drug delivery to the brain has become a subject of recent studies (167). Sphenopalatine ganglion stimulation is a novel technique for transient (4 h) BBB disruption via neural stimulation (57). Sphenopalatine ganglion stimulation caused downregulation of TJ proteins, similar to that seen in hyperosmolar disruption, and resulted in ipsilateral, hemispheric extravasation of a 70-kDa FLS-labeled dextran in a rat model (57). The safety and clinical efficacy of this method, especially compared to the more focused MEUS, is yet to be established.

Photodynamic Method

Photodynamic opening of the BBB using 5-ALA has been described in a mouse model (169). Irradiation with a 635-nm laser, 30 min after IV administration of 5-ALA resulted in a transient (4 h) increased BBB permeability to Evans blue dye, 70-kDa FITC-dextrans, and intravascular solutes. Histological analysis demonstrated complete recovery from the induced perivascular edema within 3 days. Implications of these findings for the current 5-ALA-based fluorescence-guided surgical techniques or photodynamic therapy should be investigated further. However, 5-ALA is mostly cleared from the blood by the time of glioma resection (~6 h after oral administration).

Clinical Applicability of BBB Disruption for Fluorescence-Guided Surgery

With regard to optically guided brain tumor resection, techniques for BBB disruption may be used to enhance the delivery of targeted optical markers, improving the sensitivity of tumor visualization, especially in low-grade gliomas and at the border of high-grade gliomas, where the BBTB remains largely intact. However, clinical procedures for BBB disruption may be too invasive and time consuming to warrant their application solely to improve fluorescence-guided surgery. Preoperative BBB disruption for delivery of targeted optical drugs should ideally be combined with therapeutic agents in order to take full advantage of transient BBB opening. Further, wider adoption of MEUS and transcranial magnetic stimulation should stimulate the clinical translation of novel combinatory drugs that include not only therapeutic agents, but also optical fluorescent tracers for better intraoperative visualization of brain tumor margins. However, major efforts are directed toward development of molecular techniques for bypassing and targeting the BBB/BBTB without destroying its integrity (170).

Bypassing the BBB

Techniques to bypass the BBB entirely are primarily surgical in nature (**Figure 4B**). These include methods such as intrathecal/intraventricular injection, transnasal administration, convection-enhanced delivery (CED), and intracerebral or topical implantation.

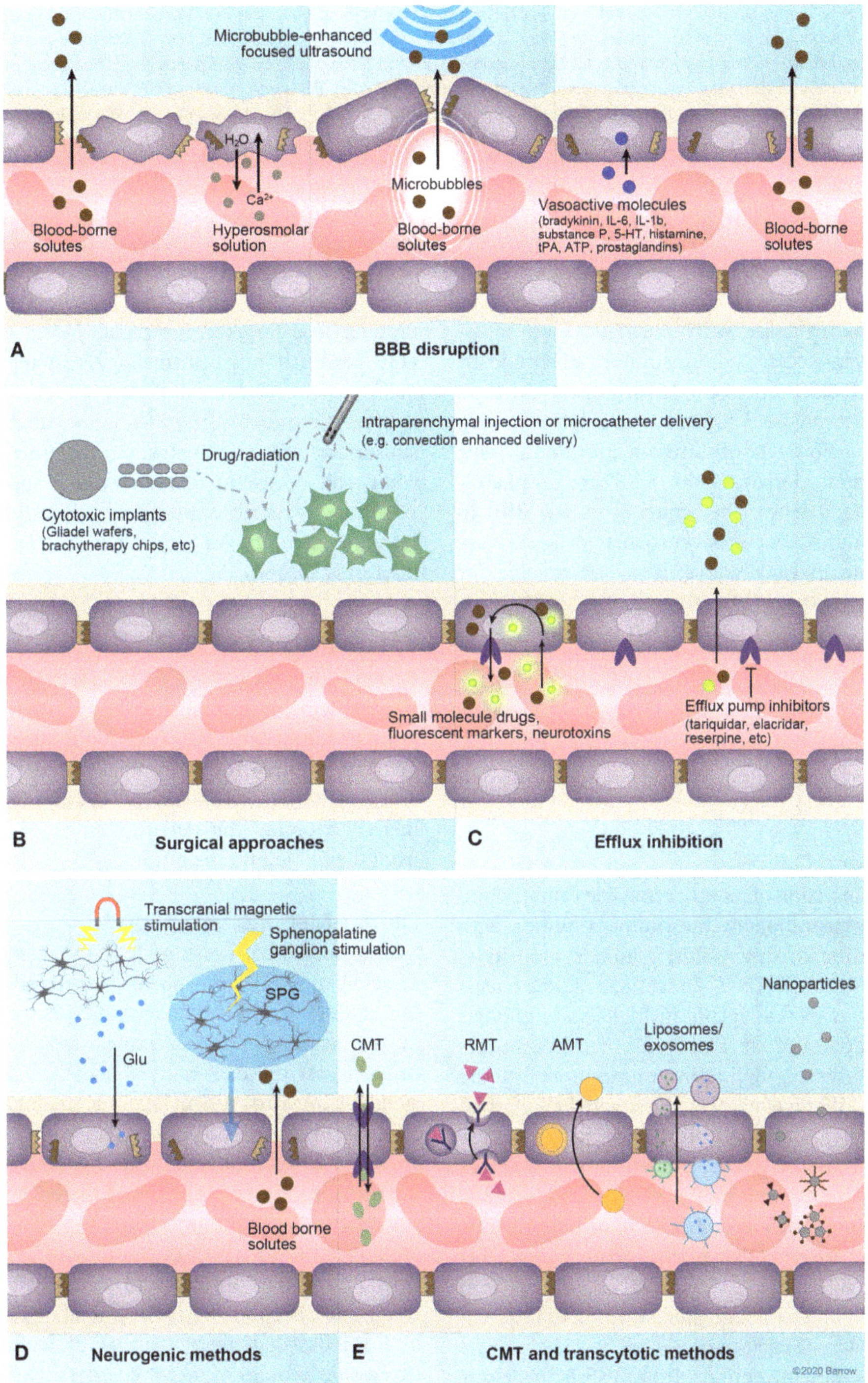

FIGURE 4 | Drug delivery to the central nervous system. **(A)** Techniques that involve coadministration of a drug coupled to disruption of the blood-brain barrier (BBB) include hyperosmolar disruption, microbubble-enhanced focused ultrasound (MEUS), and administration of vasoactive substances. The intravascular injection of a hyperosmolar solution dehydrates endothelial cells, shrinking them and causing strain at tight junctions, and ultimately causing tight-junction protein displacement and BBB disruption. MEUS involves the intravascular administration of small (~1 μm) bubbles that are targeted by focused ultrasound to induce cavitation, creating tight-junction strain and resulting in BBB permeation. Finally, vasoactive molecules including bradykinin, interleukins 6 and 1β, substance P, serotonin, histamine, tissue plasminogen activator, adenosine triphosphate, and prostaglandins, alter the expression of tight-junction proteins, affecting BBB permeability. **(B)** Surgical approaches deliver drugs by circumventing the BBB entirely. These approaches include the implantation of a polymer with delayed drug release [for example, radioactive brachytherapy (157) or chemotherapeutic-loaded implants (157, 158)] into the brain or the injection of a drug into the brain via microcatheter. **(C)** Efflux inhibition aims to augment the diffusion of a drug across the BBB via the inhibition of efflux pumps that mediate its active removal from the brain. Examples of known efflux pump

(Continued)

FIGURE 4 | inhibitors include tariquidar, elacridar, and reserpine (159). **(D)** Neurogenic methods of increasing BBB permeability include transcranial magnetic stimulation and sphenopalatine ganglion stimulation. Transcranial magnetic stimulation is thought to increase BBB permeability through the endothelial binding of glutamate released from magnetically excited neurons. The exact mechanisms of sphenopalatine-mediated BBB permeability are currently unknown, but likely involve sympathetic innervation of intracranial vasculature provided through the sphenopalatine ganglion. **(E)** Carrier-mediated and transcytotic methods involve the targeted binding of drug-bearing molecules to structures expressed on the luminal surface of the endothelium. This delivery system includes freely soluble drug molecules that bind to expressed transporters or surface molecules, drug-delivery vehicles such as liposomes or exosomes, or nanoparticles. Importantly, these drug-delivery methods often incorporate transporter or receptor substrates or molecular probes for targeting to specific structures at the BBB/BBTB. 5-HT, serotonin; AMT, adsorption-mediated transport; ATP, adenosine triphosphate; BBB, blood-brain barrier; CMT, carrier-mediated transport; Glu, glutamate; IL, interleukin; RMT, receptor-mediated transport; SPG, sphenopalatine ganglion; tPA, tissue plasminogen activator. *Used with permission from Barrow Neurological Institute, Phoenix, Arizona.*

Intrathecal or Intraventricular Administration

Intrathecal or intraventricular administration theoretically bypasses the BBB, but diffusion from the cerebrospinal fluid (CSF) to the brain parenchyma is limited by a relatively rapid bulk flow of CSF and a slow rate of diffusion into brain tissue (87). Thus, drugs administered to the CSF are ultimately redistributed to the blood where they must cross the BBB to be effective. While intrathecal or intraventricular drug delivery is effective for leptomeningeal diseases, it is not suitable for parenchymal brain tumors (64, 171).

Transnasal Drug Administration

Transnasal drug administration and mucosal engrafting (172, 173) techniques initially avoid the BBB, but the drug must still cross into the subarachnoid space, where it will face the same obstacles as intrathecally administered drugs while providing only limited focal drug distribution.

Convection-Enhanced Delivery

CED involves surgical insertion of a semipermeable catheter into the area of drug administration in the brain or tumor with a constant administration of drug solution under a positive-pressure gradient (174, 175). Over 20 clinical studies used CED for delivery of therapeutic agents in high-grade gliomas and showed moderate clinical efficiency (158). A few studies have used coinfusion with gadolinium to monitor infusate distribution (176, 177). Wang et al. (93) investigated CED of an ^{18}[F]-positron-emitting, fluorescent derivative of the Abl-kinase inhibitor dasatinib in a mouse glioma model. Similar to other studies (178, 179), the main purpose of coadministration of the fluorescent agent is to monitor drug distribution in experimental settings. As trials for the delivery of novel therapeutics using CED are still being conducted (180, 181), the utilization of CED with fluorescent markers for optical image guidance, for example in recurrent gliomas, is yet to be explored.

Another method for circumvention of the BBB is to deliver drug directly into the resection cavity intraoperatively. This technique has seen relative success with current therapeutic agents, such as an implantable, biodegradable polyanhydride polymer infused with the alkylating agent carmustine (Gliadel) (182–184) or a collagen wafer embedded with x-ray-emitting cesium-131 (94). Such administration promotes delayed diffusion of the drug that creates areas of increased drug concentration and CED in the peritumoral bed over time. Direct intracavitary delivery of optical imaging agents, especially "activatable" fluorescence probes that turn on upon specific binding to a targeted molecular motif, is also being explored (185, 186). Although promising, local application of fluorescent markers to the surface of a resection cavity is inherently limited in that it requires some incubation time and would leave any subsurface tumor unlabeled. On the other hand, topical staining could still be useful to identify any apparent residual tumor. Furthermore, such staining could be used for a small-field, intraoperative, digital biopsy assessment of selected regions of interest (187, 188).

Targeting the BBB

Recent technologies have adopted a strategy of targeting existing transporters, receptors or other molecules expressed on the luminal surface of the CNS endothelium to facilitate drug delivery (**Figures 4C,E**). Importantly, these techniques allow for crossing of the BBB without disrupting interendothelial TJs, thereby avoiding the potential efflux of neurotoxic substances from the blood into the brain.

Carrier-Mediated Transport

Carrier-mediated transport (CMT) takes advantage of an array of small-molecule transporters expressed at the BBB. Through the conjugation of small-molecule drugs to or the mimicking of the ligands of these transporters, selective movement of drugs across the BBB may be achieved. Classically, drugs such as L-3,4-dihydroxyphenylalanine, melphalan, and gabapentin take advantage of CMT for CNS activity. Singh and Subudhi (116) have demonstrated this by delivering a methotrexate-lysine conjugate prodrug across the BBB via L-type amino acid transporter 1. In a similar approach, Peura et al. (117) synthesized amino acid prodrugs of dopamine to increase uptake across the BBB via the large amino acid transporter 1. While these early results have been successful in animal models, clinical application of CMT-based delivery may be difficult. Examination of the expression profiles of these receptors in a given tumor or BBTB might be needed prior to determination of a therapeutic target. Further, CMT-based strategies are limited to small-molecule drugs or prodrugs, as transporters will not support the passage of larger molecules.

Receptor-Mediated Transport

Receptor-mediated transport (RMT) strategies target receptors expressed on the luminal surface of CNS endothelium in order to initiate endocytosis or transcytosis for transport of the molecule to the abluminal surface. Often, these strategies involve the linking of an effector molecule to a receptor ligand or antibody that can bind and initiate endocytosis.

An example of a molecule used successfully for RMT is angiopep-2 (ANG2), a synthetic peptide that targets LRP1 at the BBB. Importantly, LRP1 is a shuttling receptor, able to mediate transcytosis while avoiding the destructive lysosomal compartment (111, 189). LRP1 has also been shown to be overexpressed on glioblastoma cells (190), giving ANG2 tumor-specific targeting capabilities. So far, ANG2 has proven capable of delivering paclitaxel to glioma and brain metastases, avoiding P-glycoprotein-mediated paclitaxel efflux (90), and is currently in Phase II clinical trials for recurrent high-grade glioma (NCT01967810) and breast cancer with recurrent brain metastases (NCT02048059).

Rajora et al. (118) reported the successful targeting of LRP-1 expressed on orthotopic U87 glioblastoma cells in mice using apolipoprotein E3 porphyrin-lipid nanoparticles. Glioblastoma cells readily took up the nanoparticles, exhibiting near-infrared fluorescence and sensitization to photodynamic therapy. In another study, Lam et al. (119) reported the success of transferrin-functionalized nanoparticles bearing temozolomide and bromodomain inhibitor JQ1 to selectively target and kill glioblastoma cells in a mouse model. These studies both demonstrate the efficacy of RMT-mediated targeting of tumors *in vivo*. Importantly, these therapies have a potential to traverse the intact portion of the BBTB for treatment of otherwise shielded tumor cells.

The Future and Caveats of Techniques for Transcellular Transport

Increasingly, CMT- and RMT-based therapeutic strategies are incorporating delivery vehicles such as nanoparticles, liposomes, or exosomes to target brain tumors. These strategies involve the assembly of a custom-built molecular vehicle, often housing an effector molecule, that is coated with receptor ligands or other targeting molecules to facilitate the precise targeting of the vehicles to the endothelium of the BBB or tumor cells. A detailed review of liposome-based drug vehicles was recently published (141), and several have been published regarding nanoparticle-based drug delivery to the brain (85, 89, 170, 191–196). The main advantage of nanoparticle technology is its customizability, as the size, composition, cargo, and target are tunable, affecting changes in BBB permeability, therapeutic effect, or drug pharmacokinetics. However, several caveats to these strategies need to be carefully considered.

Bypassing the endothelial barrier with an optical or other diagnostic agent only informs about the location and degree of BBB disruption and not necessarily about the tumor cells themselves. In order to achieve better selectivity and ability to target tumor cells beyond the competent BBTB, the agent should dissociate from the encapsulating vehicle, travel through the extracellular space and, ideally, label the tumor cells. Given the complexity of the underlying mechanisms of drug delivery, many obstacles must be overcome. If the vehicle is too stable, the drug is not released and does not react with the target (197, 198). However, if the drug has low molecular weight, it risks diffusion back to the circulation upon dissociation from the large carrier (197, 199, 200). Large molecular constructs, and especially micelles, should additionally withstand shear stress of the microvascular circulation (201). For example, it has been demonstrated that a significant amount of doxorubicin has leaked out of encapsulating micelles within a few hours after administration because of shear stress (200). These problems are only a few considerations that hinder the safety and efficacy of these therapies, but nonetheless, they must be reconciled before clinical application.

MECHANISMS OF FLUORESCENT LABELING OF BRAIN TUMORS

5-Aminolevulinic Acid

General Characteristics

5-ALA ($C_5H_9NO_3$, 131.13 Da), is an endogenous metabolite and a precursor for the biosynthesis of heme *in vivo* (**Figure 5A**). Under the action of intracellular enzymes in the heme biosynthetic pathway, 5-ALA is converted to an endogenous fluorophore, protoporphyrin IX (PpIX) (excitation: 405 nm; emission: 635 nm, with a minor emission peak at 710 nm). Intraoperatively, the blue excitation light contrasts well with the red fluorescence of PpIX, facilitating tumor margin delineation. 5-ALA was initially investigated for use in photodynamic therapy (202–205), whereby absorption of light by PpIX mediates the production of tumor-killing reactive oxygen species, but became a drug for improved visualization of high-grade gliomas during resection (206, 207) approved by the US Food and Drug Administration (FDA) (208). The mechanisms of 5-ALA passage through the BBTB (209) and intracellular metabolism (127, 210) have been previously reviewed in detail, so here we provide a brief summary of the key steps.

5-ALA Delivery Across the BBTB

The oral bioavailability of 5-ALA is around 60% in healthy subjects (127). Plasma half-life of 5-ALA after oral administration is about 45 min and plasma concentration approaches zero after about 6.5 h (211, 212). Experiments with radioactive 5-ALA in mice showed that 5-ALA does not penetrate an intact BBB but accumulates and undergoes conversion to PpIX in brain regions with a diminished BBB, such as the ependyma, choroid plexus, arcuate nucleus, and median eminence. (213, 214) PpIX visualization in high-grade gliomas correlates well with gadolinium-enhanced MRI (215), suggesting that the main mechanism of accumulation of PpIX in glioma is leakage of free 5-ALA through the altered BBTB. The lack of PpIX accumulation in low-grade gliomas is likely due to the presence of a more competent BBTB that prevents 5-ALA delivery and a lack of severe alterations in heme metabolism that would result in PpIX accumulation. So far, it is hard to elucidate which mechanism is most determinate of 5-ALA accumulation. Observed foci of fluorescence in low-grade gliomas were correlated with anaplastic transformation and increased cellularity (216, 217), which in turn may result in a less competent BBTB that is permeable to 5-ALA but not to gadolinium-based contrast.

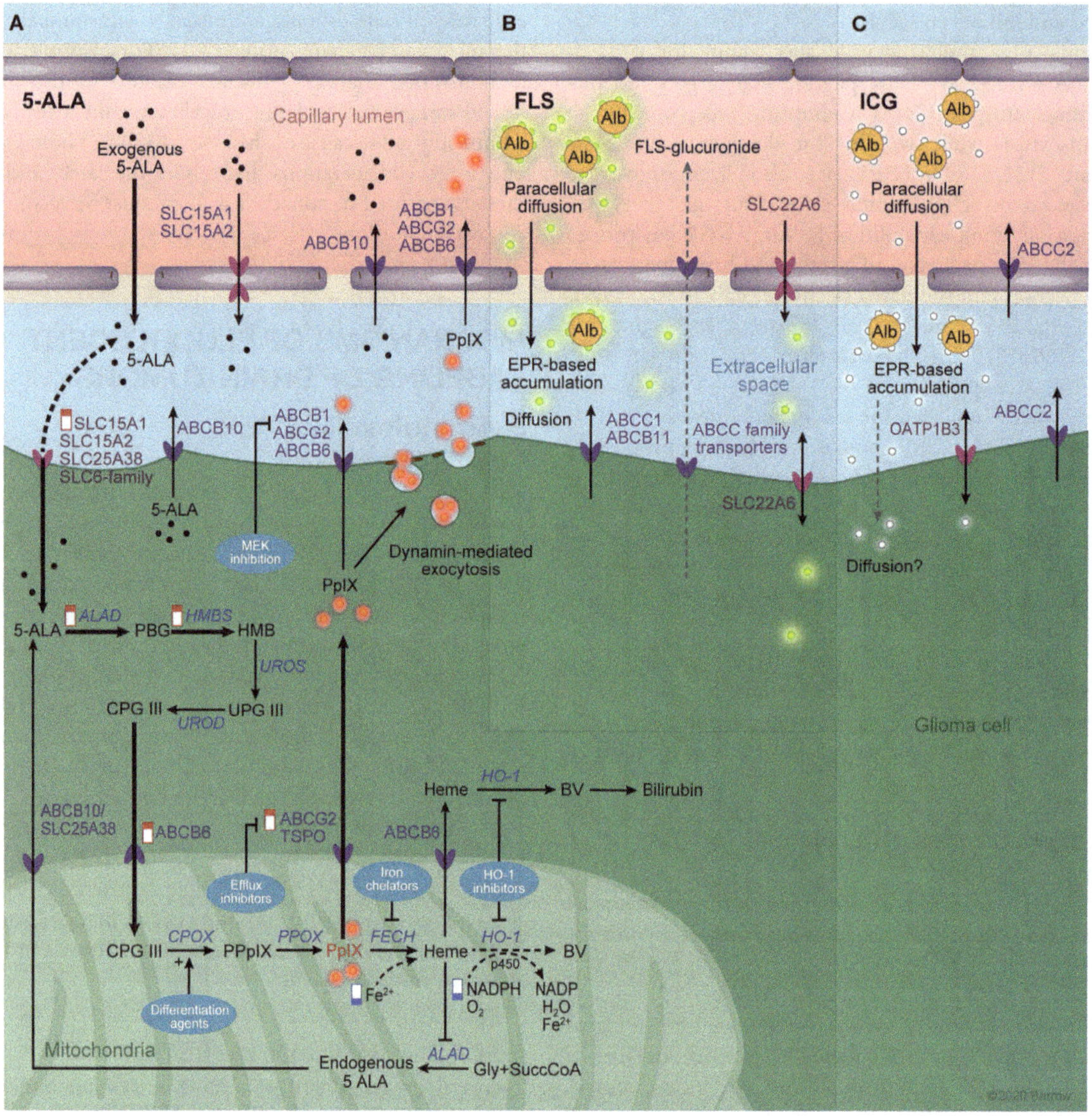

FIGURE 5 | Interaction between imaging agents and the blood-brain barrier. **(A)** The known transporters of 5-aminolevulinic acid (5-ALA) and protoporphyrin IX (PpIX) at the blood brain barrier and glioma cell membrane are shown schematically. The heme biosynthetic pathway is shown in the glioma cell cytoplasm and mitochondrial matrix. Alterations in the heme biosynthesis pathway responsible for increased PpIX accumulation in the tumor are indicated by "low" (blue) and "high" (red) signs. Thick arrows represent increased rate reactions after exogenous 5-ALA administration that contribute to the excess PpIX accumulation. Dotted arrows represent reduced rate reactions contributing to PpIX accumulation. Techniques for augmenting 5-ALA-mediated PpIX accumulation are shown in blue bubbles and include MEK inhibition, efflux inhibitors, differentiation agents, iron chelators, and heme oxygenase 1 inhibitors. **(B)** The known transporters of fluorescein and **(C)** indocyanine green are shown similarly. Active efflux pumps of the ATP-binding cassette family are depicted in dark violet and solute carrier family transporters in pink. Alb, albumin; ABC, ATP-binding cassette; ALAD, aminolevulinic acid dehydrogenase; BV, biliverdin; CPG III, coproporphyrinogen III; CPOX, CPG III oxidase; FECH, ferrochelatase; Gly, glycine; HO-1, Heme Oxygenase 1; HMB, hydroxymethylbilane; HMBS, HMB synthase; PBG, porphobilinogen; PpIX, protoporphyrinogen IX; PPOX, PpIX oxidase; SLC, solute carrier; SuccCoA, Succinyl Coenzyme A; UPG III, uroporphyrinogen III; UROD, UPG III decarboxylase; UROS, UPG III synthase. *Used with permission from Barrow Neurological Institute, Phoenix, Arizona*.

5-ALA Metabolism

Once inside the cell, 5-ALA enters the heme biosynthetic pathway, where it is converted sequentially to porphobilinogen, hydroxymethylbilane, uroporphyrinogen III, coproporphyrinogen III, protoporphyrinogen IX, PpIX, and heme (**Figure 5A**). Peak fluorescence intensity of PpIX in the tumor core is observed about 7 to 8 h after oral 5-ALA administration, while in the marginal tumor area the peak of weaker fluorescence is observed after about 8 to 9 h (218, 219).

In normal non-erythroid cells, heme biosynthesis is regulated by negative feedback mechanisms, mainly negative feedback of heme on the enzyme ALA synthase, controlling the intracellular levels of PpIX (220). In cancer cells, however, these systems are dysregulated, leading to PpIX accumulation and fluorescence. A recent examination of various human tumor samples suggests that the kinetics of PpIX accumulation are determined primarily by alterations in PpIX efflux, conversion of PpIX to heme, and PpIX biosynthesis (221). Interestingly, fluorescence was not shown to be dependent on the rate of 5-ALA uptake (221).

Heterogeneity in tumor cell signaling, protein expression, and metabolism are responsible for variations in PpIX accumulation. In this way, differential expression of transporters for elements of the heme biosynthetic pathway at the BBTB or tumor cell membrane is a source of modulation of the accumulation of PpIX. Notably, 5-ALA is a substrate of SLC15A1 and SLC15A2 (222), SLC36A1 (223), SLC6A6 and SLC6A13 (224), and ABCB10 (210), while PpIX is a substrate of ABCB6, ABCG2 (225) and ABCB1 (126). Of these, SLC15A1, SLC15A2, ABCB10, ABCB1, ABCG2, and ABCB6 are known to be expressed at the BBB (226), and therefore likely influence levels of PpIX accumulation. Kitajima et al. (227) showed that dynamin 2-mediated exocytosis plays a role in PpIX efflux from cancer cell lines in the JFCR39 panel, which includes six brain tumor lines. Interestingly, they failed to show a correlation between ABCG2 expression levels and PpIX efflux, although ABCG2 inhibition led to enhanced PpIX accumulation. This is in contrast to previous results by Hagiya et al. (228) that showed ABCG2 expression to be a major determinant of PpIX fluorescence in gastric cancer cell lines *in vitro*.

PpIX Excretion

PpIX may be converted to heme in mitochondria via the action of ferrochelatase or may be subject to active efflux from the cell by the ABCG2 efflux pump. Once in the blood, the plasma half-life of PpIX is around 8 h (229). If not further metabolized to heme, PpIX is taken up and excreted into bile by the liver (210).

Approaches to Augment PpIX Accumulation

The complex metabolism and transport of PpIX precursors create opportunities for the pharmacologic augmentation of PpIX accumulation in tumors that bear relevance for photodiagnostic and photodynamic applications of PpIX. At least five mechanisms have been identified (**Figure 5A**).

Mitogen-Activated Protein Kinase Kinase (MEK) inhibition

Yoshioka et al. (126) demonstrated enhancement of PpIX accumulation in a murine mammary tumor model via the inhibition of oncogenic Ras/MEK. MEK inhibition decreased expression of the ABCB1 efflux pump and reduced activity of ferrochelatase, the enzyme responsible for converting PpIX to non-fluorescent heme. Importantly, these changes were not observed in normal tissues, highlighting a targetable difference in regulatory mechanisms for heme biosynthesis between tumor and normal cells.

Efflux inhibition

Efflux pump inhibition relies on the principle that a known set of targetable transporters are responsible for the efflux of PpIX or its precursors from the brain or tumor tissues (**Figure 4C**). Kawai et al. (230) demonstrated that expression of the efflux pump ABCG2 was associated with a cancer stem cell phenotype and decreased 5-ALA fluorescence in a human pancreatic cancer cell line. Studies in peripheral tumors (127, 128) and with tumor cells *in vitro* (129, 130) share these results, showing an increase in 5-ALA-mediated PpIX accumulation in tumor tissue when combined with ABCG2 inhibitors. However, these studies do not necessarily account for the added heterogeneity of transporter expression at the BBB or within tumors *in vivo*.

Iron chelators

Augmentation of PpIX fluorescence by ferrochelatase inhibition using iron chelators has been demonstrated *in vitro* in glioma cell cultures (131–133). Wang et al. (134) showed that glioma stem cell escape from PpIX fluorescence could be overcome with the use of iron chelation to inhibit ferrochelatase, but not with administration of an ABCG2 inhibitor. In fact, contrary to the abovementioned reports, ABCG2 inhibition was shown to slightly decrease PpIX accumulation in these cells. The authors suggest that these results are likely due to the off-target inhibition of ABCB6, required for trafficking of coproporphyrinogen III across the mitochondrial membrane, leading to decreased PpIX synthesis overall. These results emphasize the importance of targeting specific transporters if efflux inhibition is to be employed and also raise questions about the viability of this approach in all tumors.

Differentiation agents

Differentiation therapy (calcitriol, vitamin E) has been shown to increase the cytotoxic effects of 5-ALA-mediated photodynamic therapy via upregulation of coproporphyrinogen oxidase in epithelial cancers (135, 137). Calcitriol was also shown to enhance 5-ALA-induced fluorescence and photodynamic therapy in human glioma cells *in vitro* (136).

Heme oxygenase 1 (HO-1) inhibition

Inhibition of HO-1 has also been shown to increase PpIX accumulation in melanoma (138). This strategy has the added benefit of disabling the cytoprotective and anti-inflammatory properties of HO-1, making tumor cells more prone to lysis by oxidative stress (139).

Opportunities and Limitations of 5-ALA Augmentation

Overall, the intricacy of cell-signaling pathways and transporter expression that governs heme biosynthesis complicates PpIX-based fluorescence visualization. Notably, elements of the heme biosynthetic pathway are substrates of a diverse set of transporters that modulate their intracellular accumulation. Furthermore, heme biosynthetic enzymes are often aberrantly expressed or active in tumor cells, hampering the reliable prediction of PpIX fluorescence status. For example, Lai et al. (231) demonstrated that selective inhibition of SLC15A1 and SLC36A1 expressed in normal but not cancerous lung and prostate cell lines allowed for augmentation of PpIX accumulation in tumor cells. This approach may actually hinder PpIX accumulation in glioma, though, as SLC15A1 is expressed at the BBB and may mediate 5-ALA accumulation in the brain (231). Nevertheless, the general approach of inhibiting transporters selectively expressed in normal cells versus tumor cells may still prove useful to augment tumor-selective accumulation of PpIX.

The described approaches provide tools for control of the selective augmentation of PpIX fluorescence in tumor cells. While these results remain to be evaluated amidst the added complexity of the BBB and BBTB in humans, they support the viability of pharmacological strategies to enhance PpIX fluorescence. Further research may one day see the ultimate translation of these approaches to the operating room, where they can help to augment the sensitivity and utility of 5-ALA-guided brain tumor resection.

Fluorescein Sodium

General Characteristics

FLS ($C_{20}H_{10}Na_2O_5$, 376.5 Da) is a yellow-green fluorescent dye (excitation 460–490 nm, emission 510–530 nm) (232) whose derivatives, such as FITC and Alexa 488, are used widely in research. The LD_{50} of IV FLS is 300 mg/kg in rabbits (233). FLS-guided resection of high-grade glioma was successful in a recent Phase II clinical trial ($n = 46$ patients) (234) and in a prospective observational study ($n = 279$ patients) (78), indicating its clinical applicability. FLS has also been used as a contrast for intraoperative assessment of tissue microstructure using confocal laser endomicroscopy (235, 236).

Pharmacokinetics

After IV administration, FLS weakly binds to serum albumin and rapidly distributes throughout the central circulation. FLS has a volume of distribution of 0.5 L/kg (237), indicating an even distribution between blood and interstitial spaces. FLS exists in the circulation in both a free unbound fraction and a serum-protein bound fraction. The small size of unbound FLS allows for rapid diffusion into the tumor due to first-pass extravasation, creating a large early peak in tumor fluorescence (**Figure 5B**). In contrast, the larger effective diameter of protein-bound FLS leads to a later smaller peak that is facilitated by the EPR effect. The unbound fraction of FLS only minimally crosses the intact BBB when administered in high doses (95) but is not readily detected within the normal brain using the operative microscope at the time of surgery. Unspecific leakage of unbound FLS through a heterogeneous and dynamic BBB/BBTB explains reports of unspecific FLS staining in peritumoral areas (238). Compared to unbound FLS, a PEGylated form of FLS with a molecular weight similar to that of gadolinium-based contrast agents (939 Da) showed improved specificity of accumulation in U251 orthotopic mouse gliomas 1 h after administration (95). An albumin-bound formulation of 5-aminofluorescein (66,950 Da) was investigated in a Phase I/II study in Germany (96, 97), where bright fluorescence was observed in 10 of 10 patients with high-grade gliomas 0.5 to 4 days after IV administration. These results highlight the utility of the EPR effect for prolonging the fluorescent staining window for small non-targeted molecules.

Optimal FLS Timing and Dosage

Increasing the dose of FLS (5 vs. 20 mg/kg human equivalent) results in an increase in unbound FLS in the blood and normal brain tissue (95). Therefore, the dose and timing of FLS administration should be considered to optimize fluorescent contrast during surgery. Thus far, the optimal strategy is to use lower doses of FLS [1–2 mg/kg (239), 3 mg/kg (240), and 5 mg/kg (234)] to minimize unspecific extravasation and to administer FLS 2 to 4 h before visualization, which corresponds to the wash-out period of the FLS from the normal brain (78).

FLS and BBTB Heterogeneity

FLS tends to accumulate in extravascular spaces and not within tumor cells. Accordingly, FLS-defined high-grade glioma margins correlate well with gadolinium-based MRI results (240). Reports on the use of FLS for the visualization of brain metastases demonstrated that the majority of them were fluorescent [90/95 (95%) (241) and 16/17 (94%) (242)]. However, surrounding normal brain also showed a low degree of fluorescence (241). Data on FLS efficacy in low- and intermediate-grade gliomas show that about half of tumors are not labeled with FLS, likely because the BBTB is not sufficiently disrupted (243). However, some non-gadolinium-enhancing gliomas can still be labeled with FLS (244, 245). These findings support the hypothesis that the unbound, low-molecular-weight fraction of FLS plays an important role in labeling tumors with minimally disrupted BBTB. Such tumors and peritumoral brain regions may allow extravasation or convection-based transport of the smaller unbound FLS molecules but not gadolinium-based contrast. Thus, a balance must be struck between dosing that creates an increased proportion of unbound FLS that is more likely to unspecifically stain normal brain but more readily stain marginal tumor and dosing in which a smaller dose of free and protein-bound FLS promotes EPR-based labeling of the tumor core but less labeling of the surrounding normal brain.

Potential Molecular Transporters and Clearance of FLS

Molecular transporters may also play a role in FLS pharmacokinetics. In the liver, FLS is conjugated to glucuronide before being excreted in the urine. FLS has a plasma half-life of 23.5 min, while minimally fluorescent FLS-glucuronide has a plasma half-life of 264 min (237). The small size and relative lipophilicity of FLS may allow for greater BBB permeability compared to ICG or gadolinium-based agents, but the activity of certain transporters at the BBB or BBTB may limit unaided extravasation. FLS is a substrate for the SLC22A6 transporter (237), the bile salt export pump, ABCB11 (246), and multidrug resistance-associated protein 1 (ABCC1) (247). Notably, SLC22A6 is involved in drug clearance from the CSF (248) and is expressed at low levels in CNS endothelium (226), and ABCC1 is expressed at the BBB (25). FLS-glucuronide is also likely a substrate of other members of the ABCC-subfamily of multidrug resistance proteins that are responsible for transporting conjugated metabolites (249), although, to our knowledge, this has not been shown. As such, these transporters likely alter the BBB permeability of unbound FLS.

Indocyanine Green

General Characteristics

ICG ($C_{43}H_{47}N_2NaO_6S_2$, 774.96 Da) is a water soluble, unstable [half-life in aqueous solution is 20 h (250)], amphiphilic fluorescent dye. The LD_{50} of IV ICG is 50 to 75 mg/kg

(251). After IV injection, ICG rapidly binds to plasma proteins and is distributed throughout the circulation with a volume of distribution of 0.035 L/kg (252), reflecting a high degree of plasma protein binding (140). The excitation and emission maximums of bound ICG exist in the near-infrared range (805 and 830 nm, respectively) thus enabling greater tissue penetration than markers that fluoresce in the visible range (253, 254).

Pharmacokinetics

ICG binding with plasma proteins increases the brightness of ICG fluorescence nearly 3-fold. Although it was initially thought that IV-injected ICG binds to albumin (255), later studies of blood samples following IV ICG injection suggested that ICG binds more intensely to high density lipoproteins (175–360 kDa, 7–14 nm) and moderately to low-density lipoproteins (256, 257). The larger size of bound ICG and the fact that, unlike FLS, ICG is almost completely bound to plasma proteins are important considerations for understanding the transport of ICG across the BBTB (**Figure 5C**).

Bound ICG gradually traverses the incompetent BBTB and accumulates in brain tumors such as high-grade gliomas and meningiomas, primarily due to the EPR effect (258). The timing of ICG accumulation in the tumor and optimal dosing of ICG was the subject of animal and human studies that could be grouped into three categories based on the imaging time: imaging immediately after ICG injection, delayed imaging within a few hours after injection, and imaging within a day after injection, termed the second-window ICG (251, 259, 260).

A study by Haglund et al. (251) investigated ICG in low- and high-grade gliomas using a charge-coupled device camera attached to a standard operating microscope within the first 10 min after IV ICG administration at 1 mg/kg. They observed progressively increased ICG signal within 10 min of recording in a high-grade glioma.

A study by Charalampaki et al. (261) demonstrated ICG accumulation in high-grade gliomas and meningiomas 1 h after IV injection of 50 mg ICG (<1 mg/kg). They used a commercially available operating microscope with a near-infrared imaging mode (ARveo Glow800, Leica microsystems, Wetzlar, Germany). In a study by Eyüpoglu et al. (262), 5 mg/kg ICG was administered intravenously at the end of high-grade glioma resection. Using this technique and a standard operating microscope (OPMI Pentero, Carl Zeiss AG, Oberkochen, Germany) the authors were able to highlight PpIX-negative, hypervascularized transitional tumor zone (262).

Several studies (98–102) assessed high-dose ICG (5 mg/kg administered IV over 1 h, 24 h prior to surgery) with a dedicated commercial near-infrared exoscope/endoscope imaging system (Iridium, VisionSense, Medtronic, Dublin, Republic of Ireland) in various brain tumors to take advantage of EPR-based drug accumulation.

ICG and BBTB Heterogeneity

It is worth noting that in all three ICG-based tumor-imaging methods described, high-grade gliomas were efficiently labeled with ICG. In low-grade gliomas, fluorescence intensity returned to the baseline within 5 min after a slight delay in clearance compared to the adjacent normal brain (251). Extravascular ICG in the tumor region does not specifically bind to brain tumor cells; however, it does penetrate certain cells, creating cytoplasmic contrast for confocal imaging and histopathologic tissue analysis (261, 263).

Potential Molecular Transporters and Clearance of ICG

ICG is rapidly and exclusively cleared by the liver. There is evidence in animal models that ICG clearance proceeds in a biphasic method, with an initial phase of rapid clearance resulting in a half-life of 2 to 4 min and a secondary phase with a half-life of more than an hour at low concentrations (264–266). Uptake into hepatocytes and excretion into bile is mediated by two members of the ABC transporter family: the canalicular multispecific organic anion transporter 1 (ABCC2) and the bile salt export pump (ABCB11) (267, 268).

There is also evidence that ICG-uptake is enhanced in peripheral hepatocellular carcinoma cells expressing organic anion transporting polypeptide 1B3 (SLCO1B3), a member of the SLC family of membrane transporters (269). Importantly, ABCC2 is expressed at the BBB (27), and so may mediate the active efflux of ICG. While SLCO1B3 and ABCB11 are not significantly expressed at the BBB, their aberrant expression in tumor cells would likely modulate the dynamics of ICG-staining, warranting investigation of their expression if ICG visualization is to be used.

OPTIMIZING DELIVERY OF OPTICAL AGENTS TO BRAIN TUMORS ACROSS THE BBB AND BBTB

Various fluorophores, including currently approved ICG and FLS, could be conjugated to other molecules or packed in molecular vehicles with two main goals: first, to improve tumor-to-normal brain contrast by increasing delivery efficiency compared to a fluorophore alone and, second, to improve the specificity of delivery by including targeting mechanisms. Here, we discuss the vehicles irrespective of the optical agent, assuming that criteria and considerations for optical agent selection are a completely separate issue mostly related to the detection methodology and tools. These optical considerations were reviewed previously (270–273). It is worth noting that any study of novel molecular vehicles, even for non-imaging purposes of brain tumor treatment, is relevant to the development of fluorescence-guided surgical technology and strategy because localization experiments are necessarily involved as part of the study. Among the available localization methods that include electron microscopy, radioactive tracers, and MRI, optical imaging methods and fluorescence microscopy are arguably among the most widely used and convenient approaches.

Creating Small-Size Molecules

Efforts in nanotechnology research have been directed toward creating molecules small enough to pass the BBB and BBTB. Even if a molecule is designed that may pass the ~6-nm pore restriction in healthy BBB endothelium, it is unlikely that such a nanoparticle could achieve targeted delivery to tumor cells, as the size restriction greatly limits targeting options. However, several nanoparticles that are <100 nm in size have shown good tumor penetration in solid orthotopic animal gliomas.

One potential solution to this problem is quantum dots (QDs). QDs are nanoscale semiconductor crystals that can be excited to emit fluorescence. A unique property of QDs is that their absorption and emission wavelengths are functions of both the size and shape of the QD, allowing for the tailoring of emission and absorption spectra for desired applications (274). Tang et al. (103) report the use of aptamer-conjugated PEGylated QDs (~20-nm size) for the fluorescent visualization of epidermal growth factor receptor (EGFR)-expressing glioma. In this study, QDs were conjugated to a deoxyribonucleic acid oligonucleotide aptamer designed to bind to EGFR variant III (EGFRvIII), which is known to be expressed specifically on glioma cells. The authors showed that the QD-aptamer probe was able to cross the BBTB to highlight tumor cells in an orthotopic mouse model *in vivo*. Whether a nanoparticle of this size could pass the competent portions of a BBTB to label invading tumor cells *in vivo* still needs to be investigated.

Although QDs represent a novel class of nanoscale, highly stable, fluorescent molecules that have been stably conjugated to antibodies, peptides, and small molecule drugs (275, 276), several issues related to QDs specifically have to be addressed for clinical translation. Namely, stability within the pH-range in normal and tumor tissues, biosafety, stability within the circulation and clearance by the reticuloendothelial system are all characteristics that must be evaluated before clinical application. Furthermore, some QDs are composed of heavy metals including cadmium, lead, or mercury, which raises biosafety questions. While such QDs have yet to be tested clinically, successful preclinical studies warrant their further investigation.

Enhancing EPR

Malignant tumors are notorious for disorganized and functionally abnormal vasculature that has sluggish blood flow, but which is a target for EPR optimization methods (142). The main strategies to improve permeability via EPR are directed toward dilating tumor vasculature, such as with nitric oxide-mediated vasodilation (angiotensin-converting-enzyme inhibitors, nitroglycerin, etc.), prostaglandin I2 agonists (105), tumor necrosis factor-a (106), or increasing systemic blood pressure by intraarterial administration of angiotensin II (107). The latter method improves tumor perfusion through unreactive tumor vessels that remain dilated while systemic vessels constrict and develop even tighter interendothelial connections. Such methods have commonalities with BBB disruption techniques and might be useful for enabling EPR through a relatively intact BBTB.

Increasing the molecular weight and size of a drug above 40 kDa by conjugating optical labels to targeting molecules or combining optical labels with large molecular vehicles would prolong drug circulation, increase the specificity of extravasation, and promote retention within high-grade gliomas and other tumors with severely disrupted BBTB for improved EPR-based drug delivery (277).

Xu et al. (104) developed silk fibroin nanoparticles loaded with ICG for imaging-guided photothermal therapy of orthotopic C6 glioma cells. Silk fibroin (200–350 kDa) is a biocompatible natural protein originating from silkworm cocoons. Conjugation with ICG created nanoparticles of about 200 nm in diameter, with improved EPR delivery in flank C6 gliomas, resulting in eight times higher intensity compared with free ICG injection 8 h after IV injection.

Nanoparticle delivery can enhance the circulation time and photostability of ICG (278) and offers a method for the specific targeting of ICG to tumor tissues. A drawback to this approach is limitation of drug delivery to the larger pores of the BBTB. Therefore, large molecules that are not targeted for transendothelial BBB or BBTB transport are unlikely to have better sensitivity in labeling glial tumors than already existing non-specific FLS, ICG, and metabolic 5-ALA.

Tumor Targeting Coupled With Passive BBTB Transport

Molecular probes are molecules that bind specifically to a second target molecule, allowing for the interrogation of the properties of that molecule. Recent experimental studies have developed fluorescent molecular probes for labeling glioma. In general, fluorescent molecular probes are made up of two components: a signaling component (label) and an affinity component. The signaling component is a contrast agent or marker, such as a radionuclide, luciferin, or a paramagnetic molecule, that can generate a detectable signal, while the affinity component is a targeting molecule, such as an oligonucleotide or antibody, that specifically binds to and labels a molecule of interest. Importantly, the affinity component of these molecules is customizable, allowing for the precise targeting of minute differences in protein or cell-surface marker expression in tumor cells, thus providing contrast between tumor and normal tissue. These probes can be additionally classified based on structure, binding affinity, or type of signaling component (279, 280). Fortunately, advances in genome sequencing have allowed for better characterization of the aberrant genetic environment of gliomas, uncovering potential probe targets. Thus, molecular probes may provide a highly targeted labeling technique for the fluorescence visualization of glioma.

Peptide-Based Labels

BLZ-100 or tozuleristide (4,766 Da) is a protein composed of chlorotoxin (CTX), a 36-residue neurotoxic peptide found in scorpion venom, conjugated to ICG. As a neurotoxin, CTX works to block small-conductance chloride channels, triggering internalization by endocytosis (281). CTX has been shown to selectively localize to gliomas via inhibitory binding of matrix metalloproteinase 2 that is frequently upregulated by glioma cells to facilitate tissue invasion (282). Thus, BLZ-100 is a high-affinity, targeted fluorescent probe that has shown specificity for glioma cells and is capable of near-infrared fluorescence, making it viable for applications of fluorescence-guided glioma resection. BLZ-100 has seen success in preclinical studies for resection of glioma (120), head and neck carcinoma (121), and soft-tissue sarcoma (122). Liposomes targeted with CTX were also tested in mouse glioblastoma (283). BLZ-100 has also passed a Phase I clinical trial, showing no toxicity for doses up to 30 mg (123). When administered in doses of >9 mg, BLZ-100 fluorescence was detected *ex vivo* or *in vivo* in 4 of 7 grade-2 gliomas and 4 of 4 grade-4 gliomas, demonstrating potential transport across the relatively competent BBTB in these tumors and optimism for sensitive and specific brain tumor labeling. Currently, BLZ-100 is undergoing a joint Phase II/III trial for fluorescence-guided resection of pediatric CNS tumors (NCT03579602).

Another fluorescent molecular probe that falls in this category is IRDye 800CW-cyclic-RGD. This probe employs a recognition motif containing a tripeptide sequence (Arg-Gly-Asp) that binds integrin receptors that are overexpressed on the tumor surface. Huang et al. (124) tested this near-infrared probe in three mouse glioblastoma models, including a transgenic glioblastoma mouse model (RCAS-PDGF-driven/tv-a glioblastoma), which mimics the infiltrative growth pattern of human glioblastomas and associated heterogeneity of the BBTB. In this model, the label demonstrated great delineation of tumor margin and tumor cells.

Affibody-Based Labels

Elliott et al. (108) reported on the simultaneous administration of an anti-EGFR affibody conjugated to a near-infrared fluorescent probe, named ABY-029 (7,914.95 Da), a marker of perfusion, IRDye680RD (927.13 Da), and 5-ALA, for the fluorescent visualization of F98 orthotopic gliomas in rats. All three labels were administered simultaneously, 3 h before imaging, thus relying on passive targeting and EPR mechanisms. The results of the study showed significant but complementary differences in staining patterns of the three markers. As measured by histological analysis, ABY-029 performed expectedly better in the visualization of EGFR-expressing tumors (91% accuracy, 80% overall accuracy), while 5-ALA performed better in the visualization of the tumor margins of non-EGFR-expressing tumors (87% accuracy, 84% overall accuracy). ABY-029 is currently undergoing a Phase I clinical trial for the fluorescent-guided resection of recurrent glioma (NCT02901925). We expect this affibody to have a good correlation with a gadolinium-based contrast imaging based on similar molecular weights and therefore expected similarity in crossing the BBTB.

Antibody-Based Labels

Martirosyan et al. (109) reported the use of an FITC-conjugated anti-EGFR antibody (~70,000 Da) for the identification of EGFR-expressing F98 tumor cells using confocal laser endomicroscopy in rats 24 h after IV administration of the FITC-conjugated antibodies. Warram et al. (110) investigated IRDye 800CW conjugated to an anti-EGFR antibody for fluorescence guidance in orthotopic mouse gliomas 3 days after IV administration. In both studies, EGFR-expressing tumor cells were readily visualized *in vivo*, confirming the viability of antibody-conjugated fluorescent tumor identification in the presence of a BBTB. While these studies are preclinical, there is significant potential for the application of this technique clinically for resection of high-grade glioma, but not for low-grade glioma, where the BBTB more closely resembles an intact BBB. Future applications of this technique may be as a part of a theranostic approach, whereby characterization of tumor protein expression guides the selection of appropriate antibodies for targeted fluorescence visualization.

Liposomal-Based Labels

Liposomes represent a class of highly modifiable nano- to micro-scale carriers that have a bi-lipid membrane. The size, composition of the lipid membrane, surface charge, mechanical properties, and anchoring of biologically active ligands can each be adjusted to optimize pharmacokinetics (141). Importantly, some liposome formulations are already FDA approved.

Jia et al. (125) investigated ICG-laden, biomimetic proteolipid liposomes (BLIPO-ICG, 104 ± 3 nm size) for the fluorescence-guided resection of C6 orthotopic mouse gliomas. These nanoparticles were infused with cell-surface proteins harvested from C6 glioma cells, enabling them to evade phagocytosis and to precisely target tumor cells via the homotypic interaction of surface proteins. Further, the authors were able to achieve complete surgical resection of tumors, guided by BLIPO-ICG and validated with histology. These results did not extend to resection guided by control nanoparticles without tumor-derived cell-surface markers, indicating that the cell-surface proteins contributed to greater tumor-specificity. Despite this, the invasiveness of C6 glioma cells in this study likely does not accurately replicate the invasiveness of high-grade human gliomas. As such, further testing is needed to evaluate the effectiveness of this nanoparticle beyond intact regions of BBTB and for further clinical applicability.

The design of fluorescent molecular probes for brain tumor visualization warrants consideration of the wide variation in structural characteristics of these molecules as they relate to interactions with the BBB. The barrier properties of the CNS endothelium severely restrict passive diffusion of molecules across the BBB, and transporters such as the neonatal Fc receptor and ABC-type efflux pumps work to actively remove antibodies and other large molecules from the brain. Absent any mechanisms for selective targeting of probes to tumor cells, accumulation via the EPR effect is likely not sufficient to stain high-grade brain tumor margins and low-grade gliomas, which are the main areas of difficulty for current fluorescent markers. As such, methods to functionalize markers for delivery across the BBB are warranted to ensure adequate BBB permeability and marker accuracy.

Functionalizing Particles for BBB Passage in Gliomas

Crucially, functionalization of nanoparticles can allow for effective extravasation despite an intact BBB, increasing the utility of fluorescence-guided glioma resection. Identifying a family of peptides with structural homology to the ligands that induce endothelial transcytosis is an important step to deliver drugs across the intact BBB and BBTB endothelium. ANG2, a member of the angiopep family of proteins, was identified to exhibit high transcytosis capacity via LRP-1 and is actively used for functionalization of various molecular vehicles that can carry therapeutic or diagnostic agents or both (112).

Hao et al. (113) demonstrated the efficacy of a combined chemo-phototherapy technique using ANG2-coated polylactide-co-glycolide (PLGA) nanoparticles loaded with ICG and the microtubule toxin docetaxel (DTX) (ANG2/PLGA/DTX/ICG probe) in a U87MG mouse orthotopic glioma model. Ni et al. (114) investigated an ANG2-targeted dual MRI-optical nanoprobe consisting of a fluorescent up-conversion nanoparticle loaded with gadolinium (ANG2/PEG-UCNP probe) in an orthotopic mouse glioblastoma model. The ANG2 coating facilitated the selective uptake of these labels across the BBB in both studies, as visualized by fluorescence imaging.

Ma et al. (115) described a fluorescent probe conjugated with TGN, a BBB targeting peptide selected from a library of phage display. In their experiments, TGN was conjugated with glioma targeting aptamer AS1411 and Cy3 orange fluorescent dye and showed some glioma cell-labeling capacity in an orthotopic C6 mouse glioma model.

These nanoparticles are examples of an extensively functionalized drug-delivery system, where a BBB-targeting motif potentially allows for better labeling of the marginal tumor zone. Unfortunately, all three studies were performed in orthotopic glioblastoma models that display disrupted BBTB, which might not fully represent the heterogeneous BBTB and especially its competent regions. The additional complexity of the probes raises further concerns about stability, toxicity, and clearance that have to be further investigated. Overall, functionalization of the labels with BBB-targeted molecules is a significant advance for trans-BBB drug delivery.

CONCLUSION

The optimal surgical treatment of invasive brain tumors requires accurate visualization of tumor margins to maximize cytoreductive resection within functionally safe borders. Optically guided brain tumor surgery is an intriguing method for improving resection and has seen a number of exciting advancements within the last few years. Despite the initial enthusiasm in some of these techniques, the diversity and heterogeneity of gliomas complicate the consistent and accurate labeling of all tumors and limit clinical success. These difficulties require visualization agents to cross the BBB or BBTB to reach target tumor tissues. Not only do these barriers physically limit passive diffusion of many therapeutics, but also the dynamic expression of a vast network of transporters and junctional proteins further complicates drug delivery to gliomas. Thus, the efficacy of labels for optically guided glioma surgery will vary depending on tumor- and patient-specific BBB and BBTB properties. In this review, we described the barrier properties of the CNS and gliomas and discussed a number of technologies that have potential in overcoming these barriers for better fluorescence-visualization of gliomas.

Many novel tumor-targeted labels that have a large molecular weight do not cross competent BBTB regions in low-grade gliomas. Given that these areas of competent BBB or BBTB are where currently used markers struggle, it is important that novel tumor labels address this impediment. Novel BBB disruption techniques could be used to improve brain tumor labeling using these labels. Alternative BBB-targeted drugs with optical imaging properties are promising new tools. While many of these technologies are still in the preclinical stages of development and, therefore, require additional time and development before they may be available clinically, these advances offer a number of solutions for BBB-mediated brain tumor labeling and therapy.

AUTHOR CONTRIBUTIONS

EB and CL: conception and design. KS, EB, VB, and CL: acquisition of data and drafting the article. All authors critically revised the article. All authors reviewed and edited the manuscript. LC and MP: supervision. All authors approved the final version of the manuscript.

ACKNOWLEDGMENTS

The authors thank the Neuroscience Publications staff at Barrow Neurological Institute for assistance with manuscript preparation.

REFERENCES

1. Ostrom QT, Cioffi G, Gittleman H, Patil N, Waite K, Kruchko C, et al. CBTRUS statistical report: primary brain and other central nervous system tumors diagnosed in the United States in 2012-2016. *Neuro Oncol.* (2019) 21:v1–100. doi: 10.1093/neuonc/noz150
2. Taylor OG, Brzozowski JS, Skelding KA. Glioblastoma multiforme: an overview of emerging therapeutic targets. *Front Oncol.* (2019) 9:963. doi: 10.3389/fonc.2019.00963
3. Deng Z, Yu H, Wang N, et al. Impact of preoperative Karnofsky Performance Scale (KPS) and American Society of Anesthesiologists (ASA) scores on perioperative complications in patients with recurrent glioma undergoing repeated operation. *J Neurorestoratol.* (2019) 7:143–52. doi: 10.26599/JNR.2019.9040015
4. Hervey-Jumper SL, Berger MS. Evidence for improving outcome through extent of resection. *Neurosurg Clin N Am.* (2019) 30:85–93. doi: 10.1016/j.nec.2018.08.005
5. Clark VE, Cahill DP. Extent of resection versus molecular classification: what matters when? *Neurosurg Clin N Am.* (2019) 30:95–101. doi: 10.1016/j.nec.2018.08.006
6. Lu VM, Goyal A, Graffeo CS, Perry A, Burns TC, Parney IF, et al. Survival benefit of maximal resection for glioblastoma reoperation in the temozolomide era: a meta-analysis. *World Neurosurg.* (2019) 127:31–7. doi: 10.1016/j.wneu.2019.03.250
7. Mampre D, Ehresman J, Pinilla-Monsalve G, Osorio MAG, Olivi A, Quinones-Hinojosa A, et al. Extending the resection beyond the contrast-enhancement for glioblastoma: feasibility, efficacy, and outcomes. *Br J Neurosurg.* (2018) 32:528–35. doi: 10.1080/02688697.2018.1498450
8. DeLong JC, Hoffman RM, Bouvet M. Current status and future perspectives of fluorescence-guided surgery for cancer. *Expert Rev Anticancer Ther.* (2016) 16:71–81. doi: 10.1586/14737140.2016.1121109
9. Gandhi S, Tayebi Meybodi A, Belykh E, Cavallo C, Zhao X, Syed MP, et al. Survival outcomes among patients with high-grade glioma treated with 5-aminolevulinic acid-guided surgery: a systematic review and meta-analysis. *Front Oncol.* (2019) 9:620. doi: 10.3389/fonc.2019.00620
10. Nduom EK, Yang C, Merrill MJ, Zhuang Z, Lonser RR. Characterization of

the blood-brain barrier of metastatic and primary malignant neoplasms. *J Neurosurg.* (2013) 119:427–33. doi: 10.3171/2013.3.JNS122226
11. Stewart DJ. A critique of the role of the blood-brain barrier in the chemotherapy of human brain tumors. *J Neuro Oncol.* (1994) 20:121–39. doi: 10.1007/BF01052723
12. Colditz MJ, Leyen Kv, Jeffree RL. Aminolevulinic acid (ALA)–protoporphyrin IX fluorescence guided tumour resection. Part 2: theoretical, biochemical and practical aspects. *J Clin Neurosci.* (2012) 19:1611–6. doi: 10.1016/j.jocn.2012.03.013
13. Roberts DW, Valdés PA, Harris BT, Hartov A, Fan X, Ji S, et al. Glioblastoma multiforme treatment with clinical trials for surgical resection (aminolevulinic acid). *Neurosurg Clin North Am.* (2012) 23:371–7. doi: 10.1016/j.nec.2012.04.001
14. Kutuzov N, Flyvbjerg H, Lauritzen M. Contributions of the glycocalyx, endothelium, and extravascular compartment to the blood-brain barrier. *Proc Natl Acad Sci USA.* (2018) 115:E9429–38. doi: 10.1073/pnas.1802155115
15. Ando Y, Okada H, Takemura G, Suzuki K, Takada C, Tomita H, et al. Brain-specific ultrastructure of capillary endothelial glycocalyx and its possible contribution for blood brain barrier. *Sci Rep.* (2018) 8:17523. doi: 10.1038/s41598-018-35976-2
16. Reitsma S, Slaaf DW, Vink H, van Zandvoort MA, oude Egbrink MG. The endothelial glycocalyx: composition, functions, and visualization. *Pflugers Archiv Eur J Physiol.* (2007) 454:345–59. doi: 10.1007/s00424-007-0212-8
17. Haeren RH, van de Ven SE, van Zandvoort MA, Vink H, van Overbeeke JJ, Hoogland G, et al. Assessment and imaging of the cerebrovascular glycocalyx. *Curr Neurovasc Res.* (2016) 13:249–60. doi: 10.2174/1567202613666160504104434
18. Sweeney MD, Sagare AP, Zlokovic BV. Blood–brain barrier breakdown in Alzheimer disease and other neurodegenerative disorders. *Nat Rev Neurol.* (2018) 14:133–50. doi: 10.1038/nrneurol.2017.188
19. Tietz S, Engelhardt B. Brain barriers: crosstalk between complex tight junctions and adherens junctions. *J Cell Biol.* (2015) 209:493–506. doi: 10.1083/jcb.201412147
20. Pardridge WM. The blood-brain barrier: bottleneck in brain drug development. *NeuroRX.* (2005) 2:3–14. doi: 10.1602/neurorx.2.1.3
21. Banks WA. From blood-brain barrier to blood-brain interface: new opportunities for CNS drug delivery. *Na Rev Drug Discov.* (2016) 15:275–92. doi: 10.1038/nrd.2015.21
22. Hitchcock SA, Pennington LD. Structure-brain exposure relationships. *J Med Chem.* (2006) 49:7559–83. doi: 10.1021/jm060642i
23. Hediger MA, Clémençon B, Burrier RE, Bruford EA. The ABCs of membrane transporters in health and disease (SLC series): introduction. *Mol Aspects Med.* (2013) 34:95–107. doi: 10.1016/j.mam.2012.12.009
24. Pardridge WM. Blood–brain barrier endogenous transporters as therapeutic targets: a new model for small molecule CNS drug discovery. *Expert Opin Ther Targets.* (2015) 19:1059–72. doi: 10.1517/14728222.2015.1042364
25. Zhao Z, Nelson AR, Betsholtz C, Zlokovic BV. Establishment and dysfunction of the blood-brain barrier. *Cell.* (2015) 163:1064–78. doi: 10.1016/j.cell.2015.10.067
26. Chen Z, Shi T, Zhang L, Zhu P, Deng M, Huang C, et al. Mammalian drug efflux transporters of the ATP binding cassette (ABC) family in multidrug resistance: a review of the past decade. *Cancer Lett.* (2016) 370:153–64. doi: 10.1016/j.canlet.2015.10.010
27. Löscher W, Potschka H. Blood-brain barrier active efflux transporters: ATP-binding cassette gene family. *NeuroRX.* (2005) 2:86–98. doi: 10.1602/neurorx.2.1.86
28. Mahringer A, Fricker G. ABC transporters at the blood–brain barrier. *Expert Opin Drug Metab Toxicoly.* (2016) 12:499–508. doi: 10.1517/17425255.2016.1168804
29. Zhang Y, Pardridge WM. Rapid transferrin efflux from brain to blood across the blood-brain barrier. *J Neurochem.* (2001) 76:1597–600. doi: 10.1046/j.1471-4159.2001.00222.x
30. Schlachetzki F, Zhu C, Pardridge WM. Expression of the neonatal Fc receptor (FcRn) at the blood-brain barrier. *J Neurochem.* (2002) 81:203–6. doi: 10.1046/j.1471-4159.2002.00840.x
31. Zhang Y, Pardridge WM. Mediated efflux of IgG molecules from brain to blood across the blood–brain barrier. *J Neuroimmunol.* (2001) 114:168–72. doi: 10.1016/S0165-5728(01)00242-9
32. Dore-Duffy P. Pericytes: pluripotent cells of the blood brain barrier. *Curr Pharm Design.* (2008) 14:1581–93. doi: 10.2174/138161208784705469
33. Mathiisen TM, Lehre KP, Danbolt NC, Ottersen OP. The perivascular astroglial sheath provides a complete covering of the brain microvessels: an electron microscopic 3D reconstruction. *GLIA.* (2010) 58:1094–103. doi: 10.1002/glia.20990
34. Abbott NJ, Rönnbäck L, Hansson E. Astrocyte–endothelial interactions at the blood–brain barrier. *Nat Rev Neurosci.* (2006) 7:41–53. doi: 10.1038/nrn1824
35. Alvarez JI, Katayama T, Prat A. Glial influence on the blood brain barrier. *GLIA.* (2013) 61:1939–58. doi: 10.1002/glia.22575
36. Armulik A, Genové G, Mäe M, Nisancioglu MH, Wallgard E, Niaudet C, et al. Pericytes regulate the blood–brain barrier. *Nature.* (2010) 468:557–61. doi: 10.1038/nature09522
37. Banerjee S, Bhat MA. Neuron-glial interactions in blood-brain barrier formation. *Annu Rev Neurosci.* (2007) 30:235–58. doi: 10.1146/annurev.neuro.30.051606.094345
38. Bauer H-C, Krizbai IA, Bauer H, Traweger A. "You Shall Not Pass" - tight junctions of the blood brain barrier. *Front Neurosci.* (2014) 8:392. doi: 10.3389/fnins.2014.00392
39. Daneman R, Zhou L, Kebede AA, Barres BA. Pericytes are required for blood–brain barrier integrity during embryogenesis. *Nature.* (2010) 468:562–6. doi: 10.1038/nature09513
40. Obermeier B, Daneman R, Ransohoff RM. Development, maintenance and disruption of the blood-brain barrier. *Nat Med.* (2013) 19:1584–96. doi: 10.1038/nm.3407
41. Daneman R, Prat A. The Blood–Brain Barrier. *Cold Spring Harbor Perspect Biol.* (2015) 7:a020412. doi: 10.1101/cshperspect.a020412
42. Komarova YA, Kruse K, Mehta D, Malik AB. Protein interactions at endothelial junctions and signaling mechanisms regulating endothelial permeability. *Circ Res.* (2017) 120:179–206. doi: 10.1161/CIRCRESAHA.116.306534
43. Luissint AC, Artus C, Glacial F, Ganeshamoorthy K, Couraud PO. Tight junctions at the blood brain barrier: physiological architecture and disease-associated dysregulation. *Fluids Barriers CNS.* (2012) 9:23. doi: 10.1186/2045-8118-9-23
44. Reinhold AK, Rittner HL. Barrier function in the peripheral and central nervous system—a review. *Pflugers Archiv Eur J Physiol.* (2017) 469:123–34. doi: 10.1007/s00424-016-1920-8
45. Arvanitis CD, Ferraro GB, Jain RK. The blood–brain barrier and blood–tumour barrier in brain tumours and metastases. *Nat Rev Cancer.* (2019) 20:26–41. doi: 10.1038/s41568-019-0205-x
46. Hardee ME, Zagzag D. Mechanisms of glioma-associated neovascularization. *Am J Pathol.* (2012) 181:1126–41. doi: 10.1016/j.ajpath.2012.06.030
47. Plate KH, Scholz A, Dumont DJ. Tumor angiogenesis and anti-angiogenic therapy in malignant gliomas revisited. *Acta Neuropathol.* (2012) 124:763–75. doi: 10.1007/s00401-012-1066-5
48. Madden SL, Cook BP, Nacht M, Weber WD, Callahan MR, Jiang Y, et al. Vascular gene expression in nonneoplastic and malignant brain. *Am J Pathol.* (2004) 165:601–8. doi: 10.1016/S0002-9440(10)63324-X
49. Ningaraj NS, Rao M, Hashizume K, Asotra K, Black KL. Regulation of blood-brain tumor barrier permeability by calcium-activated potassium channels. *J Pharmacol Exp Ther.* (2002) 301:838–51. doi: 10.1124/jpet.301.3.838
50. Nishio S, Ohta M, Abe M, Kitamura K. Microvascular abnormalities in ethylnitrosourea (ENU)-induced rat brain tumors: structural basis for altered blood-brain barrier function. *Acta Neuropathol.* (1983) 59:1–10. doi: 10.1007/BF00690311
51. Phoenix TN, Patmore DM, Boop S, Boulos N, Jacus MO, Patel YT, et al. Medulloblastoma genotype dictates blood brain barrier phenotype. *Cancer Cell.* (2016) 29:508–22. doi: 10.1016/j.ccell.2016.03.002
52. Zhan C, Lu W. The blood-brain/tumor barriers: challenges and chances for malignant gliomas targeted drug delivery. *Curr Pharm Biotechnol.* (2012) 13:2380–7. doi: 10.2174/138920112803341798
53. Hobbs SK, Monsky WL, Yuan F, Roberts WG, Griffith L, Torchilin VP, et al. Regulation of transport pathways in tumor vessels: role of tumor type and microenvironment. *Proc Natl Acad Sci U.S.A.* (1998) 95:4607–12. doi: 10.1073/pnas.95.8.4607
54. Hoffmann A, Bredno J, Wendland M, Derugin N, Ohara P, Wintermark M. High and low molecular weight fluorescein isothiocyanate (fitc)–dextrans to

assess blood-brain barrier disruption: technical considerations. *Transl Stroke Res.* (2011) 2:106–11. doi: 10.1007/s12975-010-0049-x
55. Mayhan WG, Heistad DD. Permeability of blood-brain barrier to various sized molecules. *Am J Physiol Heart Circ Physiol.* (1985) 17:H712–8. doi: 10.1152/ajpheart.1985.248.5.H712
56. Natarajan R, Northrop N, Yamamoto B. Fluorescein isothiocyanate (FITC)-dextran extravasation as a measure of blood-brain barrier permeability. *Curr Protoc Neurosci.* (2017) 9.58.51-59.58.15. doi: 10.1002/cpns.25
57. Schmidt RF, Theofanis TN, Lang MJ, Stricsek GP, Lin R, Lebrun A, et al. Sphenopalatine ganglion stimulation is a reversible and frequency-dependent modulator of the blood-brain barrier. *Brain Res.* (2019) 1718:231–41. doi: 10.1016/j.brainres.2019.04.030
58. Yuan W, Lv Y, Zeng M, Fu BM. Non-invasive measurement of solute permeability in cerebral microvessels of the rat. *Microvasc Res.* (2009) 77:166–73. doi: 10.1016/j.mvr.2008.08.004
59. Sarin H, Kanevsky AS, Wu H, Brimacombe KR, Fung SH, Sousa AA, et al. Effective transvascular delivery of nanoparticles across the blood-brain tumor barrier into malignant glioma cells. *J Transl Med.* (2008) 6:80. doi: 10.1186/1479-5876-6-80
60. Firth JA. Endothelial barriers: from hypothetical pores to membrane proteins. *J Anat.* (2002) 200:541–8. doi: 10.1046/j.1469-7580.2002.00059.x
61. Aird WC. Phenotypic heterogeneity of the endothelium. *Circ Res.* (2007) 100:158–73. doi: 10.1161/01.RES.0000255691.76142.4a
62. Nir I, Levanon D, Iosilevsky G. Permeability of blood vessels in experimental gliomas: uptake of 99mTc-glucoheptonate and alteration in blood-brain barrier as determined by cytochemistry and electron microscopy. *Neurosurgery.* (1989) 25:523-31; discussion 531–22. doi: 10.1227/00006123-198910000-00004
63. Blasberg RG, Nakagawa H, Bourdon MA, Groothuis DR, Patlak CS, Bigner DD. Regional localization of a glioma-associated antigen defined by monoclonal antibody 81c6 *in vivo*: kinetics and implications for diagnosis and therapy. *Cancer Res.* (1987) 47:4432–43.
64. Groothuis DR. The blood-brain and blood-tumor barriers: A review of strategies for increasing drug delivery. *Neuro Oncol.* (2000) 2:45–59. doi: 10.1215/15228517-2-1-45
65. Schlageter KE, Molnar P, Lapin GD, Groothuis DR. Microvessel organization and structure in experimental brain tumors: microvessel populations with distinctive structural and functional properties. *Microvasc Res.* (1999) 58:312–28. doi: 10.1006/mvre.1999.2188
66. Machein MR, Kullmer J, Fiebich BL, Plate KH, Warnke PC. Vascular endothelial growth factor expression, vascular volume, and capillary permeability in human brain tumors. *Neurosurgery.* (1999) 44:732–40. doi: 10.1097/00006123-199904000-00022
67. Guo H, Kang H, Tong H, Du X, Liu H, Tan Y, et al. Microvascular characteristics of lower-grade diffuse gliomas: investigating vessel size imaging for differentiating grades and subtypes. *Eur Radiol.* (2019) 29:1893–902. doi: 10.1007/s00330-018-5738-y
68. Dhermain FG, Hau P, Lanfermann H, Jacobs AH, van den Bent MJ. Advanced MRI and PET imaging for assessment of treatment response in patients with gliomas. *Lancet Neurol.* (2010) 9:906–20. doi: 10.1016/S1474-4422(10)70181-2
69. Groothuis DR, Molnar P, Blasberg RG. Regional blood flow and blood-to-tissue transport in five brain tumor models. Implications for chemotherapy. *Prog Exp Tumor Res.* (1984) 27:132–53. doi: 10.1159/000408227
70. Wesseling P, van der Laak JA, de Leeuw H, Ruiter DJ, Burger PC. Quantitative immunohistological analysis of the microvasculature in untreated human glioblastoma multiforme. *J Neurosurg.* (1994) 81:902–9. doi: 10.3171/jns.1994.81.6.0902
71. Watkins S, Robel S, Kimbrough IF, Robert SM, Ellis-Davies G, Sontheimer H. Disruption of astrocyte-vascular coupling and the blood-brain barrier by invading glioma cells. *Nat Commun.* (2014) 5:1–15. doi: 10.1038/ncomms5196
72. Hambardzumyan D, Bergers G. Glioblastoma: defining tumor niches. *Trends Cancer.* (2015) 1:252–65. doi: 10.1016/j.trecan.2015.10.009
73. la Fougère C, Suchorska B, Bartenstein P, Kreth FW, Tonn JC. Molecular imaging of gliomas with PET: opportunities and limitations. *Neuro Oncol.* (2011) 13:806–19. doi: 10.1093/neuonc/nor054
74. Kushchayev SV, Sankar T, Eggink LL, Kushchayeva YS, Wiener PC, Hoober JK, et al. Monocyte galactose/N-acetylgalactosamine-specific C-type lectin receptor stimulant immunotherapy of an experimental glioma. Part II: combination with external radiation improves survival. *Cancer Manage Res.* (2012) 4:325–34. doi: 10.2147/CMAR.S33355
75. Kushchayev SV, Sankar T, Eggink LL, Kushchayeva YS, Wiener PC, Hoober JK, et al. Monocyte galactose/N-acetylgalactosamine-specific C-type lectin receptor stimulant immunotherapy of an experimental glioma. Part 1: stimulatory effects on blood monocytes and monocyte-derived cells of the brain. *Cancer Manage Res.* (2012) 4:309–23. doi: 10.2147/CMAR.S33248
76. Kushchayev SV, Kushchayeva YS, Wiener PC, Scheck AC, Badie B, Preul MC. Monocyte-derived cells of the brain and malignant gliomas: the double face of janus. *World Neurosurg.* (2014) 82:1171–86. doi: 10.1016/j.wneu.2012.11.059
77. Underwood JL, Murphy CG, Chen J, Franse-Carman L, Wood I, Epstein DL, et al. Glucocorticoids regulate transendothelial fluid flow resistance and formation of intercellular junctions. *Am J Physiol Cell Physiol.* (1999) 277:C330–42. doi: 10.1152/ajpcell.1999.277.2.C330
78. Falco J, Cavallo C, Vetrano IG, de Laurentis C, Siozos L, Schiariti M, et al. Fluorescein application in cranial and spinal tumors enhancing at preoperative mri and operated with a dedicated filter on the surgical microscope: preliminary results in 279 patients enrolled in the FLUOCERTUM prospective study. *Front Surg.* (2019) 6:49. doi: 10.3389/fsurg.2019.00049
79. Yuan F, Salehi HA, Boucher Y, Vasthare US, Tuma RF, Jain RK. Vascular permeability and microcirculation of gliomas and mammary carcinomas transplanted in rat and mouse cranial windows. *Cancer Res.* (1994) 54:4564–8.
80. Claes A, Idema AJ, Wesseling P. Diffuse glioma growth: a guerilla war. *Acta Neuropathol.* (2007) 114:443–58. doi: 10.1007/s00401-007-0293-7
81. Eidel O, Burth S, Neumann JO, Kieslich PJ, Sahm F, Jungk C, et al. Tumor infiltration in enhancing and non-enhancing parts of glioblastoma: a correlation with histopathology. *PLOS ONE.* (2017) 12:e0169292. doi: 10.1371/journal.pone.0169292
82. Dong X. Current strategies for brain drug delivery. *Theranostics.* (2018) 8:1481–93. doi: 10.7150/thno.21254
83. Ha D, Yang N, Nadithe V. Exosomes as therapeutic drug carriers and delivery vehicles across biological membranes: current perspectives and future challenges. *Acta Pharm Sin B.* (2016) 6:287–96. doi: 10.1016/j.apsb.2016.02.001
84. Hendricks BK, Cohen-Gadol AA, Miller JC. Novel delivery methods bypassing the blood-brain and blood-tumor barriers. *Neurosurg Focus.* (2015) 38:E10. doi: 10.3171/2015.1.FOCUS14767
85. Juillerat-Jeanneret L. The targeted delivery of cancer drugs across the blood–brain barrier: chemical modifications of drugs or drug-nanoparticles? *Drug Discov Today.* (2008) 13:1099–106. doi: 10.1016/j.drudis.2008.09.005
86. Mäger I, Meyer AH, Li J, Lenter M, Hildebrandt T, Leparc G, et al. Targeting blood-brain-barrier transcytosis – perspectives for drug delivery. *Neuropharmacology.* (2017) 120:4–7. doi: 10.1016/j.neuropharm.2016.08.025
87. Pardridge WM. CSF, blood-brain barrier, and brain drug delivery. *Expert Opin Drug Deliv.* (2016) 13:963–75. doi: 10.1517/17425247.2016.1171315
88. Pardridge WM. Drug transport across the blood–brain barrier. *J Cereb Blood Flow Metab.* (2012) 32:1959–72. doi: 10.1038/jcbfm.2012.126
89. Parveen S, Misra R, Sahoo SK. Nanoparticles: a boon to drug delivery, therapeutics, diagnostics and imaging. *Nanomed Nanotechnol Biol Med.* (2012) 8:147–66. doi: 10.1016/j.nano.2011.05.016
90. Pulgar VM. Transcytosis to cross the blood brain barrier, new advancements and challenges. *Front Neurosci.* (2019) 12:1019. doi: 10.3389/fnins.2018.01019
91. van Tellingen O, Yetkin-Arik B, de Gooijer MC, Wesseling P, Wurdinger T, de Vries HE. Overcoming the blood–brain tumor barrier for effective glioblastoma treatment. *Drug Resist Updates.* (2015) 19:1–12. doi: 10.1016/j.drup.2015.02.002
92. Zhu Z, Kalyan BS, Chen L. Therapeutic potential role of exosomes for ischemic stroke. *Brain Sci Adv.* (2020) 5:128–43. doi: 10.1177/2096595820902588
93. Wang M, Kommidi H, Tosi U, Guo H, Zhou Z, Schweitzer ME, et al. A murine model for quantitative, real-time evaluation of convection-enhanced delivery (RT-CED) using an 18[F]-positron

emitting, fluorescent derivative of dasatinib. *Mol Cancer Ther.* (2017) 16:2902–12. doi: 10.1158/1535-7163.MCT-17-0423
94. Brachman DG, Youssef E, Dardis CJ, Sanai N, Zabramski JM, Smith KA, et al. Resection and permanent intracranial brachytherapy using modular, biocompatible cesium-131 implants: results in 20 recurrent, previously irradiated meningiomas. *J Neurosurg.* (2019) 2019:1–10. doi: 10.3171/2018.7.JNS18656
95. Folaron M, Strawbridge R, Samkoe KS, Filan C, Roberts DW, Davis SC. Elucidating the kinetics of sodium fluorescein for fluorescence-guided surgery of glioma. *J Neurosurg.* (2019) 131:724–34. doi: 10.3171/2018.4.JNS172644
96. Ding R, Frei E, Fardanesh M, Schrenk HH, Kremer P, Haefeli WE. Pharmacokinetics of 5-aminofluorescein-albumin, a novel fluorescence marker of brain tumors during surgery. *J Clin Pharmacol.* (2011) 51:672–8. doi: 10.1177/0091270010372626
97. Kremer P, Fardanesh M, Ding R, Pritsch M, Zoubaa S, Frei E. Intraoperative fluorescence staining of malignant brain tumors using 5-aminofluorescein-labeled albumin. *Oper Neurosurg.* (2009) 64:ons53–61. doi: 10.1227/01.NEU.0000335787.17029.67
98. Cho SS, Jeon J, Buch L, Nag S, Nasrallah M, Low PS, et al. Intraoperative near-infrared imaging with receptor-specific versus passive delivery of fluorescent agents in pituitary adenomas. *J Neurosurg.* (2018) 1:1–11. doi: 10.3171/2018.7.JNS181642
99. Jeon JW, Cho SS, Nag S, Buch L, Pierce J, Su YS, et al. Near-Infrared Optical Contrast of Skull Base Tumors During Endoscopic Endonasal Surgery. *Oper Neurosurg.* (2019) 17:32–42. doi: 10.1093/ons/opy213
100. Lee JY, Thawani JP, Pierce J, Zeh R, Martinez-Lage M, Chanin M, et al. Intraoperative near-infrared optical imaging can localize gadolinium-enhancing gliomas during surgery. *Neurosurgery.* (2016) 79:856–71. doi: 10.1227/NEU.0000000000001450
101. Lee JYK, Pierce JT, Zeh R, Cho SS, Salinas R, Nie S, et al. Intraoperative near-infrared optical contrast can localize brain metastases. *World Neurosurg.* (2017) 106:120–30. doi: 10.1016/j.wneu.2017.06.128
102. Lee JYK, Pierce JT, Thawani JP, Zeh R, Nie S, Martinez-Lage M, et al. Near-infrared fluorescent image-guided surgery for intracranial meningioma. *J Neurosurg.* (2018) 128:380–90. doi: 10.3171/2016.10.JNS161636
103. Tang J, Huang N, Zhang X, Zhou T, Tan Y, Pi J, et al. Aptamer-conjugated PEGylated quantum dots targeting epidermal growth factor receptor variant III for fluorescence imaging of glioma. *Int J Nanomedicine.* (2017) 12:3899–911. doi: 10.2147/IJN.S133166
104. Xu HL, ZhuGe DL, Chen PP, Tong MQ, Lin MT, Jiang X, et al. Silk fibroin nanoparticles dyeing indocyanine green for imaging-guided photo-thermal therapy of glioblastoma. *Drug Deliv.* (2018) 25:364–75. doi: 10.1080/10717544.2018.1428244
105. Tanaka S, Akaike T, Wu J, Fang J, Sawa T, Ogawa M, et al. Modulation of tumor-selective vascular blood flow and extravasation by the stable prostaglandin 12 analogue beraprost sodium. *J Drug Target.* (2003) 11:45–52. doi: 10.1080/1061186031000086072
106. Seki T, Carroll F, Illingworth S, Green N, Cawood R, Bachtarzi H, et al. Tumour necrosis factor-alpha increases extravasation of virus particles into tumour tissue by activating the Rho A/Rho kinase pathway. *J Controlled Release.* (2011) 156:381–9. doi: 10.1016/j.jconrel.2011.08.022
107. Nagamitsu A, Greish K, Maeda H. Elevating blood pressure as a strategy to increase tumor-targeted delivery of macromolecular drug SMANCS: cases of advanced solid tumors. *Jpn J Clin Oncol.* (2009) 39:756–66. doi: 10.1093/jjco/hyp074
108. Elliott JT, Marra K, Evans LT, Davis SC, Samkoe KS, Feldwisch J, et al. Simultaneous *in vivo* fluorescent markers for perfusion, protoporphyrin metabolism, and EGFR expression for optically guided identification of orthotopic glioma. *Clin Cancer Res.* (2017) 23:2203–12. doi: 10.1158/1078-0432.CCR-16-1400
109. Martirosyan NL, Georges J, Kalani MY, Nakaji P, Spetzler RF, Feuerstein BG, et al. Handheld confocal laser endomicroscopic imaging utilizing tumor-specific fluorescent labeling to identify experimental glioma cells *in vivo*. *Surg Neurol Int.* (2016) 7:995. doi: 10.4103/2152-7806.195577
110. Warram JM, de Boer E, Korb M, Hartman Y, Kovar J, Markert JM, et al. Fluorescence-guided resection of experimental malignant glioma using cetuximab-IRDye 800CW. *Br J Neurosurg.* (2015) 29:850–8. doi: 10.3109/02688697.2015.1056090
111. Demeule M, Currie JC, Bertrand Y, Ché C, Nguyen T, Régina A, et al. Involvement of the low-density lipoprotein receptor-related protein in the transcytosis of the brain delivery vector Angiopep-2. *J Neurochem.* (2008) 106:1534–44. doi: 10.1111/j.1471-4159.2008.05492.x
112. Demeule M, Régina A, Ché C, Poirier J, Nguyen T, Gabathuler R, et al. Identification and design of peptides as a new drug delivery system for the brain. *Jf Pharmacol Exp Ther.* (2008) 324:1064–72. doi: 10.1124/jpet.107.131318
113. Hao Y, Wang L, Zhao Y, Meng D, Li D, Li H, et al. Targeted imaging and chemo-phototherapy of brain cancer by a multifunctional drug delivery system. *Macromol Biosci.* (2015) 15:1571–85. doi: 10.1002/mabi.201500091
114. Ni D, Zhang J, Bu W, Xing H, Han F, Xiao Q, et al. Dual-targeting upconversion nanoprobes across the blood-brain barrier for magnetic resonance/fluorescence imaging of intracranial glioblastoma. *ACS Nano.* (2014) 8:1231–42. doi: 10.1021/nn406197c
115. Ma H, Gao Z, Yu P, Shen S, Liu Y, Xu B. A dual functional fluorescent probe for glioma imaging mediated by blood-brain barrier penetration and glioma cell targeting. *Biochem Biophys Res Commun.* (2014) 449:44–8. doi: 10.1016/j.bbrc.2014.04.148
116. Singh VK, Subudhi BB. Development and characterization of lysine-methotrexate conjugate for enhanced brain delivery. *Drug Deliv.* (2014) 23:1–11. doi: 10.3109/10717544.2014.984369
117. Peura L, Malmioja K, Huttunen K, Leppänen J, Hämäläinen M, Forsberg MM, et al. Design, synthesis and brain uptake of LAT1-targeted amino acid prodrugs of dopamine. *Pharm Res.* (2013) 30:2523–37. doi: 10.1007/s11095-012-0966-3
118. Rajora MA, Ding L, Valic M, Jiang W, Overchuk M, Chen J, et al. Tailored theranostic apolipoprotein E3 porphyrin-lipid nanoparticles target glioblastoma. *Chem Sci.* (2017) 8:5371–84. doi: 10.1039/C7SC00732A
119. Lam FC, Morton SW, Wyckoff J, Vu Han TL, Hwang MK, Maffa A, et al. Enhanced efficacy of combined temozolomide and bromodomain inhibitor therapy for gliomas using targeted nanoparticles. *Nat Commun.* (2018) 9:1991. doi: 10.1038/s41467-018-04315-4
120. Butte PV, Mamelak A, Parrish-Novak J, Drazin D, Shweikeh F, Gangalum PR, et al. Near-infrared imaging of brain tumors using the Tumor Paint BLZ-100 to achieve near-complete resection of brain tumors. *Neurosurg Focus.* (2014) 36:E1. doi: 10.3171/2013.11.FOCUS13497
121. Baik FM, Hansen S, Knoblaugh SE, Sahetya D, Mitchell RM, Xu C, et al. Fluorescence identification of head and neck squamous cell carcinoma and high-risk oral dysplasia with BLZ-100, a chlorotoxin-indocyanine green conjugate. *JAMA Otolaryngol Head Neck Surg.* (2016) 142:330. doi: 10.1001/jamaoto.2015.3617
122. Fidel J, Kennedy KC, Dernell WS, Hansen S, Wiss V, Stroud MR, et al. Preclinical validation of the utility of BLZ-100 in providing fluorescence contrast for imaging spontaneous solid tumors. *Cancer Res.* (2015) 75:4283–91. doi: 10.1158/0008-5472.CAN-15-0471
123. Patil CG, Walker DG, Miller DM, Butte P, Morrison B, Kittle DS, et al. Phase 1 Safety, pharmacokinetics, and fluorescence imaging study of tozuleristide (BLZ-100) in adults with newly diagnosed or recurrent gliomas. *Neurosurgery.* (2019) 2019:1–9. doi: 10.1093/neuros/nyz125
124. Huang R, Vider J, Kovar JL, Olive DM, Mellinghoff IK, Mayer-Kuckuk P, et al. Integrin αvβ3-targeted IRDye 800CW near-infrared imaging of glioblastoma. *Clin Cancer Res.* (2012) 18:5731–40. doi: 10.1158/1078-0432.CCR-12-0374
125. Jia Y, Wang X, Hu D, Wang P, Liu Q, Zhang X, et al. Phototheranostics: active targeting of orthotopic glioma using biomimetic proteolipid nanoparticles. *ACS Nano.* (2019) 13:386–98. doi: 10.1021/acsnano.8b06556
126. Yoshioka E, Chelakkot VS, Licursi M, Rutihinda SG, Som J, Derwish L, et al. Enhancement of cancer-specific protoporphyrin ix fluorescence by targeting oncogenic ras/MEK pathway. *Theranostics.* (2018) 8:2134–46. doi: 10.7150/thno.22641
127. Yang X, Palasuberniam P, Kraus D, Chen B. Aminolevulinic acid-based tumor detection and therapy: molecular mechanisms and strategies for enhancement. *Int J Mol Sci.* (2015) 16:25865–80. doi: 10.3390/ijms161025865
128. Palasuberniam P, Yang X, Kraus D, Jones P, Myers KA, Chen B ABCG2 transporter inhibitor restores the sensitivity of triple negative breast cancer cells to aminolevulinic acid-mediated photodynamic therapy. *Sci Rep.* (2015) 5:13298. doi: 10.1038/srep13298

129. Sun W, Kajimoto Y, Inoue H, Miyatake S, Ishikawa T, Kuroiwa T. Gefitinib enhances the efficacy of photodynamic therapy using 5-aminolevulinic acid in malignant brain tumor cells. *Photodiagn Photodyn Ther.* (2013) 10:42–50. doi: 10.1016/j.pdpdt.2012.06.003
130. Liu W, Baer MR, Bowman MJ, Pera P, Zheng X, Morgan J, et al. The tyrosine kinase inhibitor imatinib mesylate enhances the efficacy of photodynamic therapy by inhibiting ABCG2. *Clin Cancer Res.* (2007) 13:2463–70. doi: 10.1158/1078-0432.CCR-06-1599
131. Blake E, Curnow A. The hydroxypyridinone iron chelator CP94 can enhance PpIX-induced PDT of cultured human glioma cells. *Photochem Photobiol.* (2010) 86:1154–60. doi: 10.1111/j.1751-1097.2010.00770.x
132. Blake E, Allen J, Curnow A. An *in vitro* comparison of the effects of the iron-chelating agents, CP94 and dexrazoxane, on protoporphyrin IX accumulation for photodynamic therapy and/or fluorescence guided resection. *Photochem Photobiol.* (2011) 87:1419–26. doi: 10.1111/j.1751-1097.2011.00985.x
133. Reinert M, Piffaretti D, Wilzbach M, Hauger C, Guckler R, Marchi F, et al. Quantitative modulation of PpIX fluorescence and improved glioma visualization. *Front Surg.* (2019) 6:41. doi: 10.3389/fsurg.2019.00041
134. Wang W, Tabu K, Hagiya Y, Sugiyama Y, Kokubu Y, Murota Y, et al. Enhancement of 5-aminolevulinic acid-based fluorescence detection of side population-defined glioma stem cells by iron chelation. *Sci Rep.* (2017) 7:42070. doi: 10.1038/srep42070
135. Anand S, Hasan T, Maytin EV. Mechanism of differentiation-enhanced photodynamic therapy for cancer: upregulation of coproporphyrinogen oxidase by C/EBP transcription factors. *Mol Cancer Ther.* (2013) 12:1638–50. doi: 10.1158/1535-7163.MCT-13-0047
136. Chen X, Wang C, Teng L, Liu Y, Chen X, Yang G, et al. Calcitriol enhances 5-aminolevulinic acid-induced fluorescence and the effect of photodynamic therapy in human glioma. *Acta Oncol.* (2014) 53:405–13. doi: 10.3109/0284186X.2013.819993
137. Kouchesfehani HM, Nabiuni M, Majlesara MH, Amini E, Irian S. Effect of vitamin E succinate as a differentiation agent on the efficacy of 5-ALA-PDT on prostate cancer cells in culture. *J Paramed Sci.* (2011) 2:16–23.
138. Frank J, Lornejad-Schäfer MR, Schöffl H, Flaccus A, Lambert C, Biesalski HK. Inhibition of heme oxygenase-1 increases responsiveness of melanoma cells to ALA-based photodynamic therapy. *Int J Oncol.* (2007) 31:1539–45. doi: 10.3892/ijo.31.6.1539
139. Podkalicka P, Mucha O, Józkowicz A, Dulak J, Łoboda A. Heme oxygenase inhibition in cancers: possible tools and targets. *Współczesna Onkol.* (2018) 2018:23–32. doi: 10.5114/wo.2018.73879
140. Maeda H, Nakamura H, Fang J. The EPR effect for macromolecular drug delivery to solid tumors: Improvement of tumor uptake, lowering of systemic toxicity, and distinct tumor imaging *in vivo*. *Adv Drug Deliv Rev.* (2013) 65:71–9. doi: 10.1016/j.addr.2012.10.002
141. Vieira DB, Gamarra LF. Getting into the brain: liposome-based strategies for effective drug delivery across the blood-brain barrier. *Int J Nanomedicine.* (2016) 11:5381–414. doi: 10.2147/IJN.S117210
142. Maeda H, Tsukigawa K, Fang J. A retrospective 30 years after discovery of the enhanced permeability and retention effect of solid tumors: next-generation chemotherapeutics and photodynamic therapy–problems, solutions, and prospects. *Microcirculation.* (2016) 23:173–82. doi: 10.1111/micc.12228
143. Matsumura Y, Maeda H. A new concept for macromolecular therapeutics in cancer chemotherapy: mechanism of tumoritropic accumulation of proteins and the antitumor agent smancs. *Cancer Res.* (1986) 46:6387–92.
144. Fang J, Nakamura H, Maeda H. The EPR effect: unique features of tumor blood vessels for drug delivery, factors involved, and limitations and augmentation of the effect. *Adv Drug Deliv Rev.* (2011) 63:136–51. doi: 10.1016/j.addr.2010.04.009
145. Maeda H. Nitroglycerin enhances vascular blood flow and drug delivery in hypoxic tumor tissues: analogy between angina pectoris and solid tumors and enhancement of the EPR effect. *J Controlled Release.* (2010) 142:296–8. doi: 10.1016/j.jconrel.2010.01.002
146. Noguchi Y, Wu J, Duncan R, Strohalm J, Ulbrich K, Akaike T, et al. Early phase tumor accumulation of macromolecules: a great difference in clearance rate between tumor and normal tissues. *Jpn J Cancer Res.* (1998) 89:307–14. doi: 10.1111/j.1349-7006.1998.tb00563.x
147. Fang J, Liao L, Yin H, Nakamura H, Shin T, Maeda H. Enhanced bacterial tumor delivery by modulating the EPR effect and therapeutic potential of *Lactobacillus casei. J Pharm Sci.* (2014) 103:3235–43. doi: 10.1002/jps.24083
148. Quarles CC, Bell LC, Stokes AM. Imaging vascular and hemodynamic features of the brain using dynamic susceptibility contrast and dynamic contrast enhanced MRI. *Neuroimage.* (2019) 187:32–55. doi: 10.1016/j.neuroimage.2018.04.069
149. Rapoport SI. Effect of concentrated solutions on blood-brain barrier. *Am J Physiol.* (1970) 219:270–4. doi: 10.1152/ajplegacy.1970.219.1.270
150. Rapoport SI, Hori M, Klatzo I. Testing of a hypothesis for osmotic opening of the blood-brain barrier. *Am J Physiol.* (1972) 223:323–31. doi: 10.1152/ajplegacy.1972.223.2.323
151. Nduom EK, Zhuang Z, Lonser RR. Blood-brain barrier. response. *J Neurosurg.* (2014) 120:291.
152. Neuwelt EA, Frenkel EP, Diehl J, Vu LH, Rapoport S, Hill S. Reversible osmotic blood-brain barrier disruption in humans. *Neurosurgery.* (1980) 7:44–52. doi: 10.1227/00006123-198007000-00007
153. Williams JA, Roman-Goldstein S, Crossen JR, D'Agostino A, Dahlborg SA, Neuwelt EA. Preirradiation osmotic blood-brain barrier disruption plus combination chemotherapy in gliomas: quantitation of tumor response to assess chemosensitivity. *Adv Exp Med Biol.* (1993) 331:273–84. doi: 10.1007/978-1-4615-2920-0_43
154. Neuwelt E, Ambady P, Muldoon L, McConnell H, Doolittle N. Outwitting the blood-brain barrier. *Oncology.*(2016) 30:963, 966–7.
155. Priest R, Ambady P, Neweult E. ACTR-23. safety of intra-arterial chemotherapy with osmotic opening of the blood-brain barrier. *Neuro Oncology.* (2018) 20:vi16. doi: 10.1093/neuonc/noy148.057
156. Oberoi RK, Parrish KE, Sio TT, Mittapalli RK, Elmquist WF, Sarkaria JN. Strategies to improve delivery of anticancer drugs across the blood–brain barrier to treat glioblastoma. *Neuro Oncology.* (2016) 18:27–36. doi: 10.1093/neuonc/nov164
157. Bartek J Jr, Alattar AA, Dhawan S, Ma J, Koga T, Nakaji P, et al. Receipt of brachytherapy is an independent predictor of survival in glioblastoma in the Surveillance, Epidemiology, and End Results database. *J Neuro Oncol.* (2019) 145:75–83. doi: 10.1007/s11060-019-03268-y
158. Shi M, Sanche L. Convection-enhanced delivery in malignant gliomas: a review of toxicity and efficacy. *J Oncol.* (2019) 2019:9342796. doi: 10.1155/2019/9342796
159. Ughachukwu P, Unekwe P. Efflux pump-mediated resistance in chemotherapy. *Ann Med Health Sci Res.* (2012) 2:191–8. doi: 10.4103/2141-9248.105671
160. Burgess A, Shah K, Hough O, Hynynen K. Focused ultrasound-mediated drug delivery through the blood–brain barrier. *Expert Rev Neurother.* (2015) 15:477–91. doi: 10.1586/14737175.2015.1028369
161. Aryal M, Fischer K, Gentile C, Gitto S, Zhang YZ, McDannold N. Effects on P-glycoprotein expression after blood-brain barrier disruption using focused ultrasound and microbubbles. *PLOS ONE.* (2017) 12:e0166061. doi: 10.1371/journal.pone.0166061
162. Zhang J, Liu H, Du X, Guo Y, Chen X, Wang S, et al. Increasing of blood-brain tumor barrier permeability through transcellular and paracellular pathways by microbubble-enhanced diagnostic ultrasound in a C6 glioma model. *Front Neurosci.* (2017) 11:86. doi: 10.3389/fnins.2017.00086
163. di Biase L, Falato E, Di Lazzaro V. Transcranial focused ultrasound (tFUS) and Transcranial unfocused ultrasound (tUS) neuromodulation: from theoretical principles to stimulation practices. *Front Neurol.* (2019) 10:549. doi: 10.3389/fneur.2019.00549
164. Lipsman N, Meng Y, Bethune AJ, Huang Y, Lam B, Masellis M, et al. Blood–brain barrier opening in Alzheimer's disease using MR-guided focused ultrasound. *Nat Commun.* (2018) 9:1–8. doi: 10.1038/s41467-018-04529-6
165. Gallay MN, Moser D, Jeanmonod D. Safety and accuracy of incisionless transcranial MR-guided focused ultrasound functional neurosurgery: single-center experience with 253 targets in 180 treatments. *J Neurosurg.* (2019) 130:1234–43. doi: 10.3171/2017.12.JNS172054
166. Krishna V, Sammartino F, Rezai A. A review of the current therapies, challenges, and future directions of transcranial focused ultrasound technology advances in diagnosis and treatment. *JAMA Neurol.* (2018) 75:246–54. doi: 10.1001/jamaneurol.2017.3129

167. Levi D, Raffa G, Periti M, Broggi G. A New possible application of transcranial magnetic stimulation: case report. *EC Neurol.* (2018) 10:1000–5.
168. Pell G, Zangen A, Roth Y, Friedman A, Vazana U, inventors; Brainsway Ltd, assignee. *Use of transcranial magnetic stimulation tomodulate permeability of the blood-brain barrier.* United States patent US 9636517B2 (2017). Available online at: https://patents.google.com/patent/US9636517B2/en
169. Semyachkina-Glushkovskaya O, Kurths J, Borisova E, Sokolovski S, Mantareva V, Angelov I, et al. Photodynamic opening of blood-brain barrier. *Biomed Optics Express.* (2017) 8:5040. doi: 10.1364/BOE.8.005040
170. Tang W, Fan W, Lau J, Deng L, Shen Z, Chen X. Emerging blood-brain-barrier-crossing nanotechnology for brain cancer theranostics. *Chem Soc Rev.* (2019) 48:2967–3014. doi: 10.1039/C8CS00805A
171. Witham TF, Fukui MB, Meltzer CC, Burns R, Kondziolka D, Bozik ME. Survival of patients with high grade glioma treated with intrathecal thiotriethylenephosphoramide for ependymal or leptomeningeal gliomatosis. *Cancer.* (1999) 86:1347–53. doi: 10.1002/(SICI)1097-0142(19991001)86:7<1347::AID-CNCR34>3.0.CO;2-M
172. Bleier BS, Kohman RE, Feldman RE, Ramanlal S, Han X. Permeabilization of the blood-brain barrier via mucosal engrafting: implications for drug delivery to the brain. *PLOS ONE.* (2013) 8:e61694. doi: 10.1371/journal.pone.0061694
173. Miyake MM, Bleier BS. Bypassing the blood-brian barrier using established skull base reconstruction techniques. *World J Otorhinolaryngol Head Neck Surg.* (2015) 1:11–6. doi: 10.1016/j.wjorl.2015.09.001
174. Stine CA, Munson JM. Convection-enhanced delivery: connection to and impact of interstitial fluid flow. *Front Oncol.* (2019) 9:966. doi: 10.3389/fonc.2019.00966
175. Platt S, Nduom E, Kent M, Freeman C, Machaidze R, Kaluzova M, et al. Canine model of convection-enhanced delivery of cetuximab-conjugated iron-oxide nanoparticles monitored with magnetic resonance imaging. *Clin Neurosurg.* (2012) 59:107–13. doi: 10.1227/NEU.0b013e31826989ef
176. Saito R, Sonoda Y, Kumabe T, Nagamatsu K, Watanabe M, Tominaga T. Regression of recurrent glioblastoma infiltrating the brainstem after convection-enhanced delivery of nimustine hydrochloride. *J Neurosurg Pediatr.* (2011) 7:522–6. doi: 10.3171/2011.2.PEDS10407
177. Sampson JH, Brady M, Raghavan R, Mehta AI, Friedman AH, Reardon DA, et al. Colocalization of gadolinium-diethylene triamine pentaacetic acid with high-molecular-weight molecules after intracerebral convection-enhanced delivery in humans. *Neurosurgery.* (2011) 69:668–76. doi: 10.1227/NEU.0b013e3182181ba8
178. Pang HH, Chen PY, Wei KC, Huang CW, Shiue YL, Huang CY, et al. Convection-enhanced delivery of a virus-like nanotherapeutic agent with dual-modal imaging for besiegement and eradication of brain tumors. *Theranostics.* (2019) 9:1752–63. doi: 10.7150/thno.30977
179. Weng KC, Hashizume R, Noble CO, Serwer LP, Drummond DC, Kirpotin DB, et al. Convection-enhanced delivery of targeted quantum dot-immunoliposome hybrid nanoparticles to intracranial brain tumor models. *Nanomedicine.* (2013) 8:1913–25. doi: 10.2217/nnm.12.209
180. Souweidane MM, Kramer K, Pandit-Taskar N, Zhou Z, Zanzonico P, Donzelli M, et al. A phase I study of convection-enhanced delivery of 124I-8H9 radio-labeled monoclonal antibody in children with diffuse intrinsic pontine glioma: An update with dose-response assessment. *J Clin Oncol.* (2019) 37:2008. doi: 10.1200/JCO.2019.37.15_suppl.2008
181. Vogelbaum MA, Brewer C, Barnett GH, Mohammadi AM, Peereboom DM, Ahluwalia MS, et al. First-in-human evaluation of the Cleveland Multiport Catheter for convection-enhanced delivery of topotecan in recurrent high-grade glioma: results of pilot trial 1. *J Neurosurg.* (2019) 130:476–85. doi: 10.3171/2017.10.JNS171845
182. Ashby LS, Smith KA, Stea B. Gliadel wafer implantation combined with standard radiotherapy and concurrent followed by adjuvant temozolomide for treatment of newly diagnosed high-grade glioma: a systematic literature review. *World J Surg Oncol.* (2016) 14:225. doi: 10.1186/s12957-016-0975-5
183. McGirt MJ, Than KD, Weingart JD, Chaichana KL, Attenello FJ, Olivi A, et al. Gliadel (BCNU) wafer plus concomitant temozolomide therapy after primary resection of glioblastoma multiforme. *J Neurosurg.* (2009) 110:583–8. doi: 10.3171/2008.5.17557
184. Westphal M, Hilt DC, Bortey E, Delavault P, Olivares R, Warnke PC, et al. A phase 3 trial of local chemotherapy with biodegradable carmustine (BCNU) wafers (Gliadel wafers) in patients with primary malignant glioma. *Neuro Oncology.* (2003) 5:79–88. doi: 10.1215/15228517-5-2-79
185. Byvaltsev VA, Bardonova LA, Onaka NR, Polkin RA, Ochkal SV, Shepelev VV, et al. Acridine orange: a review of novel applications for surgical cancer imaging and therapy. *Front Oncol.* (2019) 9:925. doi: 10.3389/fonc.2019.00925
186. Kitagawa Y, Tanaka S, Kuriki Y, Yamamoto K, Ogasawara A, Nejo T, et al. Spray fluorescent probes for fluorescence-guided neurosurgery. *Front Oncol.* (2019) 9:727. doi: 10.3389/fonc.2019.00727
187. Cutter JL, Cohen NT, Wang J, Sloan AE, Cohen AR, Panneerselvam A, et al. Topical application of activity-based probes for visualization of brain tumor tissue. *PLOS ONE.* (2012) 7:e33060. doi: 10.1371/journal.pone.0033060
188. Martirosyan NL, Georges J, Eschbacher JM, Cavalcanti DD, Elhadi AM, Abdelwahab MG, et al.MPotential application of a handheld confocal endomicroscope imaging system using a variety of fluorophores in experimental gliomas and normal brain. *Neurosurg Focus.* (2014) 36:E16. doi: 10.3171/2013.11.FOCUS13486
189. Candela P, Gosselet F, Miller F, Buee-Scherrer V, Torpier G, Cecchelli R, et al. Physiological pathway for low-density lipoproteins across the blood-brain barrier: transcytosis through brain capillary endothelial cells *in vitro*. *Endothelium J Endothelial Cell Res.* (2008) 15:254–64. doi: 10.1080/10623320802487759
190. Yamamoto M, Ikeda K, Ohshima K, Tsugu H, Kimura H, Tomonaga M. Increased expression of low density lipoprotein receptor-related protein/alpha2-macroglobulin receptor in human malignant astrocytomas. *Cancer Res.* (1997) 57:2799–805.
191. Blasi P, Giovagnoli S, Schoubben A, Ricci M, Rossi C. Solid lipid nanoparticles for targeted brain drug delivery. *Adv Drug Deliv Rev.* (2007) 59:454–77. doi: 10.1016/j.addr.2007.04.011
192. Gao H. Progress and perspectives on targeting nanoparticles for brain drug delivery. *Acta Pharm Sin B.* (2016) 6:268–86. doi: 10.1016/j.apsb.2016.05.013
193. Harilal S, Jose J, Parambi DGT, Kumar R, Mathew GE, Uddin MS, et al. Advancements in nanotherapeutics for Alzheimer's disease: current perspectives. *J Pharm Pharmacol.* (2019) 71:1370–83. doi: 10.1111/jphp.13132
194. Masserini M. Nanoparticles for brain drug delivery. *ISRN Biochem.* (2013) 2013:238428. doi: 10.1155/2013/238428
195. Saraiva C, Praça C, Ferreira R, Santos T, Ferreira L, Bernardino L. Nanoparticle-mediated brain drug delivery: overcoming blood-brain barrier to treat neurodegenerative diseases. *J Control Release.* (2016) 235:34–47. doi: 10.1016/j.jconrel.2016.05.044
196. Nduom EK, Bouras A, Kaluzova M, Hadjipanayis CG. Nanotechnology applications for glioblastoma. *Neurosurg Clin N Am.* (2012) 23:439–49. doi: 10.1016/j.nec.2012.04.006
197. Hollis CP, Weiss HL, Leggas M, Evers BM, Gemeinhart RA, Li T. Biodistribution and bioimaging studies of hybrid paclitaxel nanocrystals: lessons learned of the EPR effect and image-guided drug delivery. *J Controlled Release.* (2013) 172:12–21. doi: 10.1016/j.jconrel.2013.06.039
198. Park K. Questions on the role of the EPR effect in tumor targeting *Controlled Release.* (2013) 172:391. doi: 10.1016/j.jconrel.2013.10.001
199. Maeda H, Khatami M. Analyses of repeated failures in cancer therapy for solid tumors: poor tumor-selective drug delivery, low therapeutic efficacy and unsustainable costs. *Clin Transl Med.* (2018) 7:11. doi: 10.1186/s40169-018-0185-6
200. Nakanishi T, Fukushima S, Okamoto K, Suzuki M, Matsumura Y, Yokoyama M, et al. Development of the polymer micelle carrier system for doxorubicin. *J Controlled Release.* (2001) 74:295–302. doi: 10.1016/S0168-3659(01)00341-8
201. Takeda KM, Yamasaki Y, Dirisala A, Ikeda S, Tockary TA, Toh K, et al. Effect of shear stress on structure and function of polyplex micelles from poly(ethylene glycol)-poly(l-lysine) block copolymers as systemic gene delivery carrier. *Biomaterials.* (2017) 126:31–8. doi: 10.1016/j.biomaterials.2017.02.012
202. Mahmoudi K, Garvey KL, Bouras A, Cramer G, Stepp H, Jesu Raj JG, et al. 5-aminolevulinic acid photodynamic therapy for the treatment of high-grade gliomas. *J Neurooncol.* (2019) 141:595–607. doi: 10.1007/s11060-019-03103-4

203. Namikawa T, Yatabe T, Inoue K, Shuin T, Hanazaki K. Clinical applications of 5-aminolevulinic acid-mediated fluorescence for gastric cancer. *World J Gastroenterol.* (2015) 21:8817–25. doi: 10.3748/wjg.v21.i29.8769
204. Lucena SR, Salazar N, Gracia-Cazaña T, Zamarrón A, González S, Juarranz Á, et al. Combined treatments with photodynamic therapy for non-melanoma skin cancer. *In J Mol Sci.* (2015) 16:25912–33. doi: 10.3390/ijms161025912
205. Lakomkin N, Hadjipanayis CG. Fluorescence-guided surgery for high-grade gliomas. *J Surg Oncol.* (2018) 118:356–61. doi: 10.1002/jso.25154
206. Hadjipanayis CG, Stummer W, Sheehan JP. 5-ALA fluorescence-guided surgery of CNS tumors. *J Neurooncol.* (2019) 141:477–8. doi: 10.1007/s11060-019-03109-y
207. Hadjipanayis CG, Widhalm G, Stummer W. What is the surgical benefit of utilizing 5-aminolevulinic acid for fluorescence-guided surgery of malignant gliomas? *Neurosurgery.* (2015) 77:663–73. doi: 10.1227/NEU.0000000000000929
208. Hadjipanayis CG, Stummer W. 5-ALA and FDA approval for glioma surgery. *J Neurooncol.* (2019) 141:479–86. doi: 10.1007/s11060-019-03098-y
209. Novotny A, Stummer W. 5-Aminolevulinic acid and the blood-brain barrier – A review. *Med Laser Appl.* (2003) 18:36–40. doi: 10.1078/1615-1615-00085
210. Sachar M, Anderson KE, Ma X. Protoporphyrin IX: the good, the bad, and the ugly. *J Pharmacol Exp Ther.* (2016) 356:267–75. doi: 10.1124/jpet.115.228130
211. Dalton JT, Yates CR, Yin D, Straughn A, Marcus SL, Golub AL, et al. Clinical pharmacokinetics of 5-aminolevulinic acid in healthy volunteers and patients at high risk for recurrent bladder cancer. *J Pharmacol Exp Ther.* (2002) 301:507–12. doi: 10.1124/jpet.301.2.507
212. Rick K, Sroka R, Stepp H, Kriegmair M, Huber RM, Jacob K, et al. Pharmacokinetics of 5-aminolevulinic acid-induced protoporphyrin IX in skin and blood. *J Photochem Photobiol B Biol.* (1997) 40:313–9. doi: 10.1016/S1011-1344(97)00076-6
213. Olivo M, Wilson BC. Mapping ALA-induced PPIX fluorescence in normal brain and brain tumour using confocal fluorescence microscopy. *Int J Oncol.* (2004) 25:37–45. doi: 10.3892/ijo.25.1.37
214. Terr L, Weiner LP. An autoradiographic study of delta-aminolevulinic acid uptake by mouse brain. *Exp Neurol.* (1983) 79:564–8. doi: 10.1016/0014-4886(83)90234-0
215. Valdés PA, Moses ZB, Kim A, Belden CJ, Wilson BC, Paulsen KD, et al. Gadolinium- and 5-aminolevulinic acid-induced protoporphyrin IX levels in human gliomas: an *ex vivo* quantitative study to correlate protoporphyrin IX levels and blood-brain barrier breakdown. *J Neuropathol Exp Neurol.* (2012) 71:806–13. doi: 10.1097/NEN.0b013e31826775a1
216. Goryaynov SA, Widhalm G, Goldberg MF, Chelushkin D, Spallone A, Chernyshov KA, et al. The role of 5-ALA in low-grade gliomas and the influence of antiepileptic drugs on intraoperative fluorescence. *Front Oncol.* (2019) 9:423. doi: 10.3389/fonc.2019.00423
217. Widhalm G, Olson J, Weller J, Bravo J, Han SJ, Phillips J, et al. The value of visible 5-ALA fluorescence and quantitative protoporphyrin IX analysis for improved surgery of suspected low-grade gliomas. *J Neurosurg.* (2019) 2019:1–10. doi: 10.3171/2019.1.JNS182614
218. Kaneko S, Suero Molina E, Ewelt C, Warneke N, Stummer W. Fluorescence-based measurement of real-time kinetics of protoporphyrin IX after 5-aminolevulinic acid administration in human *in situ* malignant gliomas. *Neurosurgery.* (2019) 85:E739–46. doi: 10.1093/neuros/nyz129
219. Tonn JC, Stummer W. Fluorescence-guided resection of malignant gliomas using 5-aminolevulinic acid: practical use, risks, and pitfalls. *Clin Neurosurg.* (2008) 55:20–6.
220. Ajioka RS, Phillips JD, Kushner JP. Biosynthesis of heme in mammals. *Biochim Biophys Acta Mol Cell Res.* (2006) 1763:723–36. doi: 10.1016/j.bbamcr.2006.05.005
221. Nakanishi T, Ogawa T, Yanagihara C, Tamai I. Kinetic evaluation of determinant factors for cellular accumulation of protoporphyrin IX induced by external 5-aminolevulinic acid for photodynamic cancer therapy. *J Pharm Sci.* (2015) 104:3092–100. doi: 10.1002/jps.24462
222. Döring F, Walter J, Will J, Föcking M, Boll M, Amasheh S, et al. Delta-aminolevulinic acid transport by intestinal and renal peptide transporters and its physiological and clinical implications. *J Clin Invest.* (1998) 101:2761–7. doi: 10.1172/JCI1909
223. Frølund S, Marquez OC, Larsen M, Brodin B, Nielsen CU. Delta-aminolevulinic acid is a substrate for the amino acid transporter SLC36A1 (hPAT1). *Br J Pharmacol.* (2010) 159:1339–53. doi: 10.1111/j.1476-5381.2009.00620.x
224. Tran TT, Mu A, Adachi Y, Adachi Y, Taketani S. Neurotransmitter transporter family including SLC6A6 and SLC6A13 contributes to the 5-aminolevulinic acid (ALA)-induced accumulation of protoporphyrin IX and photodamage, through uptake of ALA by cancerous cells. *Photochem Photobiol.* (2014) 90: 1136–43. doi: 10.1111/php.12290
225. Krishnamurthy P, Schuetz JD. The role of ABCG2 and ABCB6 in porphyrin metabolism and cell survival. *Curr Pharm Biotechnol.* (2011) 12:647–55. doi: 10.2174/138920111795163995
226. Geier EG, Chen EC, Webb A, Papp AC, Yee SW, Sadee W, et al. Profiling solute carrier transporters in the human blood–brain barrier. *Clin Pharmacol Ther.* (2013) 94:636–9. doi: 10.1038/clpt.2013.175
227. Kitajima Y, Ishii T, Kohda T, Ishizuka M, Yamazaki K, Nishimura Y, et al. Mechanistic study of PpIX accumulation using the JFCR39 cell panel revealed a role for dynamin 2-mediated exocytosis. *Sci Rep.* (2019) 9:8666. doi: 10.1038/s41598-019-44981-y
228. Hagiya Y, Endo Y, Yonemura Y, Takahashi K, Ishizuka M, Abe F, et al. Pivotal roles of peptide transporter PEPT1 and ATP-binding cassette (ABC) transporter ABCG2 in 5-aminolevulinic acid (ALA)-based photocytotoxicity of gastric cancer cells *in vitro*. *Photodiagn Photodyn Ther.* (2012) 9:204–14. doi: 10.1016/j.pdpdt.2011.12.004
229. Webber J, Kessel D, Fromm D. Plasma levels of protoporphyrin IX in humans after oral administration of 5-aminolevulinic acid. *J Photochem Photobiol B Biol.* (1997) 37:151–3. doi: 10.1016/S1011-1344(96)07348-4
230. Kawai N, Hirohashi Y, Ebihara Y, Saito T, Murai A, Saito T, et al. ABCG2 expression is related to low 5-ALA photodynamic diagnosis (PDD) efficacy and cancer stem cell phenotype, and suppression of ABCG2 improves the efficacy of PDD. *PLOS ONE.* (2019) 14:e0216503. doi: 10.1371/journal.pone.0216503
231. Lai HW, Sasaki R, Usuki S, Nakajima M, Tanaka T, Ogura SI. Novel strategy to increase specificity of ALA-Induced PpIX accumulation through inhibition of transporters involved in ALA uptake. *Photodiagn Photodyn Ther.* (2019) 27:327–35. doi: 10.1016/j.pdpdt.2019.06.017
232. Li Y, Rey-Dios R, Roberts DW, Valdés PA, Cohen-Gadol AA. Intraoperative fluorescence-guided resection of high-grade gliomas: a comparison of the present techniques and evolution of future strategies. *World Neurosurg.* (2014) 82:175–85. doi: 10.1016/j.wneu.2013.06.014
233. Emerson GA, Andersen HH. Toxicity of certain proposed antileprosy dyes: fluorescein, eosin, erythrosin and others. *Int J Leprosy.* (1934) 2:257–63.
234. Acerbi F, Broggi M, Schebesch KM, Höhne J, Cavallo C, De Laurentis C, et al. Fluorescein-guided surgery for resection of high-grade gliomas: a multicentric prospective phase II study (FLUOGLIO). *Clin Cancer Res.* (2018) 24:52–61. doi: 10.1158/1078-0432.CCR-17-1184
235. Belykh E, Miller EJ, Carotenuto A, Patel AA, Cavallo C, Martirosyan NL, et al. Progress in confocal laser endomicroscopy for neurosurgery and technical nuances for brain tumor imaging with fluorescein. *Front Oncol.* (2019) 9:554. doi: 10.3389/fonc.2019.00554
236. Martirosyan NL, Eschbacher JM, Kalani MY, Turner JD, Belykh E, Spetzler RF, et al. Prospective evaluation of the utility of intraoperative confocal laser endomicroscopy in patients with brain neoplasms using fluorescein sodium: experience with 74 cases. *Neurosurg Focus.* (2016) 40:E11. doi: 10.3171/2016.1.FOCUS15559
237. Blair NP, Evans MA, Lesar TS, Zeimer RC. Fluorescein and fluorescein glucuronide pharmacokinetics after intravenous injection. *Invest Ophthalmol Vis Sci.* (1986) 27:1107–14.
238. Stummer W. Fluorescein in brain metastasis and glioma surgery. *Acta Neurochir.* (2015) 157:2199–200. doi: 10.1007/s00701-015-2576-4
239. Fan C, Jiang Y, Liu R, Wu G, Wu G, Xu K, et al. Safety and feasibility of low-dose fluorescein-guided resection of glioblastoma. *Clin Neurol Neurosurg* (2018) 175:57–60. doi: 10.1016/j.clineuro.2018.10.011
240. Diaz RJ, Dios RR, Hattab EM, Burrell K, Rakopoulos P, Sabha N, et al. Study of the biodistribution of fluorescein in glioma-infiltrated mouse brain and histopathological correlation of intraoperative findings in high-grade gliomas resected under fluorescein fluorescence guidance. *J Neurosurg* (2015) 122:1360–9. doi: 10.3171/2015.2.JNS132507

241. Höhne J, Hohenberger C, Proescholdt M, Riemenschneider MJ, Wendl C, Brawanski A, et al. Fluorescein sodium-guided resection of cerebral metastases-an update. *Acta Neurochir.* (2017) 159:363–7. doi: 10.1007/s00701-016-3054-3
242. Xiao SY, Zhang J, Zhu ZQ, Li YP, Zhong WY, Chen JB, et al. Application of fluorescein sodium in breast cancer brain-metastasis surgery. *Cancer Manage Res.* (2018) 10:4325–31. doi: 10.2147/CMAR.S176504
243. Xiang Y, Zhu XP, Zhao JN, Huang GH, Tang JH, Chen HR, et al. Blood-brain barrier disruption, sodium fluorescein, and fluorescence-guided surgery of gliomas. *Br J Neurosurg.* (2018) 32:141–8. doi: 10.1080/02688697.2018.1428731
244. Schebesch KM, Rosengarth K, Brawanski A, Proescholdt M, Wendl C, Höhne J, et al. Clinical benefits of combining different visualization modalities in neurosurgery. *Front Surg.* (2019) 6:56. doi: 10.3389/fsurg.2019.00056
245. Schebesch KM, Brawanski A, Doenitz C, Rosengarth K, Proescholdt M, Riemenschneider MJ, et al. Fluorescence-guidance in non-Gadolinium enhancing, but FET-PET positive gliomas. *Clin Neurol Neurosurg.* (2018) 172:177–82. doi: 10.1016/j.clineuro.2018.07.011
246. Wang EJ, Casciano CN, Clement RP, Johnson WW. Fluorescent substrates of sister-P-glycoprotein (BSEP) evaluated as markers of active transport and inhibition: evidence for contingent unequal binding sites. *Pharm Res* (2003) 20:537–44. doi: 10.1023/a:1023278211849
247. Sun H, Johnson DR, Finch RA, Sartorelli AC, Miller DW, Elmquist WF. Transport of fluorescein in MDCKII-MRP1 transfected cells and mrp1-knockout mice. *Biochem Biophy Res Commun.* (2001) 284:863–9. doi: 10.1006/bbrc.2001.5062
248. Zhang Z, Tachikawa M, Uchida Y, Terasaki T. Drug clearance from cerebrospinal fluid mediated by organic anion transporters 1 (Slc22a6) and 3 (Slc22a8) at arachnoid membrane of rats. *Mol Pharm.* (2018) 15:911–22. doi: 10.1021/acs.molpharmaceut.7b00852
249. Barar J, Rafi MA, Pourseif MM, Omidi Y. Blood-brain barrier transport machineries and targeted therapy of brain diseases. *Bioimpacts.* (2016) 6:225–48. doi: 10.15171/bi.2016.30
250. Saxena V, Sadoqi M, Shao J. Degradation kinetics of indocyanine green in aqueous solution. *J Pharm Sci.* (2003) 92:2090–7. doi: 10.1002/jps.10470
251. Haglund MM, Berger MS, Hochman DW. Enhanced optical imaging of human gliomas and tumor margins. *Neurosurgery.* (1996) 38:308–17. doi: 10.1097/00006123-199602000-00015
252. Obach RS, Lombardo F, Waters NJ. Trend analysis of a database of intravenous pharmacokinetic parameters in humans for 670 drug compounds. *Drug Metab Dispos.* (2008) 36:1385–405. doi: 10.1124/dmd.108.020479
253. Desmettre T, Devoisselle JM, Mordon S. Fluorescence properties and metabolic features of indocyanine green (ICG) as related to angiography. *Surv Ophthalmol.* (2000) 45:15–27. doi: 10.1016/S0039-6257(00)00123-5
254. Yoneya S, Noyori K. Improved visualization of the choroidal circulation with indocyanine green angiography. *Archiv Ophthalmol.* (1993) 111:1165. doi: 10.1001/archopht.1993.01090090015002
255. Cherrick GR, Stein SW, Leevy CM, Davidson CS. Indocyanine green: observations on its physical properties, plasma decay, and hepatic extraction*. *J Clin Invest.* (1960) 39:592–600. doi: 10.1172/JCI104072
256. Baker KJ. Binding of sulfobromophthalein (BSP) sodium and indocyanine green (ICG) by plasma 1 lipoproteins. *Exp Biol Med.* (1966) 122:957–63. doi: 10.3181/00379727-122-31299
257. Yoneya S, Saito T, Komatsu Y, Koyama I, Takahashi K, Duvoll-Young J. Binding properties of indocyanine green in human blood. *Invest Ophthalmol Vis Sci.* (1998) 39:1286–90.
258. Schaafsma BE, Mieog JS, Hutteman M, van der Vorst JR, Kuppen PJ, Löwik CW, et al. The clinical use of indocyanine green as a near-infrared fluorescent contrast agent for image-guided oncologic surgery. *J Surg Oncol.* (2011) 104:323–32. doi: 10.1002/jso.21943
259. Haglund MM, Hochman DW, Spence AM, Berger MS. Enhanced optical imaging of rat gliomas and tumor margins. *Neurosurgery.* (1994) 35:930–40; discussion 940–31. doi: 10.1097/00006123-199411000-00019
260. Hansen DA, Spence AM, Carski T, Berger MS. Indocyanine green (ICG) staining and demarcation of tumor margins in a rat glioma model. *Surg Neurol.* (1993) 40:451–6. doi: 10.1016/0090-3019(93)90046-4
261. Charalampaki P, Nakamura M, Athanasopoulos D, Heimann A. Confocal-assisted fluorescent microscopy for brain tumor surgery. *Front Oncol.* (2019) 9:583. doi: 10.3389/fonc.2019.00583
262. Eyüpoglu IY, Hore N, Fan Z, Buslei R, Merkel A, Buchfelder M, et al. Intraoperative vascular DIVA surgery reveals angiogenic hotspots in tumor zones of malignant gliomas. *Sci Rep.* (2015) 5:7958. doi: 10.1038/srep07958
263. Martirosyan NL, Cavalcanti DD, Eschbacher JM, Delaney PM, Scheck AC, Abdelwahab MG, et al. Use of *in vivo* near-infrared laser confocal endomicroscopy with indocyanine green to detect the boundary of infiltrative tumor. *J Neurosurg.* (2011) 115:1131–8. doi: 10.3171/2011.8.JNS11559
264. Hollins B, Noe B, Henderson JM. Fluorometric determination of indocyanine green in plasma. *Clin Chem.* (1987) 33:765–8. doi: 10.1093/clinchem/33.6.765
265. Ott P, Keiding S, Johnsen AH, Bass L. Hepatic removal of two fractions of indocyanine green after bolus injection in anesthetized pigs. *Am J Physiol Gastrointest Liver Physiol.* (1994) 266:G1108–22. doi: 10.1152/ajpgi.1994.266.6.G1108
266. Song W, Tang Z, Zhang D, Burton N, Drissen W, Chen X. Comprehensive studies of pharmacokinetics and biodistribution of indocyanine green and liposomal indocyanine green by multispectral optoacoustic tomography. *RSC Adv.* (2015) 5:3807–13. doi: 10.1039/C4RA09735A
267. Jansen PL, van Klinken JW, van Gelder M, Ottenhoff R, Elferink RP. Preserved organic anion transport in mutant TR-rats with a hepatobiliary secretion defect. *Am J Physiol.* (1993) 265:G445–52. doi: 10.1152/ajpgi.1993.265.3.G445
268. Pedersen JM, Matsson P, Bergström CA, Hoogstraate J, Norén A, LeCluyse EL, et al. Early identification of clinically relevant drug interactions with the human bile salt export pump (BSEP/ABCB11). *Toxicol Sci.* (2013) 136:328–43. doi: 10.1093/toxsci/kft197
269. Shibasaki Y, Sakaguchi T, Hiraide T, Morita Y, Suzuki A, Baba S, et al. Expression of indocyanine green-related transporters in hepatocellular carcinoma. *J Surg Res.* (2015) 193:567–76. doi: 10.1016/j.jss.2014.07.055
270. Belykh E, Miller EJ, Hu D, Martirosyan NL, Woolf EC, Scheck AC, et al. Scanning fiber endoscope improves detection of 5-aminolevulinic acid-induced protoporphyrin IX fluorescence at the boundary of infiltrative glioma. *World Neurosurg.* (2018) 113:e51–69. doi: 10.1016/j.wneu.2018.01.151
271. Valdés PA, Roberts DW, Lu FK, Golby A. Optical technologies for intraoperative neurosurgical guidance. *Neurosurg Focus.* (2016) 40:E8. doi: 10.3171/2015.12.FOCUS15550
272. Vasefi F, MacKinnon N, Farkas DL, Kateb B. Review of the potential of optical technologies for cancer diagnosis in neurosurgery: a step toward intraoperative neurophotonics. *Neurophotonics.* (2016) 4:011010. doi: 10.1117/1.NPh.4.1.011010
273. Wei L, Roberts DW, Sanai N, Liu JTC. Visualization technologies for 5-ALA-based fluorescence-guided surgeries. *J Neuro Oncol.* (2019) 141:495–505. doi: 10.1007/s11060-018-03077-9
274. Murray CB, Kagan CR, Bawendi MG. synthesis and characterization of monodisperse nanocrystals and close-packed nanocrystal assemblies. *Annu Rev Mater Sci.* (2000) 30:545–610. doi: 10.1146/annurev.matsci.30.1.545
275. Akerman ME, Chan WC, Laakkonen P, Bhatia SN, Ruoslahti E. Nanocrystal targeting *in vivo*. *Proc Natl Acad Sci USA.* (2002) 99:12617–21. doi: 10.1073/pnas.152463399
276. Matea CT, Mocan T, Tabaran F, Pop T, Mosteanu O, Puia C, et al. Quantum dots in imaging, drug delivery and sensor applications. *Int J Nanomedicine.* (2017) 12:5421–31. doi: 10.2147/IJN.S138624
277. Greish K. Enhanced permeability and retention (EPR) effect for anticancer nanomedicine drug targeting. *Methods Mol Biol.* (2010) 624:25–37. doi: 10.1007/978-1-60761-609-2_3
278. Saxena V, Sadoqi M, Shao J. Enhanced photo-stability, thermal-stability and aqueous-stability of indocyanine green in polymeric nanoparticulate systems. *J Photochem Photobiol B Biol.* (2004) 74:29–38. doi: 10.1016/j.jphotobiol.2004.01.002

279. Massoud TF, Gambhir SS. Molecular imaging in living subjects: seeing fundamental biological processes in a new light. *Genes Dev.* (2003) 17:545–80. doi: 10.1101/gad.1047403

280. Weissleder R, Mahmood U. Molecular Imaging. *Radiology.* (2001) 219:316–33. doi: 10.1148/radiology.219.2.r01ma19316

281. McFerrin MB, Sontheimer H. A role for ion channels in glioma cell invasion. *Neuron Glia Biol.* (2006) 2:39–49. doi: 10.1017/S1740925X06000044

282. Deshane J, Garner CC, Sontheimer H. Chlorotoxin inhibits glioma cell invasion via matrix metalloproteinase-2. *J Biol Chem.* (2003) 278:4135–44. doi: 10.1074/jbc.M205662200

283. Xiang Y, Liang L, Wang X, Wang J, Zhang X, Zhang Q. Chloride channel-mediated brain glioma targeting of chlorotoxin-modified doxorubicine-loaded liposomes. *J Controlled Release.* (2011) 152:402–10. doi: 10.1016/j.jconrel.2011.03.014

10

Survival Outcomes Among Patients with High-Grade Glioma Treated with 5-Aminolevulinic Acid–Guided Surgery

Sirin Gandhi[1], *Ali Tayebi Meybodi*[1], *Evgenii Belykh*[1,2], *Claudio Cavallo*[1], *Xiaochun Zhao*[1], *Masood Pasha Syed*[3], *Leandro Borba Moreira*[1], *Michael T. Lawton*[1], *Peter Nakaji*[1] *and Mark C. Preul*[1*]

[1] *Department of Neurosurgery, St. Joseph's Hospital and Medical Center, Barrow Neurological Institute, Phoenix, AZ, United States,* [2] *Department of Neurosurgery, Irkutsk State Medical University, Irkutsk, Russia,* [3] *Department of Medicine, Saint Vincent Hospital, Worcester, MA, United States*

***Correspondence:**
Mark C. Preul
neuropub@barrowneuro.org

Background: High-grade glioma (HGG) is associated with a dismal prognosis despite significant advances in adjuvant therapies, including chemotherapy, immunotherapy, and radiotherapy. Extent of resection continues to be the most important independent prognosticator of survival. This underlines the significance of increasing gross total resection (GTR) rates by using adjunctive intraoperative modalities to maximize resection with minimal neurological morbidity. 5-aminolevulinic acid (5-ALA) is the only US Food and Drug Administration–approved intraoperative optical agent used for fluorescence-guided surgical resection of gliomas. Despite several studies on the impact of intra-operative 5-ALA use on the extent of HGG resection, a clear picture of how such usage affects patient survival is still unavailable.

Methods: A systematic review was conducted of all relevant studies assessing the GTR rate and survival outcomes [overall survival (OS) and progression-free survival (PFS)] in HGG. A meta-analysis of eligible studies was performed to assess the influence of 5-ALA-guided resection on improving GTR, OS, and PFS. GTR was defined as >95% resection.

Results: Of 23 eligible studies, 19 reporting GTR rates were included in the meta-analysis. The pooled cohort had 998 patients with HGG, including 796 with newly diagnosed cases. The pooled GTR rate among patients with 5-ALA–guided resection was 76.8% (95% confidence interval, 69.1–82.9%). A comparative subgroup analysis of 5-ALA–guided vs. conventional surgery (controlling for within-study covariates) showed a 26% higher GTR rate in the 5-ALA subgroup (odds ratio, 3.8; $P < 0.001$). There were 11 studies eligible for survival outcome analysis, 4 of which reported PFS. The pooled mean difference in OS and PFS was 3 and 1 months, respectively, favoring 5-ALA vs. control ($P < 0.001$).

Conclusions: This meta-analysis shows a significant increase in GTR rate with 5-ALA–guided surgical resection, with a higher weighted GTR rate (~76%) than the pivotal phase III study (~65%). Pooled analysis showed a small yet significant increase in survival measures associated with the use of 5-ALA. Despite the statistically significant results, the low level of evidence and heterogeneity across these studies make it difficult to conclusively report an independent association between 5-ALA use and survival outcomes in HGG. Additional randomized control studies are required to delineate the role of 5-ALA in survival outcomes in HGG.

Keywords: 5-aminolevulinic acid, fluorescence-guided surgery, glioblastoma multiforme, gross total resection, high-grade glioma, meta-analysis, survival outcome

INTRODUCTION

High-grade gliomas (HGGs), including World Health Organization (WHO) grade III and grade IV gliomas, are the most common subtype of primary adult malignant cerebral neoplasms with a poor prognosis. Current management strategies include maximal safe surgical resection along with a combination of chemotherapy and fractionated radiotherapy. Complete resection of enhancing tumor (CRET) or gross total resection (GTR) have been demonstrated to be independent prognosticators of increased progression-free survival (PFS) and overall survival (OS) (1). However, true delineation of the tissue boundaries of HGGs is extremely difficult. Gadolinium enhancement on magnetic resonance imaging (MRI) is conventionally used to determine the tumor boundaries and postoperative resection analysis. In recent years, fluorescence image-guided resection using agents like fluorescein sodium (2), indocyanine green (3, 4), and 5-aminolevulinic acid (5-ALA) (5, 6) has gained significant traction in the treatment of HGGs. These optical agents can augment visual differentiation of the tumor border zone intraoperatively by selective fluorescence of the abnormal diseased tissue (7, 8).

5-ALA is currently approved in many countries, with US Food and Drug Administration (FDA) approval obtained a decade after European Medical Agency (EMA) approval (9). Selective accumulation of protoporphyrin IX (PpIX), which is an endogenous fluorophore and a downstream metabolite of 5-ALA in the heme synthesis pathway, occurs in the malignant glioma cells in HGGs (10). PpIX-fluorescence is best visualized using filtered xenon light with blue-violet light 375–440 nm wavelength and an emission filter for red fluorescence of 635–704 nm (8, 11). The standard dose of 5-ALA oral administration is 20 mg/kg dissolved in 50 mL of water given 3 h prior to surgery with a peak visible fluorescence at 6–8 h after consumption (12). However, photobleaching effects have been observed in this tumor-specific fluorescence, with 36% fluorescence decay in 25 min at an excitation wavelength of 405 nm and after 87 min under unfiltered wide-field illumination (8, 13).

Several studies have suggested that intraoperative PpIX accumulates even in the absence of contrast enhancement on MRI and supersedes the margins of contrast-enhancing tumor in the gadolinium-enhancing tumor subtypes (14, 15). Thus, it is imperative to determine the added surgical benefit of resection of this residual non-enhancing fluorescent tissue while minimizing any postoperative neurological morbidity. This particular question was examined in 50 patients with GBM who underwent operations with 5-ALA-based fluorescence guidance with matched non-surgical prognostic markers, such as age, location, O^6-methylguanine-DNA-methyltransferase status, and Karnofsky Performance Scale score (14). The mean OS was significantly worse in the CRET subgroup (17 months; 95% confidence interval [CI]: 22.4–31.6 months) if patients had persistent residual fluorescence in comparison with maximal safe fluorescent tissue resection (27 months; 95% CI: 12.5–22.5 months) (14). This study demonstrated discrepancy between intraoperative tissue fluorescence and gadolinium contrast enhancement. Use of adjunctive tools like navigation with tractography, somatosensory evoked potential or motor evoked potential mapping, confocal endomicroscopy, intraoperative MRI (iMRI), ultrasound, or awake craniotomy may be beneficial in conjunction with fluorescence-guided surgical resection of aggressive HGGs in eloquent locations. In the current age of personalized and precision medicine, 5-ALA seems to have been identified as a tool in surgical theranostics, with benefits seen during photodynamic therapy using 5-ALA in experimental studies and patients with glioma (16–18).

The current standard of care for HGGs, including GBM, includes the Stupp protocol, which calls for maximal safe surgical resection with concomitant temozolomide and radiation therapy (19). The largest systematic review to date with quantitative analysis of the influence of extent of resection (EOR) on survival outcomes in patients with GBM observed a substantial improvement in PFS and OS in patients undergoing GTR (1). Since 5-ALA has been shown to significantly improve EOR and GTR/CRET in patients with HGG, this would indirectly imply an enhanced survival benefit for this subset of patients. However, there is a paucity of quantitative data analysis in reported systematic reviews owing to the heterogeneity of the patient population and low levels of scientific evidence based on study designs (10, 20–22).

Despite the previous systematic reviews assessing the value of 5-ALA for the treatment of HGG (10, 20, 21), the benefit of 5-ALA to patients (e.g., improvements in neurological outcomes, quality of life, and overall survival) remain inconclusive. The benefit of 5-ALA has so far been demonstrated only indirectly by showing increased GTR rates when using fluorescence guidance. We attempted to bridge the gap and investigate the evidence for 5-ALA benefits on the basis of patient outcome–based metrics. The objective of this study was to conduct a systematic review

Abbreviations: CRET, complete resection of enhancing tumor; EOR, extent of resection; FDA, US Food and Drug Administration; GBM, glioblastoma multiforme; GTR, gross total resection; HGG, high-grade glioma; iMRI, intraoperative magnetic resonance imaging; LGG, low-grade glioma; MRI, magnetic resonance imaging; OS, overall survival; PFS, progression-free survival; PpIX, protoporphyrin IX; RCT, randomized control trial; WHO, World Health Organization; 5-ALA, 5 aminolevulinic acid.

of the literature and perform a quantitative pooled evaluation of survival outcomes and GTR rates of 5-ALA-guided surgical resection in HGGs. Since our pooled cohort included patients with recurrent HGG, a subgroup outcomes analysis among patients with primary HGG was also performed to assess the survival outcomes.

METHODS

This systematic review was conducted in accordance with the Preferred Reporting Items for Systematic Reviews and Meta-Analyses (PRISMA) guidelines. This study was exempt from institutional review board approval as it was a meta-analytical review of literature.

Search Strategy

PubMed, MEDLINE, and EMBASE electronic databases were searched to identify studies from the database inception through December 31, 2018, regarding the use of intraoperative 5-ALA for fluorescence-guided resection of HGGs. No studies were excluded on the basis of publication type or date of publication. However, preclinical and *in vitro* studies involving animals were excluded. MeSH and EMTREE terms relevant to 5-ALA and HGGs were used to search the PubMed, MEDLINE, and EMBASE databases. These terms included "aminolevulinic acid," "levulinic acid," "5ALA" or "5-ALA," "glioma," "high grade glioma," "malignant glioma," and "glioblastoma." The bibliography of all articles meeting the inclusion criteria was examined to identify any missing additional studies. All articles from this search were added to an Endnote library X 8.2 (Clarivate Analytics, Philadelphia, PA). Non-English literature was excluded from this study.

Systematic Review Protocol and Data Extraction

Titles and abstracts were screened by two independent reviewers (SG, ATM) with input from the senior author (MCP) in case of ambiguity. Inclusion criteria for this meta-analysis were as follows: (1) all patients with histopathologically confirmed (WHO grade III and grade IV) HGG including recurrent gliomas and (2) all studies reporting on the GTR or CRET rate and survival outcomes (OS and PFS) pertinent to the use of 5-ALA in the surgical resection of HGGs in adult patients. Laboratory studies, technical reports, review articles including systematic reviews, editorials, commentaries, conference proceedings, and abstracts were excluded from the analyses. Studies were also excluded if there was a lack of clear reporting of HGG type (i.e., whether HGG was primary or recurrent), if they had a small sample size ($n < 10$), if they included overlapping patient populations, and if we were unable to extract analyzable data points.

Full-text review of the studies shortlisted using the above methodology was conducted by two reviewers in an independent fashion, and the relevant data were subsequently extracted from each study for further statistical analyses. The variables of interest included first-author name, year of publication, study design, sample size, demographic distribution, follow-up duration, survival data, EOR, and subtypes and location of glioma. The study design was used as a surrogate marker for assessing any biases. Studies were analyzed quantitatively for three major parameters: GTR (defined as >95% tumor volume resection), PFS, and OS rates. In studies that reported a 95% CI and no standard deviation (SD) in their results, the SD value was obtained from a formula using the standard errors and 95% CI values as follows:

$$\mathrm{SD} = \sqrt{N} \times \frac{(\mathrm{UL} - \mathrm{LL})}{3.92}$$

where N is the number of subjects, UL is the upper limit and LL is the lower limit of the 95% CI.

Additionally, in studies with a lower sample size ($n < 50$), the denominator of 3.92 was replaced with a manual t distribution calculation using the degree of freedom (23). This calculation allowed for inclusion of a few studies in our final analyses that have been excluded in the previously reported studies.

Statistical Analysis of Data

After obtaining the proportional values of GTR >95% and the mean (SD) values for OS and PFS as described above, the statistical analysis was conducted using an open-source meta-analytical software, Open MetaAnalyst for Mac OS Sierra 10.12 (Brown University, Providence, RI). Heterogeneity across the various studies included for the meta-analyses was determined using an I^2 statistical test for inconsistency with an arbitrary cutoff value of $I^2 \geq 50\%$ with a $P < 0.05$ representing significant heterogeneity. A fixed-effect model was used for conducting the meta-analysis in the absence of substantial heterogeneity, and a random-effect model was used for significant heterogeneity across the various combined studies. The random-effect model utilized the DerSimonian-Laird method to evaluate within-study variance (24).

RESULTS

The initial screening using the search strategy described in the Methods section yielded 864 articles, commentaries, and conference proceedings. After removal of duplicates and screening for non-English and non-relevant articles, 88 full-text articles remained. Each full-text article was checked by two independent reviewers to confirm that it met the inclusion criteria (**Figure 1**). Sixty-five articles were excluded because they did not meet the aforementioned eligibility criteria for this study. Twenty-three studies were included in the final meta-analysis of the pooled GTR and survival outcomes analysis.

5-ALA and Gross Total Resection

Of the 23 studies included in the analyses, 19 reported a GTR or CRET rate (5, 25–42). The number of participants who underwent 5-ALA–guided resection in these studies ranged from 10 to 139, with the GTR ranging from 47.6 to 98.5%. The I^2 statistics showed a significant heterogeneity level (90.09%; $P < 0.001$). Therefore, a random-effect model was used for the pooled estimate of these data. In pooled analysis of all HGGs, including

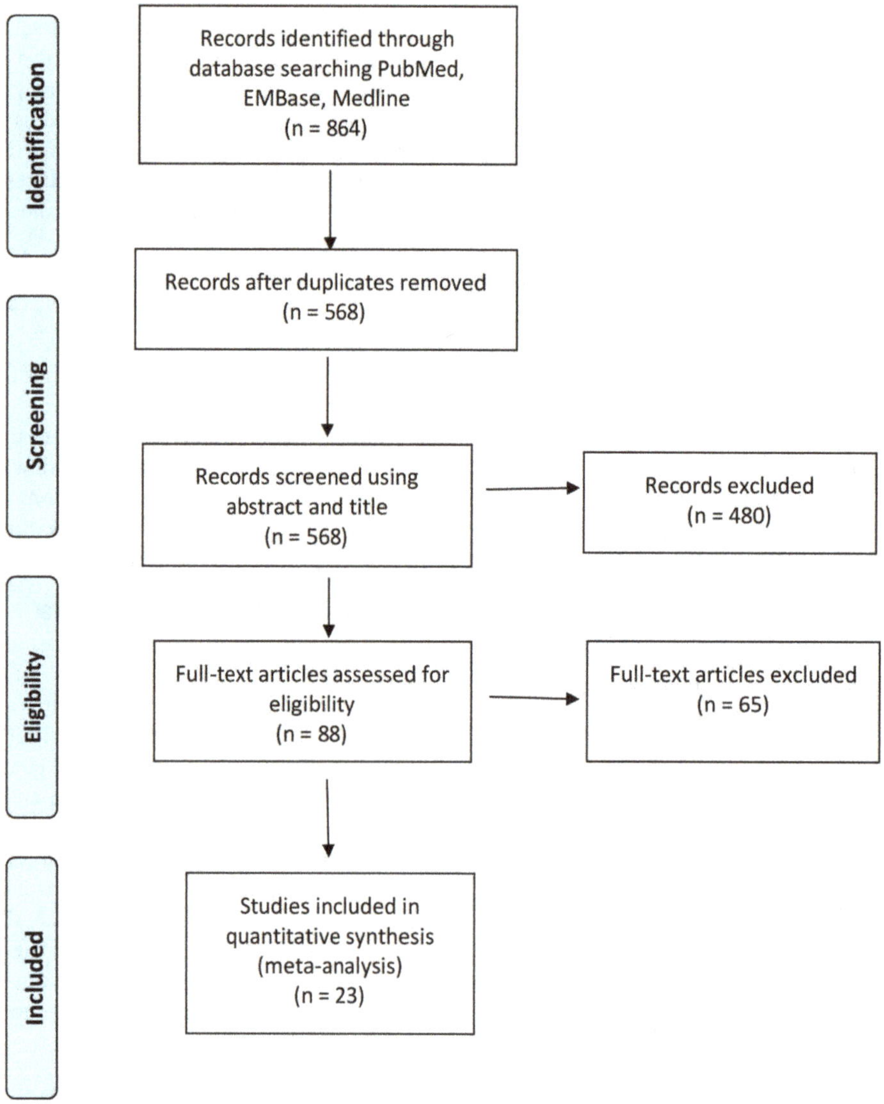

FIGURE 1 | Preferred Reporting Items for Systematic Reviews and Meta-Analyses (PRISMA) flow diagram of the studies included in the meta-analysis of resection and survival outcomes among patients with 5-aminolevulinic acid–guided resection of high-grade glioma. Used with permission from Barrow Neurological Institute, Phoenix, Arizona.

primary and recurrent subtypes, GTR was achieved in 759 of 998 patients, resulting in an overall GTR rate of 76% (95% CI, 69–83%; $P < 0.001$) (**Figure 2**). In the subgroup analysis of primary GBM alone, GTR was achieved in 599 of 796 patients, resulting in a similar GTR rate of 76.8% (95% CI, 68–85%, $P < 0.001$) (**Figure 3**).

Four case-controlled studies were found to be eligible for a meta-analysis of GTR with 5-ALA ($n = 382$) vs. conventional resection ($n = 326$) (31, 34, 37, 43). All other covariates (e.g., use of intraoperative MRI, postoperative treatment with specific chemotherapeutic agents) remained the same within each study but were variable across the studies. However, there was no significant statistical heterogeneity across these studies ($I^2 = 0\%$; $P = 0.57$); hence, we used a fixed-effect model for analysis. GTR was achieved in 302 of 382 (79.1%) patients in the 5-ALA group vs. 172 of 326 (52.8%) patients in the control group. In the pooled estimate of all HGGs (primary and recurrent), 5-ALA was associated with a 26% increase in GTR rate compared with the control group in which surgeries were performed without 5-ALA, resulting in OR = 3.79 (95% CI, 2.65–5.41; $P < 0.001$) for achieving GTR (**Figure 4**).

Overall Survival Data for 5-ALA–Guided Glioma Resection

Of the 23 studies, 9 reported a mean OS period in months ranging from 10 to 22 months (5, 25, 26, 31, 34, 44–47). One of the studies, by Stummer et al. (31), stratified the survival analysis by age (55 years of age and younger vs. older than 55 years). Hence, these

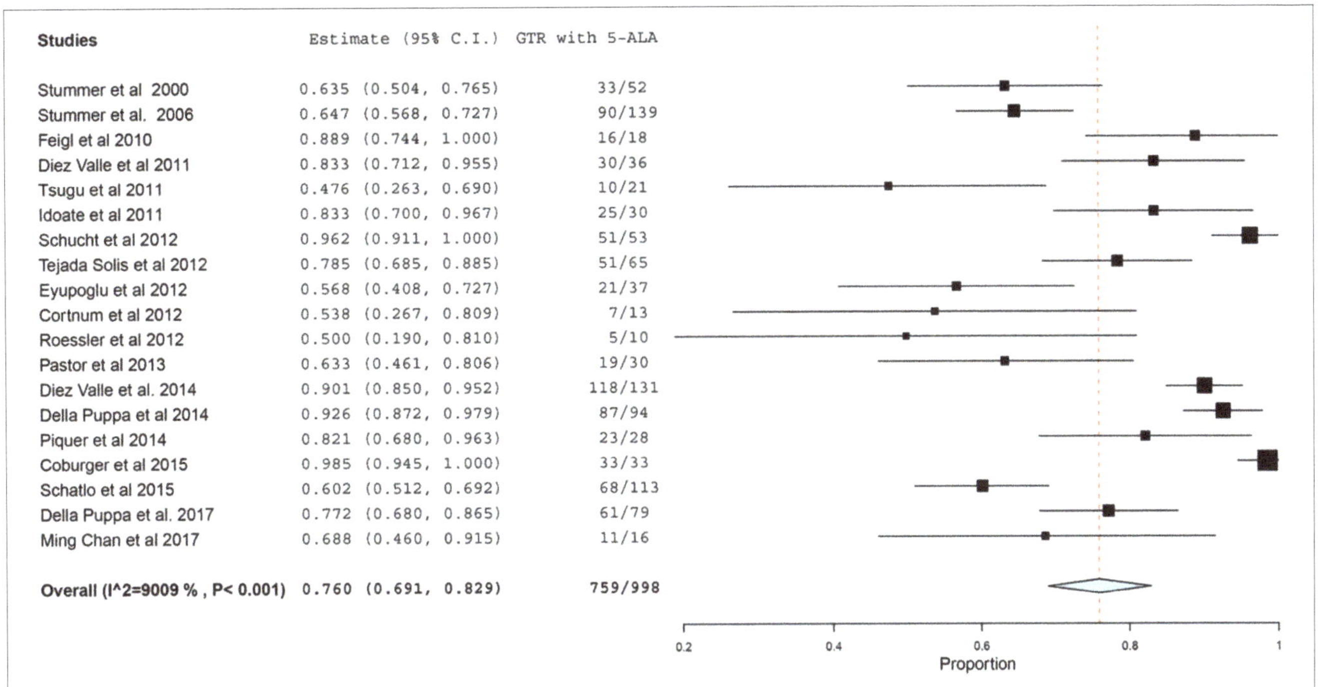

FIGURE 2 | Forest plot graph representing the meta-analysis of gross total resection (GTR) rate (95% confidence interval [CI]) among patients with high-grade glioma, including primary and recurrent cases, treated using 5-aminolevulinic acid (5-ALA)–guided surgical resection. Used with permission from Barrow Neurological Institute, Phoenix, Arizona.

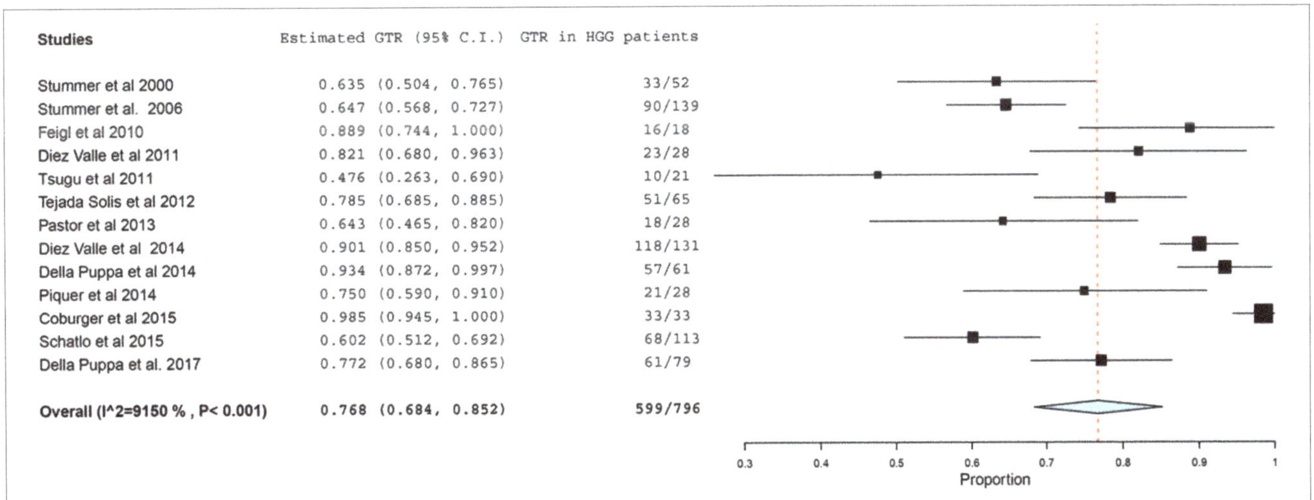

FIGURE 3 | Forest plot graph representing the meta-analysis of gross total resection (GTR) rate (95% confidence interval [CI]) among patients with primary high-grade glioma (HGG) treated using 5-aminolevulinic acid–guided surgical resection. Used with permission from Barrow Neurological Institute, Phoenix, Arizona.

patients were included in our analysis as two independent patient groups conducted by the same methodology used by this phase III randomized control trial (RCT) (31). Similarly, another study had subdivided its patients into two treatment groups (treated using 5-ALA) and one control group (treated without the use of 5-ALA).Thus, we treated the two treatment arms as independent patient groups in our analysis for OS (25). Therefore, 11 distinct groups of patients who underwent 5-ALA–guided resection of primary HGG were extracted for analysis. There was significant heterogeneity across these groups ($I^2 = 96.3\%$; $P < 0.001$); therefore, a random-effects model for continuous variable was used. The meta-analysis in the group of patients with primary HGG who underwent 5-ALA–guided resection showed a mean OS of 16.3 months (95% CI, 14.1–18.5 months; $P < 0.001$) (**Figure 5**). Five studies (seven distinct 5-ALA groups) were available for comparison of OS (measured as a mean survival

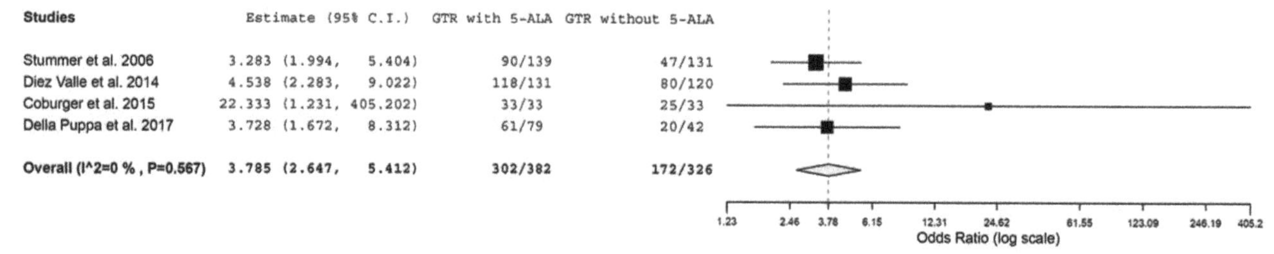

FIGURE 4 | Forest plot graph representing the meta-analysis of the odd ratio (95% confidence interval [CI]) of gross total resection (GTR) among patients with primary high-grade gliomas treated using 5-aminolevulinic acid (5-ALA)–guided surgical resection vs. conventional microsurgical resection. Used with permission from Barrow Neurological Institute, Phoenix, Arizona.

difference) between 5-ALA vs. control groups (25, 31, 34, 46, 47). No significant heterogeneity was noted across these groups ($I^2 = 0\%$; $P = 0.47$); hence, we used a fixed-effects model. The meta-analysis yielded a pooled OS difference of 3.05 months (95% CI, 2.43–3.68 months; $P < 0.001$) favoring 5-ALA-guided resection compared with control groups without 5-ALA (**Figures 6, 7**).

Progression Free Survival Data for 5-ALA Guided Glioma Resection

Of the 23 papers, three studies reported PFS ranging from 5.1 to 11 months. From these 3 studies, 4 distinct groups of patients who underwent 5-ALA–guided resection of primary HGG were extracted for analysis. Significant heterogeneity was noted across these groups ($I^2 = 96.3\%$; $P < 0.001$), with use of a random-effects model for continuous variables. The meta-analysis of patients with primary HGG who underwent 5-ALA–guided resection showed a mean PFS of 8.4 months (95% CI, 5.9–10.9 months; $P < 0.001$) (**Figure 8**). The mean PFS difference was 1.03 months (95% CI, 0.61–1.45 months; $P < 0.001$) favoring 5-ALA when compared with matched control groups (**Figures 9, 10**).

DISCUSSION

Interpretation of the Meta-Analytic Data

This meta-analysis was conducted to evaluate the potential survival advantage gained, if any, with the use of 5-ALA–guided resection of HGGs. The pooled analysis of 998 patients with HGG who underwent 5-ALA–guided surgical resection showed a higher rate of GTR in the cohort of all patients with HGG (~76%) as well as in the subgroup of patients with primary HGG (~77%), as compared with the phase III RCT conducted by Stummer et al. (31) that reported a GTR rate of 65%. The pooled analysis of the eligible case-controlled studies demonstrated that the estimated GTR rate was significantly higher with the intraoperative use of 5-ALA compared with conventional white light technique surgery (79 vs. 53%; OR = 3.78; $P < 0.001$). As GTR is the most significant independent prognostic marker of survival in patients with HGG (1), these results encourage the utilization of fluorescence-guided resection of these lesions. There was a high level of heterogeneity across the studies included in this pooled GTR analysis, attributable to the observational nature of some of these studies and a multitude of other factors that are difficult to control for. For example, invasion of eloquent cortical tissue by an aggressive lesion, determined by preoperative imaging or intraoperatively, is a critical reason for planned subtotal resection, irrespective of the use of 5-ALA. However, inclusion of such preplanned subtotal resection can contribute to an underestimation of the rate of GTR truly attributable to the use of fluorescence guidance. Unfortunately, owing to the lack of specific data in these studies regarding GTR rate in eloquent cortical locations, an analysis could not be performed on this specific population.

The collated survival analysis demonstrated an overall survival advantage (~3-months higher mean OS; $P < 0.001$) with the use of 5-ALA. This has been represented using a cumulative meta-analysis that shows a positive trend in the increase in mean survival difference across the studies published over time (**Figure 7**). However, OS is not the most convenient study endpoint owing to the vast heterogeneity and lack of control on the various postoperative adjuvant therapies that can influence the overall survival. Additionally, in recent years, there seems to be an increase in survival for all patients with HGG that is perhaps attributable to the standardization of the Stupp protocol (19), constant evolution of chemotherapeutic agents and radiotherapy modalities, and introduction of immunotherapy and targeted genetic therapies (48, 49). PFS is a better primary study endpoint for survival analysis than OS because of shorter follow-up period, controlling for the effects of non-study-related therapies in influencing survival and avoiding confusion from the multiple reasons for death. Unfortunately, the amount of data available on PFS in controlled studies is limited, as shown by the cumulative meta-analysis (**Figure 10**). Of the three studies included in PFS analysis, a statistically significant delay of 1 month in time to progression was noted in our pooled cohort (25, 26, 31, 34).

Evolution of Evidence on Benefits of 5-ALA–Guided HGG Surgery

The first clinical study on 5-ALA was reported in 1998, which led to the development of the pivotal randomized, multicenter phase III clinical trial in 5-ALA by Stummer et al. (31) in 2006. The study reported a 29% difference in CRET (65% in 5-ALA vs. 36% using white light surgery; $P < 0.001$). This study demonstrated superior clinical outcomes, significantly

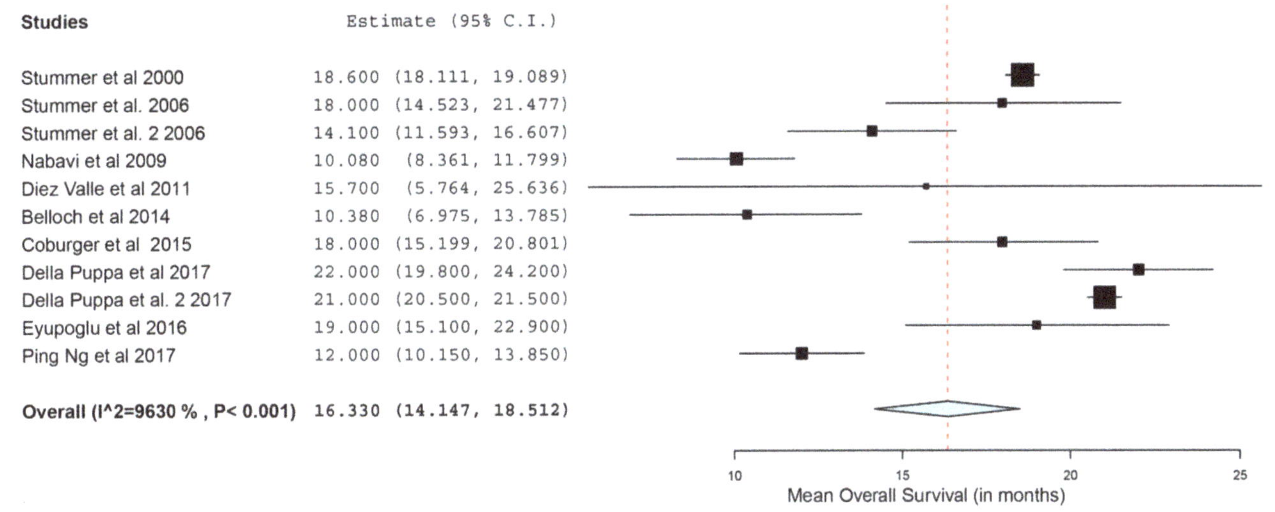

FIGURE 5 | Forest plot graph representing the meta-analysis of mean overall survival (95% confidence interval [CI]) among patients with primary high-grade gliomas treated using 5-aminolevulinic acid–guided surgical resection. Used with permission from Barrow Neurological Institute, Phoenix, Arizona.

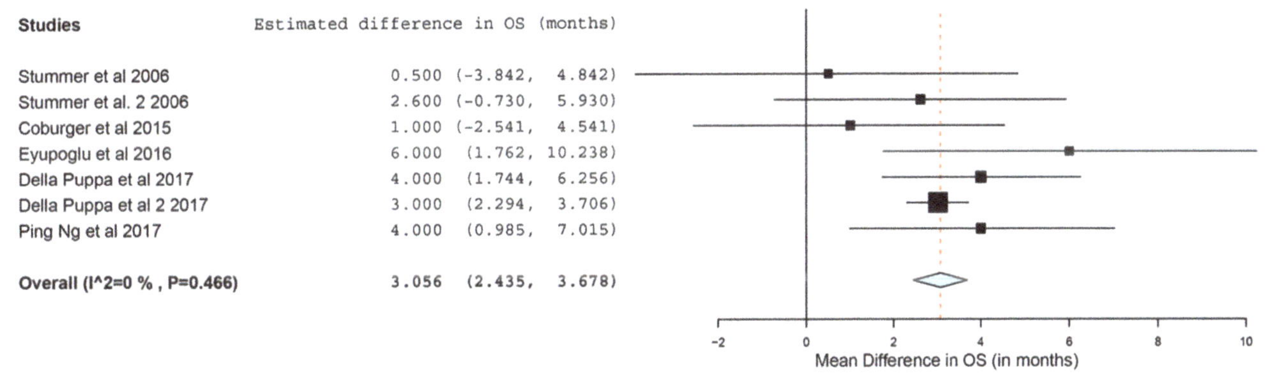

FIGURE 6 | Forest plot graph representing the meta-analysis of mean difference in overall survival (95% confidence interval [CI]) among patients with primary high-grade glioma treated using 5-aminolevulinic acid–guided surgical resection vs. conventional microsurgical resection. Used with permission from Barrow Neurological Institute, Phoenix, Arizona.

higher rates of CRET, and significant improvement in PFS at 6 months using fluorescence-guided surgery vs. the conventional wide-field microsurgical resection (31). In 2007, on the basis of the results of the aforementioned trial, EMA approved the use of 5-ALA. Thereafter, the drug was approved by various countries. In 2011, an FDA request for approval of 5-ALA was filed. The conceptualization of this drug as a therapeutic agent rather than an intraoperative diagnostic tool led to significant delay in the approval of 5-ALA in the United States (9). The drug received FDA approval in June 2017 and became the first optical agent approved by the FDA for use as an intraoperative imaging resource for the resection of HGGs. It is critical to treat 5-ALA and other optical agents as diagnostic markers or tools and not as a means of therapeutic intervention. 5-ALA fluorescence guidance is a modality that is associated with a direct benefit of improving GTR rates and an indirect effect on survival outcomes by increasing maximal safe surgical resection. This is the reason our study chose to assess GTR rates and survival outcomes (OS, PFS) in our final analysis. Concurrently, since the early 2000s, various preclinical and a few clinical studies have investigated the potential therapeutic role of 5-ALA for photodynamic therapy for malignant gliomas with what appear to be advantageous preliminary results (16, 18, 50–59).

Previous Systematic Reviews and Meta-Analyses on 5-ALA–Guided Surgical Resection

Several systematic literature reviews have evaluated the role of fluorescence-guided surgery grouping several optical agents (e.g., fluorescein, 5-ALA, indocyanine green) in terms of GTR, diagnostic metrics (sensitivity and specificity), and survival outcomes (18, 21, 22, 60, 61). Because fluorescein, 5-ALA,

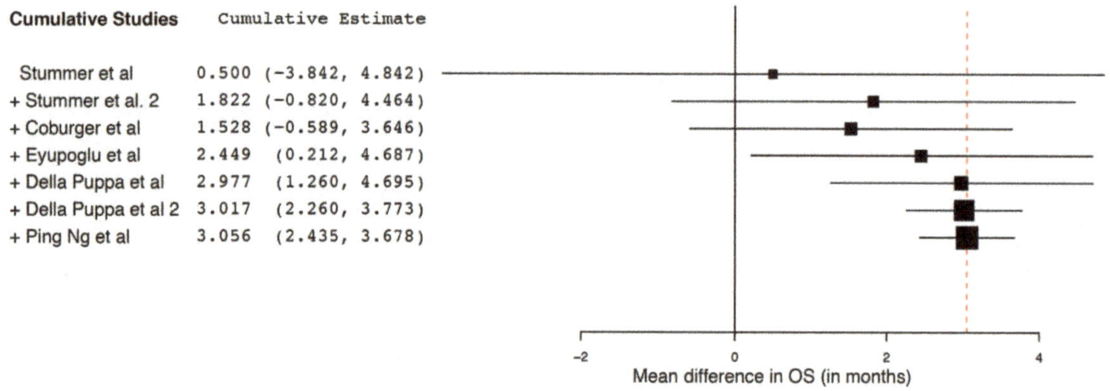

FIGURE 7 | Cumulative regression analysis demonstrating the temporal trend of mean difference (95% confidence interval [CI]) in overall survival among patients with primary high-grade glioma treated using 5-aminolevulinic acid–guided surgical resection vs. conventional microsurgical resection. Used with permission from Barrow Neurological Institute, Phoenix, Arizona.

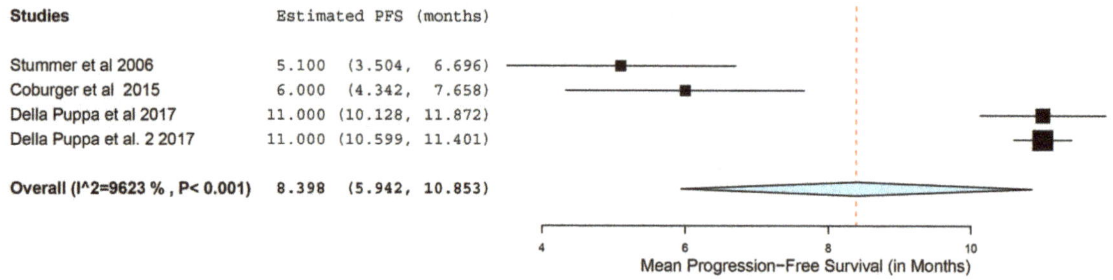

FIGURE 8 | Forest plot graph representing the meta-analysis of mean progression-free survival (95% confidence interval [CI]) among patients with primary high-grade glioma treated using 5-aminolevulinic acid–guided surgical resection. Used with permission from Barrow Neurological Institute, Phoenix, Arizona.

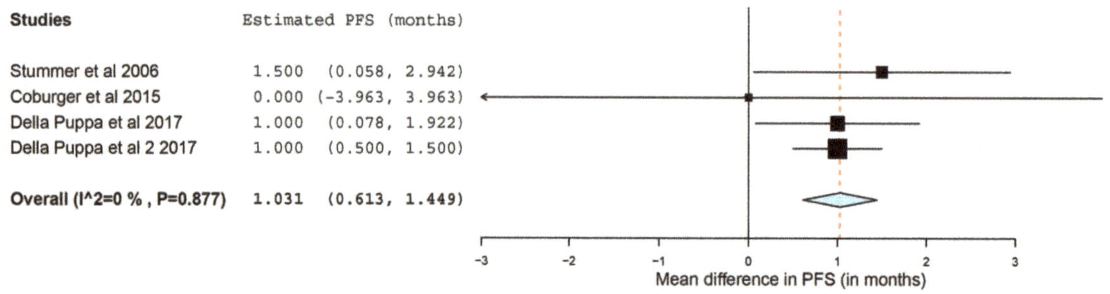

FIGURE 9 | Forest plot graph representing the meta-analysis of mean difference in progression-free survival (95% confidence interval [CI]) among patients with primary high-grade glioma treated using 5-aminolevulinic acid–guided surgical resection vs. conventional microsurgical resection. Used with permission from Barrow Neurological Institute, Phoenix, Arizona.

and indocyanine green have substantially different fluorescent properties and mechanistic behaviors, our study focused on the evaluation of these important study endpoints with the use of 5-ALA as a fluorophore. Eljamel et al. (20) conducted a meta-analysis of 5-ALA–guided resection of GBMs and reported a high sensitivity (82.6%) and specificity (88.9%). The 75% mean GTR rate was in congruence with our results that included a higher sample size. The mean PFS reported in that study was also similar to the PFS reported in our study (~8 months). In contrast with that study, we calculated the measures of continuous outcomes (e.g., SD) as mentioned in the Methods and included several observational studies that were excluded in the previous analyses.

Mansouri et al. (10) conducted a systematic review of literature to assess the adjunctive intraoperative role of 5-ALA in HGGs. The study included 43 articles (1 RCT, 28

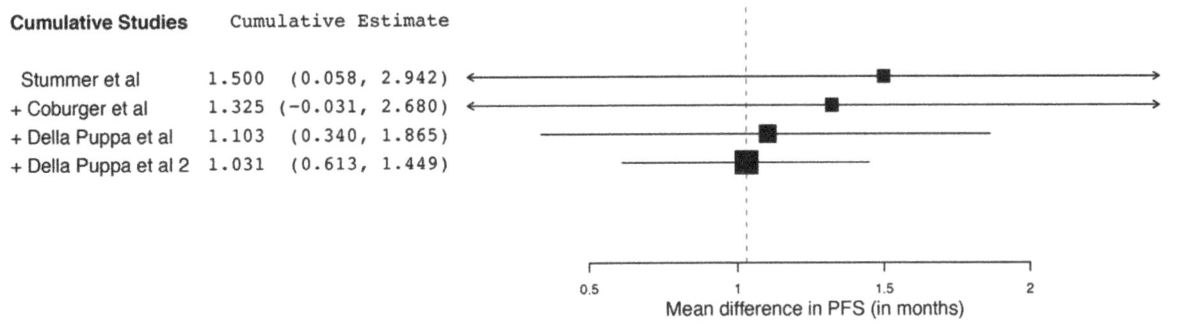

FIGURE 10 | Cumulative regression analysis demonstrating the temporal trend of mean difference in progression-free survival (95% confidence interval [CI]) among patients with primary high-grade glioma treated using 5-aminolevulinic acid–guided surgical resection vs. conventional microsurgical resection. Used with permission from Barrow Neurological Institute, Phoenix, Arizona.

prospective studies, and 14 retrospective studies) and concluded that 5-ALA was associated with improved tumor visualization with a diagnostic accuracy >80%, enabling a greater EOR, that could be indirectly linked to increased survival. Our study had similar inclusion criteria to the aforementioned study. However, we added the quantitative data analyses to objectively evaluate the added benefit of using 5-ALA in HGG surgery.

Potential Limitations of 5-ALA

Fluorophores for intraoperative *in vivo* use in the brain are limited (62). Like other fluorophores in use, 5-ALA has certain drawbacks for its use in a clinical setting. Exogenous administration of 5-ALA leads to selective accumulation of PpIX in the malignant cells of HGG tumors, as mentioned previously (8, 11, 12). From a metabolomic perspective, the molecular mechanism of action of 5-ALA leading to a differential fluorescence of malignant cells can be attributed to the turnover rate of PpIX rather than its accumulation. For instance, in a study of WHO Grade III glioma patients with an *IDH-1* mutation, a depletion of nicotinamide adenine dinucleotide phosphate was hypothesized to mediate the differential temporary accumulation of PpIX (a downstream product of 5-ALA in heme synthesis pathway) in the malignant cells (63). Numerous studies have reported on the potential molecular mechanism for 5-ALA fluorescence properties in malignant cells (63–66). An in-depth analysis of this is beyond the scope of this article.

Blood brain barrier disruption is essential for the accumulation of PpIX in the malignant cells, which is hypothesized to be the cause for lower or negligible fluorescence in LGG cases (8). In addition, the visual PpIX fluorescence signal can be vague or inhomogeneous in appearance with various areas of high and low signal intensity even in HGGs (67, 68). This patchy appearance may be attributed to inhomogeneous tumor growth, glioma cell diversity, overall tissue component heterogeneity (e.g., cysts and necrotic tissue), and differential tumor cellular metabolism. Another level of complexity in accurate detection of fluorescence signal strength originates with the optical detection equipment (e.g., operating microscopes) (7). Limitations of wide-field operating microscopy imaging can, in turn, lead to reduced accuracy of tumor detection at the marginal infiltrative border, especially in eloquent cortical locations. Adjunctive tools that can improve fluorescence detection and provide intraoperative cellular or near-cellular resolution of PpIX fluorescence include the confocal laser endomicroscope (69) and the scanning fiber endoscope (67), whereas implicational or indirect indication of such fluorescent labeling can be correlated with spectroscopy (70–75) and other intraoperative diagnostic adjuncts, such as brain mapping, neuronavigation, ultrasound navigation, and intraoperative MRI (10, 41, 62, 75). These technologies, alone or synergistically, may help to alleviate these limitations and increase the overall EOR.

Photobleaching, defined as the degradation of fluorescence signal of PpIX with prolonged light exposure, is an important limiting phenomenon of which the neurosurgeon should be aware. PpIX photobleaching is directly related to the intensity of the operating microscope light as well as the duration of exposure (7). Photobleaching of PpIX is usually not of major concern during resection of high-grade gliomas, because new tissue layers with unbleached PpIX are exposed with the advancement of resection (11). However, photobleaching may impact accurate quantification or detection of any pathology with low fluorescence signal strength (7). Stummer et al. (11) and Belykh et al. (7) have discussed the potential reasons for insufficient or absent fluorescence and how to circumvent the technical issues, including but not limited to the presence of blood products or overlying soft tissue, photobleaching, improper 5-ALA administration, and incorrect microscope settings. Additionally, the use of 5-ALA requires intermittent switching between the blue light and the white light modes of the neurosurgical operating microscope. Use of 5-ALA likely increases operative time and certainly increases pharmaceutical procedure costs.

Use of Intraoperative MRI in Conjunction With 5-ALA

In addition to neuronavigation and intraoperative cortical (sensory/motor) monitoring, several studies investigated the use of iMRI with 5-ALA guidance. As gadolinium enhancement on MRI is still the most reliable radiological marker of the EOR, these data are important to consider. Tsugu et al. (42) emphasized the utility of iMRI in patients with negative fluorescence, increasing the GTR to 55.6% from zero. However, the study did not show significant resection benefit with the adjunctive use of iMRI in patients with strong PpIX fluorescence signal. A retrospective study by Roder et al. (76) showed higher CRET rates in patients with iMRI plus 5-ALA vs. 5-ALA alone (74% vs. 45%; $P = 0.02$). Another study with 99 patients with malignant glioma undergoing 5-ALA–guided surgery in conjunction with iMRI reported a mean resection rate of 95% and suggested that 5-ALA allowed marginal tumor identification of the tumor extension beyond its radiological borders on iMRI (77). A recent systematic review by Coburger et al. concluded that the simultaneous use of 5-ALA in conjunction with iMRI can provide superior resection margins beyond radiological contrast enhancement (78). Obvious drawbacks of iMRI would be the added surgical time and significant increase in facilities and procedural costs. Although the assessment of iMRI in conjunction with 5-ALA was beyond the scope of this study, it may play a role in improving EOR and GTR in brain tumors with minimal or negative 5-ALA fluorescence.

Potential Therapeutic Role of 5-ALA

Recent years have witnessed a surge in the institution of novel adjuvant therapies in the management of HGGs, including photodynamic therapy (18, 79). Photodynamic therapy causes direct cytotoxicity by activating cellular death via apoptosis, necrosis, autophagy, and paraptosis through various intrinsic intracellular mechanisms. Several *in vitro* and *in vivo* studies have evaluated the role of 5-ALA as a therapeutic agent for intraoperative photodynamic therapy of the residual tumor (50, 52, 57, 79). Early *in vivo* studies have shown promising results. Because 5-ALA is not cytotoxic on systemic administration and has a better adverse effect profile than the other photosensitizer therapies, it has the potential to function beyond its role as a diagnostic tool by becoming a part of the future armamentarium of adjuvant therapies for aggressive gliomas.

Other Agents for Fluorescence Image-Guided Surgery

Apart from 5-ALA, fluorescein sodium has been used for intraoperative fluorescence-guided resection of HGGs. Fluorescein is an intravenous dye with selective accumulation through a damaged blood-brain barrier in malignant gliomas. A multicenter, controlled, Phase II trial showed complete resection of tumor in 82.6% patients with a 6-month PFS of 56.6%. However, the fluorescence characteristics of fluorescein are different than 5-ALA (2). Both exhibit variable fluorescence signal strength toward the periphery of the tumor, but, while 5-ALA stains cells, fluorescein is a non-specific dye leaked into the extravascular space by means of abnormal tumor vasculature or cortical trauma, with minor uptake by some cells (80). Thus, identification of the tumor marginal zone may be more difficult with fluorescein using wide-field fluorescence detection of the operating microscope, although it presents unique background staining of all cells visualized using confocal laser endomicroscopy (2, 67, 81). An advantage of fluorescein is that dosing can be repeated to a limited degree in the operating room. A pilot study recently investigated the synergistic use of 5-ALA and fluorescein in primary GBM. The complementary properties of these agents were used to capitalize on the advantages of each fluorophore to identify the tumor border zone in these patients (82). There are fewer studies on the use of fluorescein sodium compared to those using 5-ALA. Additional controlled comparative studies with a larger patient cohort are needed to establish the role of other fluorophores in image-guided resection of malignant gliomas.

Study Limitations and Potential Biases

There have been a few publications that have systematically documented the various aspects of the role of 5-ALA in HGGs, as discussed above (10, 20–22). Our study focused on the quantitative data synthesis of EOR, OS, and PFS in HGGs. However, there is a high degree of heterogeneity in the data based on factors such as tumor location, radiological assessment of residual or recurrent tumor, different protocols for neoadjuvant or adjuvant therapy, differential resources or utilization of adjunctive intraoperative tools discussed above, and so on (37, 41, 46, 76). Additionally, the studies were performed at various institutions internationally, imparting a greater degree of diversity in management strategy. The level of evidence supporting the benefit of fluorescence-guided surgery using 5-ALA in HGG is very low to low quality in nature, with the exception of one RCT (31). Therefore, these data must be interpreted with caution. Since 5-ALA is already approved in most of the countries, conducting an additional controlled study might present an ethical problem. Further blinded multicenter RCTs will aid in generating class I level of evidence for the survival outcomes associated with 5-ALA and comparing 5-ALA to the other available intraoperative adjuncts (e.g., iMRI, ultrasound, confocal laser endomicroscopy, and scanning fiber endoscopy) to improve maximal safe EOR (8, 67, 83). Although we attempted careful selection of studies, we cannot control for the inherent limitations and potential risks of surgical trial and retrospective study biases in this pooled analysis of data.

CONCLUSION

Our systematic review and meta-analysis show a modest survival benefit associated with the use of 5-ALA–guided surgery for HGGs. Unfortunately, at this time, the small number of studies and the low level of evidence of the available studies limit the ability to draw firm conclusions about the impact of 5-ALA–guided HGG resection on the OS and PFS of these patients. More high-quality studies with better controlling of confounding factors, such as adjuvant therapies, are needed to delineate the role of 5-ALA–guided surgery in improving survival of patients with these daunting tumors.

AUTHOR CONTRIBUTIONS

SG: literature review and study selection, statistical analysis, figures, manuscript draft, revision, and final draft approval. AT and LB: manuscript draft, review of final draft. EB: manuscript draft, figures, review of final draft. CC: literature review and study selection, review of final draft. XZ: statistical analysis, review of final draft. MS: table for summary of studies, statistical analysis, review of final draft. ML, PN, and MP: study supervision, review and revision of final draft. MP: generation of the topic, approval of final draft.

ACKNOWLEDGMENTS

The authors thank the staff of Neuroscience Publications at Barrow Neurological Institute for assistance with manuscript preparation.

REFERENCES

1. Brown TJ, Brennan MC, Li M, Church EW, Brandmeir NJ, Rakszawski KL, et al. Association of the extent of resection with survival in glioblastoma: a systematic review and meta-analysis. *JAMA Oncol.* (2016) 2:1460–9. doi: 10.1001/jamaoncol.2016.1373
2. Acerbi F, Broggi M, Schebesch KM, Hohne J, Cavallo C, De Laurentis C, et al. Fluorescein-guided surgery for resection of high-grade gliomas: a multicentric prospective phase II study (FLUOGLIO). *Clin Cancer Res.* (2018) 24:52–61. doi: 10.1158/1078-0432.CCR-17-1184
3. Li C, Sullivan PZ, Cho S, Nasrallah MP, Buch L, Isaac Chen HC, et al. Intraoperative molecular imaging with second window ICG facilitates confirmation of contrast-enhancing tissue during intracranial stereotactic needle biopsy: a case series. *World Neurosurg.* (2019). 126:e1211–8 doi: 10.1016/j.wneu.2019.02.231
4. Zeh R, Sheikh S, Xia L, Pierce J, Newton A, Predina J, et al. The second window ICG technique demonstrates a broad plateau period for near infrared fluorescence tumor contrast in glioblastoma. *PLoS ONE.* (2017) 12:e0182034. doi: 10.1371/journal.pone.0182034
5. Stummer W, Novotny A, Stepp H, Goetz C, Bise K, Reulen HJ. Fluorescence-guided resection of glioblastoma multiforme by using 5-aminolevulinic acid-induced porphyrins: a prospective study in 52 consecutive patients. *J Neurosurg.* (2000) 93:1003–13. doi: 10.3171/jns.2000.93.6.1003
6. Diez Valle R, Hadjipanayis CG, Stummer W. Established and emerging uses of 5-ALA in the brain: an overview. *J Neuro Oncol.* (2019) 141:487–94. doi: 10.1007/s11060-018-03087-7
7. Belykh E, Miller EJ, Patel AA, Bozkurt B, Yagmurlu K, Robinson TR, et al. Optical characterization of neurosurgical operating microscopes: quantitative fluorescence and assessment of PpIX photobleaching. *Sci Reports.* (2018) 8:12543. doi: 10.1038/s41598-018-30247-6
8. Belykh E, Martirosyan NL, Yagmurlu K, Miller EJ, Eschbacher JM, Izadyyazdanabadi M, et al. Intraoperative fluorescence imaging for personalized brain tumor resection: current state and future directions. *Front Surg.* (2016) 3:55. doi: 10.3389/fsurg.2016.00055
9. Hadjipanayis CG, Stummer W. 5-ALA and FDA approval for glioma surgery. *J Neurooncol.* (2019) 141:479–86. doi: 10.1007/s11060-019-03098-y
10. Mansouri A, Mansouri S, Hachem LD, Klironomos G, Vogelbaum MA, Bernstein M, et al. The role of 5-aminolevulinic acid in enhancing surgery for high-grade glioma, its current boundaries, and future perspectives: a systematic review. *Cancer.* (2016) 122:2469–78. doi: 10.1002/cncr.30088
11. Stummer W, Suero Molina E. Fluorescence imaging/agents in tumor resection. *Neurosurg Clin North Am.* (2017) 28:569–83. doi: 10.1016/j.nec.2017.05.009
12. Stummer W, Stocker S, Novotny A, Heimann A, Sauer O, Kempski O, et al. *In vitro* and *in vivo* porphyrin accumulation by C6 glioma cells after exposure to 5-aminolevulinic acid. *J Photochem Photobiol B Biol.* (1998) 45:160–9. doi: 10.1016/S1011-1344(98)00176-6
13. Stummer W, Stocker S, Wagner S, Stepp H, Fritsch C, Goetz C, et al. Intraoperative detection of malignant gliomas by 5-aminolevulinic acid-induced porphyrin fluorescence. *Neurosurgery.* (1998) 42:518–25; discussion 25–6.
14. Aldave G, Tejada S, Pay E, Marigil M, Bejarano B, Idoate MA, et al. Prognostic value of residual fluorescent tissue in glioblastoma patients after gross total resection in 5-aminolevulinic Acid-guided surgery. *Neurosurgery.* (2013) 72:915–20; discussion 20–1. doi: 10.1227/NEU.0b013e31828c3974
15. Jaber M, Wolfer J, Ewelt C, Holling M, Hasselblatt M, Niederstadt T, et al. The value of 5-aminolevulinic acid in low-grade gliomas and high-grade gliomas lacking glioblastoma imaging features: an analysis based on fluorescence, magnetic resonance imaging, 18F-fluoroethyl tyrosine positron emission tomography, and tumor molecular factors. *Neurosurgery.* (2016) 78:401–11; discussion 11. doi: 10.1227/NEU.0000000000001020
16. Fisher CJ, Niu C, Foltz W, Chen Y, Sidorova-Darmos E, Eubanks JH, et al. ALA-PpIX mediated photodynamic therapy of malignant gliomas augmented by hypothermia. *PLoS ONE.* (2017) 12:e0181654. doi: 10.1371/journal.pone.0181654
17. Kimura S, Kuroiwa T, Ikeda N, Nonoguchi N, Kawabata S, Kajimoto Y, et al. Assessment of safety of 5-aminolevulinic acid-mediated photodynamic therapy in rat brain. *Photodiagn Photodyn Ther.* (2018) 21:367–74. doi: 10.1016/j.pdpdt.2018.02.002
18. Mahmoudi K, Garvey KL, Bouras A, Cramer G, Stepp H, Jesu Raj JG, et al. 5-aminolevulinic acid photodynamic therapy for the treatment of high-grade gliomas. *J Neuro Oncol.* (2019) 141:595–607. doi: 10.1007/s11060-019-03103-4
19. Stupp R, Mason WP, van den Bent MJ, Weller M, Fisher B, Taphoorn MJ, et al. Radiotherapy plus concomitant and adjuvant temozolomide for glioblastoma. *N Engl J Med.* (2005) 352:987–96. doi: 10.1056/NEJMoa043330
20. Eljamel S. 5-ALA Fluorescence image guided resection of glioblastoma multiforme: a meta-analysis of the literature. *Int J Mol Sci.* (2015) 16:10443–56. doi: 10.3390/ijms160510443
21. Barone DG, Lawrie TA, Hart MG. Image guided surgery for the resection of brain tumours. *Cochrane Database System Rev.* (2014) 2014:Cd009685. doi: 10.1002/14651858.CD009685.pub2
22. Jenkinson MD, Barone DG, Bryant A, Vale L, Bulbeck H, Lawrie TA, et al. Intraoperative imaging technology to maximise extent of resection for glioma. *Cochrane Database System Rev.* (2018) 1:Cd012788. doi: 10.1002/14651858.CD012788.pub2
23. Higgins JPTGS. *Cochrane Handbook for Systematic Reviews.* The Cochrane Collaboration. Hoboken, NJ: Wiley-Blackwell (2011).
24. DerSimonian R, Laird N. Meta-analysis in clinical trials. *Controlled Clin Trials.* (1986) 7:177–88. doi: 10.1016/0197-2456(86)90046-2
25. Della Puppa A, Lombardi G, Rossetto M, Rustemi O, Berti F, Cecchin D, et al. Outcome of patients affected by newly diagnosed glioblastoma undergoing surgery assisted by 5-aminolevulinic acid guided resection followed by BCNU wafers implantation: a 3-year follow-up. *J Neuro Oncol.* (2017) 131:331–40. doi: 10.1007/s11060-016-2301-z
26. Diez Valle R, Tejada Solis S, Idoate Gastearena MA, Garcia de Eulate R, Dominguez Echavarri P, Aristu Mendiroz J. Surgery guided by 5-aminolevulinic fluorescence in glioblastoma: volumetric analysis of extent of resection in single-center experience. *J Neuro Oncol.* (2011) 102:105–13. doi: 10.1007/s11060-010-0296-4
27. Eyupoglu IY, Hore N, Savaskan NE, Grummich P, Roessler K, Buchfelder M, et al. Improving the extent of malignant glioma resection by dual intraoperative visualization approach. *PLoS ONE.* (2012) 7:e44885. doi: 10.1371/journal.pone.0044885
28. Feigl GC, Ritz R, Moraes M, Klein J, Ramina K, Gharabaghi A, et al. Resection of malignant brain tumors in eloquent cortical areas: a new multimodal approach combining 5-aminolevulinic acid and intraoperative monitoring. *J Neurosurg.* (2010) 113:352–7. doi: 10.3171/2009.10.JNS09447
29. Idoate MA, Diez Valle R, Echeveste J, Tejada S. Pathological characterization

of the glioblastoma border as shown during surgery using 5-aminolevulinic acid-induced fluorescence. *Neuropathology.* (2011) 31:575–82. doi: 10.1111/j.1440-1789.2011.01202.x
30. Schucht P, Beck J, Abu-Isa J, Andereggen L, Murek M, Seidel K, et al. Gross total resection rates in contemporary glioblastoma surgery: results of an institutional protocol combining 5-aminolevulinic acid intraoperative fluorescence imaging and brain mapping. *Neurosurgery.* (2012) 71:927–35; discussion 35–6. doi: 10.1227/NEU.0b013e31826d1e6b
31. Stummer W, Pichlmeier U, Meinel T, Wiestler OD, Zanella F, Reulen HJ, et al. Fluorescence-guided surgery with 5-aminolevulinic acid for resection of malignant glioma: a randomised controlled multicentre phase III trial. *Lancet Oncol.* (2006) 7:392–401. doi: 10.1016/S1470-2045(06)70665-9
32. Tejada-Solis S, Aldave-Orzaiz G, Pay-Valverde E, Marigil-Sanchez M, Idoate-Gastearena MA, Diez-Valle R. Prognostic value of ventricular wall fluorescence during 5-aminolevulinic-guided surgery for glioblastoma. *Acta Neurochirurg.* (2012) 154:1997–2002. doi: 10.1007/s00701-012-1475-1
33. Chan DTM, Yi-Pin Sonia H, Poon WS. 5-Aminolevulinic acid fluorescence guided resection of malignant glioma: Hong Kong experience. *Asian J Surg.* (2018) 41:467–72. doi: 10.1016/j.asjsur.2017.06.004
34. Coburger J, Hagel V, Wirtz CR, Konig R. Surgery for Glioblastoma: Impact of the Combined Use of 5-Aminolevulinic Acid and Intraoperative MRI on Extent of Resection and Survival. *PLoS ONE.* (2015) 10:e0131872. doi: 10.1371/journal.pone.0131872
35. Cortnum S, Laursen RJ. Fluorescence-guided resection of gliomas. *Danish Med J.* (2012) 59:A4460.
36. Della Puppa A, Ciccarino P, Lombardi G, Rolma G, Cecchin D, Rossetto M. 5-Aminolevulinic acid fluorescence in high grade glioma surgery: surgical outcome, intraoperative findings, and fluorescence patterns. *BioMed Res Int.* (2014) 2014:232561. doi: 10.1155/2014/232561
37. Diez Valle R, Slof J, Galvan J, Arza C, Romariz C, Vidal C. Observational, retrospective study of the effectiveness of 5-aminolevulinic acid in malignant glioma surgery in Spain (The VISIONA study). *Neurologia.* (2014) 29:131–8. doi: 10.1016/j.nrleng.2013.05.004
38. Pastor J, Pulido-Rivas P, Sola RG. Neurophysiological assisted transsulcal approach to a high grade glioma without affect neither motor nor somatosensory function. *Rev Neurol.* (2013) 56:370–4. doi: 10.33588/rn.5607.2013008
39. Piquer J, Llacer JL, Rovira V, Riesgo P, Rodriguez R, Cremades A. Fluorescence-guided surgery and biopsy in gliomas with an exoscope system. *BioMed Res Int.* (2014) 2014:207974. doi: 10.1155/2014/207974
40. Roessler K, Becherer A, Donat M, Cejna M, Zachenhofer I. Intraoperative tissue fluorescence using 5-aminolevolinic acid (5-ALA) is more sensitive than contrast MRI or amino acid positron emission tomography ((18)F-FET PET) in glioblastoma surgery. *Neurol Res.* (2012) 34:314–7. doi: 10.1179/1743132811Y.0000000078
41. Schatlo B, Fandino J, Smoll NR, Wetzel O, Remonda L, Marbacher S, et al. Outcomes after combined use of intraoperative MRI and 5-aminolevulinic acid in high-grade glioma surgery. *Neuro Oncol.* (2015) 17:1560–7. doi: 10.1093/neuonc/nov049
42. Tsugu A, Ishizaka H, Mizokami Y, Osada T, Baba T, Yoshiyama M, et al. Impact of the combination of 5-aminolevulinic acid-induced fluorescence with intraoperative magnetic resonance imaging-guided surgery for glioma. *World Neurosurg.* (2011) 76:120–7. doi: 10.1016/j.wneu.2011.02.005
43. Della Puppa A, Rustemi O, Rampazzo E, Persano L. Letter: combining 5-aminolevulinic acid fluorescence and intraoperative magnetic resonance imaging in glioblastoma surgery: a histology-based evaluation. *Neurosurgery.* (2017) 80:E188–e90. doi: 10.1093/neuros/nyw033
44. Nabavi A, Thurm H, Zountsas B, Pietsch T, Lanfermann H, Pichlmeier U, et al. Five-aminolevulinic acid for fluorescence-guided resection of recurrent malignant gliomas: a phase ii study. *Neurosurgery.* (2009) 65:1070–6; discussion 6–7. doi: 10.1227/01.NEU.0000360128.03597.C7
45. Belloch JP, Rovira V, Llacer JL, Riesgo PA, Cremades A. Fluorescence-guided surgery in high grade gliomas using an exoscope system. *Acta Neurochirurg.* (2014) 156:653–60. doi: 10.1007/s00701-013-1976-6
46. Eyupoglu IY, Hore N, Merkel A, Buslei R, Buchfelder M, Savaskan N. Supra-complete surgery via dual intraoperative visualization approach (DiVA) prolongs patient survival in glioblastoma. *Oncotarget.* (2016) 7:25755–68. doi: 10.18632/oncotarget.8367
47. Ng WP, Liew BS, Idris Z, Rosman AK. Fluorescence-guided versus conventional surgical resection of high grade glioma: a single-centre, 7-year, comparative effectiveness study. *Malays J Med Sci.* (2017) 24:78–86. doi: 10.21315/mjms2017.24.2.10
48. Stupp R, Taillibert S, Kanner A, Read W, Steinberg D, Lhermitte B, et al. Effect of tumor-treating fields plus maintenance temozolomide vs maintenance temozolomide alone on survival in patients with glioblastoma: a randomized clinical trial. *JAMA.* (2017) 318:2306–16. doi: 10.1001/jama.2017.18718
49. Weller M, Butowski N, Tran DD, Recht LD, Lim M, Hirte H, et al. Rindopepimut with temozolomide for patients with newly diagnosed, EGFRvIII-expressing glioblastoma (ACT IV): a randomised, double-blind, international phase 3 trial. *Lancet Oncol.* (2017) 18:1373–85. doi: 10.1016/S1470-2045(17)30517-X
50. Fujishiro T, Nonoguchi N, Pavliukov M, Ohmura N, Kawabata S, Park Y, et al. 5-Aminolevulinic acid-mediated photodynamic therapy can target human glioma stem-like cells refractory to antineoplastic agents. *Photodiagn Photodyn Ther.* (2018) 24:58–68. doi: 10.1016/j.pdpdt.2018.07.004
51. Kamoshima Y, Terasaka S, Iwasaki Y. [Photodynamic therapy mediated with 5-aminolevulinic acid for C6 glioma spheroids.] *Hokkaido J Med Sci.* (2008) 83:167–73. [Article in Japanese].
52. Leroy HA, Vermandel M, Vignion-Dewalle AS, Leroux B, Maurage CA, Duhamel A, et al. Interstitial photodynamic therapy and glioblastoma: light fractionation in a preclinical model. *Lasers Surg Med.* (2017) 49:506–15. doi: 10.1002/lsm.22620
53. Madsen SJ, Angell-Petersen E, Spetalen S, Carper SW, Ziegler SA, Hirschberg H. Photodynamic therapy of newly implanted glioma cells in the rat brain. *Lasers Surg Med.* (2006) 38:540–8. doi: 10.1002/lsm.20274
54. Schwake M, Nemes A, Dondrop J, Schroeteler J, Schipmann S, Senner V, et al. In-Vitro Use of 5-ALA for photodynamic therapy in pediatric brain tumors. *Neurosurgery.* (2018) 83:1328–37. doi: 10.1093/neuros/nyy054
55. Tetard MC, Vermandel M, Leroy HA, Leroux B, Maurage CA, Lejeune JP, et al. Interstitial 5-ALA photodynamic therapy and glioblastoma: preclinical model development and preliminary results. *Photodiagn Photodyn Ther.* (2016) 13:218–24. doi: 10.1016/j.pdpdt.2015.07.169
56. Wu SM, Ren QG, Zhou MO, Peng Q, Chen JY. Protoporphyrin IX production and its photodynamic effects on glioma cells, neuroblastoma cells and normal cerebellar granule cells *in vitro* with 5-aminolevulinic acid and its hexylester. *Cancer Lett.* (2003) 200:123–31. doi: 10.1016/S0304-3835(03)00271-4
57. Yamamoto T, Ishikawa E, Miki S, Sakamoto N, Zaboronok A, Matsuda M, et al. Photodynamic diagnosis using 5-aminolevulinic acid in 41 biopsies for primary central nervous system lymphoma. *Photochem Photobiol.* (2015) 91:1452–7. doi: 10.1111/php.12510
58. Yi W, Xu HT, Tian DF, Wu LQ, Zhang SQ, Wang L, et al. Photodynamic therapy mediated by 5-aminolevulinic acid suppresses gliomas growth by decreasing the microvessels. *J Huazhong Univ Sci Technol Med Sci.* (2015) 35:259–64. doi: 10.1007/s11596-015-1421-6
59. Lakomkin N, Hadjipanayis CG. Fluorescence-guided surgery for high-grade gliomas. *J Surg Oncol.* (2018) 118:356–61. doi: 10.1002/jso.25154
60. Zhao S, Wu J, Wang C, Liu H, Dong X, Shi C, et al. Intraoperative fluorescence-guided resection of high-grade malignant gliomas using 5-aminolevulinic acid-induced porphyrins: a systematic review and meta-analysis of prospective studies. *PLoS ONE.* (2013) 8:e63682. doi: 10.1371/journal.pone.0063682
61. Su X, Cheng K, Wang C, Xing L, Wu H, Cheng Z. Image-guided resection of malignant gliomas using fl uorescent nanoparticles. *Wiley Interdiscipl Rev Nanomed Nanobiotechnol.* (2013) 5:219–32. doi: 10.1002/wnan.1212
62. Martirosyan NL, Georges J, Eschbacher JM, Cavalcanti DD, Elhadi AM, Abdelwahab MG, et al. Potential application of a handheld confocal endomicroscope imaging system using a variety of fluorophores in experimental gliomas and normal brain. *Neurosurg Focus.* (2014) 36:E16. doi: 10.3171/2013.11.FOCUS13486
63. Kim JE, Cho HR, Xu WJ, Kim JY, Kim SK, Kim SK, et al. Mechanism for enhanced 5-aminolevulinic acid fluorescence in isocitrate dehydrogenase 1 mutant malignant gliomas. *Oncotarget.* (2015) 6:20266–77. doi: 10.18632/oncotarget.4060
64. Kitagawa T, Yamamoto J, Tanaka T, Nakano Y, Akiba D, Ueta K, et al. 5-Aminolevulinic acid strongly enhances delayed intracellular production of reactive oxygen species (ROS) generated by ionizing irradiation: quantitative analyses and visualization of intracellular ROS production in glioma cells *in vitro*. *Oncol Rep.* (2015) 33:583–90. doi: 10.3892/or.2014.3618

65. Ju D, Yamaguchi F, Zhan G, Higuchi T, Asakura T, Morita A, et al. Hyperthermotherapy enhances antitumor effect of 5-aminolevulinic acid-mediated sonodynamic therapy with activation of caspase-dependent apoptotic pathway in human glioma. *Tumour Biol.* (2016) 37:10415–26. doi: 10.1007/s13277-016-4931-3
66. Coupienne I, Fettweis G, Rubio N, Agostinis P, Piette J. 5-ALA-PDT induces RIP3-dependent necrosis in glioblastoma. *Photochem Photobiol Sci.* (2011) 10:1868–78. doi: 10.1039/c1pp05213f
67. Belykh E, Miller EJ, Hu D, Martirosyan NL, Woolf EC, Scheck AC, et al. Scanning fiber endoscope improves detection of 5-aminolevulinic acid-induced protoporphyrin IX fluorescence at the boundary of infiltrative glioma. *World Neurosurg.* (2018) 113:e51–69. doi: 10.1016/j.wneu.2018.01.151
68. Motekallemi A, Jeltema HR, Metzemaekers JD, van Dam GM, Crane LM, Groen RJ. The current status of 5-ALA fluorescence-guided resection of intracranial meningiomas-a critical review. *Neurosurg Rev.* (2015) 38:619–28. doi: 10.1007/s10143-015-0615-5
69. Wei L, Chen Y, Yin C, Borwege S, Sanai N, Liu JTC. Optical-sectioning microscopy of protoporphyrin IX fluorescence in human gliomas: standardization and quantitative comparison with histology. *J Biomed Optics.* (2017) 22:46005. doi: 10.1117/1.JBO.22.4.046005
70. Valdes PA, Leblond F, Kim A, Harris BT, Wilson BC, Fan X, et al. Quantitative fluorescence in intracranial tumor: implications for ALA-induced PpIX as an intraoperative biomarker. *J Neurosurg.* (2011) 115:11–7. doi: 10.3171/2011.2.JNS101451
71. Potapov AA, Goryaynov SA, Okhlopkov VA, Shishkina LV, Loschenov VB, Savelieva TA, et al. Laser biospectroscopy and 5-ALA fluorescence navigation as a helpful tool in the meningioma resection. *Neurosurg Rev.* (2016) 39:437–47. doi: 10.1007/s10143-015-0697-0
72. Potapov AA, Goryaynov SA, Okhlopkov VA, Pitskhelauri DI, Kobyakov GL, Zhukov VY, et al. [Clinical guidelines for the use of intraoperative fluorescence diagnosis in brain tumor surgery]. *Zh Vopr Neirokhir Im N N Burdenko.* (2015) 79:91–101. doi: 10.17116/neiro201579591-101
73. Stummer W, Tonn JC, Goetz C, Ullrich W, Stepp H, Bink A, et al. 5-Aminolevulinic acid-derived tumor fluorescence: the diagnostic accuracy of visible fluorescence qualities as corroborated by spectrometry and histology and postoperative imaging. *Neurosurgery.* (2014) 74:310–9; discussion 9–20. doi: 10.1227/NEU.0000000000000267
74. Utsuki S, Oka H, Sato S, Suzuki S, Shimizu S, Tanaka S, et al. Possibility of using laser spectroscopy for the intraoperative detection of nonfluorescing brain tumors and the boundaries of brain tumor infiltrates. Technical note. *J Neurosurg.* (2006) 104:618-20. doi: 10.3171/jns.2006.104.4.618
75. Haj-Hosseini N, Richter J, Andersson-Engels S, Wardell K. Optical touch pointer for fluorescence guided glioblastoma resection using 5-aminolevulinic acid. *Lasers Surg Med.* (2010) 42:9–14. doi: 10.1002/lsm.20868
76. Roder C, Bisdas S, Ebner FH, Honegger J, Naegele T, Ernemann U, et al. Maximizing the extent of resection and survival benefit of patients in glioblastoma surgery: high-field iMRI versus conventional and 5-ALA-assisted surgery. *Eur J Surg Oncol.* (2014) 40:297–304. doi: 10.1016/j.ejso.2013.11.022
77. Yamada S, Muragaki Y, Maruyama T, Komori T, Okada Y. Role of neurochemical navigation with 5-aminolevulinic acid during intraoperative MRI-guided resection of intracranial malignant gliomas. *Clin Neurol Neurosurg.* (2015) 130:134–9. doi: 10.1016/j.clineuro.2015.01.005
78. Coburger J, Wirtz CR. Fluorescence guided surgery by 5-ALA and intraoperative MRI in high grade glioma: a systematic review. *J Neuro Oncol.* (2019) 141:533–46. doi: 10.1007/s11060-018-03052-4
79. Shimizu K, Nitta M, Komori T, Maruyama T, Yasuda T, Fujii Y, et al. Intraoperative photodynamic diagnosis using talaporfin sodium simultaneously applied for photodynamic therapy against malignant glioma: a prospective clinical study. *Front Neurol.* (2018) 9:24. doi: 10.3389/fneur.2018.00024
80. Belykh E, Miller EJ, Patel AA, Yazdanabadi MI, Martirosyan NL, Yagmurlu K, et al. Diagnostic accuracy of a confocal laser endomicroscope for *in vivo* differentiation between normal injured and tumor tissue during fluorescein-guided glioma resection: laboratory investigation. *World Neurosurg.* (2018) 115:e337–48. doi: 10.1016/j.wneu.2018.04.048
81. Martirosyan NL, Eschbacher JM, Kalani MY, Turner JD, Belykh E, Spetzler RF, et al. Prospective evaluation of the utility of intraoperative confocal laser endomicroscopy in patients with brain neoplasms using fluorescein sodium: experience with 74 cases. *Neurosurg Focus.* (2016) 40:E11. doi: 10.3171/2016.1.FOCUS15559
82. Della Puppa A, Munari M, Gardiman MP, Volpin F. Combined fluorescence using 5-aminolevulinic acid and fluorescein sodium at glioblastoma border: intraoperative findings and histopathologic data about 3 newly diagnosed consecutive cases. *World Neurosurg.* (2019) 122:e856–63. doi: 10.1016/j.wneu.2018.10.163
83. Duffau H. The necessity of preserving brain functions in glioma surgery: the crucial role of intraoperative awake mapping. *World Neurosurg.* (2011) 76:525–7. doi: 10.1016/j.wneu.2011.07.040

11

Novel Visualization Methods Assisted Transurethral Resection for Bladder Cancer

Honglin Li[1,2†], *Yubin Cao*[1,3†], *Pingchuan Ma*[1,2], *Zhongkai Ma*[1,2], *Chunjie Li*[1,2,4], *Wenbin Yang*[1,3,4*] and *Lingyun Zhou*[5*]

[1] State Key Laboratory of Oral Diseases, National Clinical Research Center for Oral Diseases, West China School of Stomatology, Sichuan University, Chengdu, China, [2] Department of Head and Neck Oncology, West China Hospital of Stomatology, Sichuan University, Chengdu, China, [3] Department of Oral and Maxillofacial Surgery, West China Hospital of Stomatology, Sichuan University, Chengdu, China, [4] Department of Medical Affairs, West China Hospital of Stomatology, Sichuan University, Chengdu, China, [5] Center of Infectious Diseases, West China Hospital of Sichuan University, Chengdu, China

Correspondence:
Wenbin Yang
yangwenbinkq@163.com
Lingyun Zhou
4423925@qq.com

†These authors have contributed equally to this work and share first authorship

Background: Photodynamic diagnosis and narrow-band imaging could help improve the detection rate in transurethral resection (TUR) of bladder cancer. It remained controversial that the novel visualization method assisted transurethral resection (VA-TUR) could elongate patients' survival compared to traditional TUR.

Methods: We performed electronic and manual searching until December 2020 to identify randomized controlled trials comparing VA-TUR with traditional TUR, which reported patients' survival data. Two reviewers independently selected eligible studies, extracted data, assessed the risk of bias. Meta-analysis was conducted according to subgroups of types of visualization methods (A) and clinical stage of participants. Publication bias was detected.

Results: We included 20 studies (reported in 28 articles) in this review. A total of 6,062 participants were randomized, and 5,217 participants were included in the analysis. Only two studies were assessed at low risk of bias. VA-TURB could significantly improve the recurrence-free survival (RFS) (HR = 0.72, 95% CI: 0.66 to 0.79, $P < 0.00001$, $I^2 = 42\%$) and progression-free survival (PFS) (HR = 0.62, 95% CI: 0.46 to 0.82, $P < 0.0008$, $I^2 = 0\%$) compared with TUR under white light. The results remain stable whatever the type of visualization method. The difference could be observed in the non-muscle-invasive bladder cancer (NMIBC) population ($P < 0.05$) but not in the mixed population with muscle-invasive bladder cancer (MIBC) participants ($P > 0.05$).

Conclusion: VA-TUR could improve RFS and PFS in NMIBC patients. No significant difference is found among different types of VA-TUR. VA-TUR may be not indicated to MIBC patients.

Keywords: narrow-band imaging, photodynamic diagnosis, hexylaminolaevulinate, 5-aminolaevulinic acid, cystectomy, cystoscopy

INTRODUCTION

Bladder cancer is the fourth most common cancer in men (1). Nine men in every 100,000, and 2.2 as many women worldwide develop bladder cancer (2). According to the invasion of the muscle layer, bladder cancer can be divided into non-muscle invasive bladder cancer (NMIBC) and (MIBC). Of newly diagnosed tumors, 70% are NMIBC comprised of stages Ta, T1 and carcinoma *in situ* (CIS) (3). Transurethral resection (TUR) after white light cystoscopy is taken as the primary treatment option for NMIBC (4). Of particular concern is the fact that despite resection assisted by the current gold standard-white light cystoscopy, patients still have a high probability of recurrence more than 50% (5, 6). It is widely shared that a complete resection plays a central role in achieving a good prognosis (7). Residual tumors are found in 33–76% of patients and are usually located at the border of the resected tumor (8, 9). Although the bladder is a perfect darkroom for white light in the TUR, the detection of tumor is still limited to the visual localization and diagnosis experience of the surgeon, particularly of the small, occult tumor lesions and CIS (10). Therefore, some new technologies are being developed to visualize the missing lesions and guide tumor resection during TUR.

There are two main types of new technologies of tumor visualization currently used in clinical practice: photodynamic diagnosis (11) (PDD) and narrow-band imaging (NBI) (12). PDD in the bladder requires intravesical instillation of an exogenous photosensitizer, 5-aminolaevulinic acid (5-ALA) (13) or hexyl-aminolaevulinate (HLA) (14), which accumulate selectively in tumor cells (15). Under the light with a given wavelength, lesions emit red fluorescence among the green areas of healthy tissue. The visual contrast between tumor and healthy tissue allows surgeons to detect the lesion sensitively which appears to be normal in the white light cystoscopy, thereby achieving complete removal of the tumor. 5-ALA currently licensed by the FDA for the photodynamic treatment increases the production of the photosensitizer, PpIX (16). It is now well established from a variety of studies, that 5-ALA-induced PpIX preferentially accumulates in many cancer cells including the bladder (16). HLA is the derivative of 5-ALA to improve its bioavailability and solubility, which means NMIBC appears brighter and lasts longer in the HLA-guided TUR (17). Narrow-band imaging (NBI) is another novel endoscopic technique applied in clinical practice. NBI enhance the contrast between the superficial mucosa and microvascular structures *via* only emitting two bandwidths of illumination, 415 nm (blue) and 540 nm (green) (18, 19). Assisted by specialized cystoscopes, surgeons could notice abnormal microvasculature and perform NBI-guided TURBT without prior instillation of dyes (20).

A previous systematic review and meta-analysis suggested that novel visualization methods assisted TUR (VA-TUR) by PDD or NBI can improve cancer detection and decrease the risk of BC recurrence in the short and long term, compared with white light (20, 21). VA-TUR have been recommended as weak evidence in the latest European Association of Urology Guidelines on NMIBC (22). However, controversies remained on whether VA-TUR could elongate patients' survival, whereas no previous studies have addressed the complete survival data of patients, to the best of our knowledge. Therefore, this systematic review and meta-analysis aimed to analyze the effects of VA-TUR on the survival of bladder cancer patients, based on the time-to-event survival data.

METHODS

This systematic review adhered to preferred reporting items for systematic review and meta-analysis (PRISMA) statement (23).

Eligibility Criteria

Types of studies: randomized controlled trials (RCTs).

Types of participants: Patients (>18 yr) with suspected bladder cancer (first diagnosis or recurrence) based on at least one documented cystoscopy.

Types of interventions: any types of VA-TUR;

Types of controls: traditional TUR under white light or other types of VA-TUR;

Types of outcome measures: recurrence-free survival (RFS), progression-free survival (PFS), overall survival (OS), cancer-specific survival (CSS).

Literature Search

We searched PubMed, Embase, Cochrane Central Register of Controlled Trials, and China National Knowledge Infrastructure from inception to December 2020. The search strategy of each database was provided in the supplemental materials. The search attempted to identify all relevant studies, irrespective of language. We translated non-English papers. Two researchers (HL and YC) independently screened the titles and abstracts and selected articles for full-text review. They then independently reviewed full-text articles for eligibility. A third researcher (WY) arbitrated any differences that could not be resolved by consensus. We also performed a manual search of the references of eligible articles and relevant systematic reviews.

Data Extraction

Two review authors (HL and YC) carried out the data extraction in duplicate. Disagreements were resolved by discussion, and an arbitrator (WY) was involved when the disagreement remained unresolved. We designed a customized data extraction form, in accordance with guidance from the Cochrane Handbook for Systematic Reviews of Interventions version (24). We pilot-tested this, using a sample of the studies focusing on this topic, and then applied it to all the included studies. We collected the following data: first author, publication time, country, participants' gender, age, study design, interventions, number of participants randomized, number of participants analyzed, clinical stage, histopathological grade, follow-up duration, recurrence state, number of tumors, size of tumors, survival data. The time-to-event survival data were extracted according to Tierney et al. if they were not reported in the full texts (25). We contacted authors for additional information regarding the survival data of individual patients.

Assessment of Methodological Quality of Included Studies

We judged the risk of bias in each of the included studies for six domains (as identified in the Cochrane 'Risk of Bias' tool): random sequence generation, allocation concealment, blinding of outcome assessment, incomplete outcome data, selective reporting, and other bias (24). As blinding of participants and personnel were impossible for all studies, we did not assess this domain. For each of the following domains, we assigned a judgment of low, high, or unclear risk of bias. Two review authors (HL and YC) independently assessed the risk of bias according to the published article and the trial authors' responses. They discussed any discrepancies, and a third review author (LZ) arbitrated when necessary.

Method of Data Analysis

For time-to-event survival data, we calculated hazard ratio (HR) and 95% confidence intervals (CIs). We conducted Intention-to-treat (ITT) analysis if there were sufficient data. If ITT could not be adopted, we planned to analyze the available data and interpret results with caution. We used the Chi^2 test for heterogeneity to examine if heterogeneity existed among the included studies. We used the I^2 statistic to estimate the impact of the heterogeneity.

We used Review Manager 5 (version 5.4.1) to conduct a random-effect model inverse-variance-method meta-analysis (24). Subgroup analysis was performed according to types of visualization methods or clinical stages of the participant population. Sensitivity was further performed to examine the origin of heterogeneity. We assessed publication bias and other reporting biases with the help of funnel plots and Begg's test if there were more than 10 trials providing results for one outcome.

Assessment of Quality of Evidence

We used the GRADE (Grading of Recommendations, Assessment, Development and Evaluation) working group classification to assess the quality of evidence for each outcome included in the umbrella review (26). The GRADE approach categorizes evidence from systematic reviews and meta-analyses into "high," "moderate," "low," or "very low" quality. Study design dictates the baseline quality of the evidence but other factors can decrease or increase the quality level.

RESULTS

Results of Search

We identified a total of 1,509 records from electronic searches and hand-searching. After removing duplicates, we screened 1,306 records by scanning the titles and abstracts. We considered 41 records to be potentially eligible and obtained the full texts for further consideration. We excluded 13 published studies. We included 20 studies (reported in 28 articles) in this review (19, 26–52). A flow diagram illustrating the study selection process is shown in **Figure 1**.

Characteristics of Included Studies

All the included studies were two-arm parallel RCTs (**Table 1**). Six studies compared 5-ALA to WL, nine studies compared HAL to WL, and nine studies compared NBI to WL. No study directly compared different visualization methods directly. A total of 6,062 participants were randomized, and 5,217 participants were included in the analysis. The participants' age ranged from 19 to 97 years old, and female: male = 1:2.6. Approximately 12 studies only included NMIBC patients (Stage Tis/Ta/T1), four studies also included T0 patients who were confirmed benign lesions by histopathology, and four studies included patients with muscle-invasive lesions (Stage ≥T2). Nine studies adopted the histopathological system of Grade 1/Grade 2/Grade 3, seven studies adopted the PUNLMP/Low Grade/High Grade system, and the others did not report the grade distribution. Patients in 15 studies received co-interventions of BCG/MMC/epirubicin/other adjuvant treatments. Ten studies followed participants up with one year, six studies with two to five years, four studies with five years or longer.

Risk of Bias

Two studies were assessed at low risk of bias in all the methodological domains (**Figure 2**). Two studies were assessed at high risk of bias due to >20% of participants lost follow-up without ITT analysis. Nine studies reported the details of random sequencing methods; Three studies reported the correct allocation concealment methods; Six studies emphasized the blinding of outcome assessment; 15 studies had <10% follow-up loss or adopted ITT analysis; All the studies reported planned outcomes in suitable formats; The studies were assessed at low risk of bias in these domains. Studies were assessed at unclear risk of bias in other domains without adequate information or details. We did not identify risk of bias due to deviations from intended interventions, co-interventions, baseline balance or other sources.

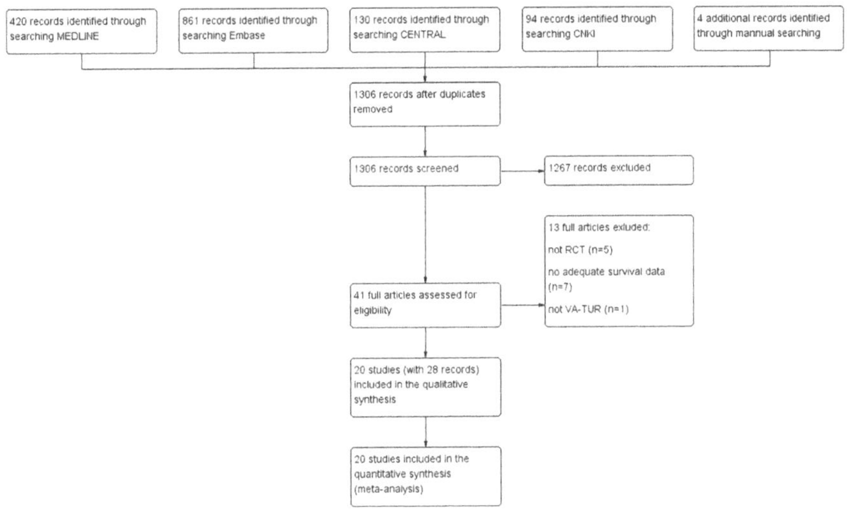

FIGURE 1 | Study flow diagram.

Effects of Interventions

RFS

RFS could be extracted from all the included studies. VA-TURB could significantly improve the RFS compared with TUR under white light (HR = 0.72, 95% CI: 0.66 to 0.79, P <0.00001, I^2 = 42%). Either 5-ALA, HAL or NBI could significantly improve the RFS (5-ALA: HR = 0.68, 95% CI: 0.58 to 0.79, P <0.00001, I^2 = 66%; HAL: HR = 0.73, 95% CI: 0.64 to 0.83, P <0.00001, I^2 = 28%; NBI: HR = 0.76, 95% CI: 0.65 to 0.90, P ≤0.001, I^2 = 29%) and no significant subgroup differences were observed (P = 0.59, I^2 = 0%) (**Figure 3**). RFS could be significantly improved by VA-TURB in the NMIBC population staged Ta/T1 (HR = 0.62, 95% CI: 0.49 to 0.78, P <0.0001, I^2 = 39%), Ta/T1/Tis (HR = 0.70, 95% CI: 0.57 to 0.87, P = 0.0009, I^2 = 37%), or T1/Ta/Tis/T0 (HR = 0.58, 95% CI: 0.46 to 0.71, P <0.00001, I^2 = 0%), but not in the mixed population of NMIBC and MIBC (HR = 0.88, 95% CI: 0.71 to 1.10, P = 0.26, I^2 = 33%). The subgroup differences were significant (P = 0.04, I^2 = 63.5%) (**Figure 4**). Sensitivity analysis excluding the mixed population of NMIBC and MIBC showed no significant subgroup differences (P = 0.42, I^2 = 0%). No publication bias was identified by funnel plot (**Figure 5**) or Begg's test (P = 0.52).

PFS

PFS could be extracted from five studies, three of 5-ALA, one of HAL, and one of NBI. VA-TURB could significantly improve the PFS compared with TUR under white light (HR = 0.62, 95% CI: 0.46 to 0.82, P <0.0008, I^2 = 0%). The subgroup analysis could not show the significant effects of either 5-ALA, HAL or NBI (P >0.05) (**Figure 6**). PFS could be significantly improved by VA-TURB in the NMIBC population staged Ta/T1/Tis (HR = 0.81, 95% CI: 0.67 to 0.99, P = 0.04, I^2 = 39%) or T1/Ta/Tis/T0 (HR = 0.56, 95% CI: 0.42 to 0.74, P <0.0001, I^2 = 0%), but not in the mixed population of NMIBC and MIBC (HR = 0.90, 95% CI: 0.62 to 1.30, P = 0.57, I^2 = 57%) (**Figure 7**). Sensitivity analysis and publication bias test were not performed due to limited included studies.

OS and CSS

Only one study reports OS and CSS. No significant benefit of OS and CSS was observed in 5-ALA assisted TUR compared with traditional white light (OS: HR = 0.69, 95% CI: 0.45 to 1.05, P = 0.09; CSS: HR = 0.55, 95% CI: 0.19 to 1.63, P = 0.28).

Quality of Evidence

Evidence of VA-TURB improving RFS was downgraded to moderate-quality evidence due to the serious risk of bias. Evidence of VA-TURB improving PFS was downgraded to low-quality of evidence due to serious risk of bias and inconsistency. Evidence for OS and CSS was downgraded to very low-quality due to serious risk of bias, very serious imprecision and a single trial.

DISCUSSION

Summary of Findings

Recent guidelines recommended that surgeons use methods to improve tumor visualization (fluorescence cystoscopy, narrow-band imaging) during TURB, but the strength was rated as weak (22). It was possibly attributed to the deficiency of firm evidence of patients' benefits. Only limited studies reported the hazard ratio of survival, but most studies reported the test results or survival curve. Our study is the first systematic review that analyzed survival data in the time-to-event form. There is moderate-quality evidence from 20 RCTs that visualization assisted TURB may lead to an increase in RFS compared to TURB in white light, and low-quality evidence from five RCTs

TABLE 1 | The characteristics of included studies.

Study	Country	Design	Age (mean, range) (Y)	Gender (F/M)	No. of participants randomized	No. of participants analyzed	ITT	pT Stage	Grade	Co-intervention	Follow-up (M)	Recurrence	No. of tumors	Size of tumors
27	Czech	RCT	68.9	40/82	WL: 62 5-ALA: 60	WL: 62 5-ALA: 60	yes	Ta: 74 T1: 47	G1:63 G2:46 G3:13	/	24	P: 48 R: 74	/	1 cm: 31 1–3 cm: 67 >3 cm: 24
28	Germany; Austria	RCT	68.5 (19–89)	29/73	WL:51 5-ALA: 51	WL: 51 5-ALA: 51	yes	Ta: 80 T1: 22	G1:16 G2:74 G3:12	/	60	/	S: 50 M: 52	/
29	Romania	RCT	60.4	34/10	WL: 22 HLA: 22	WL: 22 HLA: 22	yes	Ta: 10 T1: 24	G1:13 G2:26 G3:5	MMC	12	/	/	1.84 ± 0.57 cm
30	Romania	RCT	59.8	25/88	WL: 56 HLA: 57	WL: 56 HLA: 57	yes	Ta: 33 T1: 80 Tis: 9	G1:41 G2:59 G3:13	BCG	60	/	S: 57 M: 56	/
31	Denmark	RCT	70.1	200/499	WL: 348 HLA: 352	WL: 346 HLA: 349	no	Ta: 666 T1: 23	/	BCG MMC	12	/	/	/
32	Germany	RCT	68.9 (31–89)	/	WL: 150 5-ALA: 151	WL: 103 5-ALA: 88	yes	Ta: 138 T1: 42 Tis: 11	G1:78 G2:74 G3:13	BCG MMC	90	/	S: 134 M: 57	/
36	Romania	RCT	64.1 (30–84)	59/161	WL: 110 NBI: 110	WL: 110 NBI: 110	no	Ta: 55 T1: 137 T2: 26 T3: 2	/	MMC; BCG	12	/	S: 73 M: 147	>3 cm: all
37	Greece	RCT	67.07	17/87	WL: 64 HLA: 66	WL: 50 HLA: 54	no	Ta: 47 T1/Tis:17	LG:51 HG:13	Epirubicin re-TUR	40	P: 46 R: 58	/	/
38	Denmark	RCT	70 (35–96)	36/109	WL: 118 HLA: 115	WL: 117 HLA: 102	no	Ta: 139 T1: 5	LG:126 HG:18	/	12	/	S: 92 M: 53	<3 cm: 111 ≥3 cm: 34
39	USA	RCT	67.5 (36–99)	71/183	WL: 127 NBI: 127	WL: 127 NBI: 127	yes	T0: 95 T1: 42 Tis: 71 Ta: 47	/	BCG	24	/	S: 34 M: 220	<2 cm: 19 2–5 cm: 194 >5 cm: 41
40	Greece	RCT	64.99 (37–88)	13/73	WL: 53 HLA: 49	WL: 46 HLA: 42	no	/	LG:53 HG:23	BCG epirubicin	25	P: 63 R: 23	S: 44 M: 42	/
19	Korea	RCT	/	36/118	WL: 97 NBI: 101	WL: 55 NBI: 72	no	T0: 24 Ta: 5 T1: 2 Tis: 6	LG:57 HG:64	/	12	P: 118 R: 34	/	<1 cm: 82 1–3 cm: 54 >3 cm: 16
41	Japan; Spain; Czech; UK; China; Canada; Netherlands	RCT	66.9 (18–94)	192/773	WL: 492 NBI: 489	WL: 481 NBI: 484	no	Tx: 51 T0: 78 T1: 432 Tis: 19 Ta: 432 T2: 77	G1:281 G2:248 G3:200	MMC BCG	48	/	S: 397 M: 346	<1 cm: 545 ≥2 m: 399
42	Italy;	RCT	/	119/29	WL: 93 NBI: 95	WL: 72 NBI: 76	yes	Ta: 110 T1: 38	LG:80 HG:68	MMC; BCG	12	P: 83 R: 65	S: 76 M: 72	<3 cm: 108 ≥3 cm: 40
44	UK	RCT	68 (21–95)	46/183	WL: 120 HLA: 129	WL: 88 HLA: 97	no	Ta: 127 T1: 55 Tis: 1	G1:99 G2:28 G3:57	MMC BCG	12	/	S: 91 M: 149	/
46	Germany	RCT	66 (18–87)	87/290	WL: 273 5-ALA: 252	WL: 203 5-ALA: 174	no	T0: 40 Ta: 145 T1: 188 Tis: 4	G1:201 G2:107 G3:17	BCG reTUR	92	P: 255 R: 122	0–1: 171 2–7: 161 ≥8: 45	<3 cm: 289 ≥3 cm: 87
47	Sweden	RCT	69.5	72/207	WL: 138 HLA: 141	WL: 138 HLA: 141	yes	T0: 33 Ta: 174 T1: 13 T2: 6 Tis: 43 Tx: 10	/	MMC BCG	12	P: 136 R: 143	S: 111 M: 127	/
48	Germany; Canada; USA; Netherlands	RCT	68.8	116/435	WL: 384 HLA: 382	WL: 280 HLA: 271	yes	Ta: 262 T1: 63 Tis: 41	G1+G2:422 G3: 156	BCG	9	P: 101 R: 170	/	/
51	Germany; Austria	RCT	66	100/259	WL: 189 5-ALA: 192	WL: 183 5-ALA: 187	no	Ta: 183 T1: 76 Tis: 47 T2: 18	G1:115 G2:104 G3:48	BCG	12	/	S: 216 M: 143	/
52	USA	RCT	76 (53–97)	33/115	WL: 300 NBI: 300	WL: 70 NBI: 78	no	Ta: 129 T1: 5 Tis: 13 T2: 1	LG:113 HG:35	/	48	P: R: 148	/	/

RCT, randomized controlled trial; WT, white light; 5-ALA, 5-aminolaevulinic acid; HAL, hexylaminolaevulinate; NBI, narrow band imaging; ITT, intention-to-treat analysis; LG, low grade; Hg, high grade; re-TUR, re-transurethral resection; BCG, Bacillus Calmette Guèrin; MMC, Mitomycin-C; P, primary; R, recurrent; S, single tumors; M, multifocal tumors.

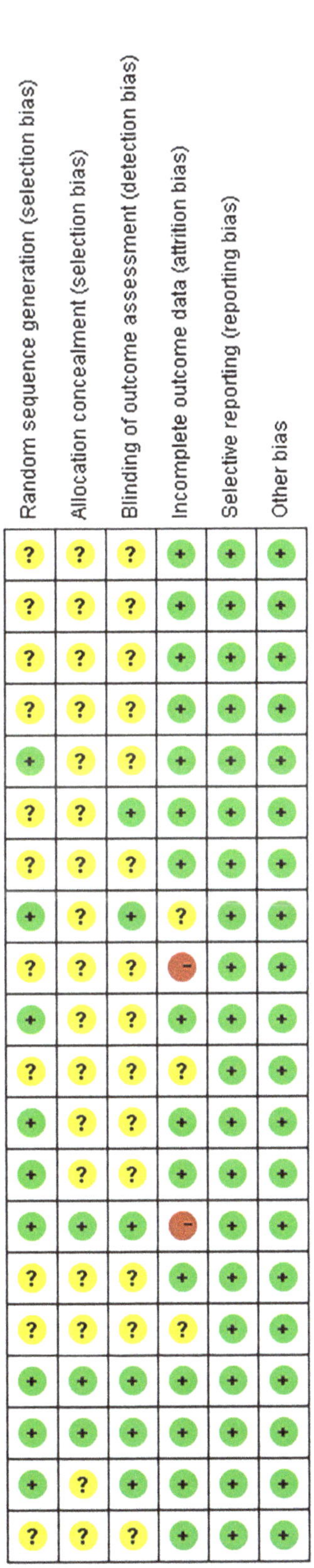

FIGURE 2 | Risk of bias summary: review authors' judgements about each risk of bias item for each included study.

suggested the benefit of VA-TURB on PFS. These results indicated that VA-TURB elongated the time to first recurrence or progression.

As we are clear that VA-TURB is recommended, the next question is which visualization method is the most recommended. We noticed that the effect size of NBI was lower than 5-ALA and HAL. However, the answer may remain unknown according to current evidence. First, no significant difference was found among subgroups of 5-ALA, HAL, and NBI. Second, we noticed that two low-risk-of-bias studies, Schumacher et al. (47) and Stenzl et al. (48), showed an insignificant or critically significant result for 5-ALA (HR = 1.06, 95% CI: 0.79 to 1.42) and HAL (HR = 0.81, 95% CI: 0.67 to 0.99) respectively. The results from low-risk-of-bias studies indicated that the effects of 5-ALA or HAL might not overwhelm NBI.

Another emerging question is whether VA-TURB did not improve survival as the high-quality studies showed. We conducted a subgroup and sensitivity analysis which might elucidate this issue. We found all the studies recruiting MIBC patients did not show a significant benefit in both RFS and PFS. For RFS, the inter-subgroup heterogeneity I^2 drastically decreased from 63.5 to 0%. These results suggested that MIBC might not be indicated to VA-TURB.

Implications for Practice and Research

Our results suggest that surgeons should use VA-TURB for all the NMIBC patients. The type of VA-TURB could be selected in accordance with the hospital's finance and clinician's preference. We recommended surgeons insist on radical cystectomy for MIBC patients rather than transurethral resection according to currently available evidence.

We identified some evidence gaps *via* this systematic review, which should be filled by future researchers. First, no low-risk-of-bias studies were performed in the NMIBC population, which should be cautiously designed and conducted by future studies for 5-ALA, HAL, and NBI respectively. If the results remain stable and promising in high-quality studies, it may be acceptable to upgrade the recommendation strength of VA-TURB to strong.

Second, there were no RCTs directly compared the efficacy of 5-ALA, HAL, and NBI. Burger et al. retrospectively reviewed the patients' records and found no difference between 5-ALA and HAL (53). A previous network meta-analysis suggested that 5-ALA might be more effective than HAL in decreasing recurrence rate (54). However, it seemed different in our study as no inter-subgroup difference was observed. Direct comparisons are needed to determine the most effective visualization method.

Third, more coefficient factors could be further explored. A post-hoc analysis by Rolevich et al. disclosed that VA-TURB might promise more patients' survival when less experienced surgeons conducted the TURB (45). Denzinger et al. analyzed the RFS stratified by prognostic risk groups, which showed that patients of all grades profit from VA-TURB, whereas the low-risk group might obtain more compared to traditional TURB (34). Future researches could address the potential correlated factors to further refine the indications of VA-TURB.

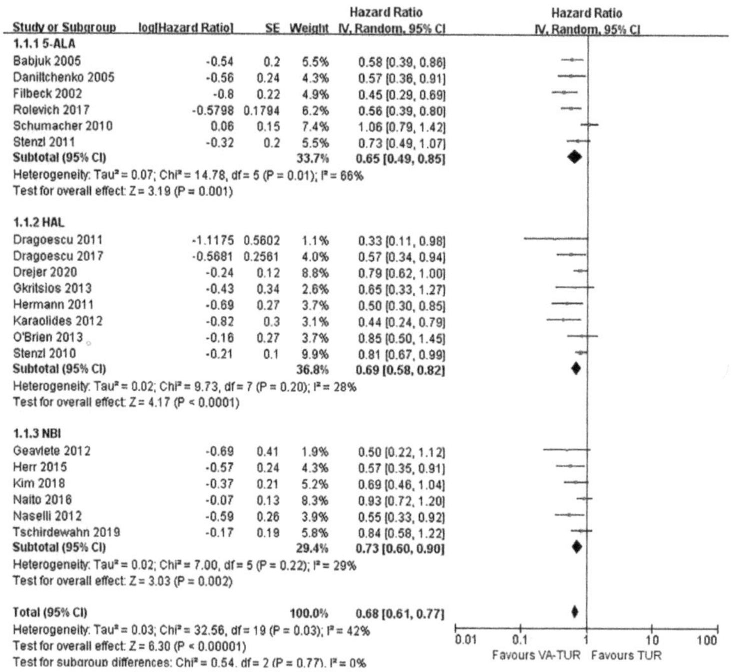

FIGURE 3 | Forest plot of RFS of VA-TUR versus TUR subgrouped by types of visualization methods.

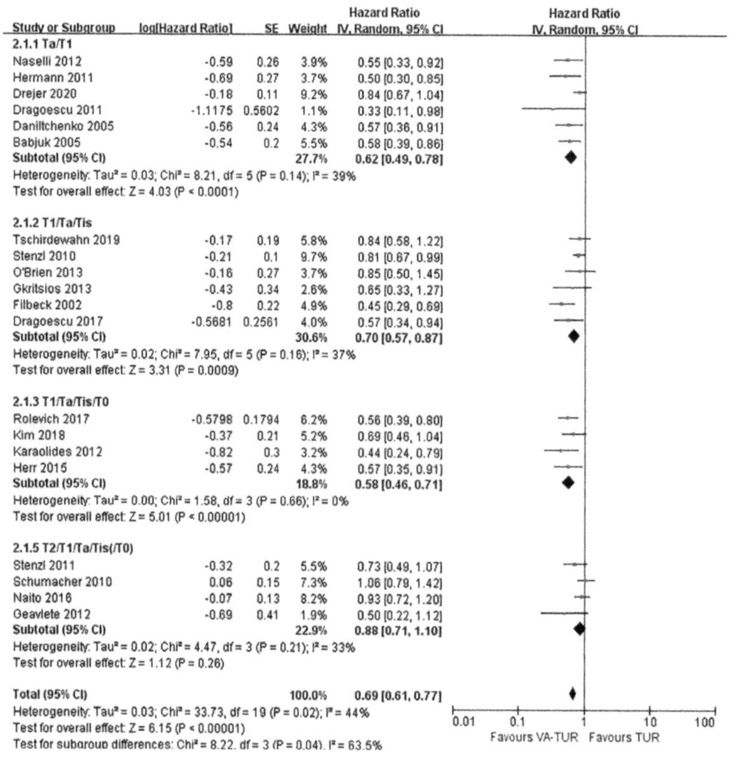

FIGURE 4 | Forest plot of RFS of VA-TUR versus TUR subgrouped by clinical stage of participants.

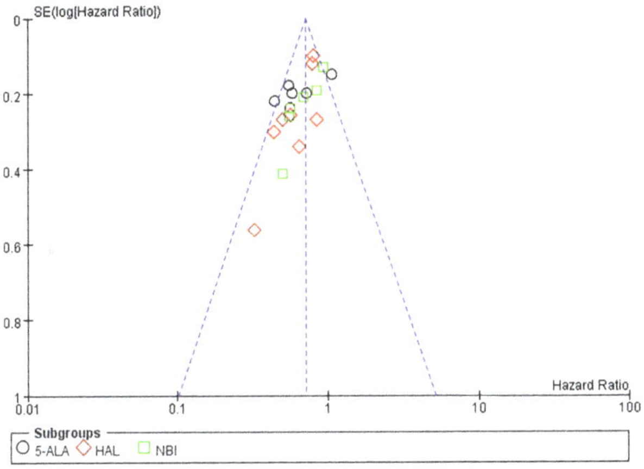

FIGURE 5 | Funnel plot of RFS of VA-TUR versus TUR.

Fourth, the effects of VA-TURB in pT2 participants still need more exploration. Our results found that VA-TURB performed similarly to traditional transurethral resection in the mixed population of NMIBC and MIBC participants. The results might have been attributable to the invalidity of transurethral resection instead of visualization methods for pT2 participants. The National Comprehensive Cancer Network guidelines list transurethral bladder tumor resection as one of the treatment options for non-cystectomy candidates (55). Moreover, a previous systematic review concluded that treatment based on a combination of resection, chemotherapy, and radiotherapy as bladder-sparing strategies may be considered as a reasonable treatment option in properly selected patients (56). However, RCTs composed with MIBC patients were very limited, this result may need further confirmation by high-quality RCTs.

In addition, although NMIBC is often recurrent, tumor progression and patient death remained to be important prognostic events. We strongly suggest researchers analyze and report the RFS, PFS, OS, and CSS completely.

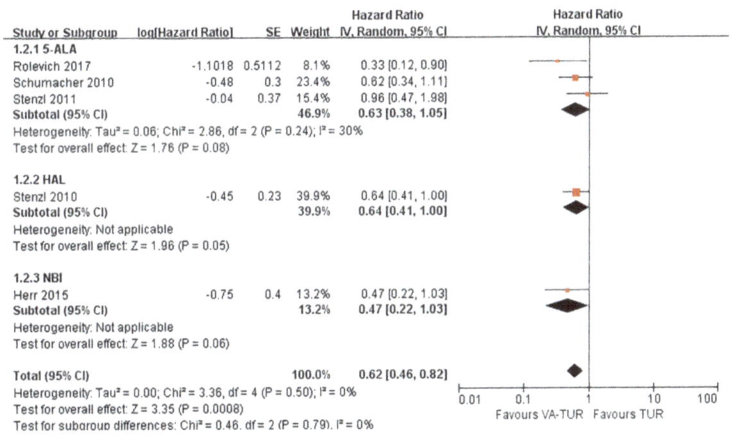

FIGURE 6 | Forest plot of PFS of VA-TUR versus TUR subgrouped by types of visualization methods.

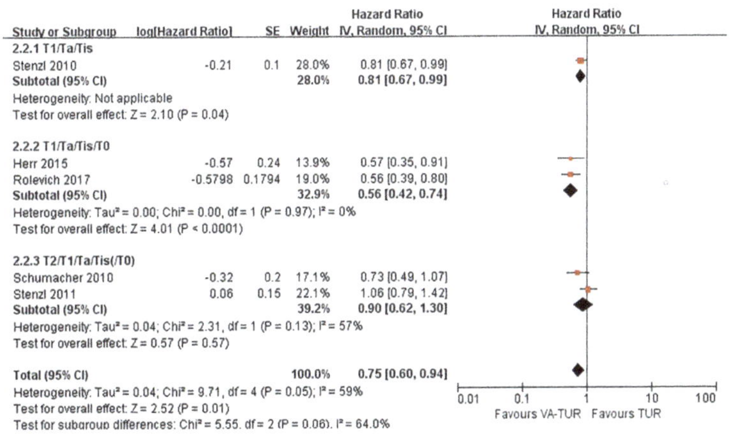

FIGURE 7 | Forest plot of PFS of VA-TUR versus TUR subgrouped by types of clinical stage of participants.

Agreements, Disagreements, and Our Strength

Previous systematic reviews or meta-analyses addressed the recurrence rate measured at 1-year follow-up, 2-year follow-up, or the longest follow-up. They all concluded that VA-TURB could reduce the recurrence rate, which was inconsistent with our study. However, in this updated systematic review, we improved the evidence credibility in several aspects. First, previous studies analyzed the recurrence as dichotomous data, which significantly sacrificed the time-to-event survival information. We extracted the time-to-event data from the survival curve or reported P values, which made meta-analysis based on survival data feasible. Second, we noticed that the inclusion of former systematic reviews was not always covered by updated review previously. Despite the comprehensive searching strategy, we manually checked the reference lists of eligible studies and relevant systematic reviews, which avoided ignoring potentially included studies. Third, previous studies did not identify the effects of staging. As the clinical staging is a significant prognostic factor of bladder cancer, we disclosed the role of staging in the survival-based analysis.

Limitations

There are some limitations in our study. First, there may be some deviations from the true values when the HR was not reported but estimated from other information. However, we strictly performed the estimation according to Tierney's instruction, which decreased the risk of severe deviations (25). Second, we did not perform a network analysis. However, all the RCTs compared a type of VA-TURB to TURB under white light, which constituted a star-like network. No closed loop formed, and no inconsistency between direct and indirect evidence existed, which decreased the necessity of network analysis. Third, we did not analyze the participants of different stages in an individual level. The conclusion about MIBC would be further confirmed if individual participant data of pT2 were available. Due to the limited data accessibility, we could not achieve the analysis. However, we believe the subgroup analysis may enlighten the future studies.

CONCLUSIONS

VA-TUR could improve RFS and PFS in NMIBC patients. No significant difference is found among different types of VA-TUR. VA-TUR may be not indicated to MIBC patients.

AUTHOR CONTRIBUTIONS

HL: Conception, data collection, data analysis, and final approval. YC: Conception, data collection, data analysis, data visualization, data interpretation, manuscript writing, manuscript revision, and final approval. PM: Data visualization, data interpretation, and final approval. ZM: Data visualization, data interpretation, and final approval. CL: Manuscript revision and final approval. WY: Conception, manuscript revision, and final approval. LZ: Conception, manuscript revision, and final approval. All authors contributed to the article and approved the submitted version.

ACKNOWLEDGMENTS

We appreciated Dr. Xia Guo (PhD, Associate Professor, College of Foreign Languages and Cultures, Sichuan University) for the assistance in English writing.

REFERENCES

1. Siegel RL, Miller KD, Jemal A. Cancer Statistics, 2019. *CA A Cancer J Clin* (2019) 69(1):7–34. doi: 10.3322/caac.21551
2. Ferlay J, Soerjomataram I, Dikshit R, Eser S, Mathers C, Rebelo M, et al. Cancer Incidence and Mortality Worldwide: Sources, Methods and Major Patterns in GLOBOCAN 2012. *Int J Cancer* (2015) 136(5):E359–86. doi: 10.1002/ijc.29210
3. Oberschmid CW. TNM Classification of Malignant Tumors 2010. *Der Pathol* (2010) 31(5):333–4, 336–8. doi: 10.1007/s00292-010-1301-6
4. Kurth KH, Bouffioux C, Sylvester R, Meijden APMVD, Oosterlinck W, Brausi M. Treatment of Superficial Bladder Tumors: Achievements and Needs. *Eur Urol* (2000) 37(1):1–9. doi: 10.1159/000052386
5. Subiela JD, Faba sR, Guerrero-Ramos F, Aumatell J, Palou J. Carcinoma *in Situ* of the Bladder: Why Is It Underdetected? *Curr Opin Urol* (2020) 30(3):1. doi: 10.1097/MOU.0000000000000758
6. Burger M, Grossman HB, Droller M, Schmidbauer J, Hermann G, Drăgoescu O, et al. Photodynamic Diagnosis of Non-Muscle Invasive Bladder Cancer With Hexaminolevulinate Cystoscopy: A Meta-Analysis. *Eur Urol Suppl* (2013) 12(1):e577. doi: 10.1016/S1569-9056(13)61060-X
7. Brausi M, Collette L, Kurth K, van der Meijden AP, Oosterlinck W, Witjes JA, et al. Variability in the Recurrence Rate at First Follow-Up Cystoscopy After TUR in Stage Ta T1 Transitional Cell Carcinoma of the Bladder: A Combined Analysis of Seven EORTC Studies. *Eur Urol* (2002) 41(5):523–31. doi: 10.1016/S0302-2838(02)00068-4
8. Zaak D, Ohlmann C, Stenzl A. Current and Established Diagnostic Modalities for Bladder Cancer. *Der Urol* (2018) 57(6):657–64. doi: 10.1007/s00120-018-0650-2
9. Cumberbatch MGK, Foerster B, Catto JWF, Kamat AM, Kassouf W, Jubber I, et al. Repeat Transurethral Resection in Non-Muscle-Invasive Bladder Cancer: A Systematic Review. *Eur Urol* (2018) 73(6):925–33. doi: 10.1016/j.eururo.2018.02.014
10. Naselli A, Hurle R, Paparella S, Buffi NM, Lughezzani G, Lista G, et al. Role of Restaging Transurethral Resection for T1 Non–Muscle Invasive Bladder Cancer: A Systematic Review and Meta-Analysis. *Eur Urol Focus* (2018) 4 (4):558–67. doi: 10.1016/j.euf.2016.12.011
11. Fukuhara H, Yamamoto S, Karashima T, Inoue K. Photodynamic Diagnosis and Therapy for Urothelial Carcinoma and Prostate Cancer: New Imaging Technology and Therapy. *Int J Clin Oncol* (2020) 26(1):18–25. doi: 10.1007/s10147-020-01704-y
12. Guyotat J, Pallud J, Armoiry X, Pavlov V, Metellus P. 5-Aminolevulinic Acid-Protoporphyrin IX Fluorescence-Guided Surgery of High-Grade Gliomas: A Systematic Review. *Adv Tech Stand Neurosurg* (2016) 43):61–90. doi: 10.1007/978-3-319-21359-0_3
13. Inoue K. 5-Aminolevulinic Acid-Mediated Photodynamic Therapy for Bladder Cancer. *Int J Urol* (2017) 24(2):97–101. doi: 10.1111/iju.13291
14. Karaolides T, Skolarikos A, Bourdoumis A, Konandreas A, Mygdalis V, Thanos A, et al. Hexaminolevulinate-Induced Fluorescence Versus White Light During Transurethral Resection of Noninvasive Bladder Tumor: Does It Reduce Recurrences? *Urology* (2012) 80(2):354 60. doi: 10.1016/j.urology.2012.03.067

15. Herceg V, Lange N, Allémann E, Babi A. Activity of Phosphatase-Sensitive 5-Aminolevulinic Acid Prodrugs in Cancer Cell Lines. *J Photochem Photobiol B Biol* (2017) 171:34. doi: 10.1016/j.jphotobiol.2017.04.029
16. Valdes PA, Millesi M, Widhalm G, Roberts DW. 5-Aminolevulinic Acid Induced Protoporphyrin IX (ALA-PpIX) Fluorescence Guidance in Meningioma Surgery. *J Neuro Oncol* (2019) 141(3):555–65. doi: 10.1007/s11060-018-03079-7
17. Bochenek K, Aebisher A, Międzybrodzka A, Cieślar G, Kawczyk-Krupka A. Methods for Bladder Cancer Diagnosis – The Role of Autofluorescence and Photodynamic Diagnosis. *Photodiagnosis Photodynamic Ther* (2019) 27:141–8. doi: 10.1016/j.pdpdt.2019.05.036
18. Kutwin P, Konecki T, Cichocki M, Falkowski P, Jabłonowski Z. Photodynamic Diagnosis and Narrow-Band Imaging in the Management of Bladder Cancer: A Review. *Photomed Laser Surg* (2017) 35(9):459–64. doi: 10.1089/pho.2016.4217
19. Kim SB, Yoon SG, Tae J, Kim JY, Shim JS, Kang SG, et al. Detection and Recurrence Rate of Transurethral Resection of Bladder Tumors by Narrow-Band Imaging: Prospective, Randomized Comparison With White Light Cystoscopy. *Investig Clin Urol* (2018) 59(2):98–105. doi: 10.4111/icu.2018.59.2.98
20. Drejer D, Béji S, Munk Nielsen A, Høyer SR, Wrist Lam G, Jensen JRB. Clinical Relevance of Narrow-Band Imaging in Flexible Cystoscopy: The DaBlaCa-7 Study. *Scand J Urol* (2017) 51(2):120–3. doi: 10.1080/21681805.2017.1295101
21. Chou R, Selph S, Buckley DI, Fu R, Griffin JC, Grusing S, et al. Comparative Effectiveness of Fluorescent Versus White Light Cystoscopy for Initial Diagnosis or Surveillance of Bladder Cancer on Clinical Outcomes: Systematic Review and Meta-Analysis. *J Urol* (2017) Part 1. 197(3):548–58. doi: 10.1016/j.juro.2016.10.061
22. Babjuk M, Burger M, Comperat EM, Gontero P, Mostafid AH, Palou J, et al. European Association of Urology Guidelines on Non-Muscle-Invasive Bladder Cancer (TaT1 and Carcinoma In Situ) - 2019 Update. *Eur Urol* (2019) 76(5):639–57. doi: 10.1016/j.eururo.2019.08.016
23. Liberati A, Altman DG, Tetzlaff J, Mulrow C, Gøtzsche PC, Ioannidis JP, et al. The PRISMA Statement for Reporting Systematic Reviews and Meta-Analyses of Studies That Evaluate Healthcare Interventions: Explanation and Elaboration. *BMJ (Clinical Res ed)* (2009) 339:b2700. doi: 10.1136/bmj.b2700
24. Higgins JPT, Sally G, eds. *Cochrane Handbook for Systematic Reviews of Interventions Version 5.1.0 [Updated March 2011]*. UK: The Cochrane Collaboration (2011).
25. Tierney JF, Stewart LA, Ghersi D, Burdett S, Sydes MR. Practical Methods for Incorporating Summary Time-to-Event Data Into Meta-Analysis. *Trials* (2007) 8:16. doi: 10.1186/1745-6215-8-16
26. Guyatt GH, Oxman AD, Vist GE, Kunz R, Falck-Ytter Y, Alonso-Coello P, et al. GRADE: An Emerging Consensus on Rating Quality of Evidence and Strength of Recommendations. *BMJ (Clinical Res ed)* (2008) 336(7650):924–6. doi: 10.1136/bmj.39489.470347.AD
27. Babjuk M, Soukup V, Petrik R, Jirsa M, Dvoracek J. 5-Aminolaevulinic Acid-Induced Fluorescence Cystoscopy During Transurethral Resection Reduces the Risk of Recurrence in Stage Ta/T1 Bladder Cancer. *BJU Int* (2005) 96 (6):798–802. doi: 10.1111/j.1464-410X.2004.05715.x
28. Daniltchenko DI, Riedl CR, Sachs MD, Koenig F, Daha KL, Pflueger H, et al. Long-Term Benefit of 5-Aminolevulinic Acid Fluorescence Assisted Transurethral Resection of Superficial Bladder Cancer: 5-Year Results of a Prospective Randomized Study. *J Urol* (2005) 174(6):2129–33, discussion 33. doi: 10.1097/01.ju.0000181814.73466.14
29. Dragoescu O, Tomescu P, Panus A, Enache M, Maria C, Stoica L, et al. Photodynamic Diagnosis of Non-Muscle Invasive Bladder Cancer Using Hexaminolevulinic Acid. *Rom J Morphol Embryol* (2011) 52(1):123–7.
30. Dragoescu PO, Tudorache S, Drocas AI, Mitroi G, Pănuş A, Drăgoescu NAM, et al. Improved Diagnosis and Long-Term Recurrence Rate Reduction for Non-Muscle-Invasive Bladder Cancer Patients Undergoing Fluorescent Hexylaminolevulinate Photodynamic Diagnosis. *Rom J Morphol Embryol* (2017) 58(4):1279–83.
31. Drejer D, Moltke AL, Nielsen AM, Lam GW, Jensen JB. DaBlaCa-11: Photodynamic Diagnosis in Flexible Cystoscopy-A Randomized Study With Focus on Recurrence. *Urology* (2020) 137:91 6. doi: 10.1016/j.urology.2019.12.002
32. Filbeck T, Pichlmeier U, Knuechel R, Wieland WF, Roessler W. Clinically Relevant Improvement of Recurrence-Free Survival With 5-Aminolevulinic Acid Induced Fluorescence Diagnosis in Patients With Superficial Bladder Tumors. *J Urol* (2002) 168(1):67–71. doi: 10.1016/S0022-5347(05)64833-1
33. Burger M, Zaak D, Stief CG, Filbeck T, Wieland WF, Roessler W, et al. Photodynamic Diagnostics and Noninvasive Bladder Cancer: Is It Cost-Effective in Long-Term Application? A Germany-Based Cost Analysis. *Eur Urol* (2007) 52(1):142–7. doi: 10.1016/j.eururo.2007.01.064
34. Denzinger S, Burger M, Walter B, Knuechel R, Roessler W, Wieland WF, et al. Clinically Relevant Reduction in Risk of Recurrence of Superficial Bladder Cancer Using 5-Aminolevulinic Acid-Induced Fluorescence Diagnosis: 8-Year Results of Prospective Randomized Study. *Urology* (2007) 69(4):675–9. doi: 10.1016/j.urology.2006.12.023
35. Denzinger S, Wieland WF, Otto W, Filbeck T, Knuechel R, Burger M. Does Photodynamic Transurethral Resection of Bladder Tumour Improve the Outcome of Initial T1 High-Grade Bladder Cancer? A Long-Term Follow-Up of a Randomized Study. *BJU Int* (2008) 101(5):566–9. doi: 10.1111/j.1464-410X.2007.07314.x
36. Geavlete B, Multescu R, Georgescu D, Stanescu F, Jecu M, Geavlete P. Narrow Band Imaging Cystoscopy and Bipolar Plasma Vaporization for Large Nonmuscle-Invasive Bladder Tumors–Results of a Prospective, Randomized Comparison to the Standard Approach. *Urology* (2012) 79(4):846–51. doi: 10.1016/j.urology.2011.08.081
37. Gkritsios P, Hatzimouratidis K, Kazantzidis S, Dimitriadis G, Ioannidis E, Katsikas V. Hexaminolevulinate-Guided Transurethral Resection of Non-Muscle-Invasive Bladder Cancer Does Not Reduce the Recurrence Rates After a 2-Year Follow-Up: A Prospective Randomized Trial. *Int Urol Nephrol* (2014) 46(5):927–33. doi: 10.1007/s11255-013-0603-z
38. Hermann GG, Mogensen K, Carlsson S, Marcussen N, Duun S. Fluorescence-Guided Transurethral Resection of Bladder Tumours Reduces Bladder Tumour Recurrence Due to Less Residual Tumour Tissue in Ta/T1 Patients: A Randomized Two-Centre Study. *BJU Int* (2011) 108(8 Pt 2): E297–303. doi: 10.1111/j.1464-410X.2011.10090.x
39. Herr HW. Randomized Trial of Narrow-Band Versus White-Light Cystoscopy for Restaging (Second-Look) Transurethral Resection of Bladder Tumors. *Eur Urol* (2015) 67(4):605–8. doi: 10.1016/j.eururo.2014.06.049
40. Karaolides T, Skolarikos A, Bourdoumis A, Konandreas A, Mygdalis V, Thanos A, et al. Hexaminolevulinate-Induced Fluorescence Versus White Light During Transurethral Resection of Noninvasive Bladder Tumor: Does it Reduce Recurrences? *Urology* (2012) 80(2):354–9. doi: 10.1016/j.urology.2012.03.067
41. Naito S, Algaba F, Babjuk M, Bryan RT, Sun YH, Valiquette L, et al. The Clinical Research Office of the Endourological Society (CROES) Multicentre Randomised Trial of Narrow Band Imaging-Assisted Transurethral Resection of Bladder Tumour (TURBT) Versus Conventional White Light Imaging-Assisted TURBT in Primary Non-Muscle-Invasive Bladder Cancer Patients: Trial Protocol and 1-Year Results. *Eur Urol* (2016) 70(3):506–15. doi: 10.1016/j.eururo.2016.03.053
42. Naselli A, Hurle R, Puppo P. The Role of Narrow-Band Imaging in the Management of Non-Muscle-Invasive Bladder Cancer. *Expert Rev Anticancer Ther* (2012) 12(12):1523–8. doi: 10.1586/era.12.137
43. Naselli A, Introini C, Bertolotto F, Spina B, Puppo P. Feasibility of Transurethral Resection of Bladder Lesion Performed Entirely by Means of Narrow-Band Imaging. *J Endourol* (2010) 24(7):1131–4. doi: 10.1089/end.2010.0042
44. O'Brien T, Ray E, Chatterton K, Khan MS, Chandra A, Thomas K. Prospective Randomized Trial of Hexylaminolevulinate Photodynamic-Assisted Transurethral Resection of Bladder Tumour (TURBT) Plus Single-Shot Intravesical Mitomycin C vs Conventional White-Light TURBT Plus Mitomycin C in Newly Presenting Non-Muscle-Invasive Bladder Cancer. *BJU Int* (2013) 112(8):1096–104. doi: 10.1111/bju.12355
45. Rolevich A, Minich A, Vasilevich V, Zhegalik A, Mokhort A, Nabebina T, et al. Efficacy of Fluorescent Cystoscopy-Assisted Transurethral Resection in Patients With Non-Muscle Invasive Bladder Cancer and Quality of Surgery: Post-Hoc Analysis of A Prospective Randomized Study. *Cent Eur J Urol* (2019) 72(4):351–6. doi: 10.5173/ceju.2019.0003
46. Rolevich AI, Zhegalik AG, Mokhort AA, Minich AA, Vasilevich VY, Polyakov SL, et al. Results of a Prospective Randomized Study Assessing the Efficacy of Fluorescent Cystoscopy-Assisted Transurethral Resection and Single Instillation of Doxorubicin in Patients With Non-Muscle-Invasive Bladder Cancer. *World J Urol* (2017) 35(5):745–52. doi: 10.1007/s00345-016-1927-y
47. Schumacher MC, Holmang S, Davidsson T, Friedrich B, Pedersen J, Wiklund NP. Transurethral Resection of non-Muscle-Invasive Bladder Transitional

Cell Cancers With or Without 5-Aminolevulinic Acid Under Visible and Fluorescent Light: Results of a Prospective, Randomised, Multicentre Study. *Eur Urol* (2010) 57(2):293–9. doi: 10.1016/j.eururo.2009.10.030

48. Stenzl A, Burger M, Fradet Y, Mynderse LA, Soloway MS, Witjes JA, et al. Hexaminolevulinate Guided Fluorescence Cystoscopy Reduces Recurrence in Patients With Nonmuscle Invasive Bladder Cancer. *J Urol* (2010) 184 (5):1907–13. doi: 10.1016/j.juro.2010.06.148
49. Grossman HB, Stenzl A, Fradet Y, Mynderse LA, Kriegmair M, Witjes JA, et al. Long-Term Decrease in Bladder Cancer Recurrence With Hexaminolevulinate Enabled Fluorescence Cystoscopy. *J Urol* (2012) 188 (1):58–62. doi: 10.1016/j.juro.2012.03.007
50. Kamat AM, Willis DL, Dickstein RJ, Anderson R, Nogueras-González G, Katz RL, et al. Novel Fluorescence *in Situ* Hybridization-Based Definition of Bacille Calmette-Guerin (BCG) Failure for Use in Enhancing Recruitment Into Clinical Trials of Intravesical Therapies. *BJU Int* (2016) 117(5):754–60. doi: 10.1111/bju.13186
51. Stenzl A, Penkoff H, Dajc-Sommerer E, Zumbraegel A, Hoeltl L, Scholz M, et al. Detection and Clinical Outcome of Urinary Bladder Cancer With 5-Aminolevulinic Acid-Induced Fluorescence Cystoscopy: A Multicenter Randomized, Double-Blind, Placebo-Controlled Trial. *Cancer* (2011) 117 (5):938 47. doi: 10.1002/cncr.25523
52. Tschirdewahn S, Harke NN, Hirner L, Stagge E, Hadaschik B, Eisenhardt A. Narrow-Band Imaging Assisted Cystoscopy in the Follow-Up of Patients With Transitional Cell Carcinoma of the Bladder: A Randomized Study in Comparison With White Light Cystoscopy. *World J Urol* (2020) 38(6):1509–15. doi: 10.1007/s00345-019-02926-0
53. Burger M, Stief CG, Zaak D, Stenzl A, Wieland WF, Jocham D, et al. Hexaminolevulinate Is Equal to 5-Aminolevulinic Acid Concerning Residual Tumor and Recurrence Rate Following Photodynamic Diagnostic Assisted Transurethral Resection of Bladder Tumors. *Urology* (2009) 74(6):1282–6. doi: 10.1016/j.urology.2009.06.088
54. Lee JY, Cho KS, Kang DH, Jung HD, Kwon JK, Oh CK, et al. A Network Meta-Analysis of Therapeutic Outcomes After New Image Technology-Assisted Transurethral Resection for Non-Muscle Invasive Bladder Cancer: 5-Aminolaevulinic Acid Fluorescence vs Hexylaminolevulinate Fluorescence vs Narrow Band Imaging. *BMC Cancer* (2015) 15:566. doi: 10.1186/s12885-015-1571-8
55. Ghandour R, Singla N, Lotan Y. Treatment Options and Outcomes in Nonmetastatic Muscle Invasive Bladder Cancer. *Trends Cancer* (2019) 5 (7):426–39. doi: 10.1016/j.trecan.2019.05.011
56. Ploussard G, Daneshmand S, Efstathiou JA, Herr HW, James ND, Rödel CM, et al. Critical Analysis of Bladder Sparing With Trimodal Therapy in Muscle-Invasive Bladder Cancer: A Systematic Review. *Eur Urol* (2014) 66(1):120–37. doi: 10.1016/j.eururo.2014.02.038

12

Clinical Benefits of Combining Different Visualization Modalities in Neurosurgery

Karl-Michael Schebesch [1], Katharina Rosengarth [1], Alexander Brawanski [1], Martin Proescholdt [1], Christina Wendl [2], Julius Höhne [1], Christian Ott [1], Hans Lamecker [3] and Christian Doenitz [1]*

[1] Department of Neurosurgery, University Medical Center Regensburg, Regensburg, Germany, [2] Department of Radiology, University Medical Center Regensburg, Regensburg, Germany, [3] 1000shapes GmbH, Berlin, Germany

Correspondence:
Karl-Michael Schebesch
karl-michael.schebesch@ukr.de

The prevailing philosophy in oncologic neurosurgery, has shifted from maximally invasive resection to the preservation of neurologic function. The foundation of safe surgery is the multifaceted visualization of the target region and the surrounding eloquent tissue. Recent advancements in pre-operative and intraoperative visualization modalities have changed the face of modern neurosurgery. Metabolic and functional data can be integrated into intraoperative guidance software, and fluorescent dyes under dedicated filters can potentially visualize patterns of blood flow and better define tumor borders or isolated tumor foci. High definition endoscopes enable the depiction of tiny vessels and tumor extension to the ventricles or skull base. Fluorescein sodium-based confocal endomicroscopy, which is under scientific evaluation, may further enhance the neurosurgical armamentarium. We aim to present our institutional workup of combining different neuroimaging modalities for surgical neuro-oncological procedures. This institutional algorithm (IA) was the basis of the recent publication by Haj et al. describing outcome and survival data of consecutive patients with high grade glioma (HGG) before and after the introduction of our Neuro-Oncology Center.

Keywords: fluorescence-guided surgery, fluorescein sodium, YELLOW 560 nm, KINEVO, tumor segmentation, confocal endomicroscopy, CONVIVO, brain tumors

INTRODUCTION

Modern oncological neurosurgery is marked by the consensus that all surgical interventions should aim to attain complete tumor resection without affecting neurological function. This dogma was finally agreed upon because low tumor burden and good neurological function has been repeatedly shown to form the basis of any successful adjuvant treatment modality and to result in prolonged progression-free and overall survival, whilst preserving good quality of life (1–3).

The combination of different imaging modalities for pre-operative planning and intraoperative guidance should always aim at clearly identifying the targeted tumor that can be extremely heterogeneous. Currently, the integration of various functional imaging data, such as functional magnetic resonance imaging (fMRI), into neuronavigation allows for increased safety when approaching vulnerable, eloquent structures. Fluorescence-guidance can further support the neurosurgeon's eye and experience in visualizing the tumor mass, scattered tumor spots, infiltrated zones and rims, and patterns of blood flow, and can ultimately confirm a tumor-free cavity (4, 5).

However, in the daily routine of a neuro-oncology center (NOC), it is always mandatory to obtain and employ the desired imaging modality in a cost-effective, fast, and uncomplicated manner. Patients must be protected from redundant assessments, and, above all, "technical overkill" in the operating theater must be avoided. Furthermore, critical self-reflection and monocentric or multicenter complication analyses should be consistently generated and published to properly outline advantages and disadvantages, as well as clinical benefits and limitations of the institutional algorithm (IA). This approach is the only way that the most important factors, namely the surgical skills and experiences of neurosurgeons, are effectively supported by innovative technical adjuncts.

In 2017, we published our outcome and survival data of consecutive patients with high grade glioma since the introduction of a certified NOC in 2009. Since 2009, all patients with HGG at our department have been treated according to our IA. The current investigation has shown clear benefits in neurological outcome, progression-free survival, and overall survival in comparison to the equivalent data collected before 2009 (6).

The impact of the NOC organization in terms of improving survival in patients with glioblastoma has been described previously (6), but the detailed description of the workflow and institutional algorithm have yet to be reported. Therefore, the aim of this paper is to present our approach of combining different visualization modalities that are pre- and post-operatively employed not solely for the intraoperative depiction of the targeted area, but also for advanced pre-operative unmasking of the tumor structure, invasiveness, environment, and adherences. This combination enables sophisticated planning of the surgical approach including positioning, craniotomy, and dissection. We strongly believe that the interaction of a visual armamentarium provides neurosurgeons with more sensitivity and purposefulness, especially in complex neuro-oncologic procedures.

RESULTS

When a new patient with a suspected brain tumor is referred to our center, structural MRI is usually initially completed (see **Table 1**). Tumors without Gadolinium enhancement are further analyzed with FET-PET, which influences the choice of intraoperative fluorescent dyes. Proximity of the tumor to eloquent areas results in a functional workup (fMRI and Diffusion Tensor Imaging, DTI). All imaging data are then pre-processed and segmented to provide the essential information of each imaging modality. The final therapeutic decision is made after 3D-visualization and demonstration of the case, followed by stereotactic biopsy, open biopsy/partial resection, or gross tumor removal. The choice of fluorescent dye depends on the level of gadolinium enhancement and the FET-PET result (see **Table 2**).

The following features of the IA (**Table 2**) were selected because of their fundamental scientific interest:

TABLE 1 | Overview of our institutional imaging workup for common intracranial lesions: magnetic resonance imaging (MRI) protocol for patients with intracranial tumors include T1 spin echo and T2 turbo spin echo sequences with 1 mm and isotropic 3D sequences (1 mm) including T1 w/gadolinium contrast (3D multiplane reformation, MPR), T2 (3D sampling perfection with application optimized contrast using different flip angle evolution, SPACE), 3D fluid attenuation inversion recovery, FLAIR, and constructive interference in steady-state (CISS MRI).

Suspected diagnosis	Low grade glioma	High grade glioma/ metastasis	Vascular lesions (aneurysms/ AVM)	Skull base tumor
MRI	SE T1 w/o CM, SE T2, 3D MPR w/contrast, 3D T2, 3D FLAIR	SE T1 w/o CM, T2, 3D MPR w/contrast, 3D T2, 3D FLAIR	SE T1 w/o CM, SE T2, 3D MPR w/contrast, 3D TOF, TWIST	SE T1 w/o CM, SE T2, 3D MPR w/contrast, 3D TOF, T2* CISS
CT thin-sliced skull base (1 mm)	*✓		✓	✓
FET-PET	✓	*✓		
fMRI, rsfMRI	✓	✓	*✓	
DTI	✓	✓	*✓	
CFD simulation			*✓	

*✓ mandatory, *✓ optional.*

3D time-of-flight (TOF) and time-resolved angiography with interleaved stochastic trajectories (TWIST) sequences are obtained in vascularized tumors. Positron emission tomography (PET) with O-(2-[^{18}F]fluoroethyl)-L-tyrosine ([^{18}F]FET) (FET-PET) is used for non-contrast enhancing and recurrent contrast-enhancing gliomas. Functional MRI (fMRI) and resting state (rs) fMRI are conducted for visualizing functional areas.

Pre-operative Workup–Completion of Structural and Metabolic Neuroimaging

When a new patient with a suspicious cranial lesion is referred to our center, neuroimaging is quickly completed according to our institutional imaging requirements (see **Table 1**) that include magnetic resonance imaging plus isotropic 3D sequences, computed tomography (CT), or 18F-fluorethyl tyrosine (FET)-/18F-fluordesoxyglucose (FDG)-positron emission tomography (PET). According to the recommendations of our daily case conference, patients are evaluated neuro-psychologically and consecutively undergo functional MRI and diffusion tensor imaging (DTI).

In 2018, we published a small series of patients with glioma that had not shown any contrast enhancement in the MRI, yet presented with distinct metabolic activity in the FET-PET (7). These patients had been suitable for fluorescence-guided surgery with Fluorescein Sodium (FL) under the YELLOW 560 nm filter (Carl Zeiss Meditec, Oberkochen, Germany). A possible correlation between FET-PET active tumors and fluorescent staining was assumed, facilitating surgical performance. Our results supported the data by Rapp et al. and Pirotte et al. who had outlined the diagnostic value of FET-PET for diagnosing hot spots inside gliomas. Clearly, FET-PET increases intraoperative diagnostic accuracy and helps to establish the most exact histopathological diagnosis (8, 9).

TABLE 2 | Institutional algorithm (IA).

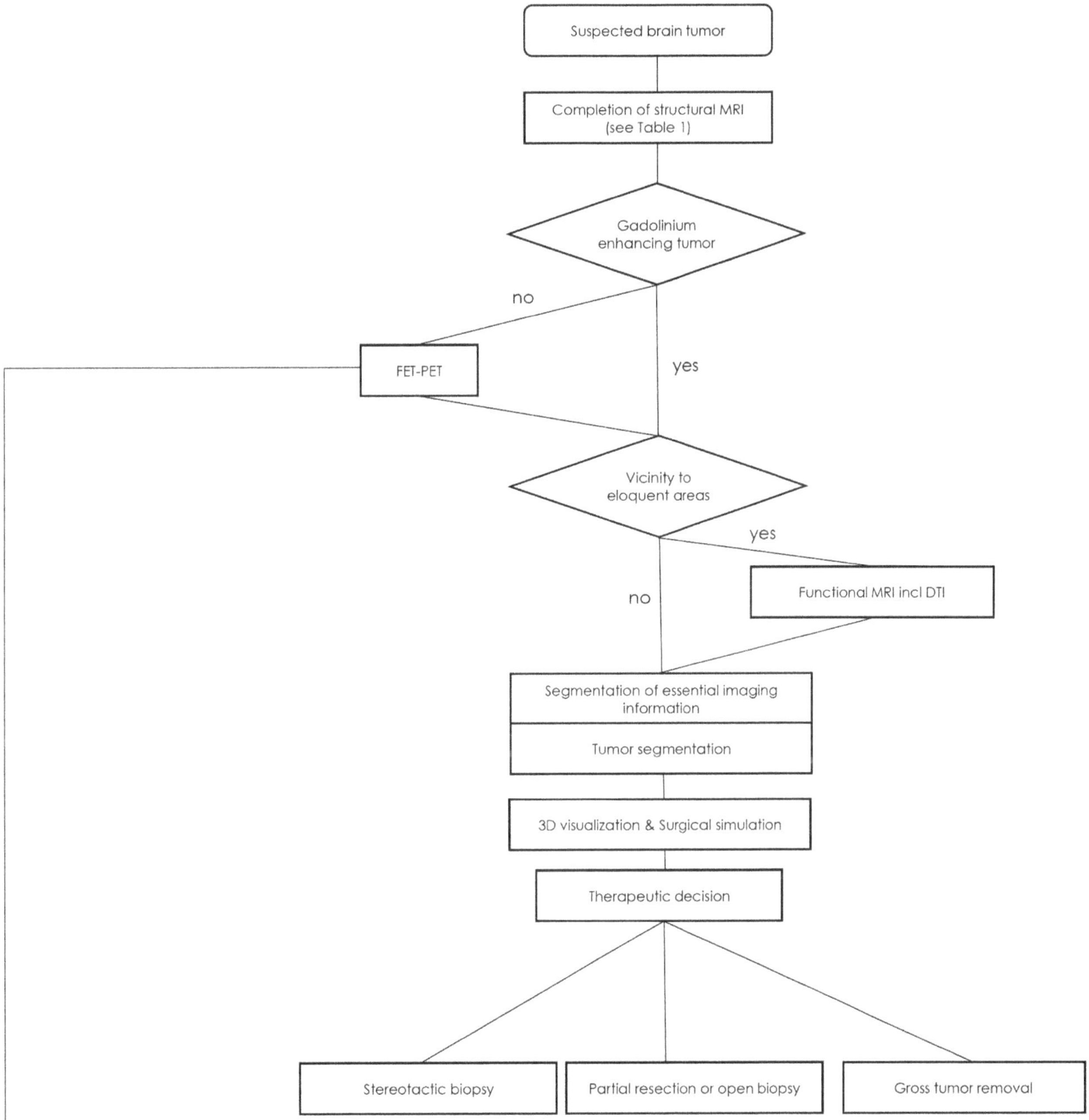

	Stereotactic biopsy	Partial resection or open biopsy / Gross tumor removal
Gadolinium enhancing tumor	FL optional	FL and/or 5-ALA
FET-PET positive tumor	FL optional	FL
FET-PET negative tumor	None	None
Neuronavigation		✓
Confocal endomicroendoscopy		optional
Ultrasound		optional
Awake surgery with direct cortical stimulation		optional
Intraoperative Monitoring		optional

Pre-operative Workup–fMRI and DTI

The aim of pre-surgical functional imaging is to maximize the resection of lesions (tumors or metastases) as well as to minimize post-operative functional deficits. Both factors increase post-operative health-related quality of life (10) and are prognostic factors for successive interventions involving radiation- and/or chemotherapy (11, 12). In our center, pre-surgical functional imaging is conducted with fMRI and resting state functional (rsf) MRI for the functional localization of cortical gray matter; diffusion-weighted imaging is used to determine subcortical white matter tracts. fMRI is exclusively carried out with 3-Tesla Siemens MRI scanners. Protocols

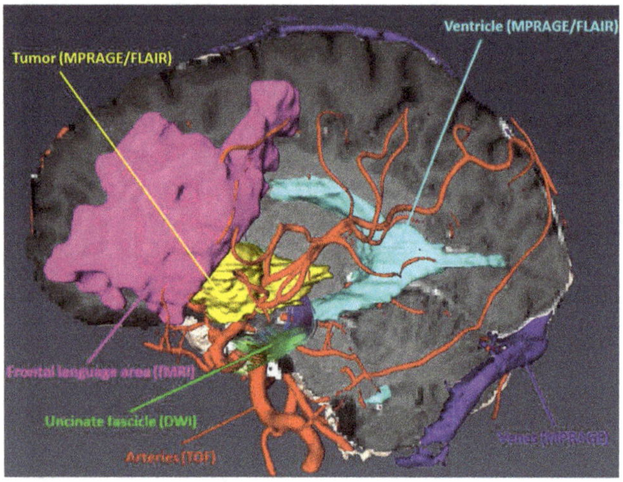

FIGURE 1 | Integration and three-dimensional display of different structural and functional modalities in AMRIA. The original imaging modality used for visualization is annotated in brackets.

for mapping the sensorimotor homunculus, language location and lateralization, and memory or retinotopic organization of the visual cortex depend on the localization of the lesion. Non-compliant or severely disabled patients may undergo rsfMRI that is also used in the case of patients with language barriers or in very young patients, awake patients with their eyes open, or in narcotized patients. fMRI data are analyzed with (S)tatistical(P)arametric(M)apping12 (www.fil.ion.ucl.ac.uk/spm/software/spm12/) including the LI-toolbox (13) and rsfMRI data with in-house generated Matlab scripts including parts of DPARSF and the GIFT-toolbox (http://mialab.mrn.org/software/gift/). According to fiber tracking, diffusion-weighted images (DWI) are acquired by means of 3T and 1.5T MRI scanners, either with 30 directions and 3 mm isotropic resolution or 64 directions with 2 mm isotropic resolution depending on the disease and patient characteristics. The following fiber tracking modeling can be done either deterministically with AMIRA (FEI Visualization Sciences, France) or probabilistically by using a modified FSL pipeline [employing Bayesian Estimation of Diffusion Parameters Obtained using Sampling Technique (BEDPOSTX)]. Fiber tracking is conducted in advance, when mainly pyramidal tracts, arcuate fascicles, uncinated fascicles, and optic tracts are shown. All functional results (fMRI, rsfMRI, and DTI) can be integrated into AMIRA (FEI Visualization Sciences, France) (see **Figure 1**).

Pre-operative Workup–Tumor Segmentation

Automatic pre-operative brain tumor segmentation is a powerful tool for surgical planning that allows the extraction of tumor characteristics (contrast-enhancing and non-contrast-enhancing compartments, edema, and necrosis) from surrounding healthy brain tissue by means of a set of MR modalities (T1 with and without contrast agent, T2, and FLAIR) (14). Such information may be very useful for guiding surgical interventions by defining the extent of resection or the area of resection. There are a number of segmentation and tumor detection algorithms, ranging from classification or clustering approaches to deep learning algorithms (15, 16). In our department, we have established a tumor segmentation pipeline based on ANSTsR [advanced normalization tools (ANTs) and the R statistical project] using random forest-derived probabilities to determine different tumor tissues (17) (see **Figure 2**).

Pre-operative Workup–3D Visualization and Surgical Simulation

Pre-operatively, a special simulation software is employed that condenses the essential information of the different imaging modalities in a 3D-viewer. This software enables the surgeon to pre-operatively envision the operative field as realistically as possible, simulating elements such as patient and head positioning in a virtual clamp, craniotomy, and corticotomy in a virtual OR setting. This software has been developed and modified by our department according to the specific needs of neurosurgeons.

Every pre-operative imaging modality provides unique information to characterize the lesion and its surroundings. For the sake of visual clarity, it is essential to condense and organize the extensive amount of anatomical and functional data. For this reason, we developed an advanced visualization software tool called NeuroVis, aimed at improving the understanding of anatomical and functional relations for pre-operative planning and intraoperative guidance in a virtual reality setting.

The essential information of every image modality is segmented and co-registered with the 3D MPR image stack by means of a semi-automated workflow with AMIRA. Segmented data are then visualized with our browser- based rendering 3D viewer NeuroVis (developed at our institute in collaboration with 1000shapes GmbH, Berlin). This tool enables neurosurgeons to plan individually tailored treatment strategies. Planning steps include skin incision, craniotomy, and intraoperative positioning of the patient and the head clamp in a realistic operative setting. We have also established an interface to a virtual reality setting using UNITY (Unity Tec., USA) and a head-mounted display (HTC, Taiwan). These tools help to pre-operatively envision the operative field as realistically as possible (see **Figure 3**). The prepared plan can also be transferred to a navigation system using the stl format for intraoperative use.

Intraoperative Workup–FET-PET Positive Non-enhancing Tumors and Fluorescence

The question of how to achieve the most effective tumor reduction without affecting relevant motor, language, and visual tracts continues to be highly controversial, particularly in non-contrast enhancing gliomas in eloquent regions of the brain. Besides the integration of functional data into neuro-navigation and conducting surgery in an awake setting, fluorescent visualization of the tumor may significantly increase the quality of resection and speed up surgery. Our recently published

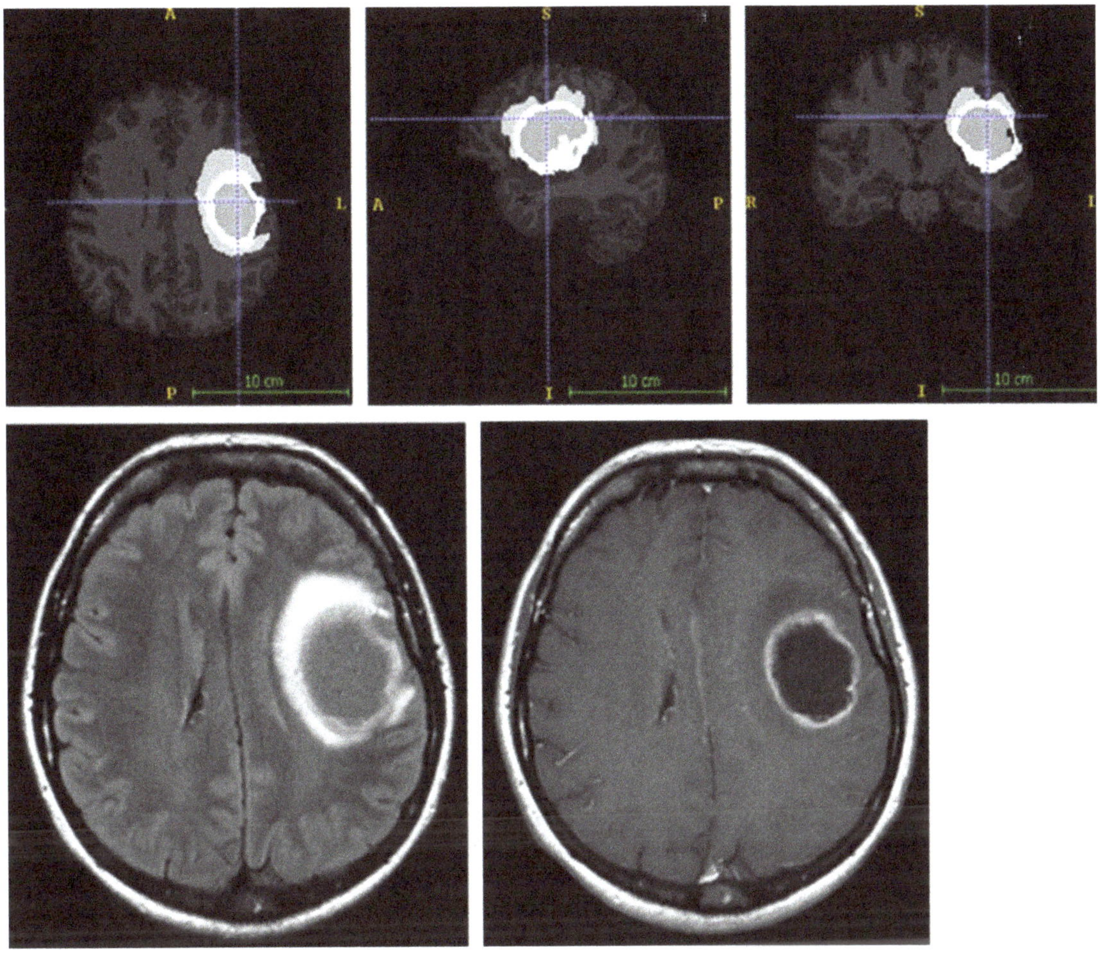

FIGURE 2 | ANTsR tumor segmentation result of glioblastoma, showing labels for contrast-enhancing tumor (very light gray), necrosis (dark gray), edema (light gray) (upper row; contrast non-enhancing tumor label is not depicted), and the corresponding FLAIR (lower row left) and T1 with contrast agency (lower row right) MR image.

experience in patients with non-enhancing gliomas with distinct metabolic activity in FET-PET and clear intraoperative fluorescent staining (7), in addition to the report by Bowden et al. (18), supports the potential supplementary role of FL in cases of low or intermediate grade glioma with high metabolic activity.

Intraoperative Workup–Fluorescein-Enhanced Confocal Endomicroscopy

Because of its unspecific accumulation in areas of disrupted blood-brain barrier (BBB), FL can be applied widely irrespective of the tumor histology in HGG (19–22), cerebral metastases (23, 24), lymphomas (25, 26), meningiomas (27), neuromas (28), and brain abscesses (29) for guiding microsurgical resection under the dedicated light filter. Furthermore, FL-based confocal endomicroscopy can be employed *in vivo* to obtain multiple digital biopsies to visualize the tissue texture, enabling distinct histological evaluation by a (remote) neuropathologist (4, 30–33). This approach circumvents having to wait for the frozen section, enabling the surgeon to rapidly identify the histological origin of the lesion and delineate the tumor border much more precisely. However, since this technique is still under scientific evaluation, clinical data are required to outline the potential significance of this approach (30).

Decision Making

This evaluation and the information provided by our neuropsychologist determine whether surgery is planned in an awake setting or under sedation. Neuro-navigation integrating all neuroimaging devices (fMRI, CT, and PET) is clinically routine.

Prior to surgery, we decide on the intraoperative visualization tools to be used, depending on the suspected etiology of the tumor, the anatomical localization, the expansion into eloquent areas and fiber tracts, and subject to the surgical approach. With the exception of intraoperative magnetic resonance imaging (iMRI), our neurosurgical department comprises all conventional technical adjuncts and personal competences of a tertiary academic neurosurgical center: (a) Fluorescence with dedicated light filters: fluorescein sodium (FL, YELLOW

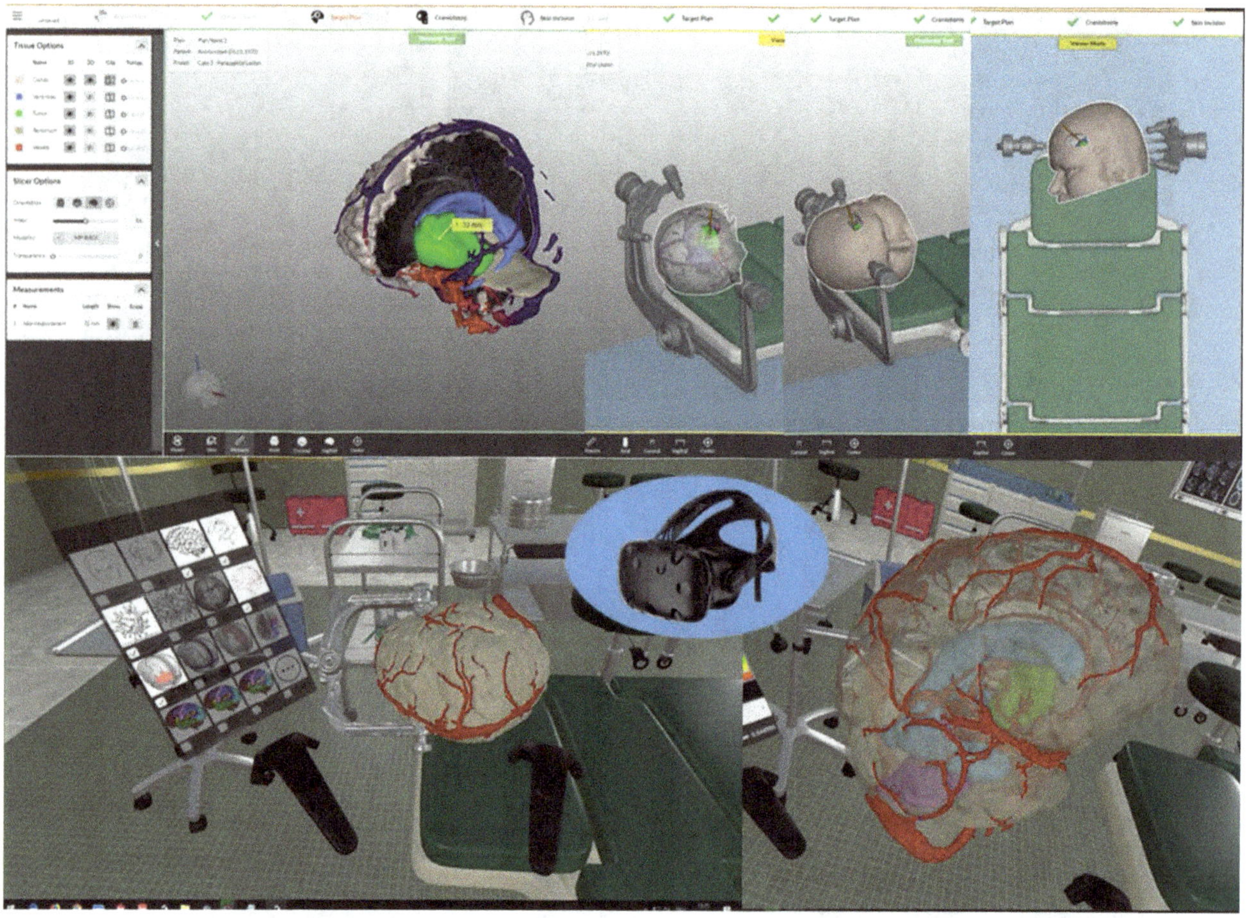

FIGURE 3 | Pre-operative visualization with NeuroVis 3D (upper row) and in a virtual reality setting (lower row) using a head-mounted display.

560 nm filter), 5-aminolevulinic acid (5-ALA, BLUE 400 nm filter), and indocyanine green (ICG, FLOW 800 module); (b) Neuronavigation, ultrasound; (c) Intraoperative monitoring (IOM); (d) Endoscopy; and (e) Confocal endomicroscopy (still under scientific evaluation).

Illustrative Cases

Case #1

This case describes our approach to the treatment of a remotely recurrent, eloquently located, contrast-enhancing astrocytoma WHO III of a 51-year-old female patient. The pre-operative neuroimage-workup consisted of conventional MRI (T1-weighted, axial sequence, **Figure 4**), FET-PET (displayed in navigational software, axial sequence, **Figure 5**), and neuronavigation with integrated fMRI, DTI, and FET-PET (**Figure 6**). The patient was surgically treated in an awake-awake setting under fluorescence-guidance with FL (5 mg/kg) and the YELLOW 560 nm filter (**Figure 7**), and the removed tumor was examined *ex vivo* with the confocal endomicroscope (**Figure 8**). Early post-operative contrast-enhanced MRI showed complete removal of the contrast-enhanced lesion that was histologically confirmed as astrocytoma WHO III.

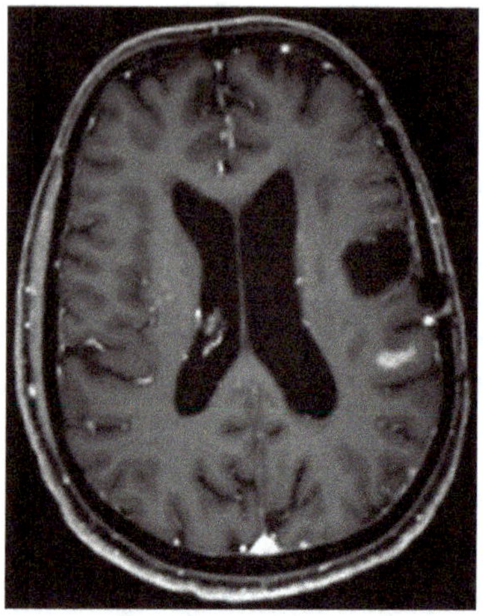

FIGURE 4 | Pre-operative MR image (T1-weighted sequence, axial plane) showing new contrast-enhancement distant to the former resection cavity.

This case was selected because the pre-operative neuroimage-workup distinctively supported the indication for surgery. The FET-PET result ruled out pseudo-progression or

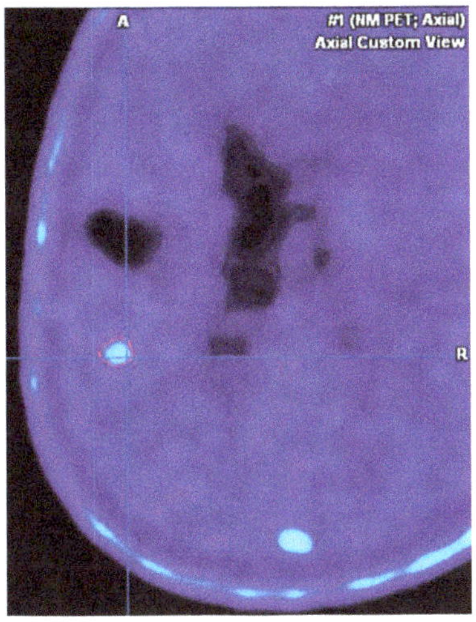

FIGURE 5 | Pre-operative FET-PET image, displayed in the navigational software, showing strong metabolic activity in the suspicious area.

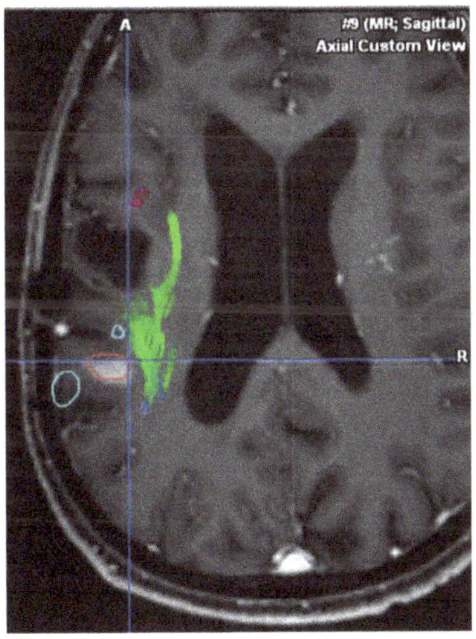

FIGURE 6 | Integration of fMRI, DTI, and FET-PET (in red) into the navigational software, unmasking the proximity to eloquent area (arcuate fasciculus in green, language-associated activation in cyan).

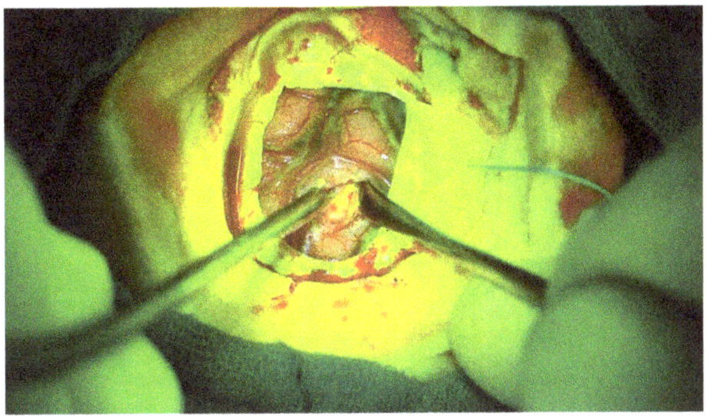

FIGURE 7 | Strong fluorescent staining of the tumor under the YELLOW 560 filter.

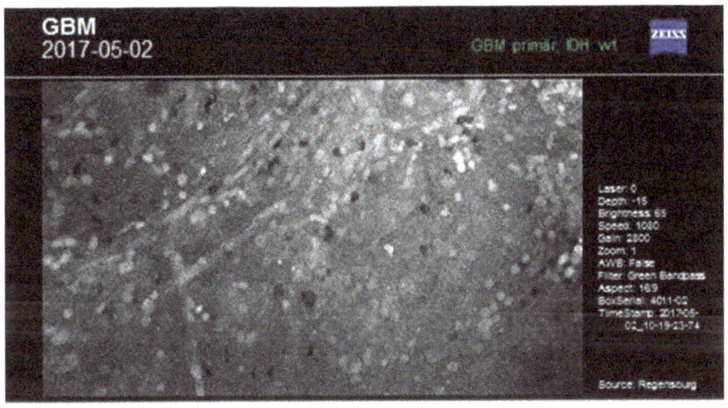

FIGURE 8 | *Ex vivo* examination of tumorous tissue with the confocal endomicroscope.

post-radiation necrosis because of the detected strong metabolic activity that could be matched to the suspicious contrast enhancement in the pre-operative MRI. The functional area was displayed by means of fMRI and DTI, clearly showing proximity but no infiltration to language-associated activation. Finally, fluorescence-guided technique with FL impressively visualized the tumor *in vivo* and *ex vivo*. Taken together, the included imaging modalities resulted in complete removal of the tumor without any functional deterioration.

Case #2

The 65-year-old female patient had a focal seizure with paresthesia of the left upper limb and the face. Initial MRI showed a contrast-enhancing lesion in the left pre- and post-central area, distant to the midline (**Figure 9**). The patient additionally received motor fMRI and DTI of the pyramidal tract that was reconstructed in 3D, including the vasculature (**Figure 10**). Consequently, we indicated awake surgery because of the proximity to the hand and upper limb area. The patient underwent awake craniotomy under fluorescence-guidance with very intensive fluorescence staining (**Figure 11**). The tumor was completely removed, and no new neurological deficits developed. Early post-operative MRI confirmed gross-total resection of the lesion (**Figure 12**), and histology showed glioblastoma WHO IV. According to our institutional algorithm, the patient did not require a PET scan because of the intense contrast-enhancement in the initial MRI; thus, we decided on administering FL (5 mg/kg) and conducting awake surgery because navigational imaging was intraoperatively equipped with functional data (**Figure 13**).

Case #3

This complex case of faintly contrast-enhancing, secondary malignantly transformed oligodendroglioma WHO III, that had been initially diagnosed as astrocytoma WHO II 11 years ago, was additionally chosen to illustrate our workflow. The

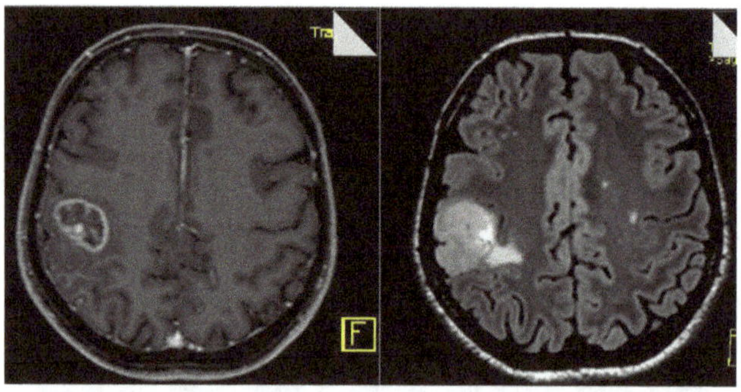

FIGURE 9 | Pre-operative MR image (T1-weighted and FLAIR sequences, axial planes) showing circular contrast-enhancement and moderate edema.

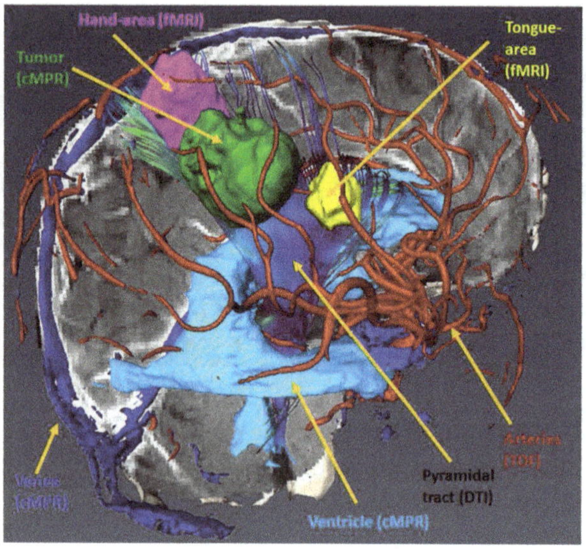

FIGURE 10 | Sagittal view of the Amira 3D-reconstruction of the cortex, the vessels, the ventricle, the tumor (green), the hand motor associations areas (magenta), the tongue motor association area (yellow), and the pyramidal tract.

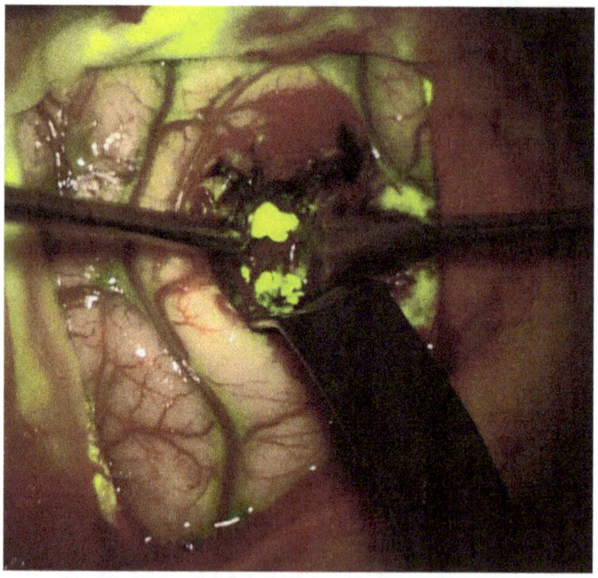

FIGURE 11 | Strong fluorescent staining of the tumor under the YELLOW 560 filter.

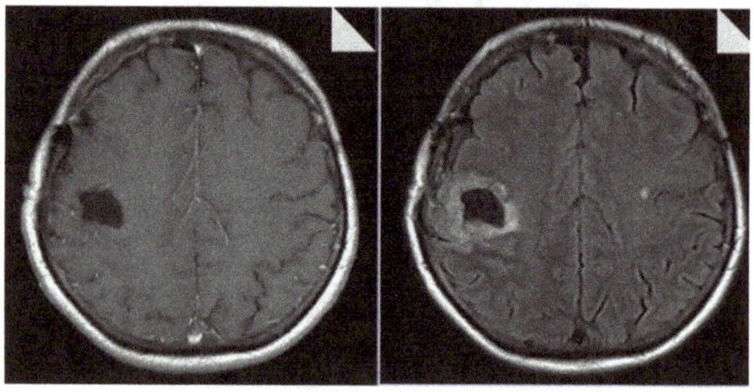

FIGURE 12 | Post-operative MR image (T1-weighted and FLAIR sequences, axial planes) confirming complete removal of the tumor.

tumor—pre-treated with surgery, radiation, and chemotherapy—had recurred, showing marginal contrast-enhancement in the T1-weighted sequence in conventional MRI (**Figure 14**). Consequently, FET-PET was conducted that also showed only marginal metabolic activity (**Figure 15**). However, because of the recent tumor progress and the near-eloquent localization of the tumor in the left frontal cortex, we recommended fMRI followed by subsequent awake craniotomy. Intraoperatively, all imaging modalities were displayed on the navigational screen (**Figure 16**), and we used fluorescence-guidance with FL (5 mg/kg) and ultrasound. Weak but still usable fluorescence was detected, allowing for complete tumor removal based on the early post-operative MRI (**Figure 17**). The neuropathological workup showed anaplastic oligodendroglioma WHO III.

Here, all possible functional and metabolic imaging modalities were included pre- and intraoperatively. Fluorescence-guidance was helpful in this patient, although the initial MRI had only indicated moderate blood brain barrier disruption and the initial PET only demonstrated weak activity.

DISCUSSION

For selected patients with a brain tumor, a detailed, sophisticated workup of different neuroimaging modalities can be of the utmost importance for the pre-operative evaluation and/or simulation of the neurosurgical approach, and for choosing the technique of dissection and removal. This way, the highest possible degree of removal of neoplastic tissue can be attempted with a significant simultaneous increase in safety. Despite pre-operative metabolic and functional visualization of the targeted area by means of PET and fMRI/rsfMRI/DTI and distinctively integrated neuro-navigation, fluorescence-guided surgery with either FL, 5-ALA, or ICG plays a key role in the majority of operations. With this technique,

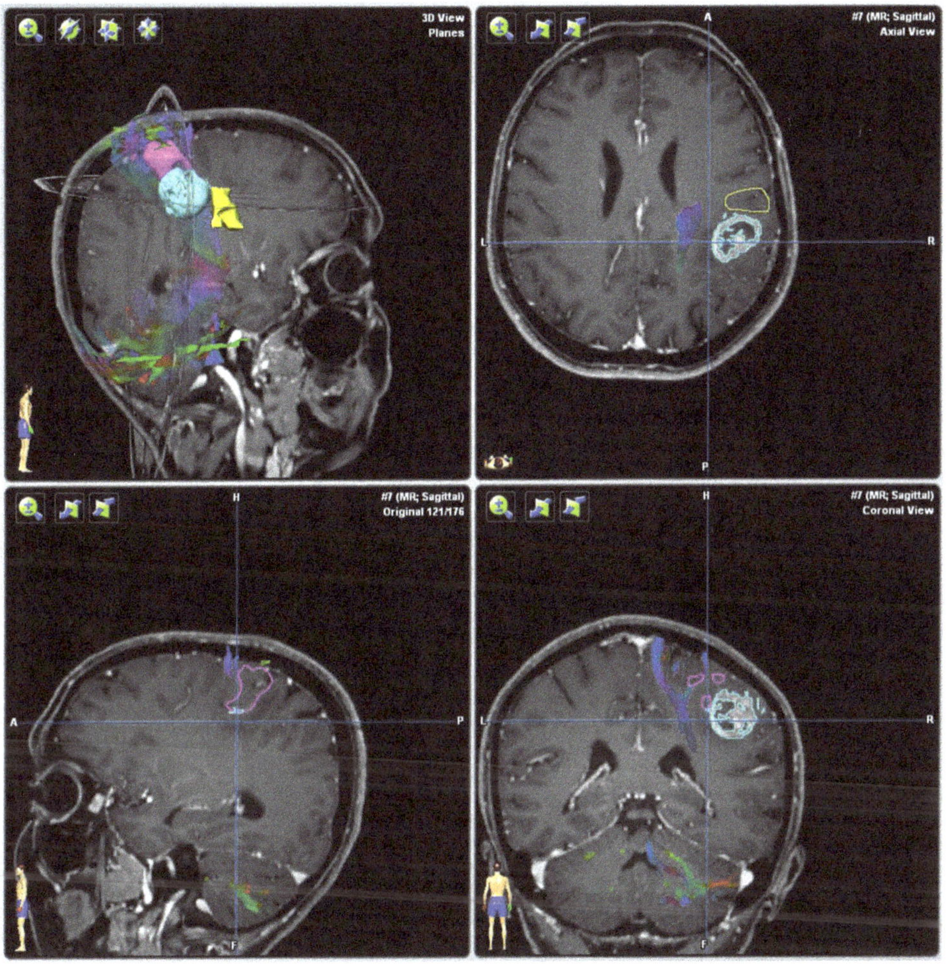

FIGURE 13 | Implementation of fMRI and DTI in the neuro-navigation system [brain tumor (light blue); tumor segmentation based on the 3d cMPR-image, the hand motor association areas (magenta), the tongue motor association area (yellow), and the pyramidal tract (darker blue)].

areas of interest are visualized in real time and according to their specific properties (tumor metabolism with 5-ALA, disrupted BBB with FL, patterns of blood flow with ICG and FL). FL-based confocal endomicroscopy, which is still under scientific evaluation, can further enhance intraoperative accuracy and efficacy.

The discussed imaging modalities, however, should not be arbitrarily applied in every patient with a brain tumor, because such application would counteract the value of an individually tailored combination of these modalities. In most neurosurgical departments, this type of imaging workup is only possible with a high standard of economic and personal competence, and in the case of well-established interdisciplinary collaboration with the departments of neuroradiology, neurology, oncology, nuclear medicine, and neuropathology. Based on this cooperation, the combination of different imaging modalities carries a huge benefit for patients in terms of preserving neurological function while creating the best possible foundation for any type of adjuvant treatment (6).

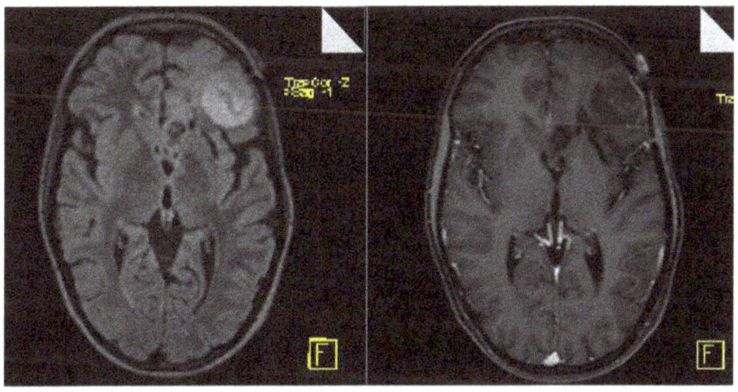

FIGURE 14 | Pre-operative MR image (T1-weighted and FLAIR sequences, axial planes) showing weak contrast-enhancement and marginal edema.

However, some limitations should be clearly stated. Like any academic institution, we can only offer the technical modalities available. For example, there is no intraoperative MRI to be integrated into our IA. Furthermore, some inter-observer bias cannot be excluded, especially in the interpretation of weak or flaw fluorescence in non-contrast enhancing gliomas. Additionally, the use of fluorescence-guided confocal endomicroscopy is still under scientific evaluation.

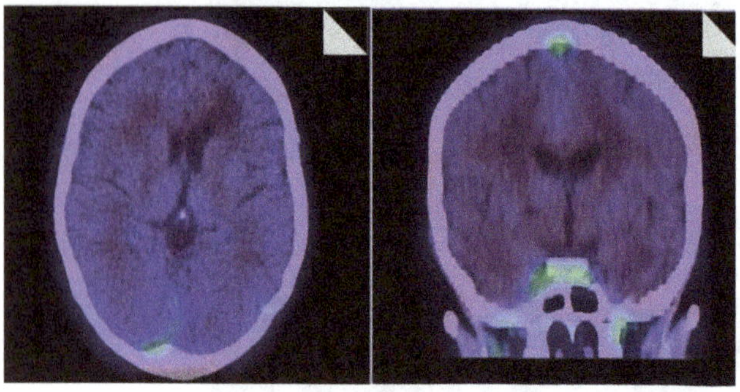

FIGURE 15 | Pre-operative FET-PET showing almost absence of metabolic activity.

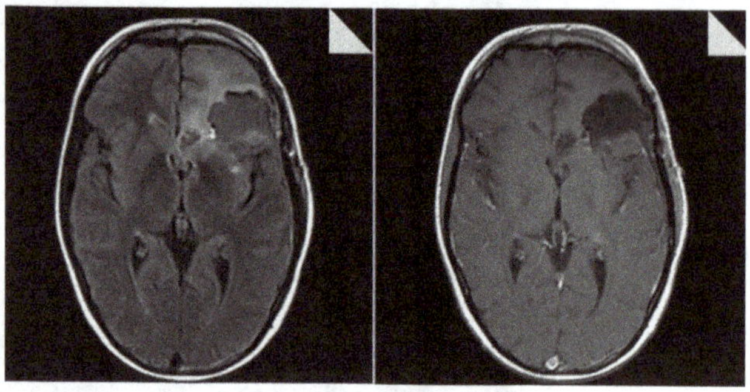

FIGURE 17 | Post-operative MR image (T1-weighted and FLAIR sequences, axial planes) confirming complete removal of the tumor.

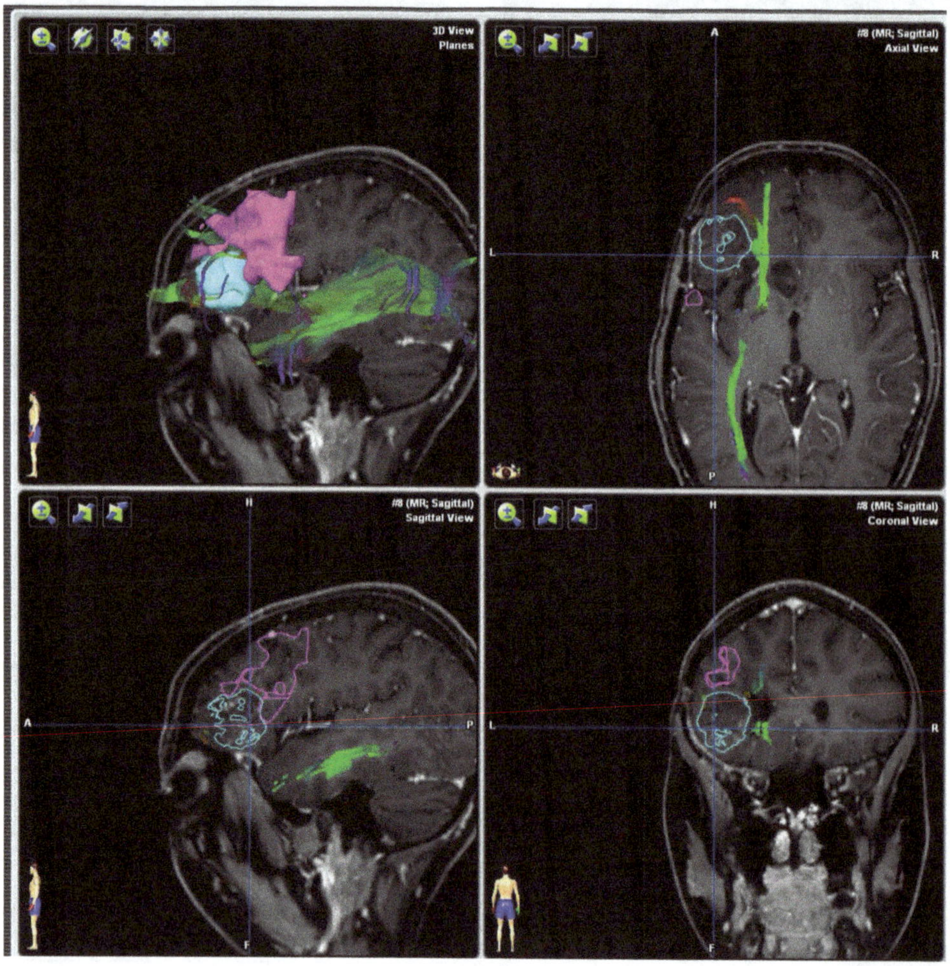

FIGURE 16 | Implementation of fMRI and DTI in the neuro-navigation system [brain tumor (light blue); tumor segmentation based on a FLAIR 3dspace image (not shown), inferior frontal language association area (magenta) and ventral language pathway including uncinate fascicle, extreme capsule, inferior longitudinal fascicle and inferior front-occipital fascicle (green)].

Our IA was established 10 years ago and has been adapted according to contemporary scientific perceptions, such as fluorescence-guided surgery and the integration of FET-PET and functional data. In 2017, we published our institutional series before and after the introduction of our IA that was established simultaneously with the opening of the certified neuro-oncologic center in 2009. This analysis confirms that the implementation of the IA has not only greatly contributed to the significantly prolonged PFS and OS, but has also clearly increased the rate of gross-total resections of HGG (6). The IA has been broadly accepted across the disciplines involved in the NOC and serves as the centerpiece of our weekly neuro-oncologic tumor board.

AUTHOR CONTRIBUTIONS

All authors listed have made a substantial, direct and intellectual contribution to the work, and approved it for publication.

REFERENCES

1. Fujii Y, Muragaki Y, Maruyama T, Nitta M, Saito T, Ikuta S, et al. Threshold of the extent of resection for WHO Grade III gliomas: retrospective volumetric analysis of 122 cases using intraoperative MRI. *J Neurosurg.* (2018) 129:1–9. doi: 10.3171/2017.3.JNS162383
2. Li YM, Suki D, Hess K, Sawaya R. The influence of maximum safe resection of glioblastoma on survival in 1229 patients: can we do better than gross-total resection? *J Neurosurg.* (2016) 124:977–88. doi: 10.3171/2015.5.JNS142087
3. Sanai N, Polley MY, McDermott MW, Parsa AT, Berger MS. An extent of resection threshold for newly diagnosed glioblastomas. *J Neurosurg.* (2011) 115:3–8. doi: 10.3171/2011.2.JNS10998
4. Belykh E, Martirosyan NL, Yagmurlu K, Miller EJ, Eschbacher JM, Izadyyazdanabadi M, et al. Intraoperative fluorescence imaging for personalized brain tumor resection: current state and future directions. *Front Surg.* (2016) 3:55. doi: 10.3389/fsurg.2016.00055
5. Valdes PA, Roberts DW, Lu FK, Golby A. Optical technologies for intraoperative neurosurgical guidance. *Neurosurg Focus.* (2016) 40:E8. doi: 10.3171/2015.12.FOCUS15550
6. Haj A, Doenitz C, Schebesch KM, Ehrensberger D, Hau P, Putnik K, et al. Extent of resection in newly diagnosed glioblastoma: impact of a specialized neuro-oncology care center. *Brain Sci.* (2017) 8:E5. doi: 10.3390/brainsci8010005
7. Schebesch KM, Brawanski A, Doenitz C, Rosengarth K, Proescholdt M, Riemenschneider MJ, et al. Fluorescence-guidance in non-Gadolinium enhancing, but FET-PET positive gliomas. *Clin Neurol Neurosurg.* (2018) 172:177–82. doi: 10.1016/j.clineuro.2018.07.011
8. Pirotte B, Goldman S, Massager N, David P, Wikler D, Vandesteene A, et al. Comparison of 18F-FDG and 11C-methionine for PET-guided stereotactic brain biopsy of gliomas. *J Nucl Med.* (2004) 45:1293–8.
9. Rapp M, Heinzel A, Galldiks N, Stoffels G, Felsberg J, Ewelt C, et al. Diagnostic performance of 18F-FET PET in newly diagnosed cerebral lesions suggestive of glioma. *J Nucl Med.* (2013) 54:229–35. doi: 10.2967/jnumed.112.109603
10. Duffau H, Mandonnet E. The "onco-functional balance" in surgery for diffuse low-grade glioma: integrating the extent of resection with quality of life. *Acta Neurochir.* (2013) 155:951–7. doi: 10.1007/s00701-013-1653-9
11. Sanai N, Berger MS. Extent of resection influences outcomes for patients with gliomas. *Rev Neurol.* (2011) 167:648–54. doi: 10.1016/j.neurol.2011.07.004
12. Stummer W, Kamp MA. The importance of surgical resection in malignant glioma. *Curr Opin Neurol.* (2009) 22:645–9. doi: 10.1097/WCO.0b013e3283320165
13. Wilke M, Lidzba K. LI-tool: a new toolbox to assess lateralization in functional MR-data. *J Neurosci Methods.* (2007) 163:128–36. doi: 10.1016/j.jneumeth.2007.01.026
14. Gordillo N, Montseny E, Sobrevilla P. State of the art survey on MRI brain tumor segmentation. *Magn Reson Imaging.* (2013) 31:1426–38. doi: 10.1016/j.mri.2013.05.002
15. Akkus Z, Galimzianova A, Hoogi A, Rubin DL, Erickson BJ. Deep learning for brain MRI segmentation: state of the art and future directions. *J Digit Imaging.* (2017) 30:449–59. doi: 10.1007/s10278-017-9983-4
16. Bauer S, Wiest R, Nolte LP, Reyes M. A survey of MRI-based medical image analysis for brain tumor studies. *Phys Med Biol.* (2013) 58:R97–129. doi: 10.1088/0031-9155/58/13/R97
17. Tustison NJ, Shrinidhi KL, Wintermark M, Durst CR, Kandel BM, Gee JC, et al. Optimal symmetric multimodal templates and concatenated random forests for supervised brain tumor segmentation (simplified) with ANTsR. *Neuroinformatics.* (2015) 13:209–25. doi: 10.1007/s12021-014-9245-2
18. Bowden SG, Neira JA, Gill BJA, Ung TH, Englander ZK, Zanazzi G, et al. Sodium fluorescein facilitates guided sampling of diagnostic tumor tissue in nonenhancing gliomas. *Neurosurgery.* (2018) 82:719–27. doi: 10.1093/neuros/nyx271
19. Acerbi F, Broggi M, Schebesch KM, Höhne J, Cavallo C, De Laurentis C, et al. Fluorescein-guided surgery for resection of high-grade gliomas: a multicentric prospective phase II study (FLUOGLIO). *Clin Cancer Res.* (2018) 24:52–61. doi: 10.1158/1078-0432.CCR-17-1184
20. Catapano G, Sgulo FG, Seneca V, Lepore G, Columbano L, di Nuzzo G. Fluorescein-guided surgery for high-grade glioma resection: an intraoperative "contrast-enhancer". *World Neurosurg.* (2017) 104:239–47. doi: 10.1016/j.wneu.2017.05.022
21. Hamamcioglu MK, Akcakaya MO, Goker B, Kasimcan MO, Kiris T. The use of the YELLOW 560 nm surgical microscope filter for sodium fluorescein-guided resection of brain tumors: our preliminary results in a series of 28 patients. *Clin Neurol Neurosurg.* (2016) 143:39–45. doi: 10.1016/j.clineuro.2016.02.006
22. Schebesch KM, Proescholdt M, Hohne J, Hohenberger C, Hansen E, Riemenschneider MJ, et al. Sodium fluorescein-guided resection under the YELLOW 560 nm surgical microscope filter in malignant brain tumor surgery–a feasibility study. *Acta Neurochir.* (2013) 155:693–9. doi: 10.1007/s00701-013-1643-y
23. Höhne J, Hohenberger C, Proescholdt M, Riemenschneider MJ, Wendl C, Brawanski A, et al. Fluorescein sodium-guided resection of cerebral metastases-an update. *Acta Neurochir.* (2017) 159:363–7. doi: 10.1007/s00701-016-3054-3
24. Xiao SY, Zhang J, Zhu ZQ, Li YP, Zhong WY, Chen JB, et al. Application of fluorescein sodium in breast cancer brain-metastasis surgery. *Cancer Manag Res.* (2018) 10:4325–31. doi: 10.2147/CMAR.S176504
25. Lin FH, Zhang XH, Zhang J, He ZQ, Duan H, Ke C, et al. Fluorescein sodium-guided biopsy or resection in primary central nervous system lymphomas with contrast-enhancing lesion in MRI. *J Neurooncol.* (2018) 139:757–65. doi: 10.1007/s11060-018-2924-3
26. Schebesch KM, Hoehne J, Hohenberger C, Acerbi F, Broggi M, Proescholdt M, et al. Fluorescein sodium-guided surgery in cerebral lymphoma. *Clin Neurol Neurosurg.* (2015) 139:125–8. doi: 10.1016/j.clineuro.2015.09.015
27. Akcakaya MO, Goker B, Kasimcan MO, Hamamcioglu MK, Kiris T. Use of sodium fluorescein in meningioma surgery performed under the YELLOW-560 nm surgical microscope filter: feasibility and preliminary results. *World Neurosurg.* (2017) 107:966–73. doi: 10.1016/j.wneu.2017.07.103
28. da Silva CE, da Silva JL, da Silva VD. Use of sodium fluorescein in skull base tumors. *Surg Neurol Int.* (2010) 1:70. doi: 10.4103/2152-7806.72247
29. Hohne J, Brawanski A, Schebesch KM. Fluorescence-guided surgery of brain abscesses. *Clin Neurol Neurosurg.* (2017) 155:36–9. doi: 10.1016/j.clineuro.2017.02.014
30. Belykh E, Cavallo C, Gandhi S, Zhao X, Veljanoski D, Izady Yazdanabadi M, et al. Utilization of intraoperative confocal laser endomicroscopy in brain tumor surgery. *J Neurosurg Sci.* (2018) 62:704–17. doi: 10.23736/S0390-5616.18.04553-8
31. Izadyyazdanabadi M, Belykh E, Mooney MA, Eschbacher JM, Nakaji P, Yang Y, et al. Prospects for theranostics in neurosurgical imaging: empowering confocal laser endomicroscopy diagnostics via deep learning. *Front Oncol.* (2018) 8:240. doi: 10.3389/fonc.2018.00240
32. Martirosyan NL, Eschbacher JM, Kalani MY, Turner JD, Belykh E, Spetzler RF, et al. Prospective evaluation of the utility of intraoperative confocal laser endomicroscopy in patients with brain neoplasms using fluorescein sodium: experience with 74 cases. *Neurosurg Focus.* (2016) 40:E11. doi: 10.3171/2016.1.FOCUS15559
33. Martirosyan NL, Georges J, Kalani MY, Nakaji P, Spetzler RF, Feuerstein BG, et al. Handheld confocal laser endomicroscopic imaging utilizing tumor-specific fluorescent labeling to identify experimental glioma cells *in vivo*. *Surg Neurol Int.* (2016) 7:S995–1003. doi: 10.4103/2152-7806.195577

13

Photodynamic Therapy for the Treatment of Glioblastoma

*Samuel W. Cramer and Clark C. Chen**

Department of Neurosurgery, University of Minnesota, Minneapolis, MN, United States

***Correspondence:**
Clark C. Chen
ccchen@umn.edu

Glioblastoma is the most common form of adult brain cancer and remains one of the deadliest of human cancers. The current standard-of-care involves maximal tumor resection followed by treatment with concurrent radiation therapy and the chemotherapy temozolomide. Recurrence after this therapy is nearly universal within 2 years of diagnosis. Notably, >80% of recurrence is found in the region adjacent to the resection cavity. The need for improved local control in this region, thus remains unmet. The FDA approval of 5-aminolevulinic acid (5-ALA) for fluorescence guided glioblastoma resection renewed interests in leveraging this agent as a means to administer photodynamic therapy (PDT). Here we review the general principles of PDT as well as the available literature on PDT as a glioblastoma therapeutic platform.

Keywords: brain tumor, photodynamic therapy (PDT), glioblastoma multiforme (GBM), tumor-targeting, neurosurgery

INTRODUCTION

Glioblastoma is a malignant central nervous system (CNS) neoplasm with histologic features resembling astrocytic cells. It is the most common form of primary brain cancer, with an incidence of 3.19 per 100,000 people in the United States (1). Glioblastomas are aggressive and infiltrative, with microscopic extension into normal brain parenchyma (2, 3). Invading tumor cells exhibit characteristic migratory patterns, including spread beneath the pial margin (subpial spread), along neurons (perineuronal spread), along cerebrovasculature (perivascular satellitosis), or along white matter tracts (intrafascicular spread) (4). Microscopic, infiltrating cells are found centimeters from the margin of the visible tumor mass (5). As such, surgical resection is not curative. The current standard-of-care involves maximal, safe surgical resection followed by concurrent chemotherapy (temozolomide) and fractionated radiotherapy (FRT) (6–9). The overall prognosis for glioblastoma patients is poor, with reported median survival of 14.6 months (7), and tumor recurrence near universal.

The observation that >80.0% of the recurrences are located adjacent to the resection cavity suggests utility for therapeutic platforms targeting this region (10–13). The recent United States Food and Drug Administration (FDA) approval of 5-aminolevulinic acid (5-ALA) for fluorescence guided resection (FGR) of tumors renewed interests in leveraging this agent as a means to administer photodynamic therapy (PDT). In principle PDT to the resection cavity can minimize the risk of local recurrence. In this article, we will review the current state of the literature as it pertains to PDT as a glioblastoma therapeutic platform.

METHODS

The goal of this article is to provide a current state of the art review of photodynamic therapies for the treatment of glioblastoma. To this end, we aim to provide an overview of the development of photodynamic therapy for glioblastoma, describe the physical mechanism of the therapeutic approach, describe known interactions between PDT and pharmacological treatments, as well as predict future developments in this field. Therefore, a comprehensive literature search was performed in PubMed (MEDLINE) using MeSH terms "photodynamic therapy gliomas" which resulted in 480 articles. The type of publications considered included clinical and pre-clinical trials, systematic reviews and case series. Relevant publications were then selected based upon validated academic metrics including journal impact factor and i10 factor.

Principle of Photodynamic Therapy (PDT)

PDT involves photo-activation of a photosensitizer molecule that is selectively incorporated into neoplastic cells. Photo-irradiation activates the photosensitizer by transfer of energy to the sensitizer resulting in excitation of molecular oxygen to a singlet or triplet state. In the singlet state the energy is converted to heat (internal conversion) or is emitted as light (fluorescence). In the triplet state, the energy generates reactive oxygen species (ROS) necessary to induce cell death (**Figure 1**). ROS rapidly react with macromolecules containing unsaturated double bonds, including proteins, unsaturated fatty acids and cholesterols. These reactions damage the membranes of intracellular organelles, such as mitochondria, lysosomes, and the endoplasmic reticulum (8), ultimately triggering necrosis, apoptosis, local ischemia (due to occlusion of neoplastic vessels) as well as subsequent immunological reactions (14).

Singlet oxygen diffuses over short distances (i.e., ~0.02–1.00 μm) and has a limited lifespan (i.e., ~0.04–4.0 μs) contributing to local tumor ablation while minimizing risk of damage to adjacent normal tissue (15). The type of photosensitizer and photo-activation determines the specific intracellular components affected as well as the degree and type of damage incurred by those components.

Like ionizing radiation, the cytotoxic effects of PDT requires the presence of molecular oxygen. Thus, the degree of oxygenation with the tumor microenvironment is a key determinant of PDT's tumoricidal activity. In this context, PDT is often delivered through multi-session treatment in order to facilitate re-oxygenation between treatments (16, 17). Pre-clinical and clinical trials of PDT performed in combination with hyperbaric oxygen demonstrate improved tumoricidal activity (18).

Though both radiation and PDT require molecular oxygen for their respective anti-neoplastic activities, their modes of action fundamentally differ. The available data suggest that ionizing radiation triggers cell death through induction of DNA damage (19). In contrast, the predominant model of cytotoxicity by PDT involves damage of cell membranes, proteins, and organelles (20). As such, PDT potentially synergizes with DNA

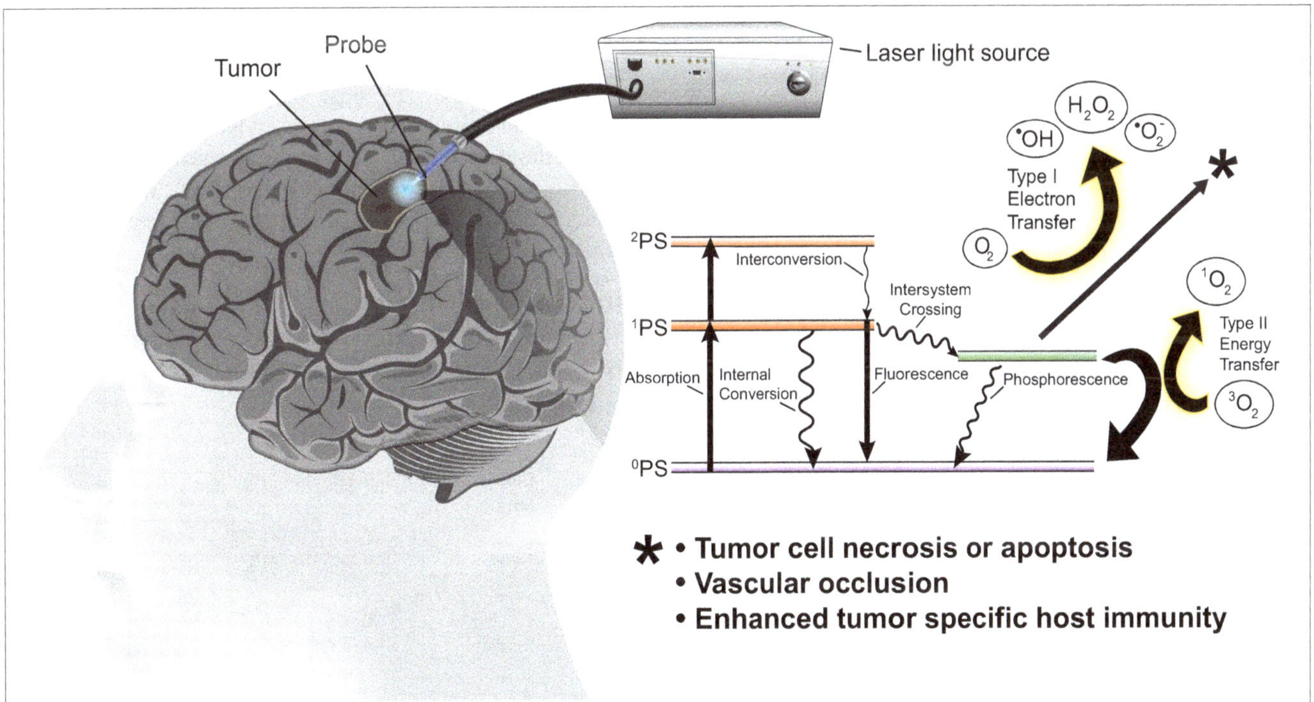

FIGURE 1 | Schematic of PDT for the treatment of glioblastoma with simplified energy diagram of the oxygen dependent photodynamic response. The photosensitizer in the ground state (^0PS) is excited to one of two states by the appropriate wavelength and power photostimulation, the first excited singlet state (^1PS) or the second excited singlet state (^2PS). The ^1PS may then convert to the excited triplet state (^3PS) via intersystem crossing. In the presence of molecular oxygen, the ^3PS may undergo Type I or Type II redox reactions producing reactive oxygen species which cause tumor cell death.

damaging agents routinely used as standard-of-care treatment for glioblastoma (21).

Photo-Activation

The light source may be incoherent or coherent (i.e., laser). The efficacy of PDT is not affected by the coherence of the light source. The emission wavelength of the light source is adjusted to the absorption spectrum of the photosensitizer. Photo-irradiation with longer wavelength light is preferred because it penetrates more deeply and delivers sufficiently energetic photons to activate the photosensitizer. Given the excitation peaks of clinically available photosensitizers and the limitations of photon propagation through biological tissues, PDT generally utilizes wavelengths between ~400 and 900 nm, with an optimal window of 600–800 nm (15). PDT stimulation may be applied in a continuous or pulsed fashion (14), with consideration that pulsed delivery may facilitate tumor re-oxygenation between pulses.

First, Second, and Third Generation Photosensitizers

First-generation photosensitizer molecules consist of naturally occurring porphyrins, including hematoporphyrin (**Table 1**). These compounds have a strong absorption around 400 nm but have limited excitation absorption at longer wavelengths of light (22). HpD is an example of a first generation photosensitizer. It consists of a proprietary combination of monomers, dimers and oligomers derived from hematoporphyrin (23). HpD is an inefficient producer of singlet oxygen requiring extended photo-stimulation to achieve adequate therapeutic effect (23).

Second-generation photosensitizers were developed to overcome the inherent limitations of first-generation sensitizers. They are usually activated by wavelengths >600 nm and are more potent in generating singlet oxygen. Chlorins (talaporfin sodium and temoporfin) and 5-Aminolevulinic acid (5-ALA) are examples of second-generation photosensitizers (15).

Talaporfin sodium and temoporfin are clinically used to treat dermatologic diseases. Talaporfin is water soluble and administered intravenously. As such, it is quickly cleared from the body. Talaporfin is activated by 664 nm light (23, 24). Temoporfin is the most potent of the clinically available photosensitizers (activated by 652 nm photostimulation). Temoporfin is generally well-tolerated but does confer photosensitivity for up to 6 weeks post-administration.

Among the commercially available photosensitizers, 5-ALA is commonly utilized (25). The clinical utility is driven by oral bioavailability and a highly favorable safety profile. Pertaining to glioblastomas, 5-ALA exhibits high selectivity in terms of preferential accumulation in malignant gliomas (15). 5-ALA is the first compound in the synthesis of porphyrin, a component required for heme synthesis. Porphyrins are assembled into porphobilinogen, which is converted to protoporphyrin IX (PpIX) by porphobilinogen deaminase. The expression of this deaminase is elevated in glioblastomas, resulting in increased synthesis of PpIX. PpIX is normally converted to heme by the enzyme ferrochelatase (26). Decreased expression of ferrochelatase in glioblastoma arrests this conversion, further augmenting the accumulation of PpIX in glioblastomas (15).

PpIX absorbs blue light (404 nm) and emits fluorescence in the red spectrum (635 nm). When excited by 635 nm light, PpIX generates triplet oxygen and produces cytotoxicity as a photosensitizer (27). Of note, there is significant inter-tumoral heterogeneity in PpIX concentration after 5-ALA administration (25). The molecular underpinning of this variation remains poorly understood though may involve inter-tumoral expression differences in ATP-binding cassette transporters (28).

Third generation photosensitizers are characterized by enhanced tumor cell selectivity achieved through the conjugation of modifiers including nanoparticles and antibodies (15, 23). Development of third generation photosensitizers has also emphasized the design of prodrugs that are only activated by neoplastic cells. The goal of rational design of third generation photosensitizers is to reduce off target effects while optimizing pharmacokinetics and excitation-absorption properties to maximize the effective PDT window while minimizing side-effects. At this time, no third generation photosensitizers are approved for PDT in humans.

Blood-Brain Barrier

In the normal brain, endothelial cells exhibit morphological specializations including the expression of tight junctions that

TABLE 1 | Properties of clinically relevant photosensitizers.

Photosensitizer	Trade name(s)	Excitation wavelength(s)	Treatment window[a]	Clearance time	Side effects
Talaporfin sodium	Laserphyrin, Aptocine™, Litx™, LS11, Photolon®	664	2–4 h	15 days	Skin sensitization for 2 weeks
HpD	Photofrin®, Photogem®	408, 510, 630[b]	24–48 h	4–6 weeks	Skin sensitization for several weeks
5-ALA (PpIX)	Levulan®	410, 510, 635[b]	4–8 h	2 days	Skin sensitization for few days, nausea, elevated liver enzymes, anemia,
Porfimer sodium	Photofrin II®	630	48–150 h	4–6 weeks	Skin sensitization for several weeks
BOPP	n/a	630	24 h	4–6 weeks	Skin sensitization for several weeks, thrombopenia
Temoporfin	Foscan®	652	4 days	2–6 weeks	Skin sensitization for several weeks

[a] *Latency after drug administration and accumulation of photosensitizer in the tumor.*
[b] *Optimal excitation wavelength for clinical application.*
HpD, Hematoporphyrin derivative; BOPP, Boronated porphyrin.

contribute to the formation of the blood-brain barrier (BBB). There is no active transport system for 5-ALA across the BBB. As such, there is little spontaneous diffusion of 5-ALA into normal brain tissue (25). Break-down in the BBB which frequently occurs in the glioblastoma microenvironment facilitates diffusion of 5-ALA into the tumor mass. In this context, 5-ALA guided surgical resection facilitates removal of the contrast enhancement, which is typically observed in these regions of BBB breakdown.

Whether 5-ALA is a true proxy for tumor mass or simply the region of BBB breakdown remains an open question. The therapeutic window for 5-ALA mediated PDT depends on the extent that PpIX is preferentially accumulated in the glioblastoma cell relative to the cellular constituents of the tumor microenvironment (29).

Medications That May Affect PDT for Glioblastoma

Glioblastoma patients are commonly prescribed anti-epileptic drugs (AEDs, such as phenytoin and levetiracetam) as well as corticosteroid therapy. There are pre-clinical data that suggests these drugs interact with 5-ALA metabolism. In pre-clinical investigation, phenytoin administration after 5-ALA infusion suppressed PpIX synthesis by 31.0% (30). In contrast, levetiracetam did not affect PpIX synthesis or the response to PDT (30).

The interaction between corticosteroid and PpIX synthesis is more complex. PpIX production in response to 5-ALA was reduced by dexamethasone administration. However, the cellular retention of PpIX retention was increased (30). The complexity is further layered in the observation that corticosteroid administration reduced BBB permeability, which may hinder uptake of 5-ALA (15). Pre-clinical studies suggest that this effect is most prominent for dexamethasone (a commonly used corticosteroid in glioblastoma patients) with doses exceeding 12 mg per day (31).

Additionally, other FDA approved medications increase PpIX accumulation in tumor cells, including iron chelators (deferoxamine and deferiprone), vitamin D, ciprofloxacin, 5-fluorouracil, and febuxostat. Combination of these drugs has been proposed as a means to augment efficacy of 5-ALA in PDT (32).

CLINICAL APPLICATIONS

Infiltrating glioblastoma cells can be found 4.0 cm beyond the border of radiologically or histologically identifiable tumor lesions (33). Infiltrating tumor growth and extent of resection is difficult to assess intraoperatively and infiltrative tumor cells are always left behind when using traditional surgical and imaging approaches. Therefore, a method that affords the visual identification of neoplastic tissue and the simultaneous ability to selectively destroy that tissue would likely improve the success of glioblastoma resection. The joint clinical application of fluorescence guided surgery (FGS) and PDT confers the ability to both visualize tumor cells and selectively destroy them.

Interstitial PDT

Interstitial PDT (iPDT) is applied via the stereotactic insertion of fiber optic cable(s) into the tumor to deliver photostimulation to the tumor mass after the patient has been administered a photosensitizer (25). The application of iPDT is similar to laser interstitial thermal therapy (LITT) for the treatment of glioblastoma as both are minimally invasive stereotactic techniques, however, iPDT has the added benefit of selective neoplastic cell targeting. Several technical considerations are unique to iPDT. For example, selecting a light diffuser with the appropriate geometry to apply optimal photostimulation to the target tumor, determining the optimal number of diffusers to insert into the tumor to maximize therapy while minimizing the harm associated with insertion of the diffuser through normal brain tissue and, finally, proper selection of tumors of the appropriate size, anatomic location, and geometry to maximize the safety and efficacy of iPDT.

A challenge of iPDT is the even delivery of photostimulation to achieve adequate fluence over a maximal volume of tumor without causing thermal injury to the normal brain tissue. Modeling experiments have examined light delivery and determined the optimal geometry of light guides for the delivery of iPDT. Cylindrical light diffusers have a larger emitting surface area with a lower fluence rate at the tissue/light emitter interface than flat cleaved fibers (34). Therefore, light delivery via cylindrical diffuser improves photon distribution with a reduced sensitivity to local tissue absorption variability thereby distributing photostimulation over a greater tissue volume than flat, cleaved fibers. However, the light fluence drops off more rapidly from the flat fiber which is useful when treating a tumor in close proximity to eloquent brain tissue. Therefore, the geometry of the light diffuser as well as the total number of diffusers needed to safely treat a tumor are factors to consider preoperatively in order to achieve optimal iPDT.

The dose of light delivered during PDT is another important consideration. A dosimetry model was developed which is specific to 5-ALA but the underlying principle must be considered for iPDT performed with any photosensitizer. To achieve the maximal therapeutic effect of PDT, the goal is to achieve "advanced photobleaching" (based on an established dosimetry model of the same name) of the photosensitizer. Advanced photobleaching is defined as the fluence rate at which causes $\geq$95% photobleaching of photosensitizer and is associated with better outcomes (35, 36). In the case of 5-ALA mediated PDT, simulations suggest advanced photobleaching is achieved to a distance of ~4 mm from the surface of a light diffuser emitting a power of 200 mW/cm for 1 h. Based upon the estimated volume of tissue affected by photo-irradiation, the optimal interfiber distance of the photo diffusers for iPDT is ~10 mm and maximum power of photostimulation should not exceed 200 mW/cm as the threshold at which the risk of increasing tissue temperatures >48°C (the threshold at which thermal side-effects become a factor) increases significantly (25, 37).

Software for optimization of iPDT delivery has been in development for several decades (31, 36). One approach utilizes the co-registration of contrasted magnetic resonance imaging and positron emission tomography imaging with stereotactic computed tomography images to allow virtual trajectory planning and positioning of light diffusers within tumors (37). The goal is to virtually plan the implantation of the optimal number of light diffusers for tumor ablation without causing injury to the adjacent vasculature or traversing eloquent cortex.

Post-resection PDT

After maximal safe tumor resection, PDT may be applied to the resection cavity in the operating room or during post-operative recovery. Cavitary PDT is commonly applied by placing a balloon filled with diffusing liquid (typically a lipid suspension) coupled to a fiber optic guide and an external light source into the intracranial resection cavity. After tumor resection, the balloon is positioned in the cavity and inflated to conform with the geometry of the cavity without causing excessive compression of surrounding brain tissue. In one photostimulation paradigm utilizing the diffuser balloon, total treatment time was derived from the volume of the diffusing media in the balloon and applied in five fractions to the tumor. Between photo-irradiation fractions, 2.0 min pauses are applied allowing brain tissue reoxygenation. All photostimulation fractions are delivered in the operating room. This is the approach being utilized in the Intraoperative Photodynamic Therapy of glioblastoma (INDYGO) clinical trial which is currently ongoing (17).

Another method for cavitary PDT is to apply fractions of photostimulation out of the operating room during the post-operative recovery period. After FGS, a balloon diffuser is placed in the resection cavity and inflated with a radio-opaque lipid emulsion until the resection cavity is filled. Fluoroscopy is used to verify balloon inflation and later complete deflation, prior to removal. The first PDT treatment is applied in the recovery area with daily PDT treatments delivered subsequently at the bedside for a total of 5 treatments. A key consideration for applying PDT over a prolonged time period is the effective half-life of the photosensitizer (in this example porfimer sodium was used). After the total number of treatments are delivered, the balloon diffuser is deflated and removed at the bedside (38, 39).

CLINICAL OUTCOMES OF PDT TREATED GLIOBLASTOMAS

Outcomes after PDT in glioblastoma patients are generally favorable compared to historical data, however, the quality of the studies is limited by the lack of randomized controlled trials. The Royal Melbourne Hospital group has the most extensive clinical experience with PDT for gliomas with a series of more than 350 patients and report overall survival rates of those with newly diagnosed and recurrent glioblastomas of 28.0 and 40.0%, at 2 years and 22.0 and 34.0% at 5 years, respectively, an improvement compared to historical controls. Similarly, a meta-analysis of more than 1,000 patients enrolled in observational studies of PDT for high-grade gliomas reported median survival of newly diagnosed and recurrent glioblastomas of 16.1 and 10.3 months, respectively (40). A summary of a summary of clinical trials evaluating PDT for the treatment of glioblastomas is found in **Table 2**.

HpD Mediated PDT for Glioblastoma

An early study evaluating the efficacy of HpD mediated PDT enrolled 18 glioblastoma patients. HpD was administered via direct arterial puncture during preoperative angiogram, IV or directly into the tumor during craniotomy for tumor resection. Cavitary PDT was applied intraoperatively after tumor resection. Patients were brought back to the operating room 3 days later for redo-craniotomy and administered another round of PDT. At publication, six patients with primary glioblastomas were surviving at 22.0 months (43).

The effects of HpD or porfimer sodium mediated PDT on glioblastomas was evaluated in 17 patients. Patients were administered the photosensitizer 18–24 h prior to undergoing maximal tumor resection and intraoperative, cavitary PDT was applied via an inflatable balloon diffuser. For glioblastoma patients that died during follow-up, mean survival was 6.3 months post-PDT (46).

HpD concentration in tumor tissue compared to survival after PDT was evaluated in 58 glioblastoma patients. Patients underwent maximal safe tumor resection, then intraoperative, cavitary PDT was administered by filling the resection cavity with a continuously circulating lipid emulsion while photostimulation was applied. There was a strong association between HpD uptake and survival among treated patients (Hazard Ratio = 0.26, $p = 0.001$) and the median overall survival for glioblastoma patients after PDT was 24.0 months (57). A similar study evaluating HpD mediated PDT for high grade gliomas including 78 glioblastoma patients was performed. Patients underwent maximal safe tumor resection followed by intra-operative photoirradiation. The median overall survival for glioblastoma patients treated with PDT was 14.3 months (58).

Porfimer Sodium Mediated PDT for Glioblastoma

A case series reports the efficacy of porfimer sodium mediated PDT for newly diagnosed and recurrent glioblastomas in 49 patients. After the maximal tumor resection, either a balloon diffuser was placed in the resection cavity or the resection cavity itself was filled with a continuous infusion of lipid emulsion and photo-irradiation was applied. The median survival of glioblastoma patients was 30 weeks, with 1- and 2-years actuarial survival of 22.0 and 2.0%, respectively (48).

A small study was conducted to evaluate porfimer sodium or temoporfin mediated PDT for malignant primary brain tumors, including 20 glioblastoma patients. Patients underwent tumor resection followed by photo-irradiation to the resection cavity. Light was delivered with a 630 nm laser with a fluence of 75 J/cm^2 in porfimer sodium patients and at 652 nm with a fluence of 20 J/cm^2 in the temoporfin patients. A continuous infusion of lipid emulsion was applied to the resection cavity during photo-irradiation to minimize the risk of thermal injury to brain tissue. Post-operatively, patients were kept in a unique ICU room with no exposure to sun-light. Sunlight was avoided for 4 weeks (porfimer sodium) or 2 weeks (temoporfin). Patients received standard temozolomide chemotherapy and FRT post-operatively. Median OS for these patients was 17 months (59).

TABLE 2 | Summary of clinical trials using PDT for the treatment of GBM.

References	Number of patients		Photosensitizer		Photo-irradiation		Median overall survival (mo)
	New GBM	rGBM	Drug	Dose, route of administration	Wavelength, nm	Energy density (J/cm^2)	
Stupp et al. (6)	287		n/a	n/a	n/a	n/a	14.6[c] newly diagnosed
Akimoto et al. (41)	6	8	Talaporfin sodium	40 mg/m^2, IV	664	27	n/a
Beck et al. (37)[a]		10	5-ALA	20 mg/kg, PO	633	100	15 rGBM
Eljamel et al. (39)	13		5-ALA and Porfimer sodium	2 mg/kg Photofrin IV; 20 mg/kg 5-ALA, PO	630	100	13.2[d] newly diagnosed
Johansson et al. (36)[a]	1	4	5-ALA	20–30 mg/kg	635	720 J/cm	n/a
Kaye et al. (42)	13	6	HpD	5 mg/kg, IV	630	70–120 or 120–230 J/cm^2	n/a
Kostron et al. (43)	18		HpD	1 mg/cm^3 of tumor IA and/or 1 mg/cm^3 into tumor and/or IV mg/cm^3	630	40–120	n/a
Kostron et al. (44)		26	Temoporfin	0.15 mg/kg, IV	652	20	8.5 rGBM
McCulloch et al. (45)	9		HpD	5 mg/kg, IV	627.8[b]	n/a	n/a
Muller and Wilson (46)	17		HpD or Porfimer sodium	1.4–2.7 mg/kg, IV	630	8–68	n/a
Muller and Wilson (47)		32	HpD or Porfimer sodium	5 mg/kg, IV; 2 mg/kg, IV	630	8–110	7.5 (29.5 from diagnosis) rGBM
Muller and Wilson (48)	12	37	Porfimer sodium	2 mg/kg, IV	n/a	58 (mean)	8.25 newly diagnosed, 7.25 rGBM
Muller and Wilson (49)	11		Porfimer sodium	2 mg/kg, IV	630	8–110	9.25 newly diagnosed
Muller et al. (50)		37	Porfimer sodium	2 mg/kg, IV	n/a	8–150	7.75 rGBM
Muragaki et al. (51)	13		Talaporfin sodium	40 mg/m^2, IV	664	27	24.8 newly diagnosed
Nitta et al. (52)	30		Talaporfin sodium	40 mg/m^2, IV	664	27	27.4 newly diagnosed
Origitano et al. (31)[a]		8	Porfimer sodium	2 mg/kg, IV	630	50 (100 J/cm interstitial)	n/a
Popovic et al. (53)	38	40	HpD	5 mg/kg, IV	628	72–260	24 newly diagnosed, 9 rGBM
Powers et al. (54)	2		Porfimer sodium	2 mg/kg, IV	630	400 J/cm	n/a
Rosenthal et al. (55)	7	9	Boronated porphyrin	0.25–8.0 mg/kg, IV	630	25–100	5 newly diagnosed, 11 rGBM
Schwartz et al. (56)[a]	15		5-ALA	20–30 mg/kg, PO	633	12.960 J	n/a
Stylli et al. (57)	58		HpD	5 mg/kg, IV	n/a[b]	240 J/cm^2 (median)	24 newly diagnosed
Stylli et al. (58)	31	55	HpD	5 mg/kg, IV	n/a[b]	230 J/cm^2 (median)	14.3 newly diagnosed, 14.9 rGBM
Vanaclocha et al. (59)	20		Porfimer sodium or temoporfin	2 mg/kg, IV; 0.15 mg/kg, IV	630; 652	20–75	17 newly diagnosed

[a]*iPDT.*
[b]*Multiple lasers used.*
[c]*Reference survival time for newly diagnosed GBM.*
[d]*Mean.*
rGBM, recurrent GBM; HpD, hematoporphyrin derivative.

A phase II study evaluated porfimer sodium mediated PDT for newly diagnosed and recurrent supratentorial gliomas including 37 recurrent and 11 newly diagnosed glioblastomas. Subjects enrolled in the study underwent tumor resection followed by intraoperative placement of expandable balloon irradiator filled with a light dispersion medium for photo-irradiation (49, 50). Those with recurrent glioblastomas who had failed prior surgical resection and FRT (with or without chemotherapy) underwent PDT while patients with newly diagnosed tumors underwent surgical resection with intraoperative PDT. The median survival for newly diagnosed glioblastoma patients was 7.75 months while those with recurrent glioblastomas had a median survival of 9.25 months.

The application of PDT as treatment for glioblastomas was first evaluated in a randomized, controlled trial by Muller and Willson (40, 48). The treatment arm enrolled 43 patients who underwent glioblastoma resection followed by porfimer sodium mediated PDT and was compared to 34 patients who underwent tumor resection alone. Post-operative FRT was administered to all patients. Median survival was 11.0 months (95% CI 6.0–14.0

months) in the treatment group compared to 8.0 months (95% CI 3.0–10.0 months) in the control group. A 38.0% increase in median survival with PDT as well as >6.0-months survival rate in the treatment group were statistically significant, but Kaplan–Meier curves crossed over at 15 months (14, 40, 48).

Eljamel et al. conducted a single-center, randomized controlled phase III trial to evaluate porfimer sodium mediated PDT after 5-ALA FGS for newly diagnosed glioblastomas. In the study, 13 patients underwent FGS for glioblastoma resection followed by intracavitary placement of a balloon diffuser to provide repetitive PDT (1 session per day, 100 J/cm^2 applied per session) for 5 days during the post-operative period. The control arm underwent FGS for tumor resection without PDT. Post-operatively, all patients underwent FRT and were followed clinically and radiographically every 3 months until death. There was no statistically significant difference in the frequency of adjuvant and salvage treatments between the two cohorts. The mean survival of patients in the PDT and surgery only groups was 52.8 weeks (95% CI 40.0–65.0 weeks) and 24.2 weeks (95% CI 18.0–30.0 weeks), respectively ($p < 0.001$). Despite an overall worse functional status in the study group prior to FGS and PDT, their functional status improved to a much higher level post-operatively compared to the surgery only group. There was no residual tumor on discharge in 10 out of 13 patients in the PDT group and in 4 out of 14 patients in the surgery only group. There was also no difference between the groups in the average length of stay in the hospital or in the complication rate.

Talaporfin Sodium Mediated PDT for Glioblastoma

Talaporfin sodium accumulates selectively in high grade gliomas and is useful for intraoperative photodiagnosis of malignant brain tumors (60). Furthermore, several small case series report the safety and efficacy of talaporfin sodium mediated PDT as glioblastoma treatment. Thirty newly diagnosed glioblastoma patients treated with PDT in addition to standard FRT and temozolomide were compared to 164 patients with newly diagnosed glioblastomas who received standard therapy alone. The median survival time was 27.4 months for PDT patients compared to 22.1 months for those receiving standard therapy (52).

Another case series reported a median survival of 26.0 months (with one patient surviving >38.0 months) for four newly diagnosed glioblastoma patients treated with maximal safe tumor resection followed by talaporfin sodium mediated PDT while six patients with recurrent glioblastomas who underwent the same treatment had a median survival of 8.5 months (41). Muragaki et al. report their experience with talaporfin sodium PDT for the treatment of newly diagnosed or recurrent malignant primary brain tumors (including 13 glioblastoma patients). Patients underwent craniotomy and tumor resection followed by intraoperative cavitary PDT. The photostimulation was targeted to regions with high risk of tumor recurrence including the genu of the corpus callosum. In total, 1-3 regions within the resection cavity were targeted with photo-irradiated. All patients with newly diagnosed glioblastomas underwent FRT and adjuvant chemotherapy with temozolomide in addition to PDT. The median overall survival for patients with newly diagnosed glioblastomas was of 24.8 months with a median progression free survival of 12.0 months (51).

5-ALA Mediated PDT for Glioblastoma

Two series report their experience with 5-ALA mediated iPDT for malignant gliomas. In a pilot study, the efficacy of 5-ALA mediated iPDT for small (maximum diameter <3 cm), circumscribed recurrent malignant gliomas was evaluated in 10 patients. Based upon 3-D photoirradiation simulations during preoperative planning, 4–6 fiber diffusers were stereotactically placed per patient to achieve complete photo-irradiation of the tumors. The 1-year survival rate was 60.0% with a median survival of 15.0 months (37). A similar series in 15 patients with small newly diagnosed (<4 cm) and unresectable glioblastomas who underwent 5-ALA iPDT and were compared to glioblastoma patients ($n = 112$) who underwent complete tumor resection alone. All patients received standard radiotherapy and temozolomide. The iPDT group demonstrated significantly longer median progression free survival of 16.0 vs. 10.2 months and a 3-years survival of 56.0 vs. 21.0% (56). Of note, 6 of the 15 patients in the iPDT group experienced progression free survival >30 months.

Boronated Porphyrin and Temoporfin Mediated PDT for Glioblastoma

A phase I trial evaluated the safety of boronated porphyrin (BOPP) for the treatment of high-grade gliomas including seven patients with newly diagnosed and 9 patients with recurrent glioblastomas. The dose of BOPP and photo-irradiation were varied incrementally with the goal of determining the maximum safe doses. The median overall survival for newly diagnosed glioblastomas was 5.0 months and the median overall survival for those with recurrent glioblastomas after PDT was 11.0 months (55).

A non-randomized controlled phase II study evaluated temoporfin mediated PDT in 26 patients with recurrent glioblastomas. Prior to enrollment, all patients had received standard surgical, chemo and radiation therapy. The PDT consisted of FGS (classified as a macroscopically total resection in 75.0% of cases) followed by the administration of intraoperative PDT. The median survival was 8.5 months, and the 2-years survival rate was 15.0%. The median survival rates for the PDT treated patients was significantly better than the survival in the control group (44).

Efficacy of PDT for Glioblastoma

Despite sample size limitations and few randomized controlled studies of PDT, the data suggest potential beneficial effect of PDT for improving survival in glioblastoma patients when compared to standard therapy. The extent of PDT's practical application is hindered by the depth of light penetration into brain and tumor tissue with an estimated effective therapeutic spatial window for PDT limited to ~0.75–1.5 cm from the light source (16, 41, 61). At this time given the above limitations of light delivery and photosensitizer properties, aggressive tumor resection is necessary prior to application of PDT except in the case of very small tumors.

Safety of PDT for the Treatment of Glioblastomas

Beyond complications associated with brain tumor resection, adverse events uniquely related to PDT include the systemic administration of a photosensitizer, the application of photostimulation and photochemical reactions. Each photosensitizer confers a slightly different safety profile. A risk common to all photosensitizers is retinal and cutaneous photosensitivity which occurs for several days in the case of 5-ALA to up to 6 weeks for temoporfin, during which time exposure to direct sunlight should be avoided (23).

A phase I–II study conducted by Kaye et al. that examined the efficacy of high-dose PDT using the photosensitizer HpD in 23 patients with malignant brain tumors found no evidence of increased cerebral edema nor any other adverse events, including hematological, hepatic and renal dysfunction (42). In another case series of 20 patients, side-effects of HpD administration included one patient with dermatotoxicity consisting of swelling of the head and hands after sun-exposure despite the application of sun blocking agents, which lasted for 1 week and three patients experienced meningeal symptoms (stiff neck, fever, headache) after direct injection of HpD into the tumors which lasted for 3 days (43). There was no mortality associated with PDT, however, three patients experienced symptomatic cerebral edema that responded to medical management. Another series reports a cerebral edema incidence of 0.04% cerebral edema after HpD PDT (58).

Reports of stereotactic iPDT suggest it is safe when applied to appropriately selected patients. One of the primary considerations is post-iPDT edema. In the experience at Kashiwaba Neurosurgical hospital with porfimer sodium mediated iPDT, cerebral edema was observed post-operatively in 46.0%, though the swelling was mild and did not require therapeutic intervention in 42.0% of cases (14).

Evaluation of 112 brain tumor patients treated with porfimer sodium mediated PDT yielded adverse events in 25.0% of cases (48). Among the adverse events were death (2.7%), post-operative hemorrhage (2.7%), neurological deficit (6.2%), deep venous thrombosis (3.6%), infection (3.6%), and light sensitivity reactions, such as hand burns, facial erythema, and facial pruritus 3.6% of patients. The majority of adverse events, however, were surgical and not directly related to photo-irradiation except for light sensitivity (48).

In a series of 365 PDT applications with 5-ALA and porfimer sodium in 150 brain tumor patients, adverse events occurred in 4.7% of patients (40). Deep venous thrombosis occurred in 2.0% of patients after administration of porfimer sodium, while no cases were observed after 5-ALA administration. Serious skin photosensitivity reactions developed in 1.3% of patients after non-adherence to light protection precautions. The photosensitivity reactions were considered avoidable had precautions been taken. Cerebral edema occurred after porfimer sodium mediated PDT in 1.3% of patients with recurrent tumors requiring intervention. In 0.7% of patients, there was rupture of the balloon diffuser used for photo-irradiation during PDT or cerebrospinal fluid leak (40).

In another series of 41 patients treated with porfimer sodium or temoporfin PDT, two patients with thalamic tumors died post-operatively due to significant post-treatment cerebral edema (59). Several adverse events were encountered during the trial. First, one scalp burn required plastic surgery with a cutaneous graft for repair. Other cutaneous toxicities were observed including blisters on the forearm and cutaneous erythema. A case of burn injury on the thumbnail from pulse oximeter was observed (59).

In another large case series of 100 patients with primary brain tumors who underwent HpD or porfimer sodium PDT, the authors report a mortality of 3.0% and combined serious morbidity-mortality rate of 8.0% (50). Of note, mean post-operative ICP is significantly higher after HpD or porfimer sodium mediated PDT compared to control patients (46).

Overall, porfimer sodium PDT has been associated with more adverse events than other photosensitizers, such as 5-ALA. For example, porfimer sodium is associated with increased risk of neurological deficits at a total photo-irradiation dose above 4,000 J (62). However, the apparent increased risk of adverse events with porfimer sodium mediated PDT compared to the use of other photosensitizers PDT may be due to the larger number of patients treated with porfimer sodium PDT.

There have been no systematic reviews of PDT safety. Overall, the common risks of PDT are retinal and cutaneous photosensitivity after administration of the photosensitizer. However, the risk of photosensitivity reactions are time limited and may be mitigated by avoidance of direct sun-light. The most serious safety risk of PDT is uncontrolled cerebral edema. The exact rate of cerebral edema after PDT is not known since it varies by photosensitizer as well as with the mode of delivery and intensity of photo-stimulation utilized during therapy.

EMERGING TECHNOLOGIES, ADVANCEMENTS IN PDT FOR GLIOBLASTOMAS

PDT Mediated Immune Response

PDT has several unique properties that induce effective anti-tumor responses, such as apoptosis, autophagy, and necrosis as well as immunogenic cell death (ICD) (8). The unique modes of cell death evoked by PDT are thought to underlie a robust tumor-specific immune response which potentially leads to sustained immune mediated surveillance and suppression of neoplastic cell growth.

A mouse model cured of brain tumor by PDT provided the first evidence for induction of a tumor-specific immune response by resisting subsequent tumor cell re-challenge a tumor-specific manner while immunosuppressed mice did not resist the re-challenge (63). Several years later, the cellular mechanism of the anti-tumor immunity was further elucidated. Among the different modes of PDT induced cell death, ICD is a type of cell death whereby neoplastic cells expose and/or release of tumor antigens molecules known as damage associated molecular patterns (DAMPs) (64, 65) which activate both innate and adaptive immune responses (66). DAMPs are integral components of cells that are only exposed on the plasma membrane and/or released in response to injury, such as the oxidative damage caused by PDT. DAMPs play a key role in cell mediated immunity by causing the activation and stimulation of antigen processing/presentation by antigen presenting cells (APCs). The activation of APCs causes their migration and proliferation in local lymph nodes where the APCs then present the tumor antigens to $CD8^+$ T cells (8). Activated $CD8^+$ T cells actively surveil the body for neoplastic cells and induce apoptosis whenever tumor cells are encountered, thereby providing long-term tumor control. Therefore, ICD induced by PDT has the potential to stimulate immune activation and surveillance, contributing to long term tumor control is observed in pre-clinical models (63, 66–69).

Overall, the survival benefit of PDT trials for malignant gliomas has been modest, thus providing the rationale for adjuvant therapies, such as further augmentation of the immune response initiated by PDT. There have been few experimental studies exploring the effects of direct PDT mediated immune response on brain tumor growth and to our knowledge no clinical studies to date.

Nanoparticle Photosensitizers

Nanoparticle technology provides several opportunities to improve upon the delivery, bio-availability, selectivity, and functionality of currently available photosensitizing molecules while reducing side-effects (70–72). Selective drug delivery using nanotechnology is an area of active research that may provide functional tumor cell type specific delivery capabilities as well as provide improved systemic pharmacokinetics of photosensitizer molecules (73–75). For example, nanoparticle-conjugated photosensitizers are in development to exploit tumor specific cell surface receptors which would deliver the photosensitizer directly to the tumor cell (76). The goal is to develop nanoparticles that are able to cross the BBB and selectively enter tumor cells. The availability of a photosensitizer capable of crossing the BBB and selectively entering tumor cells would broaden the spectrum of brain tumor targets to lower grade tumors for PDT as the requisite tumor mediated disruption of the BBB would be eliminated.

Upconverting nanoparticles, nanoparticles that convert multiple incident photons (generally in the infrared range) into an emitted photon (in the visible light range) of higher energy for PDT is an area of active research (77, 78). Another shortcoming of clinically available photosensitizers is the peak excitation wavelength necessary for activation requires wavelengths of light that poorly penetrate brain tissue. To address this limitation, nanoparticles are in development that are activated by deeper-penetrating near infrared light which causes the nanoparticles to release photons at the photosensitizer excitation wavelengths (78). The goal is to achieve a higher degree of tumor cell specificity (even in regions with intact BBB) while being able to apply PDT at greater distances from the light source and, therefore, over a larger tissue volume than can be achieved using current PDT techniques.

CONCLUSION

Following on the heels of the recent FDA approval of 5-ALA for fluorescent guided glioblastoma resection, there is emerging interest in leveraging this agent toward administering photodynamic therapy (PDT) to the resection cavity. Review of the available literatures suggests that such PDT can be safely delivered to prevent local tumor recurrence. However, it is difficult to extrapolate the efficacy of the regimen given significant heterogeneity in study design, patient cohort, and PDT agents. This review provides data spanning over 25 years of technological sophistication of PDT, hence overlaps with extension in life expectancy and quality of life parameters conferred to glioblastoma patients by optimization of their multispecialistic care are difficult to evaluate. However, lack of clear efficacy of PDT in overall survival has limited the wide-spread adaption of this technology and implementation as a standard treatment of glioblastoma. Furthermore, technical limitations in light delivery and photosensitizer design have blunted the impact that this technology might have in the treatment of glioblastoma.

The immunological effects of PDT is of particular interest given recent studies demonstrating the importance of these processes in glioblastoma. Further studies of PDT in glioblastoma after stratification of pertinent molecular biomarkers, including isocitrate dehydrogenase mutation status and methyl-guanine-methyl transferase (MGMT) promoter methylation status is warranted. Incorporation of PDT into the current standard-of-care therapy should be explored in this context. Furthermore, exploration of next generation photosensitizer agents with increased specificity to glioblastoma is equally warranted.

AUTHOR CONTRIBUTIONS

All authors listed have made a substantial, direct and intellectual contribution to the work, and approved it for publication.

ACKNOWLEDGMENTS

We thank Alexander Cramer for generating graphics.

REFERENCES

1. Tamimi AF, Juweid M. Epidemiology and outcome of glioblastoma. In: De VleeSchouwer S, editor. *Glioblastoma*. Brisbane, QLD: Codon Publications (2017). p. 143–53. doi: 10.1016/B978-0-323-47660-7.00006-9
2. Claes A, Idema AJ, Wesseling P. Diffuse glioma growth: a guerilla war. *Acta Neuropathol.* (2007) 114:443–58. doi: 10.1007/s00401-007-0293-7
3. Sahm F, Capper D, Jeibmann A, Habel A, Paulus W, Troost D, et al. Addressing diffuse glioma as a systemic brain disease with single-cell analysis. *Arch Neurol.* (2012) 69:523–6. doi: 10.1001/archneurol.2011.2910

4. Scherer HJ. The forms of growth in gliomas and their practical significance. *Brain.* (1940) 63:1–35. doi: 10.1093/brain/63.1.1
5. Kelly PJ, Daumas-Duport C, Kispert DB, Kall BA, Scheithauer BW, Illig JJ. Imaging-based stereotaxic serial biopsies in untreated intracranial glial neoplasms. *J Neurosurg.* (1987) 66:865–74. doi: 10.3171/jns.1987.66.6.0865
6. Stupp R, Mason WP, van den Bent MJ, Weller M, Fisher B, Taphoorn MJB, et al. Radiotherapy plus concomitant and adjuvant temozolomide for glioblastoma. *N Engl J Med.* (2005) 352:987–96. doi: 10.1056/NEJMoa043330
7. Stupp R, Hegi ME, Mason WP, van den Bent MJ, Taphoorn MJB, Janzer RC, et al. Effects of radiotherapy with concomitant and adjuvant temozolomide versus radiotherapy alone on survival in glioblastoma in a randomised phase III study: 5-year analysis of the EORTC-NCIC trial. *Lancet Oncol.* (2009) 10:459–66. doi: 10.1016/S1470-2045(09)70025-7
8. Hirschberg H, Berg K, Peng Q. Photodynamic therapy mediated immune therapy of brain tumors. *Neuroimmunol Neuroinflamm.* (2018) 5:27. doi: 10.20517/2347-8659.2018.31
9. Pellerino A, Franchino F, Soffietti R, Rudà R. Overview on current treatment standards in high-grade gliomas. *Q J Nucl Med Mol Imaging.* (2018) 62:225–38. doi: 10.23736/S1824-4785.18.03096-0
10. Petrecca K, Guiot MC, Panet-Raymond V, Souhami L. Failure pattern following complete resection plus radiotherapy and temozolomide is at the resection margin in patients with glioblastoma. *J Neurooncol.* (2013) 111:19–23. doi: 10.1007/s11060-012-0983-4
11. Ganau M, Foroni RI, Gerosa M, Zivelonghi E, Longhi M, Nicolato A. Radiosurgical options in neuro-oncology: a review on current tenets and future opportunities. Part I: therapeutic strategies. *Tumori.* (2014) 100:459–65. doi: 10.1700/1636.17912
12. Ganau M, Foroni RI, Gerosa M, Ricciardi GK, Longhi M, Nicolato A. Radiosurgical options in neuro-oncology: a review on current tenets and future opportunities. Part II: adjuvant radiobiological tools. *Tumori.* (2015) 101:57–63. doi: 10.5301/tj.5000215
13. Thon N, Tonn JC, Kreth FW. The surgical perspective in precision treatment of diffuse gliomas. *Onco Targets Ther.* (2019) 12:1497–508. doi: 10.2147/OTT.S174316
14. Kaneko S, Fujimoto S, Yamaguchi H, Yamauchi T, Yoshimoto T, Tokuda K. Photodynamic therapy of malignant gliomas. *Prog Neurol Surg.* (2018) 32:1–13. doi: 10.1159/000469675
15. Mahmoudi K, Garvey KL, Bouras A, Cramer G, Stepp H, Jesu Raj JG, et al. 5-Aminolevulinic acid photodynamic therapy for the treatment of high-grade gliomas. *J Neurooncol.* (2019) 141:595–607. doi: 10.1007/s11060-019-03103-4
16. Bechet D, Mordon SR, Guillemin F, Barberi-Heyob MA. Photodynamic therapy of malignant brain tumours: a complementary approach to conventional therapies. *Cancer Treat Rev.* (2014) 40:229–41. doi: 10.1016/j.ctrv.2012.07.004
17. Dupont C, Vermandel M, Leroy HA, Quidet M, Lecomte F, Delhem N, et al. INtraoperative photoDYnamic Therapy for GliOblastomas (INDYGO): study protocol for a phase I clinical trial. *Neurosurgery.* (2019) 84:E414–9. doi: 10.1093/neuros/nyy324
18. Al-Waili NS, Butler GJ, Beale J, Hamilton RW, Lee BY, Lucas P. Hyperbaric oxygen and malignancies: a potential role in radiotherapy, chemotherapy, tumor surgery and phototherapy. *Med Sci Monit.* (2005) 11:RA279–89. Available online at: https://www.medscimonit.com/abstract/index/idArt/428463
19. Maier P, Hartmann L, Wenz F, Herskind C. Cellular pathways in response to ionizing radiation and their targetability for tumor radiosensitization. *Int J Mol Sci.* (2016) 17:E102. doi: 10.3390/ijms17010102
20. Robertson CA, Evans DH, Abrahamse H. Photodynamic therapy (PDT): a short review on cellular mechanisms and cancer research applications for PDT. *J Photochem Photobiol B.* (2009) 96:1–8. doi: 10.1016/j.jphotobiol.2009.04.001
21. Zhang X, Guo M, Shen L, Hu S. Combination of photodynamic therapy and temozolomide on glioma in a rat C6 glioma model. *Photodiagnosis Photodyn Ther.* (2014) 11:603–12. doi: 10.1016/j.pdpdt.2014.10.007
22. de Paula LB, Primo FL, Tedesco AC. Nanomedicine associated with photodynamic therapy for glioblastoma treatment. *Biophys Rev.* (2017) 9:761–73. doi: 10.1007/s12551-017-0293-3
23. Allison RR, Sibata CH. Oncologic photodynamic therapy photosensitizers: a clinical review. *Photodiagnosis Photodyn Ther.* (2010) 7:61–75. doi: 10.1016/j.pdpdt.2010.02.001
24. Wang S, Bromley E, Xu L, Chen JC, Keltner L. Talaporfin sodium. *Expert Opin Pharmacother.* (2010) 11:133–40. doi: 10.1517/14656560903463893
25. Stepp H, Stummer W. 5-ALA in the management of malignant glioma. *Lasers Surg Med.* (2018) 50:399–419. doi: 10.1002/lsm.22933
26. Lakomkin N, Hadjipanayis CG. Fluorescence-guided surgery for high-grade gliomas. *J Surg Oncol.* (2018) 118:356–61. doi: 10.1002/jso.25154
27. Ewelt C, Nemes A, Senner V, Wölfer J, Brokinkel B, Stummer W, et al. Fluorescence in neurosurgery: its diagnostic and therapeutic use. Review of the literature. *J Photochem Photobiol B Biol.* (2015) 148:302–9. doi: 10.1016/j.jphotobiol.2015.05.002
28. Kawai N, Hirohashi Y, Ebihara Y, Saito T, Murai A, Saito T, et al. ABCG2 expression is related to low 5-ALA photodynamic diagnosis (PDD) efficacy and cancer stem cell phenotype, and suppression of ABCG2 improves the efficacy of PDD. *PLoS ONE.* (2019) 14:e0216503. doi: 10.1371/journal.pone.0216503
29. Hirschberg H, Uzal FA, Chighvinadze D, Zhang MJ, Peng Q, Madsen SJ. Disruption of the blood-brain barrier following ALA-mediated photodynamic therapy. *Lasers Surg Med.* (2008) 40:535–42. doi: 10.1002/lsm.20670
30. Lawrence JE, Steele CJ, Rovin RA, Belton RJ, Winn RJ. Dexamethasone alone and in combination with desipramine, phenytoin, valproic acid or levetiracetam interferes with 5-ALA -mediated PpIX production and cellular retention in glioblastoma cells. *J Neurooncol.* (2016) 127:15–21. doi: 10.1007/s11060-015-2012-x
31. Origitano TC, Karesh SM, Henkin RE, Halama JR, Reichman OH. Photodynamic therapy for intracranial neoplasms: investigations of photosensitizer uptake and distribution using indium-111 Photofrin-II single photon emission computed tomography scans in humans with intracranial neoplasms. *Neurosurgery.* (1993) 32:357–63; discussion 363–4. doi: 10.1227/00006123-199303000-00004
32. Kast RE, Skuli N, Sardi I, Capanni F, Hessling M, Frosina G, et al. Augmentation of 5-aminolevulinic acid treatment of glioblastoma by adding ciprofloxacin, deferiprone, 5-fluorouracil and febuxostat: the CAALA regimen. *Brain Sci.* (2018) 8:E203. doi: 10.3390/brainsci8120203
33. Silbergeld DL, Chicoine MR. Isolation and characterization of human malignant glioma cells from histologically normal brain. *J Neurosurg.* (1997) 86:525–31. doi: 10.3171/jns.1997.86.3.0525
34. Baran TM, Foster TH. Comparison of flat cleaved and cylindrical diffusing fibers as treatment sources for interstitial photodynamic therapy. *Med Phys.* (2014) 41:1–8. doi: 10.1118/1.4862078
35. Johansson A, Palte G, Schnell O, Tonn JC, Herms J, Stepp H. 5-aminolevulinic acid-induced protoporphyrin IX levels in tissue of human malignant brain tumors. *Photochem Photobiol.* (2010) 86:1373–8. doi: 10.1111/j.1751-1097.2010.00799.x
36. Johansson A, Faber F, Kniebühler G, Stepp H, Sroka R, Egensperger R, et al. Protoporphyrin IX fluorescence and photobleaching during interstitial photodynamic therapy of malignant gliomas for early treatment prognosis. *Lasers Surg Med.* (2013) 45:225–34. doi: 10.1002/lsm.22126
37. Beck TJ, Kreth FW, Beyer W, Mehrkens JH, Obermeier A, Stepp H, et al. Interstitial photodynamic therapy of nonresectable malignant glioma recurrences using 5-aminolevulinic acid induced protoporphyrin IX. *Lasers Surg Med.* (2007) 39:386–93. doi: 10.1002/lsm.20507
38. Eljamel MS. Photodynamic assisted surgical resection and treatment of malignant brain tumours technique, technology and clinical application. *Photodiagnosis Photodyn Ther.* (2004) 1:93–8. doi: 10.1016/S1572-1000(04)00014-6
39. Eljamel MS, Goodman C, Moseley H. ALA and Photofrin® fluorescence-guided resection and repetitive PDT in glioblastoma multiforme: a single centre phase III randomised controlled trial. *Lasers Med Sci.* (2008) 23:361–7. doi: 10.1007/s10103-007-0494-2
40. Eljamel S. Photodynamic applications in brain tumors: a comprehensive review of the literature. *Photodiagnosis Photodyn Ther.* (2010) 7:76–85. doi: 10.1016/j.pdpdt.2010.02.002
41. Akimoto J, Haraoka J, Aizawa K. Preliminary clinical report on safety and efficacy of photodynamic therapy using talaporfin sodium for malignant gliomas. *Photodiagnosis Photodyn Ther.* (2012) 9:91–9. doi: 10.1016/j.pdpdt.2012.01.001
42. Kaye AH, Morstyn G, Brownbill D. Adjuvant high-dose photoradiation therapy in the treatment of cerebral glioma: a phase 1-2 study. *J Neurosurg.* (1987) 67:500–5. doi: 10.3171/jns.1987.67.4.0500

43. Kostron H, Fritsch E, Grunert V. Photodynamic therapy of malignant brain tumours: a phase I/II trial. *Br J Neurosurg.* (1988) 2:241–8. doi: 10.3109/02688698808992675
44. Kostron H, Fiegele T, Akatuna E. Combination of FOSCAN® mediated fluorescence guided resection and photodynamic treatment as new therapeutic concept for malignant brain tumors. *Med Laser Appl.* (2006) 21:285–90. doi: 10.1016/j.mla.2006.08.001
45. McCulloch GA, Forbes IJ, See KL, Cowled PA, Jacka FJ, Ward AD. Phototherapy in malignant brain tumors. *Prog Clin Biol Res.* (1984). 170:709–17.
46. Muller PJ, Wilson BC. Photodynamic therapy of malignant primary brain tumours: clinical effects, post-operative ICP, and light penetration of the brain. *Photochem Photobiol.* (1987) 46:929–35. doi: 10.1111/j.1751-1097.1987.tb04871.x
47. Muller PJ, Wilson BC. Photodynamic therapy for recurrent supratentorial gliomas. *Semin Surg Oncol.* (1995) 11:346–54. doi: 10.1002/ssu.2980110504
48. Muller PJ, Wilson BC. Photodynamic therapy of brain tumors–a work in progress. *Lasers Surg Med.* (2006) 38:384–9. doi: 10.1002/lsm.20338
49. Muller PJ, Wilson BC. Photodynamic therapy of supratentorial gliomas. In: *Proceedings of SPIE 2972, Optical Methods for Tumor Treatment and Detection: Mechanisms and Techniques in Photodynamic Therapy VI, 8 May 1997* (San Jose, CA) (1997). doi: 10.1117/12.273505
50. Muller PJ, Wilson BC, Lilge LD, Yang VX, Hetzel FW, Chen Q, et al. Photofrin photodynamic therapy for malignant brain tumors. *Opt Methods Tumor Treat Detect Mech Tech Photodyn Ther X.* (2001) 4248:34. doi: 10.1117/12.424454
51. Muragaki Y, Akimoto J, Maruyama T, Iseki H, Ikuta S, Nitta M, et al. Phase II clinical study on intraoperative photodynamic therapy with talaporfin sodium and semiconductor laser in patients with malignant brain tumors. *J Neurosurg.* (2013) 119:845–52. doi: 10.3171/2013.7.JNS13415
52. Nitta M, Muragaki Y, Maruyama T, Iseki H, Komori T, Ikuta S, et al. Role of photodynamic therapy using talaporfin sodium and a semiconductor laser in patients with newly diagnosed glioblastoma. *J Neurosurg.* (2018) 1–8. doi: 10.3171/2018.7.JNS18422. [Epub ahead of print].
53. Popovic EA, Kaye AH, Hill JS. Photodynamic therapy of brain tumors. *Semin Surg Oncol.* (1995) 11:335-45. doi: 10.1002/ssu.2980110503
54. Powers SK, Cush SS, Walstad DL, Kwock L. Stereotactic intratumoral photodynamic therapy for recurrent malignant brain tumors. *Neurosurgery.* (1991) 29:688-95; discussion: 695–6. doi: 10.1097/00006123-199111000-00008
55. Rosenthal MA, Kavar B, Uren S, Kaye AH. Promising survival in patients with high-grade gliomas following therapy with a novel boronated porphyrin. *J Clin Neurosci.* (2003) 10:425–7. doi: 10.1016/S0967-5868(03)00062-6
56. Schwartz C, Ruhm A, Tonn J-C, Kreth S, Kreth F-W. Interstital photodynamic therapy of *de-novo* glioblastoma multiforme WHO IV. *Neurooncology.* (2015) 17:v214–20. doi: 10.1093/neuonc/nov235.25
57. Stylli SS, Howes M, MacGregor L, Rajendra P, Kaye AH. Photodynamic therapy of brain tumours: Evaluation of porphyrin uptake versus clinical outcome. *J Clin Neurosci.* (2004) 11:584–96. doi: 10.1016/j.jocn.2004.02.001
58. Stylli SS, Kaye AH, MacGregor L, Howes M, Rajendra P. Photodynamic therapy of high grade glioma–long term survival. *J Clin Neurosci.* (2005) 12:389–98. doi: 10.1016/j.jocn.2005.01.006
59. Vanaclocha V, Sureda M, Azinovic I, Rebollo J, Cañón R, Sapena NS, et al. Photodynamic therapy in the treatment of brain tumours. A feasibility study. *Photodiagnosis Photodyn Ther.* (2015) 12:422–7. doi: 10.1016/j.pdpdt.2015.05.007
60. Akimoto J, Fukami S, Ichikawa M, Mohamed A, Kohno M. Intraoperative photodiagnosis for malignant glioma using photosensitizer talaporfin sodium. *Front Surg.* (2019) 6:12. doi: 10.3389/fsurg.2019.00012
61. Akimoto J, Fukami S, Suda T, Ichikawa M, Haraoka R, Kohno M, et al. First autopsy analysis of the efficacy of intra-operative additional photodynamic therapy for patients with glioblastoma. *Brain Tumor Pathol.* (2019) 36:144–51. doi: 10.1007/s10014-019-00351-0
62. Krishnamurthy S, Powers SK, Witmer P, Brown T. Optimal light dose for interstitial photodynamic therapy in treatment for malignant brain tumors. *Lasers Surg Med.* (2000) 27:224–34. doi: 10.1002/1096-9101(2000)27:3<224::AID-LSM4>3.0.CO;2-#
63. Canti G, Lattuada D, Nicolin A, Taroni P, Valentini G, Cubeddu R. Antitumor immunity induced by photodynamic therapy with aluminum disulfonated phthalocyanines and laser light. *Anticancer Drugs.* (1994) 5:443–7. doi: 10.1097/00001813-199408000-00009
64. Krysko DV, Garg AD, Kaczmarek A, Krysko O, Agostinis P, Vandenabeele P. Immunogenic cell death and DAMPs in cancer therapy. *Nat Rev Cancer.* (2012) 12:860–75. doi: 10.1038/nrc3380
65. Kroemer G, Galluzzi L, Kepp O, Zitvogel L. Immunogenic cell death in cancer therapy. *Annu Rev Immunol.* (2013) 31:51–72. doi: 10.1146/annurev-immunol-032712-100008
66. Castano AP, Mroz P, Hamblin MR. Photodynamic therapy and anti-tumour immunity. *Nat Rev Cancer.* (2006) 6:535–45. doi: 10.1038/nrc1894
67. Garg AD, Nowis D, Golab J, Agostinis P. Photodynamic therapy: illuminating the road from cell death towards anti-tumour immunity. *Apoptosis.* (2010) 15:1050–71. doi: 10.1007/s10495-010-0479-7
68. Yi W, Xu HT, Tian DF, Wu LQ, Zhang SQ, Wang L, et al. Photodynamic therapy mediated by 5-aminolevulinic acid suppresses gliomas growth by decreasing the microvessels. *J Huazhong Univ Sci Technol Med Sci.* (2015) 35:259–64. doi: 10.1007/s11596-015-1421-6
69. Shibata S, Shinozaki N, Suganami A, Ikegami S, Kinoshita Y, Hasegawa R, et al. Photo-immune therapy with liposomally formulated phospholipid-conjugated indocyanine green induces specific antitumor responses with heat shock protein-70 expression in a glioblastoma model. *Oncotarget.* (2019) 10:175–83. doi: 10.18632/oncotarget.26544
70. Ganau L, Prisco L, Ligarotti G, Ambu R, Ganau M. Understanding the pathological basis of neurological diseases through diagnostic platforms based on innovations in biomedical engineering: new concepts and theranostics perspectives. *Medicines.* (2018) 5:22. doi: 10.3390/medicines5010022
71. Ganau M. Tackling gliomas with nanoformulated antineoplastic drugs: suitability of hyaluronic acid nanoparticles. *Clin Transl Oncol.* (2014) 16:220–3. doi: 10.1007/s12094-013-1114-1
72. Ganau M, Syrmos NC, D'Arco F, Ganau L, Chibbaro S, Prisco L, et al. Enhancing contrast agents and radiotracers performance through hyaluronic acid-coating in neuroradiology and nuclear medicine. *Hell J Nucl Med.* (2017) 20:166–8. doi: 10.1967/s002449910558
73. Huang X, Wu J, He M, Hou X, Wang Y, Cai X, et al. Combined cancer chemo-photodynamic and photothermal therapy based on ICG/PDA/TPZ-loaded nanoparticles. *Mol Pharm.* (2019) 16:2172–83. doi: 10.1021/acs.molpharmaceut.9b00119
74. Yang Y, Tu J, Yang D, Raymond JL, Roy RA, Zhang D. Photo- and sono-dynamic therapy: a review of mechanisms and considerations for pharmacological agents used in therapy incorporating light and sound. *Curr Pharm Des.* (2019) 25:401–12. doi: 10.2174/1381612825666190123114107
75. Zhang H, Wang T, Liu H, Ren F, Qiu W, Sun Q, et al. Second near-infrared photodynamic therapy and chemotherapy of orthotopic malignant glioblastoma with ultra-small Cu^{2-}: X Se nanoparticles. *Nanoscale.* (2019) 11:7600–8. doi: 10.1039/c9nr01789e
76. Kruger CA, Abrahamse H. Utilisation of targeted nanoparticle photosensitiser drug delivery systems for the enhancement of photodynamic therapy. *Molecules.* (2018) 23:E2628. doi: 10.3390/molecules23102628
77. Tang XL, Wu J, Lin BL, Cui S, Liu HM, Yu RT, et al. Near-infrared light-activated red-emitting upconverting nanoplatform for T1-weighted magnetic resonance imaging and photodynamic therapy. *Acta Biomater.* (2018) 74:360–73. doi: 10.1016/j.actbio.2018.05.017
78. Tsai YC, Vijayaraghavan P, Chiang WH, Chen HH, Liu TI, Shen MY, et al. Targeted delivery of functionalized upconversion nanoparticles for externally triggered photothermal/photodynamic therapies of brain glioblastoma. *Theranostics.* (2018) 8:1435–48. doi: 10.7150/thno.22482

14

Near-Infrared Fluorescence Imaging and Photodynamic Therapy for Liver Tumors

Masaki Kaibori, Hisashi Kosaka, Kosuke Matsui, Morihiko Ishizaki, Hideyuki Matsushima, Takumi Tsuda, Hidehiko Hishikawa, Tadayoshi Okumura and Mitsugu Sekimoto*

Department of Surgery, Kansai Medical University, Osaka, Japan

***Correspondence:**
Masaki Kaibori
kaibori@hirakata.kmu.ac.jp

Surgery with fluorescence equipment has improved to treat the malignant viscera, including hepatobiliary and pancreatic neoplasms. In both open and minimally invasive surgeries, optical imaging using near-infrared (NIR) fluorescence is used to assess anatomy and function in real time. Here, we review a variety of publications related to clinical applications of NIR fluorescence imaging in liver surgery. We have developed a novel nanoparticle (indocyanine green lactosome) that is biocompatible and can be used for imaging cancer tissues and also as a drug delivery system. To date, stable particles are formed in blood and have an ~10–20 h half-life. Particles labeled with a NIR fluorescent agent have been applied to cancer tissues by the enhanced permeability and retention effect in animals. Furthermore, this article reviews recent developments in photodynamic therapy with NIR fluorescence imaging, which may contribute and accelerate the innovative treatments for liver tumors.

Keywords: near-infrared fluorescence imaging, liver surgery navigation, photodynamic therapy, liver tumors, indocyanine green lactosome

INTRODUCTION

Many imaging tools, including ultrasonography (US), positron emission tomography, computed tomography (CT), and magnetic resonance imaging (MRI), are used and necessary for recent hepatic surgery. However, these imaging treatments can be insufficient for detecting smaller tumors, which require more high spatial resolution than these methods have. For clinical use, real-time cancer detection with fluorescence probes, such as indocyanine green (ICG) and the porphyrin precursor, 5-aminolevulinic acid (5-ALA), is an important topic. ICG and 5-ALA are appropriated as fluorescence imaging (FI) agents, but their application is inadequate for certain diseases. After ICG injection, intraoperative fluorescent angiography has been performed to evaluate the patency of coronary artery bypass grafts (1–4). The use of intraoperative FI can reportedly allow better visualization during hepatobiliary surgery (5). ICG can bind to plasma proteins and affect its fluorescence, emitting near-infrared (NIF) light (6, 7). Proteins in human bile also bind to ICG (8). Prior to hepatic surgery, ICG is administered to measure the ICG retention time (ICGR15; at 15 min), estimating the maximum hepatic volume that can be safely resected (9, 10). Many high-volume hepatectomy centers in Japan are beginning to use ICG FI for intraoperative navigation, such as visualizing small liver tumors, cholangiography, and imaging hepatic segments.

Remarkable advances in photodynamic therapy (PDT) for liver tumors have also been reported. Development of molecular probes based on nanoparticles, polymer micelles that use the characteristics of neovascularization, is currently underway. By including various signaling agents (e.g., radioisotopes, fluorescent agents, magnetic substances) in the nanoparticles, diagnosis can be made by molecular imaging of new vascular tissue. If a therapeutic agent is included, this method may also provide a drug delivery system. Theranostics (a fusion of "diagnostics" and "therapy") can be realized (11) and may lead to ultra-early cancer diagnosis and treatment.

We used the enhanced permeability and retention characteristics of neovascularization (12), which are prominent in inflammatory diseases such as rheumatoid arthritis, ischemic diseases such as arteriosclerosis, and initial cancer growth. Here, we review features of NIF FI and photodynamic therapy for liver tumors.

NEAR-INFRARED FLUORESCENCE IMAGING DURING LIVER SURGERY NAVIGATION

Tumor Visualization

Gotoh et al. (13) and Ishizawa et al. (14) reported the novel technics for liver cancers with ICG fluorescence image (FI) navigation, which is based on the capacity of hepatocellular carcinoma (HCC) to accumulate ICG. ICG was injected several days before surgery. ICG FI found the HCC tumors that were completely removed, with negative margins, using the FI as a guide. It is essential to detect small HCCs for curative resection and improvement of patient outcomes. Further strong definition between tumor and non-tumor cells is essential for obtaining safe surgical margins. The authors showed that FI following pre-operative intravenous injection of ICG confirmed HCCs and colorectal liver metastases (CRLM) on cut surfaces of resected specimens in 37 patients with HCC and 12 with CRLM (14). There were three types of fluorescence patterns in tumors: (i) total, all tumor tissue showed uniform fluorescence; (ii) partial, some showed fluorescence; and (iii) rim, the surrounding liver parenchyma except cancer tissues showed fluorescence. Total-type tumors contained all well-differentiated HCCs, while rim-type tumors contained poorly differentiated HCCs and CRLM. In addition to detecting the small HCCs, ICG-FI was reportedly useful for the detection of CRLM (15, 16), peritoneal dissemination (17, 18), and lymph node metastasis from HCC (19).

The mechanism of ICG-FI for HCC has been revealed by gene expression and histochemical staining analyses (20). The expression of portal uptake transporters of ICG, which are organic anion-transporting polypeptide-8 and Na^+/taurocholate cotransporting polypeptide (21), were well-maintained in differentiated HCC tissues. However, functional biliary excretion was disordered, which was followed by ICG retention in cancerous tissues at the time of surgery. In contrast, portal uptake transporters were downregulated in poorly differentiated HCCs and biliary excretion of ICG by surrounding non-cancerous hepatic parenchyma was disordered, resulting in rim-type fluorescence. In CRLM, the rim-type fluorescence signal is reportedly found by immature hepatocytes with reduced bile excretion (22).

We reported that ICG FI for HCC is effective for both assessing tumor differentiation and detecting fibrosis in non-cancerous liver parenchyma (23). We evaluated ICG FI of resected specimens from 190 HCC patients. This system (fluorescence image; using Clairvivo OPT, Shimadzu, Kyoto, Japan) consisted of a horizontal sample table, excitation light sources, charge-coupled device camera, camera lens, optical filter, and white laser-emitting diode light sources that illuminated the sample from four angles. They were classified into two groups: high cancerous [HC] and high surrounding [HS] groups, according to FI (**Figure 1**). These groups were further sub-classified into whole and partial types (**Figures 1A,B**), and whole and ring types (**Figures 1C,D**), respectively. The patients in the HC group had a higher prevalence of esophageal or gastric varices, and worse liver function than those in the HS group. The HC group also had a higher percentage of limited resection cases as compared with the HS group. Cirrhotic liver histology was more common in the HC group than in the HS group. In multivariate analysis, HC status was a predictive factor for cirrhosis in HCC patients. In the HC group, a higher number of well-differentiated HCC cases was seen in the partial-type subgroup [23/48 (48%), **Figure 1A**] than in the whole-type subgroup [7/68 (10%), **Figure 1B**]. In the HS group, a higher number of poorly differentiated HCC cases was seen in the ring-type subgroup [6/37 (16%), **Figure 1C**] than in the whole-type subgroup [0/37 (0%), **Figure 1D**]. Tumor differentiation and fibrosis in non-cancerous liver parenchyma could affect ICG FI in HCC. ICG FI may be a good indicator of fibrosis stage.

Intraoperative ICG-FI in hepatic tumors is useful for identifying subcapsular lesions for removal during laparoscopic hepatectomy, in which visual inspection and palpation are limited compared with open surgery (24). This technique has potential drawbacks, however, including a relatively high false-positive rate (14, 20). Lesions that are newly detected by ICG-FI should be resected only when other modalities, such as palpation and intraoperative US, identify them as tumors to be removed. The incidence of false positives can be reduced by not administering ICG on the day before surgery, especially in patients with decreased liver function due to cirrhosis or pre-operative chemotherapy (14). Detecting liver tumors through ICG FI involves visualizing cholestasis inside or around liver cancer because ICG FI does not truly image cancer cells. When new fluorescent regions are visualized during surgery, palpation and US for liver tumors should be performed. Additional resection should be considered if these extra methods suggest malignancies. As ICG FI is also limited in its observation depth

---

Abbreviations: 5-ALA, 5-aminolevulinic acid; CLRM, colorectal liver metastasis; CT, computed tomography; FI, fluorescence imaging; HC, high cancerous (fluorescence in cancerous tissue); HS, high surrounding (fluorescence in surrounding tissue); ICG, indocyanine green; ICG-L, ICG-lactosome; ICGR15, ICG retention rate at 15 min; MRI, magnetic resonance imaging; NIR, near-infrared; PDT, photodynamic therapy; US, ultrasonography.

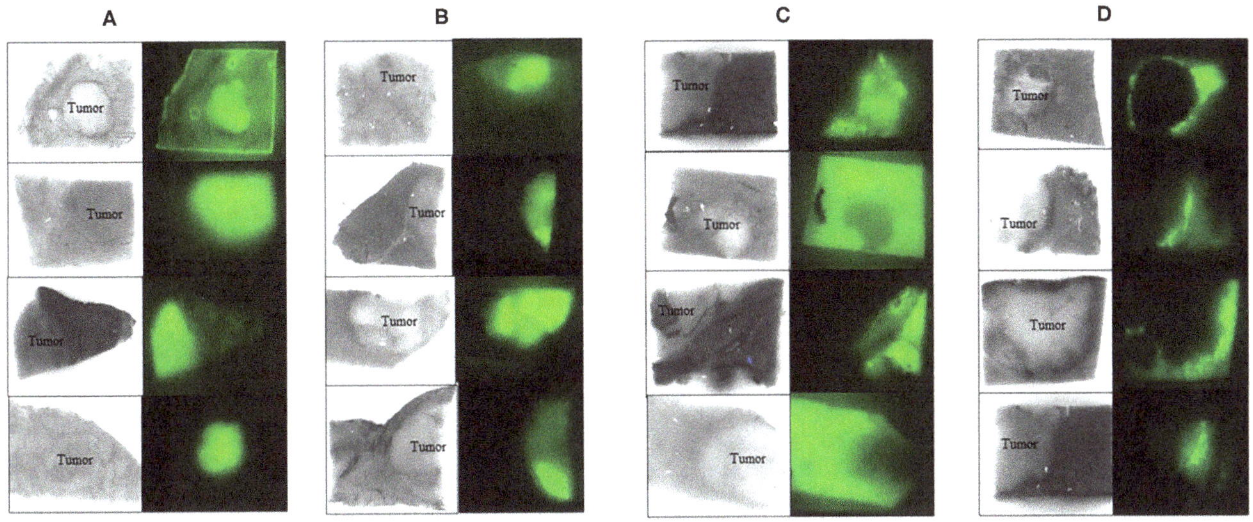

FIGURE 1 | ICG fluorescence image in cancerous liver tissue. Whole **(A)** and partial **(B)** fluorescence image (FI) in cancer. Whole **(C)** and ring **(D)** FI in the surrounding non-cancerous liver tissue. ICG FI in resected liver specimens could confirm HCC. FI; filter excitation: 785 nm, emission: 845 nm, using Clairvivo OPT, Shimadzu, Kyoto, Japan.

(up to about 8 mm), intraoperative US is required to confirm findings that lie deeper in the liver.

By using ICG and 5-ALA FI, the latent, superficial, and small liver tumors were detected and treated pre-operatively and/or intraoperatively, as we reported previously (25). 5-ALA is a natural precursor of heme, and is accumulated and converted to protoporphyrin IX, which emits red fluorescence in cancer cells (26). Thus, 5-ALA is used as a photosensitizer in photodynamic diagnostics for neurosurgery and urology (27–30). Imaging with ICG or 5-ALA detected small latent liver tumors (**Figure 2**) and peritoneal dissemination (**Figure 3**). We conducted a study with 48 patients who had primary liver tumors within 5 mm of the liver surface. With ICG, the sensitivity, specificity, and accuracy for detecting the pre-operatively identified primary tumors were 96, 50, and 94%, respectively. Twelve latent, small tumors were newly detected on the liver surface using ICG. Five of these tumors were determined to be carcinomas. With 5-ALA, the sensitivity, specificity, and accuracy for detecting the primary tumors were 57, 100, and 58%, respectively. Five latent, small tumors were newly detected using 5-ALA; all were carcinomas. Overall, five new tumors were detected by both ICG and 5-ALA FI: two were HCCs and three were metastases of colorectal cancer. The sensitivity and specificity of ICG FI for primary tumor detection were relatively high and low, respectively, but the opposite was true for 5-ALA imaging. In another study, Inoue et al. reported that there was 100% sensitivity for detecting HCC, 86% for colorectal liver metastases, and 100% for liver tumors of various etiologies. 5-ALA showed an overall sensitivity of 93% for detection in their experience with a series of 70 patients who underwent hepatic resection (31). However, Boogerd et al. reported that their study was designed to compare FI and conventional imaging modalities for laparoscopic detection of both primary and metastatic tumors in the liver (32). Sensitivity for various modalities was 80% (CT), 84% (MRI), 62% (inspection), 86% (laparoscopic ultrasonography), and 92% (ICG-FI). All 26 malignancies that were examined could be detected by combining laparoscopic ultrasonography and ICG-FI (100% sensitivity). To the best of our knowledge, our study is the first to detect liver tumors using both ICG and 5-ALA FI. FI using both ICG and 5-ALA may provide greater specificity in detecting surface-invisible liver tumors than using ICG FI alone. Both imaging methods may help improve treatment strategies for patients with liver tumors.

Cholangiography

Cholangiography is used to visualize the biliary tract intraoperatively to avoid damage to the bile ducts (33). Routine cholangiography is recommended for cholecystectomy (34, 35). A multicenter randomized controlled trial confirmed the superiority of extrahepatic bile-duct identification using ICG fluorescent cholangiography in laparoscopic cholecystectomy (36). Because ICG binds to human bile proteins, such as albumin and lipoproteins (8), intra-bile-duct injection of ICG enables FI of the biliary tract (37). The fluorescent intensity of ICG bound to these proteins was ∼0.25 mg/mL and correlates with its concentration. However, it was found to decrease at high concentrations from the absorption of near-infrared light by the ICG (5). Therefore, a diluted ICG solution (∼0.025 mg/mL) should be injected into the bile duct to obtain a clear fluorescent image of the bile duct (31). ICG was detected in the bile duct 20 min after injection and maintained for up to 2 h in patients who underwent laparoscopic cholecystectomy (38, 39). In donor hepatectomy and laparoscopic hepatectomy, ICG cholangiography has been reported (40, 41). Recently, Hong et al. reported that ICG fluorescent cholangiography was successful in delineating the biliary system around the

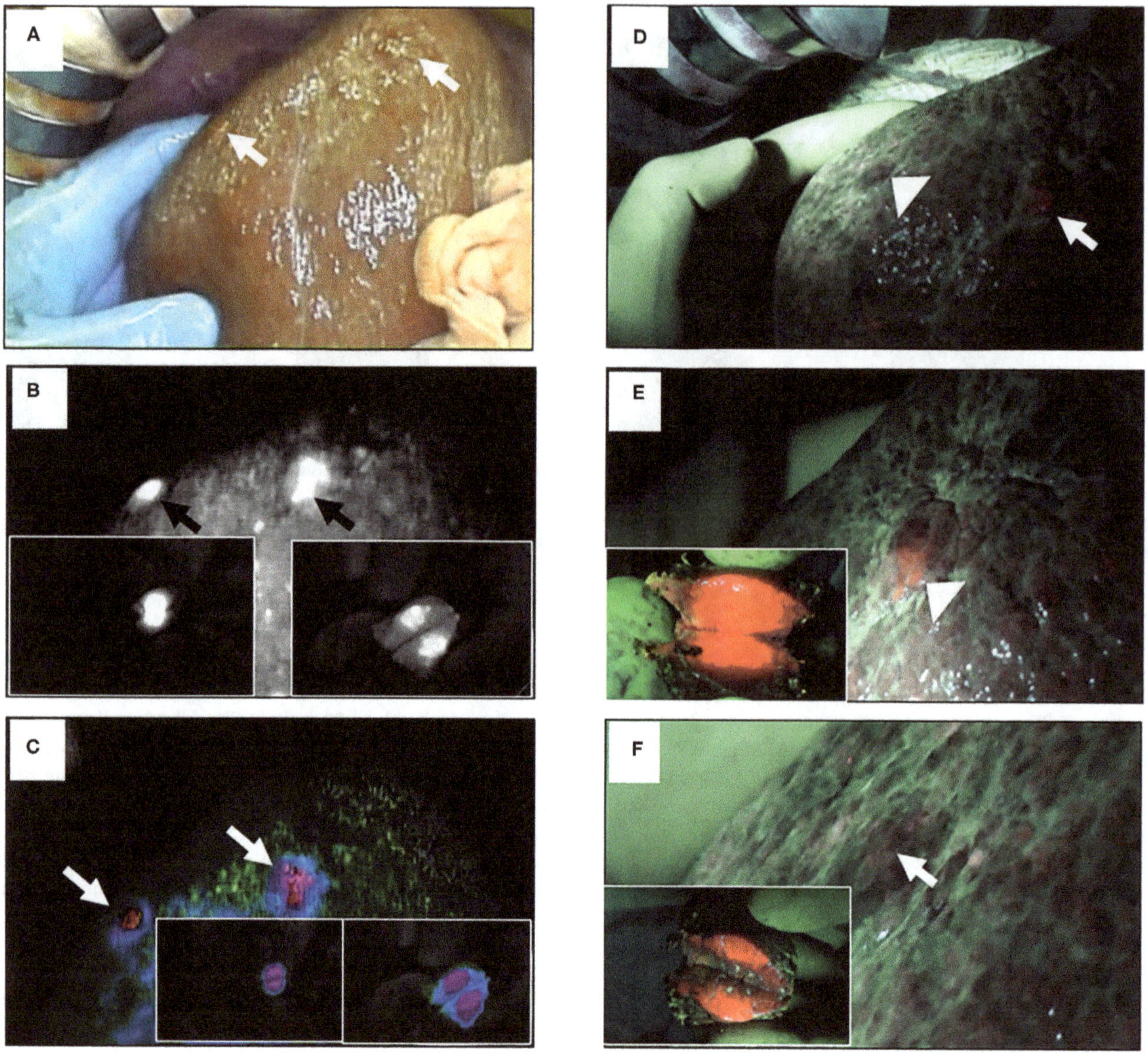

FIGURE 2 | ICG and 5-ALA fluorescence images of superficial malignant liver tumors. **(A)** Two superficial malignant liver tumors with serosa (arrows); conventional white light. **(B)** ICG FI of the same tumors (arrows); insets show the incised lesions. **(C)** ICG FI of the same tumors using color mode (arrows). **(D)** The same tumors (arrowhead and arrow); blue light. **(E)** 5-ALA FI of the same tumors (arrowhead); inset shows the incised lesion. **(F)** 5-ALA FI of the other tumor (arrow); inset shows incised lesion.

hilar plate and in determining optimal bile duct division points during laparoscopic donor hepatectomy in their ten patients. They suggest that this technique may be particularly useful in laparoscopic surgery, during which intraoperative cholangiography and probing through the divided bile duct opening or cystic duct opening is relatively difficult (42). ICG fluorescent cholangiography is also useful for real-time detection of bile leaks during hepatectomy (43, 44).

We have performed a randomized controlled trial with ICG fluorescence cholangiography in 102 patients who underwent hepatic resection without biliary reconstruction. The patients were divided into two groups: with or without ICG fluorescence cholangiography. In the control group, five patients developed post-operative bile leakage, but in the ICG cholangiography group, no bile leakage was observed in any patient (10 vs. 0%, $P = 0.019$; **Figure 4**) (44). Thus, ICG cholangiography may help prevent bile leakage. ICG cholangiography also prevented bile leakage and bile duct stenosis in bile duct anastomosis in living-donor liver transplantation (42, 45).

Imaging of Hepatic Segments

Fusion ICG FI, which displays both fluorescence images and macroscopic views on a single screen, provides clear demarcation lines for more accurate parenchymal dissection (46). Nishino et al. showed that the projection mapping with ICG fluorescence detected anatomical landmarks for parenchymal dissection in

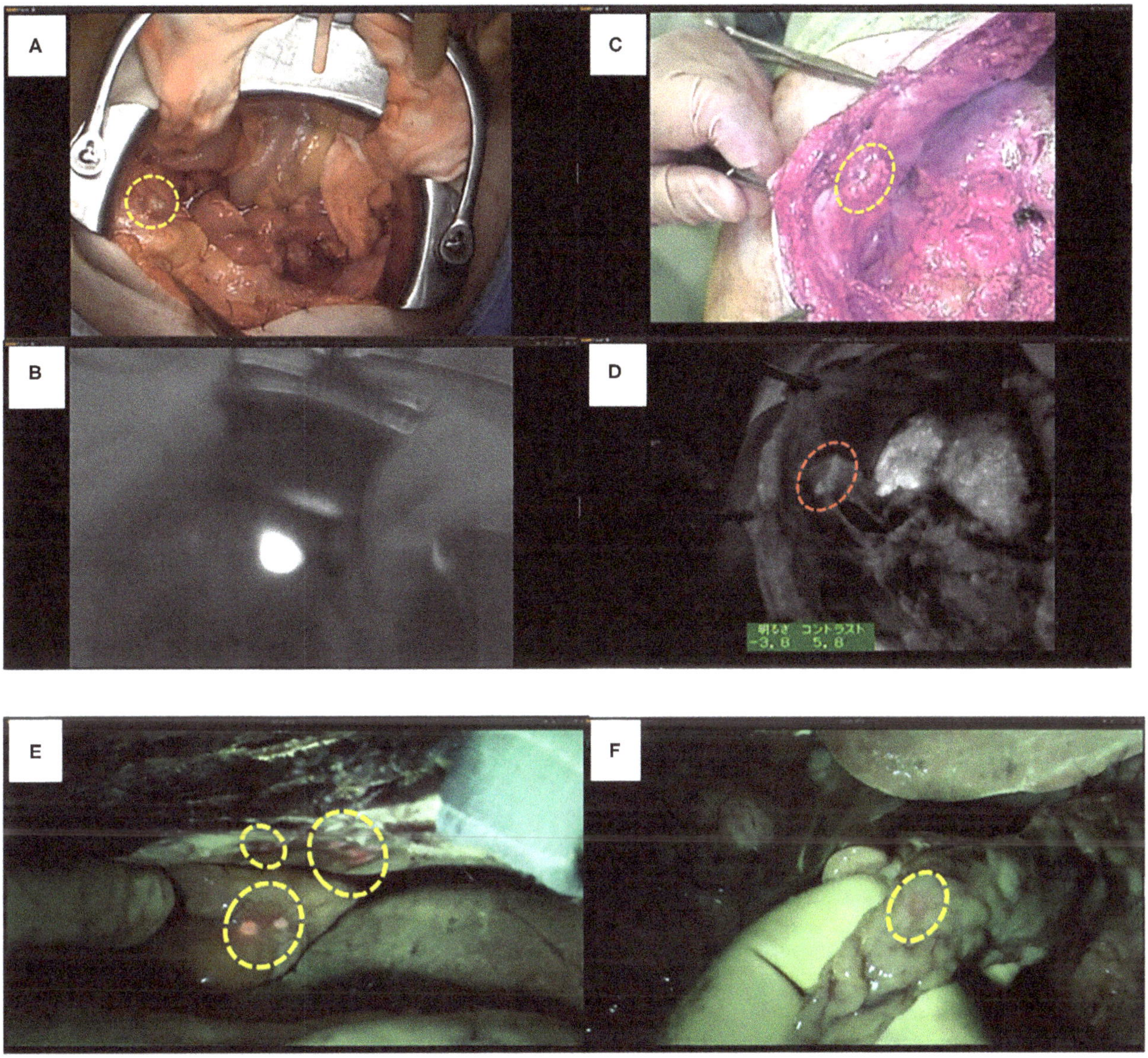

FIGURE 3 | ICG and 5-ALA fluorescence images of metastases through HCC. **(A)** Ovarian and peritoneal metastases (yellow circle); conventional white light. **(B)** ICG FI of peritoneal metastasis. **(C)** Peritoneal metastasis (yellow circle); conventional white light. **(D)** ICG FI of peritoneal metastasis (red circle). **(E)** 5-ALA FI of peritoneal and colon metastases of intrahepatic cholangiocellular carcinoma (yellow circles). **(F)** 5-ALA FI of omental metastasis (yellow circle).

clinical utility (47). Makuuchi et al. first reported anatomical liver resection (48), injecting indigo-carmine into the portal vein, which was followed by some studies of anatomical liver resection using non-anatomical liver resection (49–52). Aoki et al. obtained fluorescence images of the liver surfaces using an infrared camera, after portal vein branches in the HCC-bearing hepatic segment were punctured by intraoperative US (53, 54). They reported that the ICG-staining technique showed the sub-segments and segments in 90% (73/81) of patients, and that there were no differences in detection rates for liver segment boundaries between non-cirrhotic and cirrhotic livers.

Laparoscopic liver resection for HCC was established and became a standard treatment for minor liver resection (55). It is also performed in specialized centers for laparoscopic liver surgery (56). Ishizawa et al. used the ICG staining technique for laparoscopic anatomical resection (57). Ueno et al. used laparoscopic liver segmentation by interventional radiology technique (58). Although the ICG FI method is a relatively simple method, in the positive staining method when there are multiple dominant portal vein branches or when it is difficult to puncture a thin vessel of 2 mm or less, it is not possible to accurately visualize the hepatic segments. In the negative staining method, prior treatment of the dominant portal vein branch is required, but it is necessary to carefully perform the peeling operation while paying sufficient attention to vascular and bile duct injury (59). Additionally, unlike indigo-carmine which disappears in a

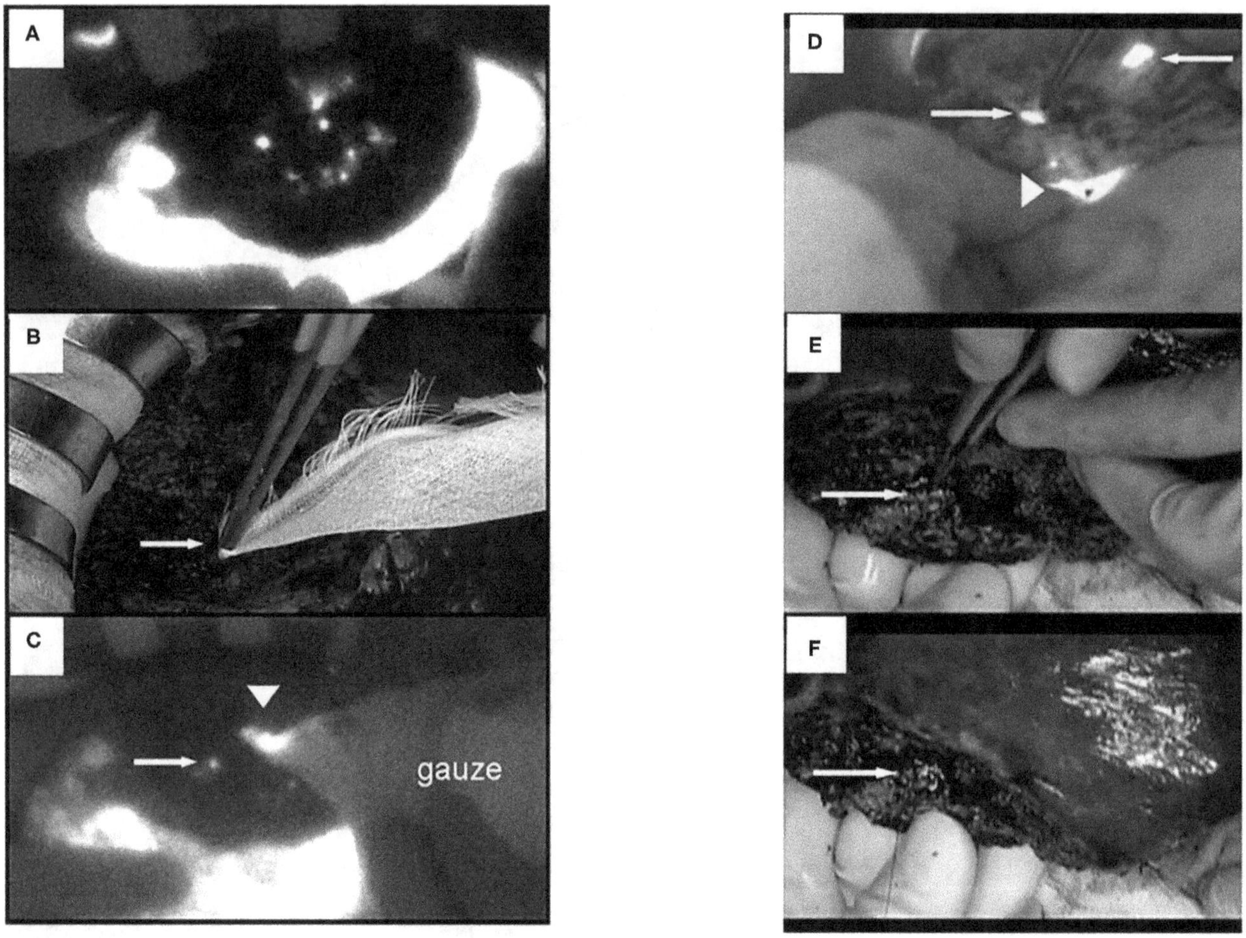

FIGURE 4 | ICG fluorescent images by the photodynamic eye system. **(A)** White spots (possible bile leakages) on cut liver surface. **(B)** Minor leak from duct is compressed with gauze, which is not visible to the surgeons (arrow). **(C)** ICG FI after gauze application reveals minor leakage on the cut liver surface (arrow); fluorescence is also detected through the gauze (arrowhead). **(D)** FI identified two fluorescing ducts on the cut liver surface (arrows). The upper bile duct is intact (upper arrow). Arrowhead: common bile duct. **(E)** The lower fluorescing lesion corresponds to a partly closed bile duct stump (arrow). **(F)** The bile duct stump was repaired (arrow, z-sutures using 6-0 non-absorbable thread).

short time, the fluorescent region from ICG is maintained for a long time, so it is difficult to correct the stained region when it is incorrect. To obtain the desired accurate ICG FI during the operation, it is important to perform sufficient simulation before surgery and carefully plan the appropriate ICG FI method for each case.

ICG FI can apparently be safe and reliable for hepatectomy at many facilities and is expected to help improve liver cancer treatment, though its usefulness should be verified in a large-scale, multicenter study.

PHOTODYNAMIC THERAPY FOR LIVER TUMORS

Indocyanine Green-Lactosome Has Anti-neoplastic Effects for HCC

We have developed a macromolecular micelle (ICG-lactosome, ICG-L) formed by self-assembly of a novel amphipathic polydepsipeptide (containing hydrophilic and hydrophobic parts). ICG-L does not accumulate very much in internal organs because of the stealth effect, but it selectively accumulates in cancer tissues with higher concentration because of the enhanced permeability and retention effect (60). In polydepsipeptide, polysarcosine constitutes the hydrophilic portion, comprises amino acids found in living tissue, and has hydrophilicity equal to or greater than that of polyethylene glycol. It is biodegradable and is widely used in industrial and medical materials. In contrast, polylactic acid is the hydrophobic portion, also biodegradable and used as a medical material, frequently in bone resorbable applications. Compared with other conventional biocompatible nanoparticles, ICG-L is easy to use in designed products. Its particle sizes can be adjusted and modified with biomaterials such as peptides; it may work as a carrier for "theranostic" diagnostic agents and pharmaceuticals (61).

For the evaluation of PDT efficacy *in vitro,* HuH-7 (human HCC cell line) cells were treated with ICG-L or ICG, followed by PDT. The cell viabilities were then measured. Laser irradiation

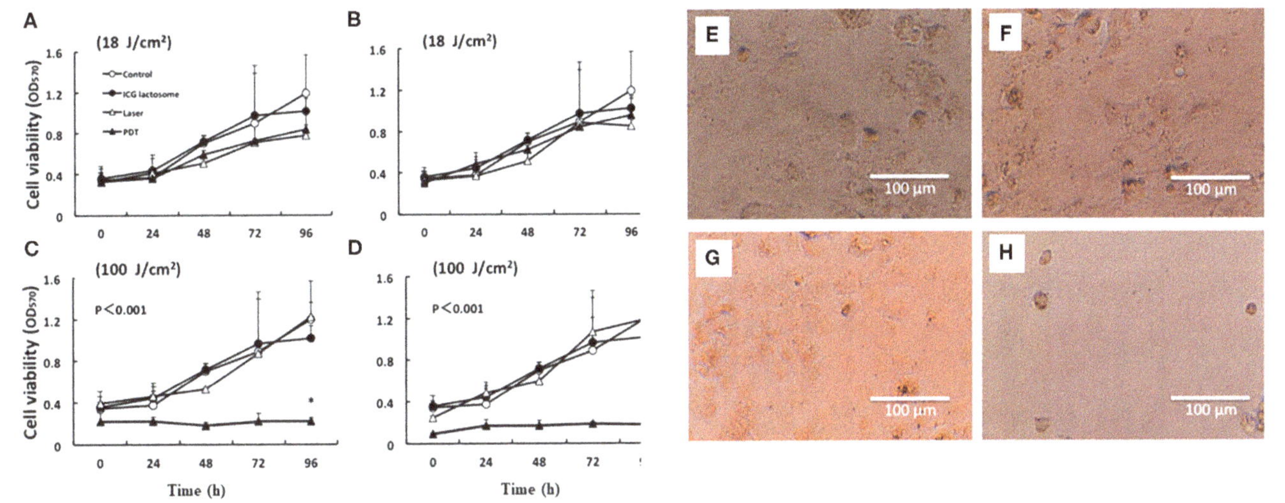

FIGURE 5 | *In vitro* PDT on cell viability and morphological changes in ICG lactosome-treated HuH-7 cells. Cells were divided into four groups: control, ICG-L, laser, and PDT (ICG-L + laser). The laser and PDT groups were irradiated with **(A)** 18 J/cm^2 (190 mW/cm^2 and 95 s), **(B)** 18 J/cm^2 (340 mW/cm^2 and 55 s), **(C)** 100 J/cm^2 (190 mW/cm^2 and 525 s), and **(D)** 100 J/cm^2 (340 mW/cm^2 and 300 s). Cell viability (OD570) was measured by the MTT assay ($n = 4$ /time/group; $^*P < 0.001$ for ICG-L vs. other groups). Morphological changes (phase-contrast microscope at 96 h). **(E)** Control, **(F)** ICG-L, **(G)** laser [100 J/cm^2 (340 mW/cm^2 and 300 s)], and **(H)** PDT (ICG-L + laser). https://doi.org/10.1371/journal.pone.0183527.g001.g002.

revealed that HuH-7 cells with ICG-L showed toxic effects, but the cells with ICG alone did not (**Figure 5**).

For NIF *in vivo*, BALB/c nude mice were subcutaneously treated with HuH-7 cells and then intravenously with ICG-L or ICG. These transplanted animals were treated with PDT and the antineoplastic effects were analyzed. Indeed, NIF imaging revealed that the tumor-area fluorescence in ICG-L-treated animals was higher than that of contralateral regions at 24 h after injection and thereafter (**Figures 6B,D**), although there was no difference between those in the tumor-area fluorescence in ICG-treated animals (**Figures 6A,C**). PDT had continuous phototoxic effects in the ICG-L group (**Figure 7A**). By laser irradiation, the median temperature in the tumor areas increased from 34 to 47.7°C and from 34.5 to 51.7°C at 0–200 s in the ICG-L and ICG groups, respectively (**Figure 6E**), where the median temperature in the ICG-L group was higher than that in the ICG group.

In the former, there was substantial apoptosis with a higher apoptotic index in the ICG-L group than in the ICG group (**Figures 7B–D**). The mechanisms involved in tumor suppression by PDT in the ICG-L group were presumably caused by singlet oxygen and ICG degradation products generated by a photochemical reaction (62). Singlet oxygen can be generated as ICG is exposed to near-infrared excitation light. The decomposition products that can be produced by ICG can further decrease cell viability (63). These products may lead to tumor cell apoptosis. PDT with ICG-L increased the tumor suppression by the heat generated from a photothermal reaction. During *in vivo* analysis of PDT with ICG-L, the temperature increased (50°C and above) relative to ICG alone, suggesting that the heat may be sufficient to damage tumor growth. In addition, optimization of ICG-L dosage and laser irradiation fluence are also necessary to prevent future tumor growth. The temperature increase is a major factor in the antitumor effect obtained in our study because PDT using ICG reportedly has a thermal effect (64). The temperature increase by PDT likely depends on various photosensitizers, including ICG. PDT using ICG can facilitate a temperature increase with antitumor effects, which supports the usefulness of ICG-L.

Our results demonstrated that tumor cells transplanted in BALB/c nude mice incorporated ICG-L and that PDT had antineoplastic effects. NIF imaging and PDT with ICG-L may be useful diagnostic and/or therapeutic strategies for HCC.

There are some limitations to ICG FI. First, ICG-L may possibly accumulate in both malignant and benign tumors, causing excessive influence in undesired areas by PDT. There is little knowledge regarding angiogenesis in benign tumors compared with in malignant tumors. Because benign tumors generally have slower growth rates and do not infiltrate into other tissues compared with malignant tumors, we believe it would be difficult to integrate ICG-L into benign tumors.

In clinical situations, Ishizawa et al. reported that ICG FI can be used to observe HCC lesions based on their tumorous fluorescence. This is because the portal uptake of ICG is preserved in well- or moderately differentiated cancer tissues, despite the lack of biliary extraction and to delineate poorly differentiated HCC as rim-fluorescing lesions because of biliary excretion disorders in the surrounding non-cancerous liver tissues that are compressed by the tumor (14).

The second limitation is that it is not clear how the PDT effect of ICG-L depends on the tumor differentiation, tumor size, and depth from the liver surface. We have only investigated the Huh-7 cell line as well-differentiated HCC. ICG-L (excitation

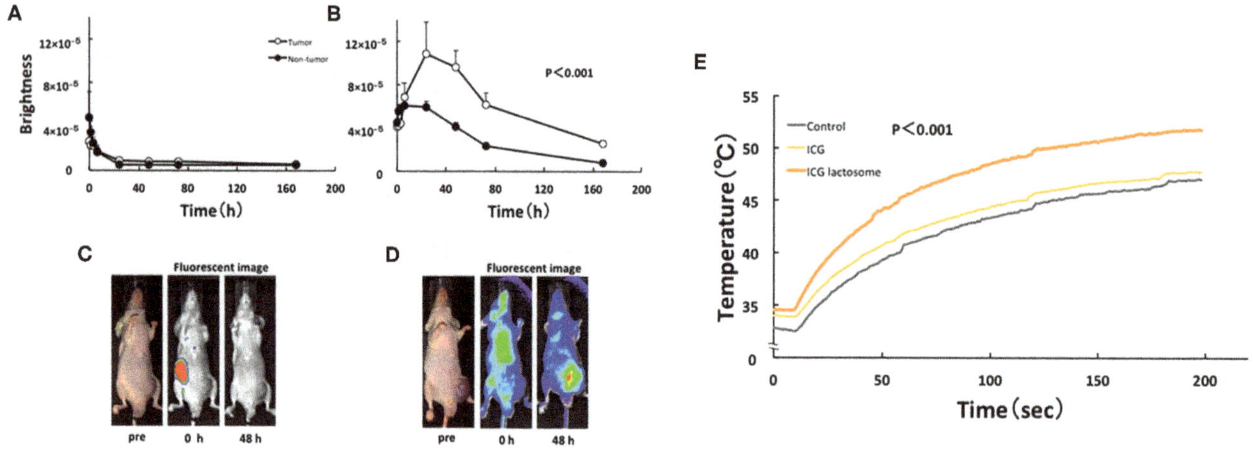

FIGURE 6 | *In vivo* fluorescence imaging in ICG lactosome-treated mice with subcutaneous tumors. After injection of ICG **(A,C)** or ICG-L **(B,D)** in mice, the brightness of the tumor (open circles) and non-tumor (contralateral inguinal, closed circles) areas was measured (IVIS system). $P < 0.001$ between the tumor and non-tumor regions in the ICG-L group; $n = 5$/group. **(E)** Effect of laser irradiation on tumor temperature. At 48 h after ICG (yellow), ICG-L (brown) or no injection (control, dark) in the tumor implanted-mice, laser irradiation (500 mW/cm^2 and 200 s, 100 J/cm^2) was initiated, and the temperatures were measured ($P < 0.001$ for ICG vs. ICG-L; $n = 6$/group). https://doi.org/10.1371/journal.pone.0183527.g004,g006.

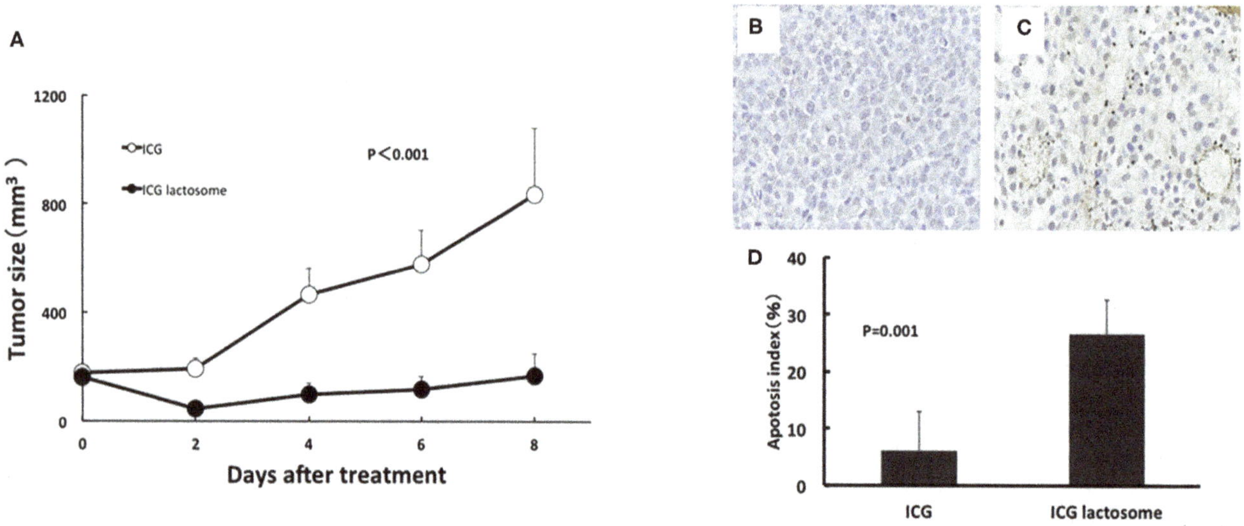

FIGURE 7 | *In vivo* PDT on tumor growth in ICG lactosome-treated mice with subcutaneous tumors. **(A)** At 48 h after ICG (open circles) or ICG-L (closed circles) injection in mice, laser irradiation (500 mW/cm^2 and 200 s, 100 J/cm^2) was carried out, and tumor volumes were measured. ($P < 0.001$ for ICG vs. ICG-L; $n = 6$/group.) **(B–D)** Effect of PDT on apoptosis of tumors. Tumors were resected at 24 h after irradiation (500 mW/cm^2 and 200 s, 100 J/cm^2) in the ICG **(B)** and ICG-L **(C)** groups and examined for apoptosis (TUNEL staining). **(D)** Apoptotic indexes in the ICG-treated and ICG L-treated groups ($P = 0.001$ for ICG vs. ICG-L; $n = 5$/group.) https://doi.org/10.1371/journal.pone.0183527.g005,g007.

wavelength: 774 nm, fluorescence wavelength: 805 nm) reaches a depth of 10–20 mm subcutaneously in the near infrared region (700–100 nm) (60, 61). Future studies are needed on the PDT effect of ICG-L on the tumor diameter and degree of HCC differentiation.

Funayama et al. (65–67) reported that PDF with ICG-L delayed the development of paralysis in rats with spinal metastases. Tsujimoto et al. (68, 69) reported that PDF with ICG-L inhibited the growth of metastases. Recently, we found an antitumor effect of PT with ICG-L on gallbladder cancer in xenograft tumors (70). In other experiments, Kaneko et al. (71, 72) reported using PDT with ICG and an NIR laser for HCC. HuH-7 cells were transplanted subcutaneously into BALB/c-*nu/nu* mice and ICG was administered 24 h before NIR irradiation (days 1 and 7). Repeated NIR increased the cell toxicity of ICG-NIR therapy. They also found that ICG-NIR therapy increased apoptosis in tumor cells through a photothermal effect and oxidative stress.

CONCLUSIONS

ICG FI has effects on fibrosis detection and tumor differentiation measurement in non-cancerous liver parenchyma in HCC. ICG FI can be a good indicator of fibrosis stage and apparently detect smaller liver tumors. FI with 5-ALA provided higher specificity in detecting surface-invisible liver tumors as compared with FI with ICG. Usage of both ICG and 5-ALA imaging can potentially improve treatment strategies for patients with liver tumors. Simply put, FI offers the benefits of a higher-resolution intraoperative navigation tool for liver cancer. ICG-L is useful as a diagnostic and therapeutic agent for HCC.

PDT using ICG-L, which is repeatedly performed, can be used in endoscopic or laparoscopic therapy for small HCC tumors. To develop PDT with FI in clinical applications, we will examine optimal drug dosages, irradiation conditions, and the effects of treatment on other carcinomas.

AUTHOR CONTRIBUTIONS

MK drafted and wrote the manuscript. HM, MI, HK, KM, TT, HH, TO, and MS participated in the study design and helped draft the manuscript. All authors contributed to the interpretation of the findings, read, and approved the final manuscript.

REFERENCES

1. Rubens FD, Ruel M, Fremes SE. A new and simplified method for coronary and graft imaging during CABG. *Heart Surg Forum*. (2002) 5:141–4.
2. Taggart DP, Choudhary B, Anastasiadis K, Abu-Omar Y, Balacumaraswani L, Pigott DW. Preliminary experience with a novel intraoperative fluorescence imaging technique to evaluate the patency of bypass grafts in total arterial revascularization. *Ann Thorac Surg*. (2003) 75:870–3. doi: 10.1016/S0003-4975(02)04669-6
3. Reuthebuch O, Haussler A, Genoni M, Tavakoli R, Odavic D, Kadner A, et al. Intraoperative quality assessment in off-pump coronary artery bypass grafting. *Chest*. (2004) 125:418–24. doi: 10.1378/chest.125.2.418
4. Balacumaraswani L, Abu-Omar Y, Choudhary B, Pigott D, Taggart DP. A comparison of transit-time flowmetry and intraoperative fluorescence imaging for assessing coronary artery bypass graft patency. *J Thorac Cardiovasc Surg*. (2005) 130:315–20. doi: 10.1016/j.jtcvs.2004.11.033
5. Mitsuhashi N, Kimura F, Shimizu H, Imamaki M, Yoshidome H, Ohtsuka M, et al. Usefulness of intraoperative fluorescence imaging to evaluate local anatomy in hepatobiliary surgery. *J Hepatobiliary Pancreat Surg*. (2008) 15:508–14. doi: 10.1007/s00534-007-1307-5
6. Landsman ML, Kwant G, Mook GA, Zijlstra WG. Light-absorbing properties, stability, and spectral stabilization of indocyanine green. *J Appl Physiol*. (1976) 40:575–83. doi: 10.1152/jappl.1976.40.4.575
7. Mordon S, Devoisselle JM, Soulie-Begu S, Desmettre T. Indocyanine green: physicochemical factors affecting its fluorescence *in vivo*. *Microvasc Res*. (1998) 55:146–52. doi: 10.1006/mvre.1998.2068
8. Mulllock BM, Shaw LJ, Fitzharris B, Peppard J, Hamilton MJ, Simpson MT, et al. Sources of proteins in human bile. *Gut*. (1985) 26:500–9. doi: 10.1136/gut.26.5.500
9. Makuuchi M, Kosuge T, Takayama T, Yamazaki S, Kakazu T, Miyagawa S, et al. Surgery for small liver cancers. *Semin Surg Oncol*. (1993) 9:298–304. doi: 10.1002/ssu.2980090404
10. Ishizawa T, Hasegawa K, Aoki T, Takahashi M, Inoue Y, Sano K, et al. Neither multiple tumors nor portal hypertension are surgical contraindications for hepatocellular carcinoma. *Gastroenterology*. (2008) 134:1908–16. doi: 10.1053/j.gastro.2008.02.091
11. Xie J, Lee S, Chen X. Nanoparticle-based theranostic agents. *Adv Drug Deliv Rev*. (2010) 62:1064–79. doi: 10.1016/j.addr.2010.07.009
12. Matsumura Y, Maeda H. A new concept for macromolecular therapeutics in cancer chemotherapy: mechanism of tumoritropic accumulation of proteins and the antitumor agent smancs. *Cancer Res*. (1986) 46:6387–92.
13. Gotoh K, Yamada T, Ishikawa O, Takahashi H, Eguchi H, Yano M, et al. A novel image-guided surgery of hepatocellular carcinoma by indocyanine green fluorescence imaging navigation. *J Surg Oncol*. (2009) 100:75–9. doi: 10.1002/jso.21272
14. Ishizawa T, Fukushima N, Shibahara J, Masuda K, Tamura S, Aoki T, et al. Real-time identification of liver cancers by using indocyanine green fluorescent imaging. *Cancer*. (2009) 115:2491–504. doi: 10.1002/cncr.24291
15. Peloso A, Franchi E, Canepa MC, Barbieri L, Briani L, Ferrario J, et al. Combined use of intraoperative ultrasound and indocyanine green fluorescence imaging to detect liver metastases from colorectal cancer. *HPB (Oxford)*. (2013) 15:928–34. doi: 10.1111/hpb.12057
16. Terasawa M, Ishizawa T, Mise Y, Inoue Y, Ito H, Takahashi Y, et al. Applications of fusion-fluorescence imaging using indocyanine green in laparoscopic hepatectomy. *Surg Endosc*. (2017) 31:5111–8. doi: 10.1007/s00464-017-5576-z
17. Miyazaki Y, Kurata M, Oshiro Y, Shimomura O, Takahashi K, Oda T, et al. Indocyanine green fluorescence-navigated laparoscopic metastasectomy for peritoneal metastasis of hepatocellular carcinoma: a case report. *Surg Case Rep*. (2018) 4:130. doi: 10.1186/s40792-018-0537-x
18. Nakamura M, Hayami S, Ueno M, Kawai M, Miyamoto A, Suzaki N, et al. Detection of needle tract implantation and peritoneal seeding after radiofrequency ablation using intraoperative near-infrared fluorescence system for recurrent hepatocellular carcinoma: a case report. *Surg Case Rep*. (2018) 4:76. doi: 10.1186/s40792-018-0485-5
19. Satou S, Ishizawa T, Masuda K, Kaneko J, Aoki T, Sakamoto Y, et al. Indocyanine green fluorescent imaging for detecting extrahepatic metastasis of hepatocellular carcinoma. *J Gastroenterol*. (2013) 48:1136–43. doi: 10.1007/s00535-012-0709-6
20. Ishizawa T, Masuda K, Urano Y, Kawaguchi Y, Satou S, Kaneko J, et al. Mechanistic background and clinical applications of indocyanine green fluorescence imaging of hepatocellular carcinoma. *Ann Surg Oncol*. (2014) 21:440–8. doi: 10.1245/s10434-013-3360-4
21. de Graaf W, Häusler S, Heger M, van Ginhoven TM, van Cappellen G, Bennink RJ, et al. Transporters involved in the hepatic uptake of (99 m)Tc-mebrofenin and indocyanine green. *J Hepatol*. (2011) 54:738–45. doi: 10.1016/j.jhep.2010.07.047
22. van der Vorst JR, Schaafsma BE, Hutteman M, Verbeek FP, Liefers GJ, Hartgrink HH, et al. Nearinfrared fluorescence-guided resection of colorectal liver metastases. *Cancer*. (2013) 119:3411–8. doi: 10.1002/cncr.28203
23. Kaibori M, Matsui K, Ishizaki M, Iida H, Sakaguchi T, Tsuda T, et al. Evaluation of fluorescence imaging with indocyanine green in hepatocellular carcinoma. *Cancer Imaging*. (2016) 16:6. doi: 10.1186/s40644-016-0064-6
24. Kudo H, Ishizawa T, Tani K, Harada N, Ichida A, Shimizu A, et al. Visualization of subcapsular hepatic malignancy by indocyanine-green fluorescence imaging during laparoscopic hepatectomy. *Surg Endosc*. (2014) 28:2504–8. doi: 10.1007/s00464-014-3468-z
25. Kaibori M, Matsui K, Ishizaki M, Iida H, Okumura T, Sakaguchi T, et al. Intraoperative detection of superficial liver tumors by fluorescence imaging using indocyanine green and 5-aminolevulinic acid. *Anticancer Res*. (2016) 36:1841–9.
26. Ohgari Y, Nakayasu Y, Kitajima S, Sawamoto M, Mori H, Shimokawa O, et al. Mechanisms involved in delta-aminolevulinic acid (ALA)-induced photosensitivity of tumor cells: relation of ferrochelatase and uptake of ALA to the accumulation of protoporphyrin. *Biochem Pharmacol*. (2005) 71:42–9. doi: 10.1016/j.bcp.2005.10.019
27. Kriegmair M, Baumgartner R, Knüchel R, Stepp H, Hofstädter F, Hofstetter A. Detection of early bladder cancer by 5-aminolevulinic acid induced porphyrin fluorescence. *J Urol*. (1996) 155:105–9. doi: 10.1016/S0022-5347(01)66559-5

28. Jichlinski P, Forrer M, Mizeret J, Glanzmann T, Braichotte D, Wagnières G, et al. Clinical evaluation of a method for detecting superficial surgical transitional cell carcinoma of the bladder by light-induced fluorescence of protoporphyrin IX following the topical application of 5-aminolevulinic acid: preliminary results. *Lasers Surg Med.* (1997) 20:402–8. doi: 10.1002/(SICI)1096-9101(1997)20:4<402::AID-LSM5>3.0.CO;2-U
29. Stummer W, Stocker S, Wagner S, Stepp H, Fritsch C, Goetz C, et al. Intraoperative detection of malignant gliomas by 5-aminolevulinic acid-induced porphyrin fluorescence. *Neurosurgery.* (1998) 42:518–26. doi: 10.1097/00006123-199803000-00017
30. Friesen SA, Hjortland GO, Madsen SJ, Hirschberg H, Engebraten O, Nesland JM, et al. 5-Aminolevulinic acid-based photodynamic detection and therapy of brain tumors. *Int J Oncol.* (2002) 21:577–82. doi: 10.3892/ijo.21.3.577
31. Inoue Y, Tanaka R, Komeda K, Hirokawa F, Hayashi M, Uchiyama K. Fluorescence detection of malignant liver tumors using 5-aminolevulinic acid-mediated photodynamic diagnosis: principles, technique, and clinical experience. *World J Surg.* (2014) 38:1786–94. doi: 10.1007/s00268-014-2463-9
32. Boogerd LS, Handgraaf HJ, Lam HD, Huurman VA, Farina-Sarasqueta A, Frangioni JV, et al. Laparoscopic detection and resection of occult liver tumors of multiple cancer types using real-time near-infrared fluorescence guidance. *Surg Endosc.* (2017) 31:952–61. doi: 10.1007/s00464-016-5007-6
33. Waage A, Nilsson M. Iatrogenic bile duct injury: a population-based study of 152 776 cholecystectomies in the Swedish inpatient registry. *Arch Surg.* (2006) 141:1207–13. doi: 10.1001/archsurg.141.12.1207
34. Rystedt JML, Tingstedt B, Montgomery F, Montgomery AK. Routine intraoperative cholangiography during cholecystectomy is a cost-effective approach when analysing the cost of iatrogenic bile duct injuries. *HPB (Oxford).* (2017) 19:881–8. doi: 10.1016/j.hpb.2017.06.004
35. Jeng KS, Huang CC, Lin CK, Lin CC, Chen KH, Chu SH. Repeated introperative cholangiography is helpful for donor safety in the procurement of right liver graft with supraportal right bile duct variants in living-donor liver transplantation. *Transplant Proc.* (2014) 46:686–8. doi: 10.1016/j.transproceed.2013.11.093
36. Dip F, LoMenzo E, Sarotto L, Phillips E, Todeschini H, Nahmod M, et al. Randomized trial of near-infrared incisionless fluorescent cholangiography. *Ann Surg.* (2019) 270:992–9. doi: 10.1097/SLA.0000000000003178
37. Ishizawa T, Tamura S, Masuda K, Aoki T, Hasegawa K, Imamura H, et al. Intraoperative fluorescent cholangiography using indocyanine green: a biliary road map for safe surgery. *J Am Coll Surg.* (2009) 208:e1–4. doi: 10.1016/j.jamcollsurg.2008.09.024
38. Schols RM, Bouvy ND, van Dam RM, Masclee AA, Dejong CH, Stassen LP. Combined vascular and biliary fluorescence imaging in laparoscopic cholecystectomy. *Surg Endosc.* (2013) 27:4511–7. doi: 10.1007/s00464-013-3100-7
39. Kaneko J, Ishizawa T, Masuda K, Kawaguchi Y, Aoki T, Sakamoto Y, et al. Indocyanine green reinjection technique for use in fluorescent angiography concomitant with cholangiography during laparoscopic cholecystectomy. *Surg Laparosc Endosc Percutan Tech.* (2012) 22:341–4. doi: 10.1097/SLE.0b013e3182570240
40. Mizuno S, Isaji S. Indocyanine green (ICG) fluorescence imaging-guided cholangiography for donor hepatectomy in living donor liver transplantation. *Am J Transplant.* (2010) 10:2725–6. doi: 10.1111/j.1600-6143.2010.03288.x
41. Kawaguchi Y, Velayutham V, Fuks D, Christidis C, Kokudo N, Gayet B. Usefulness of indocyanine green-fluorescence imaging for visualization of the bile duct during laparoscopic liver resection. *J Am Coll Surg.* (2015) 221:e113–7. doi: 10.1016/j.jamcollsurg.2015.09.001
42. Hong SK, Lee KW, Kim HS, Yoon KC, Ahn SW, Choi JY, et al. Optimal bile duct division using real-time indocyanine green near-infrared fluorescence cholangiography during laparoscopic donor hepatectomy. *Liver Transpl.* (2017) 23:847–52. doi: 10.1002/lt.24686
43. Diana M, Usmaan H, Legner A, Yin LY, D'Urso A, Halvax P, et al. Novel laparoscopic narrow band imaging for real-time detection of bile leak during hepatectomy: proof of the concept in a porcine model. *Surg Endosc.* (2016) 30:3128–32. doi: 10.1007/s00464-015-4569-z
44. Kaibori M, Ishizaki M, Matsui K, Kwon AH. Intraoperative indocyanine green fluorescent imaging for prevention of bile leakage after hepatic resection. *Surgery.* (2011) 150:91–8. doi: 10.1016/j.surg.2011.02.011
45. Mizuno S, Inoue H, Tanemura A, Murata Y, Kuriyama N, Azumi Y, et al. Biliary complications in 108 consecutive recipients with duct-to-duct biliary reconstruction in living-donor liver transplantation. *Transplant Proc.* (2014) 46:850–5. doi: 10.1016/j.transproceed.2013.11.035
46. Inoue Y, Arita J, Sakamoto T, Ono Y, Takahashi M, Takahashi Y, et al. Anatomical liver resections guided by 3-dimensional parenchymal staining using fusion indocyanine green fluorescence imaging. *Ann Surg.* (2015) 262:105–11. doi: 10.1097/SLA.0000000000000775
47. Nishino H, Hatano E, Seo S, Nitta T, Saito T, Nakamura M, et al. Real-time navigation for liver surgery using projection mapping with indocyanine green fluorescence: development of the novel medical imaging projection system. *Ann Surg.* (2018) 267:1134–40. doi: 10.1097/SLA.0000000000002172
48. Makuuchi M, Hasegawa H, Yamazaki S. Ultrasonically guided subsegmentectomy. *Surg Gynecol Obstet.* (1985) 161:346–50.
49. Jung DH, Hwang S, Lee YJ, Kim KH, Song GW, Ahn CS, et al. Small hepatocellular carcinoma with low tumor marker expression benefits more from anatomical resection than tumors with aggressive biology. *Ann Surg.* (2019) 269:511–9. doi: 10.1097/SLA.0000000000002486
50. Shindoh J, Makuuchi M, Matsuyama Y, Mise Y, Arita J, Sakamoto Y, et al. Complete removal of the tumor-bearing portal territory decreases local tumor recurrence and improves disease-specific survival of patients with hepatocellular carcinoma. *J Hepatol.* (2016) 64:594–600. doi: 10.1016/j.jhep.2015.10.015
51. Kaibori M, Kon M, Kitawaki T, Kawaura T, Hasegawa K, Kokudo N, et al. Comparison of anatomic and non-anatomic hepatic resection for hepatocellular carcinoma. *J Hepatobiliary Pancreat Sci.* (2017) 24:616–26. doi: 10.1002/jhbp.502
52. Kaibori M, Yoshii K, Hasegawa K, Ariizumi S, Kobayashi T, Kamiyama T, et al. Impact of systematic segmentectomy for small hepatocellular carcinoma. *J Hepatobiliary Pancreat Sci.* (2020) 27:331–41. doi: 10.1002/jhbp.720
53. Aoki T, Yasuda D, Shimizu Y, Odaira M, Niiya T, Kusano T, et al. Image-guided liver mapping using fluorescence navigation system with indocyanine green for anatomical hepatic resection. *World J Surg.* (2008) 32:1763–7. doi: 10.1007/s00268-008-9620-y
54. Aoki T, Murakami M, Yasuda D, Shimizu Y, Kusano T, Matsuda K, et al. Intraoperative fluorescent imaging using indocyanine green for liver mapping and cholangiography. *J Hepatobiliary Pancreat Sci.* (2010) 17:590–4. doi: 10.1007/s00534-009-0197-0
55. Ciria R, Cherqui D, Geller DA, Briceno J, Wakabayashi G. Comparative short-term benefits of laparoscopic liver resection: 9000 cases and climbing. *Ann Surg.* (2016) 263:761–77. doi: 10.1097/SLA.0000000000001413
56. Wakabayashi G, Cherqui D, Geller DA, Buell JF, Kaneko H, Han HS, et al. Recommendations for laparoscopic liver resection: a report from the second international consensus conference held in Morioka. *Ann Surg.* (2015) 261:619–29. doi: 10.1097/SLA.0000000000001184
57. Ishizawa T, Zuker NB, Kokudo N, Gayet B. Positive and negative staining of hepatic segments by use of fluorescent imaging techniques during laparoscopic hepatectomy. *Arch Surg.* (2012) 147:393–4. doi: 10.1001/archsurg.2012.59
58. Ueno M, Hayami S, Sonomura T, Tanaka R, Kawai M, Hirono S, et al. Indocyanine green fluorescence imaging techniques and interventional radiology during laparoscopic anatomical liver resection (with video). *Surg Endosc.* (2018) 32:1051–5. doi: 10.1007/s00464-017-5997-8
59. Aoki T, Koizumi T, Mansour DA, Fujimori A, Kusano T, Matsuda K, et al. Ultrasound-guided preoperative positive percutaneous indocyanine green fluorescence staining for laparoscopic anatomical liver resection. *J Am Coll Surg.* (2020) 230:e7–12. doi: 10.1016/j.jamcollsurg.2019.11.004
60. Butcher NJ, Mortimer GM, Minchin RF. Unravelling the stealth effect. *Nat Nanotechnol.* (2016) 11:310–1. doi: 10.1038/nnano.2016.6
61. Tsuda T, Kaibori M, Hishikawa H, Nakatake R, Okumura T, Ozeki E, et al. Near-infrared fluorescence imaging and photodynamic therapy with indocyanine green lactosome has antineoplastic effects for hepatocellular carcinoma. *PLoS ONE.* (2017) 12:e0183527. doi: 10.1371/journal.pone.0183527
62. Engel E, Schraml R, Maisch T, Kobuch K, Konig B, Szeimies R, et al. Light-induced decomposition of indocyanine green. *Invest Ophthalmol Vis Sci.* (2008) 49:1777–83. doi: 10.1167/iovs.07-0911

63. Hirano T, Kohno E, Gohto Y, Obana A. Singlet oxygen generation by irradiation of indocyanine green (ICG) and its effect to tissues. *J Jpn Soc Laser Surg Med.* (2007) 28:122–8. doi: 10.2530/jslsm.28.122
64. Lee YH, Lai YH. Synthesis, characterization, and biological evaluation of anti-HER2 indocyanine green-encapsulated PEG-coated PLGA nanoparticles for targeted phototherapy of breast cancer cells. *PLoS ONE.* (2016) 11:e0168192.0689760. doi: 10.1371/journal.pone.0168192
65. Funayama T, Sakane M, Abe T, Ochiai N. Photodynamic therapy with indocyanine green injection and near-infrared light irradiation has phototoxic effects and delays paralysis in spinal metastasis. *Photomed Laser Surg.* (2012) 30:47–53. doi: 10.1089/pho.2011.3080
66. Funayama T, Sakane M, Abe T, Hara I, Ozeki E, Ochiai N. Intraoperative near-infrared fluorescence imaging with novel indocyanine green-loaded nanocarrier for spinal metastasis: a preliminary animal study. *Open Biomed Eng.* (2012) 6:80–4. doi: 10.2174/1874120701206010080
67. Funayama T, Tsukanishi T, Hara I, Ozeki E, Sakane M. Tumor-selective near-infrared photodynamic therapy with novel indocyanine green-loaded nanocarrier delays paralysis in rats with spinal metastasis. *Photodiagnosis Photodyn Ther.* (2013) 10:374–8. doi: 10.1016/j.pdpdt.2013.03.002
68. Tsujimoto H, Morimoto Y, Takahata R, Nomura S, Yoshida K, Horiguchi H, et al. Photodynamic therapy using nanoparticle loaded with indocyanine green for experimental peritoneal dissemination of gastric cancer. *Cancer Sci.* (2014) 105:1626–30. doi: 10.1111/cas.12553
69. Tsujimoto H, Morimoto Y, Takahata R, Nomura S, Yoshida K, Hiraki S, et al. Theranostic photosensitive nanoparticles for lymph node metastasis of gastric cancer. *Ann Surg Oncol.* (2015) 22:S923–8. doi: 10.1245/s10434-015-4594-0
70. Hishikawa H, Kaibori M, Tsuda T, Matsui K, Okumura T, Ozeki E, et al. Near-infrared fluorescence imaging and photodynamic therapy with indocyanine green lactosomes has antineoplastic effects for gallbladder cancer. *Oncotarget.* (2019) 10:5622–31. doi: 10.18632/oncotarget.27193
71. Kaneko J, Inagaki Y, Ishizawa T, Jianjun G, Wei T, Aoki T, et al. Photodynamic therapy for human hepatoma-cell-line tumors utilizing biliary excretion properties of indocyanine green. *J Gastroenterol.* (2014) 49:110–6. doi: 10.1007/s00535-013-0775-4
72. Shirata C, Kaneko J, Inagaki Y, Kokudo T, Sato M, Kiritani S, et al. Near-infrared photothermal/photodynamic therapy with indocyanine green induces apoptosis of hepatocellular carcinoma cells through oxidative stress. *Sci Rep.* (2017) 7:13958. doi: 10.1038/s41598-017-14401-0

15

Acridine Orange: A Review of Novel Applications for Surgical Cancer Imaging and Therapy

Vadim A. Byvaltsev [1,2], Liudmila A. Bardonova [1], Naomi R. Onaka [3], Roman A. Polkin [1], Sergey V. Ochkal [1], Valerij V. Shepelev [1], Marat A. Aliyev [1] and Alexander A. Potapov [4]*

[1] Neurosurgery and Innovative Medicine Department, Irkutsk State Medical University, Irkutsk, Russia, [2] Irkutsk Scientific Center of Surgery and Traumatology, Irkutsk, Russia, [3] University of Arizona College of Medicine, Phoenix, AZ, United States, [4] Federal State Autonomous Institution "N. N. Burdenko National Scientific and Practical Center for Neurosurgery" of the Ministry of Healthcare of the Russian Federation, Moscow, Russia

Correspondence:
Vadim A. Byvaltsev
byval75vadim@yandex.ru

Introduction: Acridine orange (AO) was first extracted from coal tar in the late nineteenth century and was used as a fluorescent dye. In this paper, we review emergent research about novel applications of AO for fluorescence surgery and cancer therapy.

Materials and methods: We performed a systematic search in the MEDLINE, PubMed, Cochrane library, Google Scholar, Embase, Web of Science, and Scopus database using combinations of the term "acridine orange" with the following: "surgical oncology," "neuropathology," "microsurgery," "intraoperative fluorescence," "confocal microscopy," "pathology," "endomicroscopy," "guidance," "fluorescence guidance," "oncology," "surgery," "neurooncology," and "photodynamic therapy." Peer-reviewed articles published in English were included in this review. We have also scanned references for relevant articles.

Results: We have reviewed studies on the various application of AO in microscopy, endomicroscopy, intraoperative fluorescence guidance, photodynamic therapy, sonodynamic therapy, radiodynamic therapy.

Conclusion: Although the number of studies on the clinical use of AO is limited, pilot studies have demonstrated the safety and feasibility of its application as an intraoperative fluorescent dye and as a novel photo- and radio-sensitizator. Further clinical studies are necessary to more definitively assess the clinical benefit AO-based fluorescence guidance, therapy for sarcomas, and to establish feasibility of this new approach for the treatment of other tumor types.

Keywords: acridine orange, radiodynamic therapy, photodynamic therapy, intraoperative fluorescence, surgical cancer imaging

INTRODUCTION

Recent advancements in optical cancer imaging have facilitated the development of novel repurposing of known molecular probes for wide-field and microscopic fluorescence-based surgical guidance that have significant potential to positively impact patient care and to transform the field of surgical oncology. Acridine orange (AO) is a common fluorescent dye that has been well known for years. It has recently regained attention as a possible innovative drug for clinical applications in the field of oncology, particularly in cancer imaging and photodynamic therapy.

Acridine orange (AO) is a member of the xanthene class of molecules and shares a common aromatic structure with multiple acridine dyes (1, 2). Acridine dyes were first extracted from coal tar at the end of the nineteenth century. And was then used for a period of time as a dye in the fabric industry as well as for biological application. In 1912, Erlich and Beneda proposed to use acridines as antimalarials, with Browning suggesting use as an antimicrobial agent about a decade on in 1922 (3, 4). During World War I and II, the acridine dyes were widely used as antimicrobials prior to the widespread use of penicillin (4). The application of AO has been studied for bacteria detection in clinical specimens with prokaryotes fluorescing bright orange in low pH buffered media, while other cells produce green background fluorescence (5).

The novel research field of acridines is focused on their application in cancer theranostics due to its unique feature of preferential accumulation in the acidic environment of the tumor tissues and strong fluorescent properties (1, 6). AO has been recently explored in several preclinical (**Figures 1A,B**) and clinical studies for specific tumor cells targeting. As the novel diagnostic and therapeutic applications of AO broaden, we thought to review the existing body of knowledge regarding its potential use in various areas of medicine and outline its place and potential future impact on the rapidly growing area of image-guided cancer management. The goal of this paper is to review the current literature on the use of AO for fluorescence-guided surgery and cancer therapy. This review is focused on the clinical and translational studies that described the use of AO-based therapeutic and relevant diagnostic imaging methods.

MATERIALS AND METHODS

Search Strategy

We performed a literature search in MEDLINE, PubMed, Cochrane library, Google Scholar, Embase, Web of Science, and Scopus databases using the combinations of the term "Acridine" with the following: "surgical oncology," "neuropathology," "microsurgery," "intraoperative fluorescence," "confocal microscopy," "pathology," "endomicroscopy," "guidance," "fluorescence guidance," "oncology," "surgery," "neurooncology," and "photodynamic therapy." Peer-reviewed articles published in English till September 2018 were included to compile this review. We have also scanned references for relevant articles. Search strategy is presented in **Supplement 1**.

RESULTS AND DISCUSSION

Chemical Properties

AO (C17H19N3) is a low molecular weight (265.36 g/mol), weakly basic dye that easily penetrates cell membranes. AO has metachromatic properties and upon excitation with blue light, ($\sim$488 nm) emits green fluorescence when in monomer form and orange fluorescence when in dimer form. AO produces orange fluorescence when it binds to RNA and green fluorescence when it binds to DNA. However, this behavior differs significantly in live, apoptotic, and fixed permeabilized cells (6).

In live cells, AO diffuses through the cytoplasmic membrane and is retained in the cellular compartments with low pH, resulting in a bright orange fluorescence of lysosomes when excited with a blue light. AO also intercalates with the cytoplasmic and nuclear RNA molecules and results in a diffuse green fluorescence within all cells (7, 8). AO does not intercalate with DNA of intact living cells (9) and does not accumulate in other non-acidic organelles, such as the mitochondria, endoplasmic reticulum, or Golgi apparatus (7).

In both fixed permeabilized cells and cells undergoing apoptosis, pH compartmentalization is lost. Therefore, AO leaks from acidic lysosomes and diffusely binds to RNA and DNA molecules, resulting in yellow-orange fluorescence in the whole cell (6).

Based on the unique spectral distinctions and differential staining of RNA and DNA molecules, AO can be used to distinguish stages of apoptosis and necroptosis (10). During apoptosis, cells stained with AO demonstrate nuclear shrinkage, cellular fragmentation, and loss of nuclear demarcation, appearing therefore as red cells. Eventually the cellular RNA and red AO emission is lost while fragmented green nucleus remains. In contrast, during necrosis or necroptosis, the orange lysosomal signal is lost due to their disruption and to loss of cellular RNA, while the green signal from smooth and shrunken nuclei remains (11).

Most malignant tumors create an acidic environment due to increased anaerobic glycolysis (Warburg effect). Malignant cells also contain increased amounts of RNA and DNA compared to normal cells. Both factors result in increased accumulation and delayed elimination of AO in tumor cells (12).

Safety

Acridine dyes have a record of a mutagenic effect on certain types of bacteria, which raises a question about AO safety in humans (13). In 1969, Van Duuren showed that AO is neither an irritant nor a carcinogen to the skin of mice after repeated application. However, three out of twenty mice with skin application of AO developed liver tumors, suggesting systemic absorption of AO (14). In the same study, subcutaneous administration of AO lead to two of thirty mice and one of twenty rats developing tumors at the injection site. (14) In1978, the International Agency for Research on Cancer published the opinion that there was insufficient data or evaluation regarding the carcinogenicity of AO (15).

Systemic administration of AO has been investigated in several animal studies. The LD_{50} for intravenous (IV) administration of AO in mice was determined to be 32 and 36 mg/kg for male and female mice, respectively (16). In determining the dose/toxicity relationship, Tatsuta et al. studied mice with gastric cancer and Tomson et al. studied subcutaneously implanted mammary carcinoma tumors treated with intraperitoneal AO application at a dose of 40 mg/kg and showed effectiveness of photodynamic therapy (PDT) without significant toxic effects (17, 18). Udovich et al. also demonstrated the absence of adverse effects of AO administered

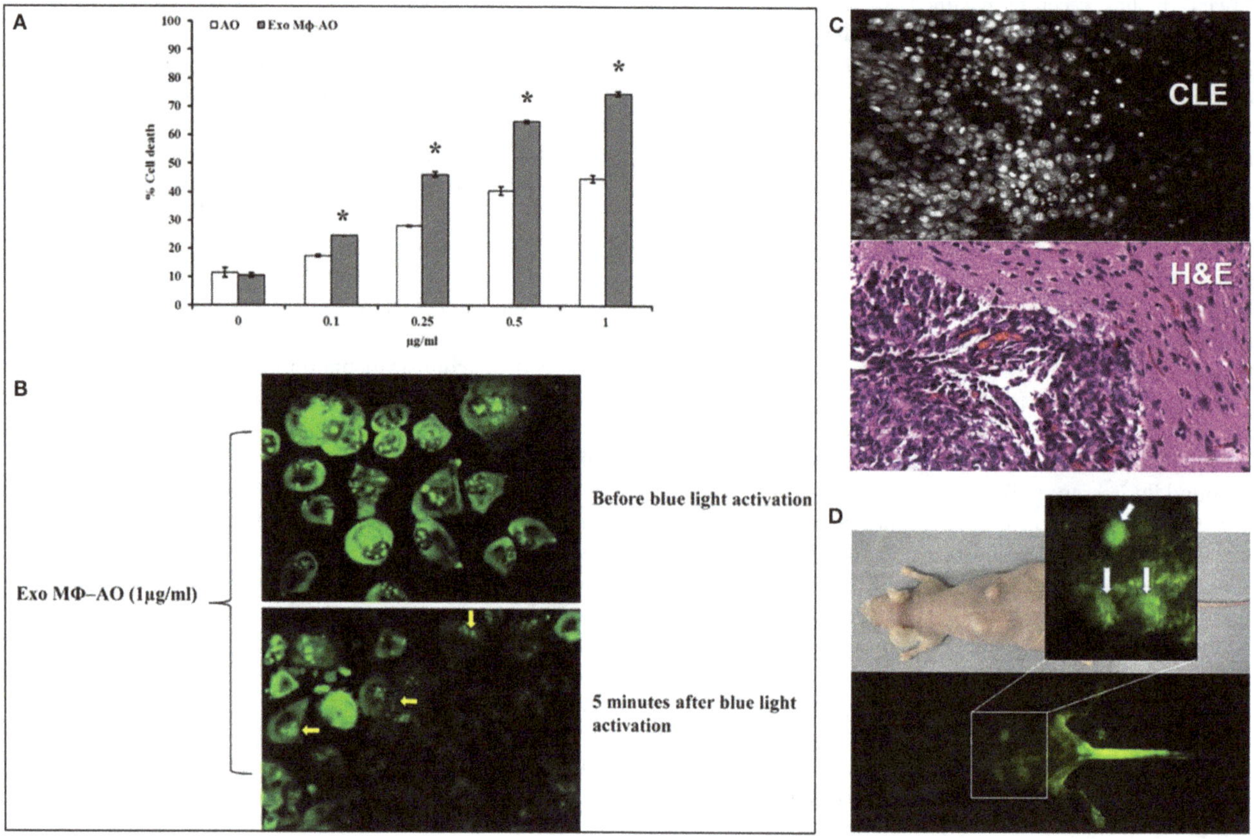

FIGURE 1 | (A) Cytotoxic effect of acridine orange (AO)-charged exosomes derived from macrophages (Exo Mϕ-AO) compared to free AO against melanoma cell monolayer by cytofluorimetry assessment. Columns, mean percentages of cell death of two independent experiments run in triplicate; bars indicate standard deviation. $p < 0.05$. Figure adapted with permission from: Iessi et al. (43) (CC BY 4.0). **(B)** Fluorescence microscopy showing the formation of membrane "blebs" in melanoma cells treated with Exo Mϕ-AO (1 Ig/ml) after 5 min of exposition to blue light. Figure adapted with permission from: Iessi et al. (43) (CC BY 4.0). **(C)** Upper image—Confocal laser endomicroscopy image of an animal glioblastoma stained with AO. Lower image—corresponding histology image. Image courtesy of Dr. Mark C. Preul. **(D)** Macroscopic fluorescence view of mouse osteosarcoma subcutaneously inoculated in the back of nude mouse after blue light excitation at 2 h after AO injection through the tail vein. Tumors emit green fluorescence (arrows). Injection site of the tail vein also emits green fluorescence Figure adapted with permission from: Kusuzaki et al. (6) (CC-BY 3.0).

intraperitoneally to mice at dose of 0.33 and 3.3 mM for confocal endomicroscopy imaging (19).

In dogs, IV administration of AO at 0.1 mg/kg showed no clinical signs of toxicity and no abnormalities were seen in the blood within 30 days (20). Serum AO levels decreased rapidly within 30 min and were below the detection limit (5 ng/ml) 2 h after intravenous administration (20). In a case report of AO-based PDT in a cat with cutaneous malignant melanoma, no side effects were reported, where AO was administered locally to the surgical site at a dose of 1 μg/ml (21).

Several human studies have demonstrated the initial safety of AO. Kusuzaki et al. reported a pilot study of eight patients with various malignant neoplasms at the terminal stages (two sarcomas, two pancreatic carcinomas, intrahepatic cholangiocarcinoma, lung, renal, and parotid carcinomas) treated with IV administration of AO at 0.5 or 1 mg/kg and low-dose (with 3 or 5 Gy) radiotherapy (RT) (13). This study did not confirm the assumptions about the toxic effects of the AO (13).

Several studies from Japan [$n = 8$ patients from Teneri, Japan (13) and $n = 51$ from Tsu City, Mie, Japan (22)] investigated the local application of AO solution to tumor cavities following tumor resection at the dosage of 1 μg/ml for 5 min. Subsequent analysis of AO-based photodiagnostics (PD), PDT and RT demonstrated no serious immediate or long-term complications (23–26).

In summary, there is still a lack of convincing data regarding the long-term safety and cancerogenic potential of AO. Future studies are needed to demonstrate if potential toxic effects of AO can be balanced by the benefits of AO-based cytoreduction therapies and diagnostics for various tissue organs, routs of administration, and doses.

Photodiagnostics

AO Use for Microscopy

AO has been extensively studied in pathology as a single dye and in combination with other dyes for specimen assessment using fluorescence microscopy. Differential staining of AO has been used to differentiate gliosis and glial neoplasms in human specimens with malignant glial cells demonstrating increased red fluorescence secondary to cytoplasmic RNA accumulation compared to reactive glial cells which remained green (27). AO has been used for mapping of GL261 mouse gliomas on 3-D reconstructed confocal imaging following tissue clearing (28). In this application, glioma regions exhibited increased intensity of fluorescence compared to the dimmer surrounding normal brain (28). Additionally, another study demonstrated the ability of AO to effectively differentiate brain tumor types using confocal microscopy of various brain tumor biopsies rapidly stained with AO (29).

Other applications of acridine orange include the simple and sensitive post-mortem detection of early myocardial infarction—normal myocardium fluoresces a golden brown color and myocardial anoxia/ischemia-damaged cells show a shift toward yellow or yellow-green (30). In the 1980's, Tejada et al. developed a specialized test with sperm AO fluorescence staining to determine male fertility (31). Krishnamurthy et al. showed that staining of breast, lung, kidney, and liver tissues with AO alone and subsequent imaging with confocal laser microscopy practically does not differ in efficiency from staining with H&E (32). Moreover, AO staining was much faster and easier than H&E (32). In yet another application, Wang et al. used AO for rapid non-destructive imaging of whole prostate biopsies using video-rate fluorescence structured illumination microscopy and demonstrated its feasibility as an alternative to destructive pathology (33).

In a study investigating surgical treatment of malignant tumors of the skin, AO was used as a nuclear dye in combination with eosin fluorescence (for labeling cytoplasm), and endogenous reflectance (for labeling collagen and keratin) for tri-modal confocal laser scanning microscopy of the skin samples (34). The authors reported that the novel staining method significantly reduced the time of surgical intervention while providing image quality similar to conventional hematoxylin and eosin staining (34). This finding corroborates with the conclusions drawn by Krishnamurthy regarding the non-inferiority of AO and CLE compared to conventional H&E. Another study reported an automatic pipeline that produces rapid, virtual H&E histology of tissue based on a fast, initial confocal staining of a tissue stained with a combination of AO and sulforhodamine 101, with the extrapolated conclusion that CLE with AO improves time to histological diagnosis over H&E (35). The intraoperative direct analysis that CLE can provide, particularly with AO as a contrast agent, has also been studied in the ophthalmological setting. The authors commented that this method provided a fast *ex vivo* preliminary diagnosis of conjunctival lesions, perhaps representing a novel tool for intraoperative as well as postsurgical management of conjunctival tumors (36).

AO is commonly used as a fluorescent dye to stain live tissues for intraoperative confocal endomicroscopy (**Figure 1C**), however, *in vivo* topical application of AO has not been investigated for all organs, and particularly in the brain up to this point due to safety concerns, with the less specific fluorescein sodium being used as a fluorescent contrast (37) In mouse brain glioma models and in fresh human biopsies *ex vivo*, AO staining and imaging with the confocal endomicroscope proved successful for differentiation of normal brain and glioma tissue (38, 39). Notably, *in vivo* AO staining was reported for confocal microlaparoscope imaging of ovarian cancer in 45 patients (40). In this study AO was used under FDA Investigational New Drug approval at a dose of ≤1 μL of 330 μM/L applied topically to the surface of the ovary just prior to imaging (40). This study concluded that trained surgeons were able to distinguish between normal and malignant ovarian surface epithelium in AO stained optical biopsies and that accuracy was similar during the *ex vivo* and *in vivo* imaging (40). There are two additional publications regarding AO application for the *in vivo* diagnosis of neoplasia in gynecology (41, 42), but currently, no *in vivo* investigation has been published for brain tissue.

AO Use in Wide-Field Fluorescence Guidance

After intravenous or topical application and soaking of the resection cavity in AO solution, researchers observed increased accumulation of AO in tumor tissue. This allowed accurate identification of the tumor regions as intense green fluorescence in wide field imaging (using specially designed fluorescence imaging operating microscope). AO fluorescence allowed for better tailoring of the resection area while maintaining the maximum amount of healthy tissue. This technology was used to remove breast tumors (35), soft tissue tumors and sarcomas (26, 44, 45), treatment of skin cancer (34, 46), conjunctival tumors (47), renal tumors, lungs, liver (32).

Considering the rapid development of intraoperative optical imaging tools and significant track of publications regarding AO-based microscopy, AO (similarly to fluorescein sodium and indocyanine green) is a promising topical contrast agent for *in vivo* pathology in humans. However, the long-term safety of topical AO should be established before such a method may be used in surgery. Alternatively, novel, dye-less *in vivo* microscopy methods like optical coherent tomography, RAMAN, and multiphoton reflectance microscopy may make any label-based methods obsolete in the future.

AO Use in PDT, SDT, and RDT

Mechanism of Action

The mechanism of AO-based PDT is based on the production of activated forms of oxygen upon AO fluorescence emission when exposed to blue light excitation (488 nm). As AO binds to the increased amount of RNA in tumor cells and also accumulates in lysosomes, released reactive oxygen species damage lipid membranes, leading to the leakage of lysosomal enzymes, and activation of apoptosis in the tumor cells (12). Myotoxicity was also suggested as another potential mechanism of AO (48).

AO can also increase the production of reactive radicals when exposed to low doses of X-ray radiation (26, 44, 49) or to the ultrasound energy (50). The principles of X-ray radiodynamic therapy (RDT) and sonodynamic therapy (SDT) have gained interest because unlike traditional light-based PDT, it has deeper tissue penetration depth. With RDT however, one energy source simultaneously activates both processes of radiotherapy and PDT, maximizing the synergetic treatment effect (49, 51). RDT with

AO shows a similar effect on tumor cells when compared to PDT (52).

Preclinical Studies

One of the earliest studies of PDT with AO by Tomson et al. in the mouse model of undifferentiated carcinoma showed tumor resolution after PDT with AO in 90% of mice (18). Another early study by Ishikawa et al. which suggested the usefulness of PDT investigated photodynamic inactivation of argon laser with topical use of AO in the treatment of bladder cancer. Human bladder cancer cells (MGH-U1) were stained with AO and irradiated with argon laser with wave length of 496.5 nm and the intensity at the sample position about 4.0 mW/cm^2. The result shows that argon laser at the low intensity and with short irradiation time has a sufficient cytocidal effect (53). Satonaka et al. studied the AO-based PDT of pulmonary metastases of osteosarcomas in mice and demonstrated its feasibility (54) (**Figure 1D**). Interestingly, AO alone and AO-PDT inhibited invasion and metastases growth (54).

AO-based PDT and RDT has been advanced to clinical studies for the treatment of sarcomas (osteosarcomas and rhabdomyosarcomas) (1, 7, 12, 23, 25, 55), while its efficacy for brain tumors has been assessed only in preclinical studies. Osman et al. investigated the efficacy of AO-based PDT of glioma cells *in vitro* (56). Treatment of cultured glioblastoma cells with AO at a concentration of 0.001 mg/mL followed by 10 or 30 min incubation with white unfiltered light from light-emitting diode bulbs demonstrated dramatic cytostatic and cytocidal effects and almost complete eradication of glioblastoma cells in 72 h (56).

Local AO Administration

Matsubara et al. investigated the combined use of AO-based PD, followed by PDT and RDT for the treatment of rhabdomyosarcoma (57). After subtotal resection of the tumor, the area of operation was filled with a solution of AO at a concentration of 1 μg/ml and after 5 min, the excess dye was washed off with saline. The first step included the use of wide-field fluorescence microscopy of the surgical area. Authors used a customized operating microscope (Carl Zeiss Co., Ltd, Oberkochen, Germany) with a xenon lamp equipped with an excitation filter (450–490 nm) resulting in a blue excitation light and a long-pass filter (>520 nm) for detection of the green fluorescence emitted by the tumor. After staining, a more thorough curettage of the area was performed until the green glow disappeared. The next step included AO-PDT, a 10 min exposure of the resection cavity to unfiltered light from a xenon lamp with a brightness of 100,000 lx mounted on an operating microscope. After that, a layer of sutures was applied to the wound without rinsing the AO solution. The patient was then transferred to the radiotherapy room where an X-ray exposure was performed (5 Gy) (57).

Matsubara et al. reported long-term results of AO-based PD followed by PDT and RDT in 18 patients from 1996 to 2008, showing that the method allows preservation of more healthy tissue during resection (26, 44). This advantage helped to preserve functionality of the limbs due to more tailored resection compared to the standard wide margin resection method without significant differences in the recurrence rate.

Systemic AO Administration

There was only one study found on the AO-based RDT with systemic administration of AO which included treatment of 8 patients with end-stage cancers. In this study, two patients had sarcomas, two had pancreatic cancer, and one patient each had intrahepatic cholangiocarcinoma, renal, lung, and parotid cancer. (13). Two hours after 1 mg/kg AO was administered IV, the patients received 3–5 Gy X-ray irradiation 3 times within a 3 week period. In 3 out of 5 patients who completed the full course of the proposed therapy, tumors reduced in size and symptoms improved. Notably, this study demonstrated the absence of a toxic effect on the body with the introduction of therapeutic doses of the drug (13).

While some patients benefited in these small pilot studies, further clinical investigation is necessary to assess if the observed cytocidal effect could be achieved in other types of cancer. However, the absence of serious side effects of AO, coupled with the likely cytolytic effect of RDT, together with the radiation, opens up new horizons for exploring its potential in other cancers.

CONCLUSIONS AND FUTURE DIRECTIONS

The use of AO in oncology represents a novel approach but the number of studies is currently limited, likely due to the historical concerns about AO safety. More studies are necessary to identify tumor types and stages where application of AO can be useful to assess its clinical value and identify potential side effects.

There are several promising areas where AO may be beneficial. First, it is worth noting the possibility of macro and confocal fluorescence microscopy for *in vivo* fluorescence guidance during surgical resection. The effect of AO fluorescence guidance has not yet been studied in brain tumors and should be tested in comparison with other fluorescence guidance techniques such as 5-aminolevulinic acid, fluorescein sodium, and indocyanine green, which are already available and have a safety record and established efficacy.

Of particular interest is the effect of intravenously administered AO on tumor cells when exposed to small doses of radiation. If successful, this could dramatically change the approach for cancer treatment. AO-based RDT treatment of distant metastasis is another promising area of application (54). AO fluorescence guidance combined with PDT, SDT, or RDT can be potentially applied to all organs for the surgical treatment of tumor lesions, including brain tumor surgery. Brain gliomas are notorious for their infiltrative growth and thus the possibility of selective killing of any residual tumor cells after surgical resection is encouraging and compelling. However, there are also considerable limitations in that the blood-tumor-brain-barrier at the periphery of the gliomas might decrease efficacy of AO delivery, decreasing its photosensitizing effect (58). It should also be noted that AO is one among many drugs (including

5-ALA) that are in development for PDT, SDA, or RDT for the treatment of various cancers and their comparative efficacy for various cancers is yet to be established (59–63). Future drug developments include nanoparticles and targeted multipurpose theranostic drugs which can be used for intraoperative guidance and subsequent precision treatment of any microscopic residual tumor (36).

AO has demonstrated utility in multiple settings up to this point in time with the majority of applications being *ex vivo*. Although use of AO is not new with practical applications from urology, gynecology, to ophthalmology detailed, repurposing AO for possible specific tumor labeling in the field of neurosurgery has been minimally explored. While there is historical evidence of potentially detrimental health effects of AO dating back to the late 1960s, there is a small body of growing literature in the time since that points to its potential uses *in vivo* without toxic systemic effects. With the evidence presented in this review regarding the role of AO in tumor identification, we are especially interested with respect to brain lesions what AO can possibly provide in terms of specific fluorescent tumor labeling. More data is needed to determine the safety of AO *in vivo* and its future applications, particularly in neurosurgery.

AUTHOR CONTRIBUTIONS

VB, LB, NO, RP, SO, VS, MA, and AP researched the data, wrote the manuscript, generated the figures, provided participation in the discussion of the content, and revised the review.

ACKNOWLEDGMENTS

LB acknowledges scholarship support #SP-2545.2018.4.

REFERENCES

1. Kusuzaki K, Murata H, Matsubara T, Satonaka H, Wakabayashi T, Matsumine A, et al. Review. Acridine orange could be an innovative anticancer agent under photon energy. *In Vivo*. (2007) 21:205–14.
2. Sharma VK, Sahare PD, Rastogi RC, Ghoshal SK, Mohan D. Excited state characteristics of acridine dyes: acriflavine and acridine orange. *Spectrochim Acta A Mol Biomol Spectrosc*. (2003) 59:1799–804. doi: 10.1016/S1386-1425(02)00440-7
3. Browning CH, Cohen JB, Gaunt R, Gulbransen R. Relationships between antiseptic action and chemical constitution with special reference to compounds of the pyridine, quinoline, acridine and phenazine series. *Proc R Soc B*. (1922) 93:329–66. doi: 10.1098/rspb.1922.0025
4. Wainwright M. Acridine–a neglected antibacterial chromophore. *J Antimicrob Chemother*. (2001) 47:1–13. doi: 10.1093/jac/47.1.1
5. Kronvall G, Myhre E. Differential staining of bacteria in clinical specimens using acridine orange buffered at low pH. *Acta Pathol Microbiol Scand B*. (1977) 85:249–54. doi: 10.1111/j.1699-0463.1977.tb01970.x
6. Kusuzaki K, Matsubara T, Satonaka H, Matsumine A, Nakamura T, Sudo A, et al. Intraoperative Photodynamic Surgery (iPDS) with acridine orange for musculoskeletal sarcomas. *Cureus*. (2014) 6:e204. doi: 10.7759/cureus.204
7. Kusuzaki K, Murata H, Takeshita H, Hashiguchi S, Nozaki T, Emoto K, et al. Intracellular binding sites of acridine orange in living osteosarcoma cells. *Anticancer Res*. (2000) 20:971–5.
8. Amagasa J. Mechanisms of photodynamic inactivation of acridine orange-sensitized transfer RNA: participation of singlet oxygen and base damage leading to inactivation. *J Radiat Res*. (1986) 27:339–51. doi: 10.1269/jrr.27.339
9. Delic J, Coppey J, Magdelenat H, Coppey-Moisan M. Impossibility of acridine orange intercalation in nuclear DNA of the living cell. *Exp Cell Res*. (1991) 194:147–53. doi: 10.1016/0014-4827(91)90144-J
10. Plemel JR, Caprariello AV, Keough MB, Henry TJ, Tsutsui S, Chu TH, et al. Unique spectral signatures of the nucleic acid dye acridine orange can distinguish cell death by apoptosis and necroptosis. *J Cell Biol*. (2017) 216:1163–81. doi: 10.1083/jcb.201602028
11. Mares I, Drevo M, Adam E, Kubatova M, Casny J. Live measles vaccine from a further attenuated strain SEVAC. *Prog Immunobiol Stand*. (1967) 3:188–91.
12. Kusuzaki K, Hosogi S, Ashihara E, Matsubara T, Satonaka H, Nakamura T, et al. Translational research of photodynamic therapy with acridine orange which targets cancer acidity. *Curr Pharm Des*. (2012) 18:1414–20. doi: 10.2174/138161212799504812
13. Kusuzaki K, Takai T, Yoshimura H, Inoue K, Takai S, Baldini N. Clinical trial of radiotherapy after intravenous injection of acridine orange for patients with cancer. *Anticancer Res*. (2018) 38:481–9. doi: 10.21873/anticanres.12248
14. Van Duuren BL, Sivak A, Katz C, Melchionne S. Tumorigenicity of acridine orange. *Br J Cancer*. (1969) 23:587–90. doi: 10.1038/bjc.1969.72
15. International Agency for Research on Cancer. Acridine orange. In: *IARC Monographs on the Evaluation of Carcinogenic Risk of Chemicals to Man*. Vol. 16. Lyon: IARC Press (1978), 145–52.
16. Nakamura T, Kusuzaki K, Matsubara T, Matsumine A, Asanuma K, Satonaka H, et al. Determination of the LD50 of acridine orange via intravenous administration in mice in preparation for clinical application to cancer therapy. *In Vivo*. (2014) 28:523–7.
17. Tatsuta M, Iishi H, Yamamura H, Yamamoto R, Okuda S. Comparison of photodynamic inactivation of experimental stomach tumors sensitized by acridine orange or hematoporphyrin derivatives. *Oncology*. (1988) 45:35–40. doi: 10.1159/000226527
18. Tomsom SH. Tumor destruction due to acridine orange photoactivation by argon laser. *Ann N Y Acad Sci*. (1976) 267:191–200. doi: 10.1111/j.1749-6632.1976.tb41608.x
19. Udovich JA, Besselsen DG, Gmitro AF. Assessment of acridine orange and SYTO 16 for *in vivo* imaging of the peritoneal tissues in mice. *J Microsc*. (2009) 234:124–9. doi: 10.1111/j.1365-2818.2009.03153.x
20. Maruo T, Shibuya K, Takahashi M, Nakayama T, Fukunaga K, Orito K. Safety of acridine orange intravenous administration in dogs. *Int J Appl Res Vet Med*. (2012) 10:164–8.
21. Hori H, Teramoto Y, Fukuyama Y, Maruo T., Marginal resection and acridine orange photodynamic therapy in a cat with recurrent cutaneous malignant melanoma. *Int J Appl Res Vet Med*. (2014) 12:181–5.
22. Matsubara T, Kusuzaki K, Matsumine A, Nakamura T, Sudo A. Can a less radical surgery using photodynamic therapy with acridine orange be equal to a wide-margin resection? *Clin Orthop Relat Res*. (2013) 471:792–802. doi: 10.1007/s11999-012-2616-9
23. Nakamura T, Kusuzaki K, Matsubara T, Matsumine A, Murata H, Uchida A. A new limb salvage surgery in cases of high-grade soft tissue sarcoma using photodynamic surgery, followed by photo- and radiodynamic therapy with acridine orange. *J Surg Oncol*. (2008) 97:523–8. doi: 10.1002/jso.21025
24. Kusuzaki K, Murata H, Matsubara T, Miyazaki S, Shintani K, Seto M, et al. Clinical outcome of a novel photodynamic therapy technique using acridine orange for synovial sarcomas. *Photochem Photobiol*. (2005) 81:705–9. doi: 10.1562/2004-06-27-RA-218.1
25. Kusuzaki K, Murata H, Matsubara T, Miyazaki S, Okamura A, Seto M, et al. Clinical trial of photodynamic therapy using acridine orange with/without low dose radiation as new limb salvage modality in musculoskeletal sarcomas. *Anticancer Res*. (2005) 25:1225–35.
26. Matsubara T, Kusuzaki K, Matsumine A, Murata H, Nakamura T, Uchida A, et al. Clinical outcomes of minimally invasive surgery using acridine orange for musculoskeletal sarcomas around the forearm, compared with conventional limb salvage surgery after wide resection. *J Surg Oncol*. (2010) 102:271–5. doi: 10.1002/jso.21602
27. Sarnat HB, Curry B, Rewcastle NB, Trevenen CL. Gliosis and glioma distinguished by acridine orange. *Can J Neurol Sci*. (1987) 14:31–5. doi: 10.1017/S0317167100026135
28. Belykh E, Miller EJ, Hu D, Martirosyan NL, Woolf EC, Scheck AC, et al. Scanning fiber endoscope improves detection of 5-aminolevulinic acid-induced protoporphyrin IX fluorescence at the boundary of infiltrative

glioma. *World Neurosurg.* (2018) 113:e51–69. doi: 10.1016/j.wneu.2018.01.151

29. Martirosyan NL, Georges J, Eschbacher JM, Belykh E, Carotenuto A, Spetzler RF, et al. Confocal scanning microscopy provides rapid, detailed intraoperative histological assessment of brain neoplasms: experience with 106 cases. *Clin Neurol Neurosurg.* (2018) 169:21–28. doi: 10.1016/j.clineuro.2018.03.015
30. Badir B, Knight B. Fluorescence microscopy in the detection of early myocardial infarction. *Forensic Sci Int.* (1987) 34:99–102. doi: 10.1016/0379-0738(87)90088-0
31. Tejada RI, Mitchell JC, Norman A, Marik JJ, Friedman S. A test for the practical evaluation of male fertility by acridine orange (AO) fluorescence. *Fertil Steril.* (1984) 42:87–91. doi: 10.1016/S0015-0282(16)47963-X
32. Krishnamurthy S, Cortes A, Lopez M, Wallace M, Sabir S, Shaw K, et al. *Ex vivo* confocal fluorescence microscopy for rapid evaluation of tissues in surgical pathology practice. *Arch Pathol Lab Med.* (2018) 142:396–401. doi: 10.5858/arpa.2017-0164-OA
33. Wang M, Kimbrell HZ, Sholl AB, Tulman DB, Elfer KN, Schlichenmeyer TC, et al. High-resolution rapid diagnostic imaging of whole prostate biopsies using video-rate fluorescence structured illumination microscopy. *Cancer Res.* (2015) 75:4032–41. doi: 10.1158/0008-5472.CAN-14-3806
34. Gareau D, Bar A, Snaveley N, Lee K, Chen N, Swanson N, et al. Tri-modal confocal mosaics detect residual invasive squamous cell carcinoma in Mohs surgical excisions. *J Biomed Opt.* (2012) 17:066018. doi: 10.1117/1.JBO.17.6.066018
35. Cahill LC, Giacomelli MG, Yoshitake T, Vardeh H, Faulkner-Jones BE, Connolly JL, et al. Rapid virtual hematoxylin and eosin histology of breast tissue specimens using a compact fluorescence nonlinear microscope. *Lab Invest.* (2018) 98:150–60. doi: 10.1038/labinvest.2017.116
36. Ni K, Lan G, Veroneau SS, Duan X, Song Y, Lin W. Nanoscale metal-organic frameworks for mitochondria-targeted radiotherapy-radiodynamic therapy. *Nat Commun.* (2018) 9:4321. doi: 10.1038/s41467-018-06655-7
37. Belykh E, Martirosyan NL, Yagmurlu K, Miller EJ, Eschbacher JM, Izadyyazdanabadi M, et al. Intraoperative fluorescence imaging for personalized brain tumor resection: current state and future directions. *Front Surg.* (2016) 3:55. doi: 10.3389/fsurg.2016.00055
38. Martirosyan NL, Georges J, Eschbacher JM, Cavalcanti DD, Elhadi AM, Abdelwahab MG, et al. Potential application of a handheld confocal endomicroscope imaging system using a variety of fluorophores in experimental gliomas and normal brain. *Neurosurg Focus.* (2014) 36:E16. doi: 10.3171/2013.11.FOCUS13486
39. Foersch S, Heimann A, Ayyad A, Spoden GA, Florin L, Mpoukouvalas K, et al. Confocal laser endomicroscopy for diagnosis and histomorphologic imaging of brain tumors *in vivo*. *PLoS ONE.* (2012) 7:e41760. doi: 10.1371/journal.pone.0041760
40. Risi MD, Rouse AR, Chambers SK, Hatch KD, Zheng W, Gmitro AF. Pilot clinical evaluation of a confocal microlaparoscope for ovarian cancer detection. *Int J Gynecol Cancer.* (2016) 26:248–54. doi: 10.1097/IGC.0000000000000595
41. Hammond DO. Fluorescence and acridine orange in the diagnosis of gynecologic neoplasia *in vivo*. *Am J Obstet Gynecol.* (1973) 115:272–3. doi: 10.1016/0002-9378(73)90299-8
42. Hoglund A, Joelsson I, Ingelman-Sundberg A, Odeblad E. Acridine orange in gynecologic cancer. I. The proton magnetic resonance spectrum of acridine orange zinc chloride. *Acta Obstet Gynecol Scand.* (1972) 51:309–13. doi: 10.3109/00016347209156864
43. Iessi E, Logozzi M, Lugini L, Azzarito T, Federici C, Spugnini EP, et al. Acridine orange/exosomes increase the delivery and the effectiveness of acridine orange in human melanoma cells: a new prototype for theranostics of tumors. *J Enzyme Inhib Med Chem.* (2017) 32:648–57. doi: 10.1080/14756366.2017.1292263
44. Matsubara T, Kusuzaki K, Matsumine A, Murata H, Marunaka Y, Hosogi S, et al. Photodynamic therapy with acridine orange in musculoskeletal sarcomas. *J Bone Joint Surg.* (2010) 92-B:760–2. doi: 10.1302/0301-620X.92B6.23788
45. Kusuzaki K, Aomori K, Suginoshita T, Minami G, Takeshita H, Murata H, et al. Total tumor cell elimination with minimum damage to normal tissues in musculoskeletal sarcomas following photodynamic therapy with acridine orange. *Oncology.* (2000) 59:174–80. doi: 10.1159/000012156
46. Jain M, Rajadhyaksha M, Nehal K. Implementation of fluorescence confocal mosaicking microscopy by "early adopter" Mohs surgeons and dermatologists: recent progress. *J Biomed Opt.* (2017) 22:24002. doi: 10.1117/1.JBO.22.2.024002
47. Iovieno A, Longo C, De Luca M, Piana S, Fontana L, Ragazzi M. Fluorescence confocal microscopy for *ex vivo* diagnosis of conjunctival tumors: a pilot study. *Am J Ophthalmol.* (2016) 168:207–16. doi: 10.1016/j.ajo.2016.06.001
48. Fotia C, Avnet S, Kusuzaki K, Roncuzzi L, Baldini N. Acridine orange is an effective anti-cancer drug that affects mitochondrial function in osteosarcoma cells. *Curr Pharm Des.* (2015) 21:4088–94. doi: 10.2174/1381612821666150918144953
49. Cline B, Delahunty I, Xie J. Nanoparticles to mediate X-ray-induced photodynamic therapy and Cherenkov radiation photodynamic therapy. *Wiley Interdiscip Rev Nanomed Nanobiotechnol.* (2018) 11:e1541. doi: 10.1002/wnan.1541
50. Suzuki N, Okada K, Chida S, Komori C, Shimada Y, Suzuki T. Antitumor effect of acridine orange under ultrasonic irradiation *in vitro*. *Anticancer Res.* (2007) 27:4179–84.
51. Wilson BC, Pogue BW. Optical and x-ray technology synergies enabling diagnostic and therapeutic applications in medicine. *J Biomed Optics.* (2018) 23:1. doi: 10.1117/1.JBO.23.12.121610
52. Hashiguchi S, Kusuzaki K, Murata H, Takeshita H, Hashiba M, Nishimura T, et al. Acridine orange excited by low-dose radiation has a strong cytocidal effect on mouse osteosarcoma. *Oncology.* (2002) 62:85–93. doi: 10.1159/000048251
53. Ishikawa S, Nemoto R, Kanoh S, Kobayashi K, Ishizaka S. Photodynamic inactivation of bladder cancer cells (MGH-U1) sensitized with acridine orange and irradiated by argon laser. *Tohoku J Exp Med.* (1984) 144:265–71. doi: 10.1620/tjem.144.265
54. Satonaka H, Kusuzaki K, Akeda K, Tsujii M, Iino T, Uemura T, et al. Acridine orange inhibits pulmonary metastasis of mouse osteosarcoma. *Anticancer Res.* (2011) 31:4163–8.
55. Matsubara T, Kusuzaki K, Matsumine A, Shintani K, Satonaka H, Uchida A. Acridine orange used for photodynamic therapy accumulates in malignant musculoskeletal tumors depending on pH gradient. *Anticancer Res.* (2006) 26:187–93.
56. Osman H, Elsahy D, Saadatzadeh MR, Pollok KE, Yocom S, Hattab EM, et al. Acridine orange as a novel photosensitizer for photodynamic therapy in glioblastoma. *World Neurosurg.* (2018) 114:e1310–5. doi: 10.1016/j.wneu.2018.03.207
57. Matsubara T, Kusuzaki K, Matsumine A, Murata H, Satonaka H, Shintani K, et al. A new therapeutic modality involving acridine orange excitation by photon energy used during reduction surgery for rhabdomyosarcomas. *Oncol Rep.* (2009) 21:89–94. doi: 10.3892/or_00000193
58. Randall EC, Emdal KB, Laramy JK, Kim M, Roos A, Calligaris D, et al. Integrated mapping of pharmacokinetics and pharmacodynamics in a patient-derived xenograft model of glioblastoma. *Nat Commun.* (2018) 9:4904. doi: 10.1038/s41467-018-07334-3
59. Costley D, Mc Ewan C, Fowley C, McHale AP, Atchison J, Nomikou N, et al. Treating cancer with sonodynamic therapy: a review. *Int J Hyperthermia.* (2015) 31:107–17. doi: 10.3109/02656736.2014.992484
60. Yoshida M, Kobayashi H, Terasaka S, Endo S, Yamaguchi S, Motegi H, et al. Sonodynamic therapy for malignant glioma using 220-kHz transcranial magnetic resonance imaging-guided focused ultrasound and 5-aminolevulinic acid. *Ultrasound Med Biol.* (2019) 45:526–38. doi: 10.1016/j.ultrasmedbio.2018.10.016
61. Suehiro S, Ohnishi T, Yamashita D, Kohno S, Inoue A, Nishikawa M, et al. Enhancement of antitumor activity by using 5-ALA-mediated sonodynamic therapy to induce apoptosis in malignant gliomas: significance of high-intensity focused ultrasound on 5-ALA-SDT in a mouse glioma model. *J Neurosurg.* (2018) 129:1416–28. doi: 10.3171/2017.6.JNS162398
62. Mahmoudi K, Garvey KL, Bouras A, Cramer G, Stepp H, Jesu Raj JG, et al. 5-aminolevulinic acid photodynamic therapy for the treatment of high-grade gliomas. *J Neurooncol.* (2019) 141:595–607. doi: 10.1007/s11060-019-03103-4
63. Takahashi J, Murakami M, Mori T, Iwahashi H. Verification of radiodynamic therapy by medical linear accelerator using a mouse melanoma tumor model. *Sci Rep.* (2018) 8:2728. doi: 10.1038/s41598-018-21152-z

16

Application of Indocyanine Green During Arteriovenous Malformation Surgery: Evidence, Techniques and Practical Pearls

Chase H. Foster[1], Peter J. Morone[2], Samuel B. Tomlinson[3] and Aaron A. Cohen-Gadol[4]*

[1] Department of Neurological Surgery, George Washington University Hospital, Washington, DC, United States, [2] Department of Neurological Surgery, Vanderbilt University Medical Center, Vanderbilt University, Nashville, TN, United States, [3] School of Medicine and Dentistry, University of Rochester Medical Center, Rochester, NY, United States, [4] Goodman Campbell Brain and Spine, Department of Neurological Surgery, Indiana University, Indianapolis, IN, United States

***Correspondence:**
Aaron A. Cohen-Gadol
acohenmd@gmail.com

Indocyanine green (ICG) is a fluorescent molecule that enables visualization of hemodynamic flow through blood vessels. The first description of its application to the resection of arteriovenous malformations (AVMs) did not occur until 2007. Since then, industry leaders have rapidly integrated this optical technology into the intraoperative microscope, and the use of ICG videoangiography (VA) has since become routine in AVM surgery among some academic centers. A number of case series have been published since the introduction of ICG VA to AVM neurosurgery. These early reports with small sample sizes were largely qualitative, assigning to the technology "usefulness" and "benefit" scores as perceived by the operators. This lack of objectivity prompted the development of FLOW 800 software, a proprietary technology of Carl Zeiss Meditec AG (Oberkochen, Germany) that can quantify relative fluorescence intensity under the microscope to generate color maps and intensity curves for *ad hoc* and *post hoc* analyses, respectively. However, subsequent case series have done little to quantify the effect of ICG VA on outcomes. The available literature predominately concludes that ICG VA, although intuitive to deploy and interpret, is limited by its dependence on direct illumination and visualization. The subcortical components of AVMs represent a natural challenge to ICG-based flow analysis, and the scope of ICG VA has therefore been limited to AVMs with a high proportion of superficial angioarchitecture. As a result, digital subtraction angiography has remained the gold standard for confirming AVM obliteration. In this review, we provide an overview of the existing literature on ICG VA in AVM resection surgery. In addition, we describe our own experiences with ICG VA and AVMs and offer the senior author's surgical pearls for optimizing the marriage of fluorescence flow technology and AVM resection surgery.

Keywords: AVM, fluorescence, indocyanine green, neurosurgery, resection, videoangiography

INTRODUCTION

A tenant of any neurosurgical operation is the maintenance of perfusion by way of avoiding undue vascular compromise. In the resection of intracerebral arteriovenous malformations (AVMs), this means the exclusion of en passage (i.e., uninvolved) vessels as well as the protection of nidal draining veins until arterial feeders have been disconnected (1). Indocyanine green (ICG) is a non-specific fluorescein-like dye that can be injected systemically to help delineate the margins of vascular anatomy under direct visualization and represents one such maneuver to successfully accomplish these goals. ICG videoangiography (VA) specifically is useful in this endeavor in that it enables the operator to directly and immediately assess the integrity of vessels under the intraoperative microscope.

Since its introduction to the field, the utility of ICG VA in optimizing the margins of safety during AVM resection has become more widely accepted. Now, some authors would posit that ICG VA is a standard component of AVM resection surgery (2). Both single-institution (3) and expert-driven (1) reports of the practicality of ICG VA as an intraoperative armament have been bolstered by larger reviews of the topic by various research cooperatives in recent years (2, 4, 5). A contemporaneous review of the topic is warranted to refresh neurosurgeons' understanding of ICG's important role in neurosurgery as it relates to AVM resection surgery and to provide an updated synthesis of available data.

HISTORY OF ICG

ICG dye was first introduced to the field of medicine after its approval by the Food and Drug Administration in 1956 (6). Providers soon discovered it to be helpful in a variety of specialties, beginning with cardiology and ending, for our purposes, in neurosurgery in 1995, when Hongo et al. (7) applied ICG to the study of cerebral hemodynamics. Their seminal work was followed by that of Raabe et al. (8), who in 2003 used ICG VA during the microsurgical clipping of intracerebral aneurysms. The use of ICG VA in neurovascular surgery has become ubiquitous, if not expected, since the subsequent introduction of an ICG VA integrated microscope to the neurosurgical operating room by Carl Zeiss Meditec. Its usefulness for excluding residual nidus in AVM resection has been endorsed repeatedly since the formative work by Takagi et al. (9) in 2007 and by Killory et al. (10) 2 years later. Part of ICG VA's appeal stems from data suggesting that it can produce results somewhat comparable to those of digital subtraction angiography (DSA) (8), which is considered the gold-standard method of assessing AVM resection completeness (11). The relatively recent development of FLOW 800 quantitative software (Carl Zeiss Meditec) has perhaps helped to mitigate some of the often-cited shortcomings of ICG VA (discussed below) by providing a measure of objectivity to this otherwise subjective auxiliary (12).

Abbreviations: AVM, arteriovenous malformation; DSA, digital subtraction angiography; ICG, indocyanine green; SMG, Spetzler-Martin grade; VA, videoangiography.

ICG PHARMACOLOGY

ICG ($C_{43}H_{47}N_2NaO_6S_2$) is a water-soluble molecule with a molecular weight of 744 g/mol (13). ICG is similar to the perhaps more familiar fluorescein in that the fluorescent properties of both are exploited to define vascular borders intraoperatively (13). Specifically, the tricarbocyanine structure of ICG is responsible for its near-infrared fluorescence, having peak excitation and emission wavelengths at 800 and 830 nm, respectively (11, 14). ICG becomes highly bound to plasma proteins such as albumin immediately after systemic intravenous injection, with a 95% rate of binding after just 1–2 s (6, 13). Physically, the molecule is too large to cross the blood–brain barrier and thus collects and concentrates only in intravascular compartments without invading surrounding parenchyma (14). ICG travels uninhibited and unfiltered through intracranial vessels after the standard 2-mL (i.e., 5 mg ICG/1 mL H_2O) bolus (15–17) is injected into a peripheral vein and appears in as little as 2–3 s under the fluorescent surgical microscope, lasting for a matter of several moments (6, 11). It also harbors favorable pharmacokinetic properties for its purpose of highlighting intraluminal flow. The biological activity of ICG is largely nil inside the body; although it is widely distributed, the liver is the only organ to actively take up ICG (6). Furthermore, the toxicity of ICG is low (2), meaning that several rounds of ICG infusion are generally well-tolerated by the majority of patients, and adverse effects occur only very rarely (17). The most likely adverse effect is allergic cross-reaction in patients with hypersensitivity to iodinated compounds; this, too, has been only very rarely documented (16). With its low side effect profile and negligible overall biologic activity (and thus, toxicity) successive rounds of ICG infusions are limited mainly by parameters such as time until already-present videoangiographic fluorescence dissipates. Practically, because ICG may accumulate in tissues where the blood-brain barrier has been disrupted, the consequential pooling of fluorescence in these areas may obfuscate nearby anatomy if multiple rounds of ICG VA are performed (14).

This combination of physical and pharmacological characteristics makes ICG an ideal choice for delineating superficial AVM anatomy and excluding intervening brain parenchyma. Although near-infrared fluoroscopy has been shown to "penetrate several centimeters into tissue" (18, 19), the obfuscation of deeper anatomy by dilated cortical vessels limits its utility during AVM resection to only real-time evaluation of superficial vascular topography (20). This limitation will be discussed further.

EVIDENCE FROM AND APPLICATIONS DURING AVM RESECTION

The 2007 report by Takagi et al. (9) is the often-cited first publicized use of ICG VA in AVM surgery. In their case report, the authors described the then-novel application of ICG to detect residual nidus during the resection of a Spetzler-Martin grade (SMG) III AVM from a 2-year-old child that was otherwise missed by intraoperative angiography. In their astute recognition of the potential that this newly integrated ICG VA technology might hold, this case report laid the foundation as the first documented use of ICG, and underscored its ancillary use as an immediately available intraoperative adjunct to the angiographic gold standard. Since 2007, several groups of seasoned operators have applied ICG VA to cohorts of patients afflicted with an AVM (1, 3, 10, 12, 15, 21–25).

Killory et al. (10) were the next to publish their experience; they reported their experience with ICG VA used in 10 consecutive AVM resections. Building on the anecdotal success of their predecessors, they effectively applied intraoperative fluorescence and found it subjectively useful for the detection of feeding arteries into the AVM nidus. They also detected a small residual nidus in 1 case. However, they were also the first to draw attention to this technique's major limitation. Namely, deeper vessels could not be visualized with ICG VA in 2 of their patients; those vessels were detected only after they resorted to DSA.

One year later, Ferroli et al. (23) published a case report detailing the use of ICG VA during microvascular decompression for trigeminal neuralgia in a 52-year-old woman in whom a micro-AVM was the unexpected etiology. In this article, they described the usefulness of ICG VA's ability to provide data about flow dynamics of visualized vessels (more specifically, to enable the operator to diagnose the malformation on the basis of an arterialized petrosal vein). Although fluorescent videoangiography did not ultimately surmount the technical challenges of completely resecting this lesion, it did provide data to help the surgeon avoid making the potentially morbid or mortal error of incorrectly ligating the vessel. Their case highlighted a major advantage of ICG VA: its availability and intuitiveness in the operating room, even when its use was not predicted a priori.

That same year, more than 500 miles away, neurosurgeons in Germany reported similar results in 15 patients with an AVM (22). The resolution of resultant videospatial output was graded by researchers in this series, who found ICG injection runs to be of "excellent" quality in the large majority of cases. In 2 of these cases, the ICG VA elucidated information that affected the operative plan, but it failed to fully visualize draining vessels in 1 case (reportedly secondary to the field depth and insufficient illumination).

Nearly 9,000 miles from their German colleagues, Khurana et al. (16) assessed the intuitiveness and usefulness of ICG VA with a "benefit" grade in 4 Australian patients undergoing 5 AVM resection surgeries. The perceived benefit grade was described as a numerical scale from 1 to 4 with the following criteria: "1" indicated that the ICG application was "not useful"; "2" indicated that the fluorescence was seen as "useful, but not affecting surgical management"; a "3" meant that ICG VA was both "useful and affected surgical management"; and a benefit grade of "4" indicated that it provided "false reassurance" (16). ICG VA received a benefit score of 3 in 3 of these patients, indicating that the surgeons found the fluorescence both useful for and influential in surgical management. However, these positive data are tempered by the outcome of the fourth patient; a 22-year-old woman who had a ruptured SMG III insular AVM. ICG VA initially falsely reassured the operators, and a repeat elective resection was necessary (benefit score of 4). In fact, of the 46 operations in which ICG VA was used (which included open aneurysm repair, bypass operations, and tumor resections), this case was the only instance of ICG VA directly misleading the researchers.

Perhaps summarizing 2010's international experience with ICG VA in AVM surgeries, Wang et al. (26) concluded, after retrospective analysis of 43 AVM resections, that no one adjunctive intraoperative modality, ICG VA included, could persistently delineate anatomy and lesional boundaries with the fidelity of DSA. Other groups, such as Taddei et al. (27) on the basis of their own success in 9 AVM operations in India, contrarily maintained that ICG VA might subvert DSA in some cases.

FLOW 800 QUANTIFICATION

The first article describing the use of FLOW 800 quantitative software was published in 2011. Just 4 years after the first publication on ICG VA and AVM surgery, Faber et al. (1) sought to address the subjectivity shortcoming of the technology. Prior to their group's contribution to the methodology, flow quantification had been attempted in several ways as far back as 1998 (28) via laser Doppler perfusion imaging in murine models (29), and diffuse optical spectroscopy with concurrent magnetic resonance correlation in both murine and porcine subjects (28, 30). These methods, however, were impractical in their complexity, requiring both sophisticated technologies and extensive time for interpretation. These obstacles made these earlier methods impractical in the operating room, in which rapid yet accurate assessment would be required. FLOW 800 software was developed to this end. The software is currently available on the OPMI Pentero and Kinevo 900 microscopes (12). FLOW 800 is an analytical software integrated into the intraoperative fluorescent microscope that transcribes the visual data obtained during ICG-laden vessel perfusion into arbitrary intensity units, which then are mathematically corrected for variance in native physiologic flow and fed through a proprietary algorithm to generate a color-coded tissue perfusion map in real time (31). The output of this process can only be considered "semi-quantitative" at best, as the arbitrary intensity units that inform the outputted data are themselves imprecise, non-real data (32). This calculated map also provides information about ICG dye intensity, time to change in intensity from 10 to 90% (i.e., "rise time"), and transit time, which is then interpreted post hoc and used to guide further surgical maneuvers (17, 32).

In the report by Faber et al. (1), this technology was applied during 2 AVM resections: an SMG I incidental malformation in a 38-year-old woman's left frontal lobe, and an epileptogenic SMG III lesion in the right temporal lobe of a 26-year-old man. It is notable that the authors specifically stated that their report was limited to these 2 cases because the lesions therein had characteristics amenable to trialing the newly developed color-encoded flow technology. Nevertheless, the authors described their inaugural experience favorably. In one respect, they commended the ergonomics of the FLOW 800 application in the operating room, even for novice users. In another, they found that quantitation of flow provided valuable insight to understanding how hemodynamics into and out of the AVM nidus were affected by ligation and resection as the procedure progressed. However, these advantages were not enough to overcome the inability of ICG VA to provide data about complex 3-dimensional structures; it remains ill-equipped to assess along the z-axis of deep-seated AVMs. As stated by Kalyvas and Spetzler (33), because FLOW 800 output is calculated from ICG VA input, it will inevitably suffer from the same lack of penetrance.

After their influential first report, Takagi et al. (15) and Kamp et al. (31) reported in 2012 on their continued experiences with 27 runs of ICG VA with FLOW 800 analysis and DSA in a series of 11 and 2 AVM resections, respectively. The researchers used ICG VA at various time points during their procedures, split roughly equally between uses before dissection, after arterial feeder clippings, and after dissection, as guided by perceived need and experience. When compared to DSA, ICG VA performed comparably, visualizing nidal filling before dissection and reliably excluding residual nidal filling after resection in 100% of cases. However, even in experienced hands, ICG VA fell short of matching the ability of DSA to visualize arterial feeding vessels (33 vs. 100%, respectively) and venous drainage vessels (89 vs. 100%, respectively). Although the authors praised ICG VA's intraoperative facility, they concluded by noting its inferiority to the DSA gold standard, particularly in regard to the detection of feeders. Furthermore, the small cohort of patients was specifically chosen for the superficial drainage patterns of their lesions, which might have further biased their opinion about the usefulness of ICG VA.

Ng et al. (21) further discussed the limitations of ICG in AVM resection in their retrospective study published the following year. Over 3 years, ICG VA with FLOW 800 quantification was performed 49 times in their cohort of 24 patients with AVMs. Their experience in many ways mirrored that of previous publications. Namely, ICG VA was useful primarily in confirming totality of resection by way of the absence of fluorescent flow through the primary draining vein. The authors found ICG VA in the detection of arterial feeders before dissection less useful than others had reported before them. In this cohort, 15% of predissection ICG runs were considered not useful by researchers because of "a thin layer of adherent clot" (21). Furthermore, although the authors endorsed FLOW 800 quantitative analysis for helping to distinguish between entering and exiting vessels on the basis of flow delay and intensity, they also lamented the need for relatively trivial maneuvers (i.e., removal of cottonoids, blood, and cerebrospinal fluid from the operative field) to prevent inaccurate ICG intensity readings during quantification. This study was unique in that it did not use concomitant DSA in validating the results of ICG VA. A study of 25 AVM surgeries by Ye et al. (25) that same year recapitulated these data closely, reporting that quantification and emulation of transit time was more useful than visualization on normal playback mode alone in differentiating pathologic from native vessels *in situ*.

In 2014, the Spetzler group published what is thought to be the largest consecutive case series of ICG VA in AVM surgery to date (3). They retrospectively reviewed data from 130 patients divided nearly equally into ICG and no-ICG groups that were otherwise similar according to patient and baseline lesion characteristics, and their results revealed no statistically significant difference between the extent of AVM resection or improvement in functional outcome as measured by the modified Rankin score at 6 weeks (12.5 vs. 14.9%, respectively) (3). Despite these equivocal data, the authors maintained that the results were at least in part attributable to the poor penetrance of direct light and consequent ICG fluorescence in deeper vasculature. The study encouraged its continued use in surgery to treat superficially seated AVMs.

A 2015 study of 7 patients who underwent ICG VA–mediated AVM resection by Fukuda et al. (34) resulted in the first detailed quantitative assessment of flow delay (measured by time to half-maximum fluorescence intensity) at various stages of the operation. Their data revealed that these calculated parameters are reliable and intuitive indicators of decreased intranidal flow after sequential and successful feeder clipping. The authors recommended FLOW 800 as reasonable inclusion in the cerebrovascular neurosurgeon's AVM armamentarium given its ability to provide data on changing hemodynamics as the resection progresses. However, a commentary on this study by Kalyvas and Spetzler (33) throttled this notion to a degree by reiterating that FLOW 800 will share the same limitations as non-quantitative ICG VA, because its output also relies on what fluorescence can be directly observed on the surface.

SPINAL AVMs

Vascular malformations of the spinal cord are grossly similar to their intracranial counterparts, yet are also distinct entities that require a specialized surgical approach. There are far fewer available data regarding the application of ICG VA techniques to these lesions in the neurosurgical library because, in part, of their overall lower incidence (35). Nevertheless, several recent case series have described institutional-specific techniques for ICG application to spinal AVMs in larger cohorts (35–37). Similar to the relationship between DSA and ICG VA of cerebral vessels, ICG VA of spinal vasculature is an increasingly employed intraoperative alternative to the "gold standard" of selective spinal angiography. ICG VA has been used adjunctively in the operating room even after preoperative selective spinal angiography was performed, particularly when the lesion of interest has multiple feeders or appears to be primarily irrigated via the indispensable Artery of Adamkiewicz (36, 37). The arguments for and against ICG VA in spinal AVMs are likewise remarkably similar, with advocates championing ICG VA's practicality and ease of rapid intraoperative interpretation to help inform safe surgical resection and preservation of uninvolved angioarchitecture (37). The technique for its infusion during surgery is also similar, and follows a regimented paradigm of a 25 mg bolus diluted in 50 mL of sterile normal saline via a peripheral vein (35, 37). The slightly modified semi-quantitative software, IR800 (also a product of Carl Zeiss Meditec), may also be readily employed through equipped intraoperative surgical microscopes to aid in the often-challenging identification of niduses and fistulas.

These published reports, though limited to single institution case series, reflect on several years of operator experience in applying ICA VA to the resection of spinal AVMs. They represent a small but apparently growing consensus on ICG VA's usefulness to these challenging operations. Although far more research is needed to address the current paucity of published data on the matter, these foundational case series are sparking innovation and unique applications of their own. In a recent study by Hamauchi et al. (38), ICG was used in combination with catheter-based intraoperative super-selective spinal angiography and high frame rate videography to help identify abnormal vasculature in a single thoracic intramedullary AVM. The slow-motion replaying of the captured video data was reportedly influential in the surgeons' resection approach, and provided crucial qualitative feedback in real-time to help guide an effective operation. This report on a single patient and lesion obviously warrants further rigorous investigation to prove its merits, but is representative of the ongoing interest in applying ICG VA to help treat challenging vascular malformations of the spinal cord.

SURGICAL PEARLS

The limitations previously discussed are perhaps unsurprising to the neurosurgical community at large. The predominately deep-to-superficial anatomical arrangement of intracranial vessels inherently limits any modality that relies on direct visualization and illumination. Today, no means to fully rectify this limitation has been found, but it still might be attenuated by a combination of operator experience and deft applications of the technology. For example, in 2017, one such experienced group published a video documenting their surgical treatment of a large, eloquently located frontoparietal SMG III AVM in a 31-year-old man who presented with hemiparesis after the malformation ruptured (24). The challenges of the case included the largely subcortical focus of the AVM and its proximity to the central sulcus. Despite these challenges, the surgeons prudently used ICG VA to detect a superficial arterialized draining vein from the lesion and simultaneously differentiated it from the nearby vein of Trolard. The authors used this finding to navigate a subcortical dissection path for the complete resection of the AVM per standard resection techniques. Aptly named the "safe sulcus" approach, this clever application of ICG VA exploits its aforementioned superficial limitation to identify an appropriate starting point for subcortical dissection. This approach has since been adopted by other groups with similar success (39). It represents a novel application of a no-longer-novel neurosurgical technology.

The senior author recently published his experience using ICG VA in a small group of patients who were undergoing cerebrovascular neurosurgery (12) (**Figure 1**). FLOW 800 software was used in 10 patients with an AVM in this case series of 23 for the purpose of guiding intraoperative planning and progression. It is the senior author's practice to use only the color maps that are output after semi-quantification because the fluorescence curves that are produced, although valuable in their own right, are not amenable to rapid intraoperative evaluation and thereby extend the patient's time in surgery. ICG was injected intravenously before dissection of the malformation to delineate the angioarchitecture of the lesion and to reliably differentiate involved structures including the feeding arteries from arterialized veins and the uninvolved *en passage* vessels. Of note, to accurately evaluate ICG VA intraoperatively, it is necessary to position the operative microscope at a predefined distance from the operative field and adjust the zoom and focus accordingly. These variables are dependent upon the microscope, and one should consult the microscope's user manual prior to the case.

In 2 of these cases, careful study of the resultant maps enabled the disconnection of an arterialized draining vein and preservation of crucial normal venous drainage. In another illustrative case of a medial parasagittal AVM, mobilization of the hemisphere was made possible after ICG VA enabled the operator to discern high-throughput cortical arterialized bridging veins from those less vigorously irrigated and therefore safe for sacrifice. To our knowledge, this application of the technology is not represented elsewhere in the literature. Although it requires a coupling of comfort with the interhemispheric approach and confidence in interpreting color map data, quantified ICG VA can be cautiously adapted for this purpose.

Nuanced quantitative ICG VA color mapping is particularly useful in a subset of AVMs with specific characteristics, as previous studies have concluded. Intraoperative fluorescent flow analysis directly influenced dissection strategies in each of the cases in the senior author's study. We find ICG VA to be most effective when judicious patient and lesion selection has occurred. For example, superficial AVM anatomy may appear obscured to the naked eye because of overlying dense arachnoid bands. In these cases, ICG VA makes an important contribution to the surgical stratagem by providing real-time data on vascular structures that would otherwise have to be dissected blindly and therefore haphazardly, guided by direct visualization alone. It is also regularly used, in our experience, when there is concern for inadvertent clip-induced *en passage* vessel stenosis. The integrated FLOW 800–capable operative microscope makes evaluation in these cases especially easy by obviating the need to rearrange surgical equipment during the operation. In fact, at least 1 study found ICG VA to be statistically significantly faster to deploy than DSA (34).

The additional time needed to perform DSA might nevertheless be warranted by the equipoise of safety in some situations. For example, in a 2013 article, Kono et al. (40) described the intra-arterial infusion of ICG into the common carotid and vertebral arteries. Although this technique successfully differentiated AVM feeding vessels from normal native arteries, we opine that the additional risk of arterial catheterization in the neck likely nullifies the benefit gained and can be performed more safely via standard DSA. For these reasons, we respectfully do not recommend this form of ICG VA technique.

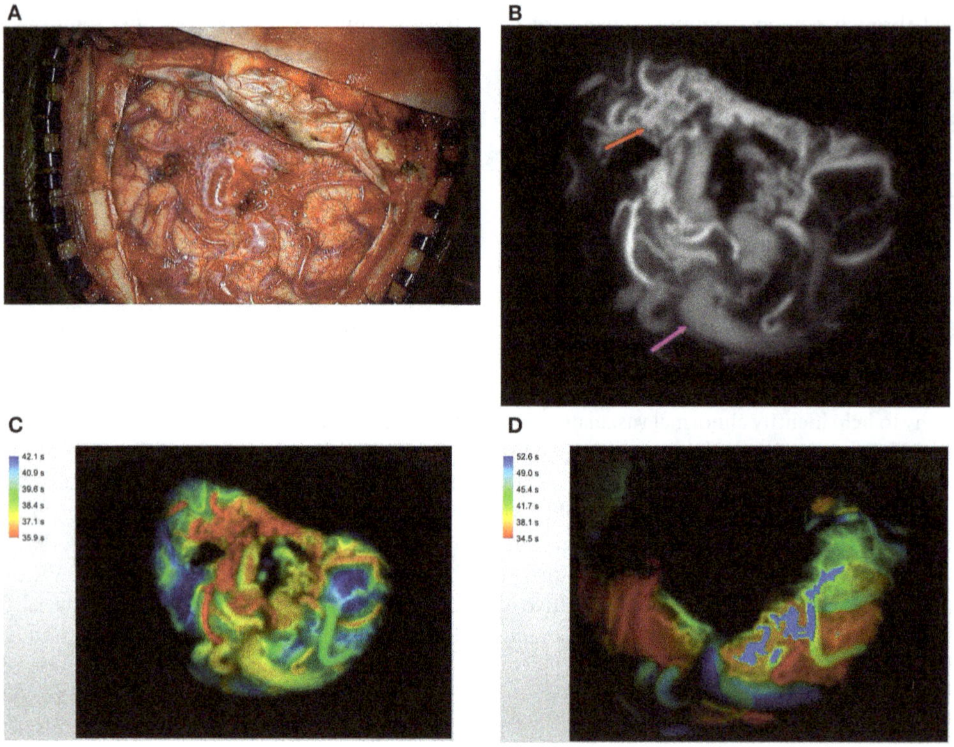

FIGURE 1 | A large right temporoparietal AVM is exposed **(A)**. ICG videoangiography **(B)** demonstrates the early filling of the arterial feeders (red arrow) and delayed filling of arterialized veins (purple arrow); this technique can confirm the identity of these vessels more accurately especially if they are covered by thick arachnoid bands. This information can also guide the early steps of disconnection to start in the area where the concentration of feeding arteries is most (red arrow). The same AVM was analyzed via the use of FLOW 800 software. Please note the feeding arteries in red, arterialized veins in yellow, and normal veins in blue **(C)**. Post-resection FLOW 800 analysis demonstrates that the primary vein is now blue **(D)**.

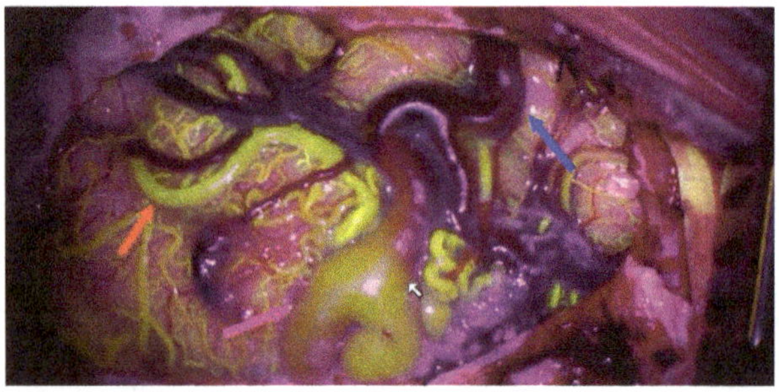

FIGURE 2 | Fluorescein videoangioram of a parietal AVM demonstrates the relative flow in different components of the AVM: feeding artery (red arrow), arterialized vein (purple arrow), and normal vein (blue arrow).

Our team has also used fluorescein in place of the ICG and has found reasonable results similar to those of the ICG (41, 42). The advantage of fluorescein over ICG is that the dye can be visualized through the microscope's binoculars (**Figure 2**) (43).

Altogether, these data make a strong argument for the role of ICG VA as an adjunct modality in AVM surgery, fulfilling a specific purpose with relative ease in a specific group of lesions. This general gestalt seems to be shared by other experienced operators at high-volume centers (3, 33). Despite the strides made toward objectifying ICG VA with FLOW 800 and the new applications being conceived by shrewd surgeons, current data suggest that ICG VA cannot emulate AVM anatomy with fidelity superior to that of DSA, especially for subcortical structures.

CONCLUSION

Studies unanimously agree that ICG VA with FLOW 800 quantitative analysis is an accurate method of delineating superficial AVM structures, but it suffers in regard to deeper structures. In our opinion and experience, it can be used effectively to guide cortical entry points for subcortical dissections and to inform the safe sacrifice of tethering secondary cortical arterialized veins in certain surgical approaches. Likewise, the generated color maps of FLOW 800 are practical, easily interpreted intraoperatively, and sufficient for guiding surgical resection. Although ICG VA has advantages over DSA in terms of deployment speed and ease of use, its inability to visualize subcortical AVM components remains a looming obstacle. Therefore, DSA remains the gold-standard method of confirming complete AVM occlusion (33).

Only 1 systematic review (4) and 2 general reviews (2, 5) of the data on ICG VA in AVM surgery exist in the neurosurgical literature. The systematic review by Scerrati et al. (4), which was published in 2014 and included 7 of the AVM studies available at the time, succinctly concluded that ICG VA might portend a "modest benefit" during AVM resection. Indeed, there is a paucity of adequately powered, prospective, multicenter studies that have investigated the true effect size that this fluorescent technology has on various outcome measures. Although current data on the topic are an amalgam of anecdotes and subjectivity, experienced groups of surgeons worldwide seem to agree that the low toxicity, non-invasiveness, intuitiveness, and real-time feedback offered by ICG VA make it a reasonable tool in the cerebrovascular neurosurgeon's repertoire for open AVM resection. Although the margins and magnitude of this role have yet to be established, it is a meritorious goal for future research.

AUTHOR CONTRIBUTIONS

CF performed literature review, synthesized data, and prepared the draft of the final manuscript. PM reviewed, edited, and augmented the drafted manuscript. ST assisted with gathering and contributing data for the drafting of the manuscript. AC-G reviewed and edited the drafted manuscript, provided expertise to technical portions of the manuscript, and provided supervisory support.

REFERENCES

1. Faber F, Thon N, Fesl G, Rachinger W, Guckler R, Tonn JC, et al. Enhanced analysis of intracerebral arterioveneous malformations by the intraoperative use of analytical indocyanine green videoangiography: technical note. *Acta Neurochir.* (2011) 153:2181–7. doi: 10.1007/s00701-011-1141-z
2. Cenzato M, Dones F, Boeris D, Marcati E, Fratianni A, Crisa FM, et al. Contemporary tools in arteriovenous malformations surgery. *J Neurosurg Sci.* (2018) 62:467–77. doi: 10.23736/S0390-5616.18.04398-9
3. Zaidi HA, Abla AA, Nakaji P, Chowdhry SA, Albuquerque FC, Spetzler RF. Indocyanine green angiography in the surgical management of cerebral arteriovenous malformations: lessons learned in 130 consecutive cases. *Neurosurgery.* (2014) 10:246–51. doi: 10.1227/NEU.0000000000000318
4. Scerrati A, Della Pepa GM, Conforti G, Sabatino G, Puca A, Albanese A, et al. Indocyanine green video-angiography in neurosurgery: a glance beyond vascular applications. *Clin Neurol Neurosurg.* (2014) 124:106–13. doi: 10.1016/j.clineuro.2014.06.032
5. Balamurugan S, Agrawal A, Kato Y, Sano H. Intra operative indocyanine green video-angiography in cerebrovascular surgery: An overview with review of literature. *Asian J Neurosur.* (2011) 6:88–93. doi: 10.4103/1793-5482.92168
6. Bervini D, Raabe A. Principles of indocyanine green videoangiography. In: Hadjipanayis CG, Stummer W, editors. *Fluorescence-Guided Neurosurgery: Neuro-oncology and Cerebrovascular Applications.* 1st ed. New York, NY: Thieme Medical Publishers, Inc. (2018). p. 125–31.
7. Hongo K, Kobayashi S, Okudera H, Hokama M, Nakagawa F. Noninvasive cerebral optical spectroscopy: depth-resolved measurements of cerebral haemodynamics using indocyanine green. *Neurol Res.* (1995) 17:89–93. doi: 10.1080/01616412.1995.11740293
8. Raabe A, Beck J, Gerlach R, Zimmermann M, Seifert V. Near-infrared indocyanine green video angiography: a new method for intraoperative assessment of vascular flow. *Neurosurgery.* (2003) 52:132–9. doi: 10.1227/00006123-200301000-00017
9. Takagi Y, Kikuta K, Nozaki K, Sawamura K, Hashimoto N. Detection of a residual nidus by surgical microscope-integrated intraoperative near-infrared indocyanine green videoangiography in a child with a cerebral arteriovenous malformation. *J Neurosurg.* (2007) 107:416–8. doi: 10.3171/PED-07/11/416
10. Killory BD, Nakaji P, Gonzales LF, Ponce FA, Wait SD, Spetzler RF. Prospective evaluation of surgical microscope-integrated intraoperative near-infrared indocyanine green angiography during cerebral arteriovenous malformation surgery. *Neurosurgery.* (2009) 65:456–62. doi: 10.1227/01.NEU.0000346649.48114.3A
11. Yeung JT, Kalani MY, Nakaji P. Applications of indocyanine green video angiography in neurovascular surgery. In: Spetzler RF, Kalani MYS, Nakaji P, editors. *Neurovascular Surgery.* 2nd ed. New York, NY: Thieme Medical Publishers, Inc. (2015). p. 194–200.
12. Shah KJ, Cohen-Gadol AA. The application of FLOW 800 ICG videoangiography color maps for neurovascular surgery and intraoperative decision making. *World Neurosurg.* (2018) 122:e186–97. doi: 10.1016/j.wneu.2018.09.195
13. Pogue BW, Gibbs-Strauss S, Valdes PA, Samkoe K, Roberts DW, Paulsen KD. Review of neurosurgical fluorescence imaging methodologies. *IEEE J Sel Top Quantum Electron.* (2010) 16:493–505. doi: 10.1109/JSTQE.2009.2034541
14. Roberts DW, Valdes PA. Indocyanine green. In: Bernstein M, Berger MS, editors. *Neuro-Oncology: The Essentials.* 3rd ed. New York, NY: Thieme Medical Publishers, Inc. (2014). p. 136–46.
15. Takagi Y, Sawamura K, Hashimoto N, Miyamoto S. Evaluation of serial intraoperative surgical microscope-integrated intraoperative near-infrared indocyanine green videoangiography in patients with cerebral arteriovenous malformations. *Neurosurgery.* (2012) 70:34–42. doi: 10.1227/NEU.0b013e31822d9749
16. Khurana VG, Seow K, Duke D. Intuitiveness, quality and utility of intraoperative fluorescence videoangiography: Australian neurosurgical experience. *Brit J Neurosurg.* (2010) 24:163–72. doi: 10.3109/02688690903518247
17. Kato N, Prinz V, Dengler J, Vajkoczy P. Blood flow assessment of arteriovenous malformations using intraoperative indocyanine green videoangiography. *Stroke Res Treat.* (2019) 2019:7292304. doi: 10.1155/2019/7292304
18. Desmettre T, Devoisselle JM, Mordon S. Fluorescence properties and metabolic features of indocyanine green (ICG) as related to angiography. *Surv Ophthalmol.* (2000) 45:15–27. doi: 10.1016/S0039-6257(00)00123-5
19. Liebert A, Wabnitz H, Obrig H, Erdmann R, Moller M, Macdonald R, et al. Non-invasive detection of fluorescence from exogenous chromophores in the adult human brain. *Neuroimage.* (2006) 31:600–8. doi: 10.1016/j.neuroimage.2005.12.046
20. Mascitelli JR, Burkhardt J-K, Lawton MT. Indocyanine green videoangiography and arteriovenous malformations. In: Hadjipanayis CG, Stummer W, editors. *Fluorescence-Guided Neurosurgery: Neuro-Oncology and Cerebrovascular Applications.* 1st ed. New York, NY: Thieme Medical Publishers, Inc. (2018). p. 133–40.
21. Ng YP, King NK, Wan KR, Wang E, Ng I. Uses and limitations of indocyanine green videoangiography for flow analysis in arteriovenous malformation surgery. *J Clin Neurosci.* (2013) 20:224–32. doi: 10.1016/j.jocn.2011.12.038
22. Hanggi D, Etminan N, Steiger HJ. The impact of microscope-integrated intraoperative near-infrared indocyanine green videoangiography on surgery of arteriovenous malformations and dural arteriovenous fistulae. *Neurosurgery.* (2010) 67:1094–103. doi: 10.1227/NEU.0b013e3181eb5049
23. Ferroli P, Acerbi F, Broggi M, Broggi G. Arteriovenous micromalformation of the trigeminal root: intraoperative diagnosis with indocyanine green videoangiography: case report. *Neurosurgery.* (2010) 67:(3 Suppl Operative):onsE309–10; discussion: onsE10. doi: 10.1227/01.NEU.0000381769.15291.4C
24. Rustemi O, Scienza R, Della Puppa A. Utility of indocyanine green videoangiography in subcortical arteriovenous malformation resection. *Neurosurg Focus.* (2017) 43:V10. doi: 10.3171/2017.7.FocusVid.1774
25. Ye X, Liu XJ, Ma L, Liu LT, Wang WL, Wang S, et al. Clinical values of intraoperative indocyanine green fluorescence video angiography with Flow 800 software in cerebrovascular surgery. *Chin Med J.* (2013) 126:4232–7. doi: 10.3760/cma.j.issn.0366-6999.20131649

26. Wang S, Liu L, Zhao YL, Zhang D, Wang R, Zhao JZ. Strategy for assisted cerebral arteriovenous malformation surgery. *Zhonghua yi xue za zhi.* (2010) 90:869–73.
27. Taddei G, Tommasi CD, Ricci A, Galzio RJ. Arteriovenous malformations and intraoperative indocyanine green videoangiography: preliminary experience. *Neurology India.* (2011) 59:97–100. doi: 10.4103/0028-3886.76878
28. Kuebler WM, Sckell A, Habler O, Kleen M, Kuhnle GE, Welte M, et al. Noninvasive measurement of regional cerebral blood flow by near-infrared spectroscopy and indocyanine green. *J Cerebral Blood Flow Metab.* (1998) 18:445–56. doi: 10.1097/00004647-199804000-00013
29. Wuestenfeld JC, Herold J, Niese U, Kappert U, Schmeisser A, Strasser RH, et al. Indocyanine green angiography: a new method to quantify collateral flow in mice. *J Vascular Surg.* (2008) 48:1315–21. doi: 10.1016/j.jvs.2008.06.049
30. Cuccia DJ, Bevilacqua F, Durkin AJ, Merritt S, Tromberg BJ, Gulsen G, et al. *In vivo* quantification of optical contrast agent dynamics in rat tumors by use of diffuse optical spectroscopy with magnetic resonance imaging coregistration. *Appl Optics.* (2003) 42:2940–50. doi: 10.1364/AO.42.002940
31. Kamp MA, Slotty P, Turowski B, Etminan N, Steiger HJ, Hanggi D, et al. Microscope-integrated quantitative analysis of intraoperative indocyanine green fluorescence angiography for blood flow assessment: first experience in 30 patients. *Neurosurgery.* (2012) 7065–73. doi: 10.1227/NEU.0b013e31822f7d7c
32. Prinz V, Hecht N, Kato N, Vajkoczy P. FLOW 800 allows visualization of hemodynamic changes after extracranial-to-intracranial bypass surgery but not assessment of quantitative perfusion or flow. *Neurosurgery.* (2014) 10(Suppl. 2):231–8; discussion: 8–9. doi: 10.1227/NEU.0000000000000277
33. Kalyvas J, Spetzler RF. Does FLOW 800 technology improve the utility of indocyanine green videoangiography in cerebral arteriovenous malformation surgery? *World Neurosurgery.* (2015) 83:147–8. doi: 10.1016/j.wneu.2014.09.010
34. Fukuda K, Kataoka H, Nakajima N, Masuoka J, Satow T, Iihara K. Efficacy of FLOW 800 with indocyanine green videoangiography for the quantitative assessment of flow dynamics in cerebral arteriovenous malformation surgery. *World Neurosurgery.* (2015) 83:203–10. doi: 10.1016/j.wneu.2014.07.012
35. Rangel-Castilla L, Russin JJ, Zaidi HA, Martinez-Del-Campo E, Park MS, Albuquerque FC, et al. Contemporary management of spinal AVFs and AVMs: lessons learned from 110 cases. *Neurosurgical Focus.* (2014) 37:E14. doi: 10.3171/2014.7.FOCUS14236
36. Walsh DC, Zebian B, Tolias CM, Gullan RW. Intraoperative indocyanine green video-angiography as an aid to the microsurgical treatment of spinal vascular malformations. *Brit J Neurosurg.* (2014) 28:259–66. doi: 10.3109/02688697.2013.829556
37. Jing L, Su W, Guo Y, Sun Z, Wang J, Wang G. Microsurgical treatment and outcomes of spinal arteriovenous lesions: learned from consecutive series of 105 lesions. *J Clin.* (2017) 46:141–7. doi: 10.1016/j.jocn.2017.09.003
38. Hamauchi S, Osanai T, Seki T, Kawabori M, Okamoto M, Hida K, et al. Intraoperative real-time identification of abnormal vessels within the bright field by superselective arterial injection of saline and its slow-motion recording using a high frame rate digital camera during surgical treatment of spinal arteriovenous shunts: technical note. *J Neurosurg Spine.* (2018) 29:576–81. doi: 10.3171/2018.3.SPINE1854
39. Muhammad S, Niemela M, Lehecka M. Utility of video indocyanine angiography to detect the cortical entry point of a draining vein with a superficial vein during arteriovenous malformation surgery. *World Neurosurgery.* (2019) 122:428. doi: 10.1016/j.wneu.2018.11.054
40. Kono K, Uka A, Mori M, Haga S, Hamada Y, Nagata S. Intra-arterial injection of indocyanine green in cerebral arteriovenous malformation surgery. *Turkish Neurosurg.* (2013) 23:676–9. doi: 10.5137/1019-5149.JTN.6420-12.0
41. Lane BC, Cohen-Gadol AA. A prospective study of microscope-integrated intraoperative fluorescein videoangiography during arteriovenous malformation surgery: preliminary results. *Neurosurg Focus.* (2014) 36:E15. doi: 10.3171/2013.11.FOCUS13483
42. Lane BC, Cohen-Gadol AA. Fluorescein fluorescence use in the management of intracranial neoplastic and vascular lesions: a review and report of a new technique. *Curr Drug Discov Technol.* (2013) 10:160–9. doi: 10.2174/1570163811310020009
43. Rey-Dios R, Cohen-Gadol AA. Technical principles and neurosurgical applications of fluorescein fluorescence using a microscope-integrated fluorescence module. *Acta Neurochir.* (2013) 155:701–6. doi: 10.1007/s00701-013-1635-y

17

Efficacy of Indocyanine Green Fluorescence Angiography in Preventing Anastomotic Leakage After McKeown Minimally Invasive Esophagectomy

Rao-Jun Luo [1], Zi-Yi Zhu [1], Zheng-Fu He [1], Yong Xu [1], Yun-Zheng Wang [1] and Ping Chen [2]*

[1] *Department of Thoracic Surgery, Sir Run Run Shaw Hospital, School of Medicine, Zhejiang University, Hangzhou, China,*
[2] *Zhejiang Provincial Key Laboratory of Laparoscopic Technology, Sir Run Run Shaw Hospital, School of Medicine, Zhejiang University, Hangzhou, China*

***Correspondence:**
Zi-Yi Zhu
zhuziyicn@zju.edu.cn

Background: Indocyanine green (ICG) fluorescence angiography (FA) was introduced to provide real-time intraoperative evaluation of the vascular perfusion of the gastric conduit during esophagectomy. However, its efficacy has not yet been proven. The aim of this study was to assess the usefulness of ICG-FA in the reduction of the rates of anastomotic leakage (AL) in McKeown minimally invasive esophagectomy (MIE).

Methods: From June 2017 to December 2019, patients aged between 18 and 80 years with esophageal carcinoma were enrolled in the study and each patient underwent McKeown MIE. Patients were divided into two groups, those with or without ICG-FA. The patient demographics and perioperative outcomes were comparable between the two groups. The primary outcome was the rate of AL.

Results: A total of 192 patients were included: 86 in the ICG-FA group and 106 in the non-ICG-FA group. Overall, 12 patients (6.3%) had AL; the rate of AL was 10.4% in the non-ICG-FA group, which was significantly higher than the 1.2% in the ICG-FA group.

Conclusions: ICG-FA has the potential to reduce the rate of AL in McKeown MIE.

Keywords: gastric conduit, McKeown, minimally invasive esophagectomy, indocyanine green fluorescence angiography, anastomotic leakage

INTRODUCTION

Esophageal cancer is the eighth most common cancer and the sixth leading cause of cancer-related death worldwide (1, 2). The incidence of esophageal cancer in China ranks fifth in terms of malignant tumors and the mortality rate ranks fourth (3, 4). Esophagectomy is still the mainstream multidisciplinary treatment for esophageal cancer in combination with chemoradiotherapy (4). Esophagectomy is an invasive and complicated procedure, and the frequency of postoperative complications is as high as 59% (5). Anastomotic leakage (AL) after esophagectomy is one of the most dreaded postoperative complications, and is responsible for higher postoperative morbidity and mortality rates, prolonged hospital stays, and the need for further surgical procedures (6, 7).

Several risk factors are involved in the development of AL; some are unchangeable, such as age, body mass index (BMI), comorbidities, and advanced tumor stage, while others, such as anastomotic tension, location of anastomosis, surgical technique, and postoperative factors, are modifiable, and many efforts have been made to decrease AL in the last decades (8–10). However, vascular perfusion to the anastomotic regions is considered to be the main driving force of AL (7, 10). In the construction of gastric conduits, it is difficult for the gastroepiploic arcade to reach the distal end of the conduit. The blood supply to the rest of the gastric tube is mainly provided by submucosal vessels. Evaluation of vascular perfusion in the area undergoing anastomosis depends largely on the objective identification of the gastric serosa by surgeons. Therefore, correctly identifying the anastomosis perfusion and selecting an appropriate anastomotic site are important to reduce AL (11).

As a means of evaluating blood flow, indocyanine green (ICG) fluorescence angiography (FA) has recently been introduced to provide real-time assessment of the anastomosis area during esophagectomy (11–13). ICG is a hydrophilic tricarbonyl cyanine dye that quickly binds to plasma proteins after intravenous injection. When the ICG binding protein is excited by a light source at 750 to 810 nm, it emits peak fluorescence around 840 nm and allows for the detection of signals as deep as 10 mm within the tissue. Therefore, ICG can be used as both a lymphatic and vascular contrast agent (14).

Although some studies have reported that ICG-FA is a potentially promising method to assess gastric vascular perfusion, these studies have limitations such as a small population study, the use of various surgical methods, or lack of a control group (10–17). Therefore, it is still unclear whether ICG-FA can decrease the rate of AL during esophagectomy. As a retrospective cohort trial, the aim of our study was to investigate the real-time perfusion of the conduit using ICG-FA during esophageal procedures. In addition, we sought to assess the efficacy of ICG-FA in the reduction of AL rates in McKeown minimally invasive esophagectomy (MIE).

MATERIALS AND METHODS

Patients

This retrospective cohort study included 192 consecutive patients with esophageal carcinoma who underwent McKeown MIE with cervical anastomosis between January 2017 and December 2019 at our hospital. Patients aged between 18 and 80 years with histologically proven primary esophageal carcinoma that was considered to be resectable were qualified. All patients underwent routine examinations, including routine blood tests, blood biochemical examinations, and electrocardiograms. Computed tomography of the chest and abdominal (CT), positron emission tomography (PET-CT), and B-ultrasound were implemented to rule out cervical lymph node metastasis. Patients with a previous history of gastrointestinal or lung cancer, severe comorbidities, other organ metastasis, combined other organ resection, or allergic hypersensitivity to ICG or iodine were excluded. The patients' treatment strategies were formulated by a multidisciplinary expert team, and all patients' operations were carried out by the same surgical team. The research protocol for this clinical study was approved by the local ethics committee. Evaluation of gastric vascular perfusion at the anastomosis sites using ICG fluorescence angiography initiated in June 2018 when an advanced laparoscopic system equipped with near-infrared camera was introduced. Since then, the ICG-FA system has been used in all patients, except for patients with allergic hypersensitivity to ICG or when the ICG-FA system was occupied by other surgical groups.

Analysis

The patients were divided into two groups: Patients who did not undergo ICG-FA were classified as the non-ICG-FA group, and patients who received ICG-FA were classified as the ICG-FA group. The collected individual and tumor-related characteristics included age, sex, BMI, comorbidities, history of smoking, history of drinking, American Society of Anesthesiologists (ASA), histopathology details, and tumor location. Information on preoperative therapies, including neoadjuvant radiotherapy (NRC), neoadjuvant chemotherapy (NAC), and endoscopic submucosal dissection (ESD), was also collected. Perioperative outcomes and complications were assessed. The primary endpoint was the rate of AL within 30 days after the initial surgery, or the rate of AL before the patient recovered from discharge. AL was defined as extravasation of contrast on postoperative CT image, presence of empyema on chest CT, or elevated drain amylase level with clinical evidence of leak (11). Postoperative electronic gastroscopy was arranged to inspect the situation around the anastomosis in suspected individuals. The secondary outcomes were operative time, blood loss, time until restoration of fluid diet, length of hospital stay, postoperative complications and oncological clearance.

Surgical Techniques

In our institution, we performed McKeown MIE with cervical anastomosis for esophageal cancer. The details of these procedures have been described previously (18). Briefly, disconnection of the azygous vein, incision of the mediastinal pleura, and dissection of the paraoesophageal and mediastinal lymph nodes was completed. The thoracic esophagus was mobilized from the azygous arch to the diaphragm hiatus while protecting the thoracic duct. The patients were then placed in a lithotomy position, and the gastrocolic ligament was separated along the greater curvature with protection of the gastroepiploic vascular arch (19). The gastric conduit was closed with an Endo-GIA stapler (ECR60, Echelon, USA) through a 5-cm mini-incision in the upper abdomen and the appropriate width of the gastric conduit was 3–4 cm based on our experience (18). Seromuscular layer sewing was routinely preferred. The cervical esophagus was mobilized after making an oblique incision on the left neck, and the gastric conduit was pulled up through the esophageal bed to the left neck incision for gastroesophageal end-to-side anastomosis (SDH 25A or SDH 21A, Ethicon Endo-Surgery, USA).

ICG Fluorescence Angiograph

The gastric conduit was created outside the abdominal cavity and placed on the anterior chest wall (**Figure 1A**). Surgeons checked the conditions of the gastric conduit, such as the color of the gastric serosa, arterial pulsation of the gastroepiploic artery, and the connection between the right and left gastroepiploic vessels (16). Subsequently, 0.5 mg/kg or a maximum of 25 mg of ICG dye (Diagnostic Green, Dandong Yichuang Pharmaceutical, Liaoning, China) was diluted in 10 cc of sterile water, and was injected as a bolus through a central venous catheter by assistant. A near-infrared camera system (Novadaq Technologies Inc. Richmond, Canada) was used for detecting the ICG fluorescence. The surgeon hold the camera 20 cm away from the gastric conduit and the evaluation with fluorescence was performed in real-time. Approximately 20 s after injection, blood flow was confirmed by ICG-FA as it passed through the right gastroepiploic vessels (**Figure 1B**). If vascular perfusion *via* ICG-FA was well visualized within 60 s, it was defined as a good perfusion zone (**Figure 1C**), while no vascular perfusion or perfusion times > 60 s were considered to indicate a poor perfusion zone (**Figure 1D**). The anastomotic perfusion result using ICG-FA was subjectively evaluated by the surgical team and the anastomosis was performed within the good perfusion zone. After the anastomosis, the poorly perfused zone of conduit was removed. The aforementioned area referred to the area where the perfusion time exceeds 60 s, such as the area at the far end of the green arrow in the figure (**Figure 1D**). We created the anastomosis in accordance with the 60 s rule.

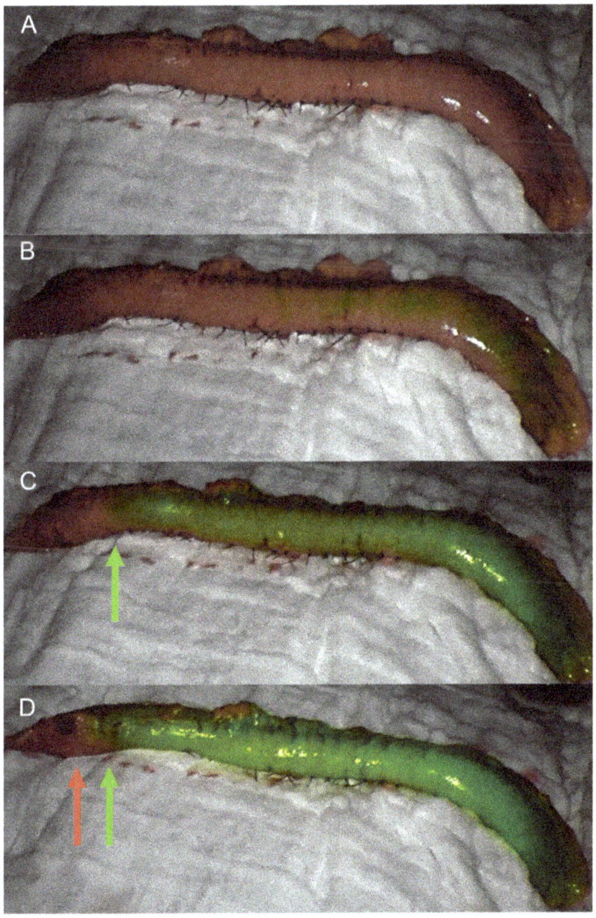

FIGURE 1 | Fluorescence evaluation during McKeown MIE. **(A)** The gastric conduit was pulled up and placed on the anterior chest wall. **(B)** Fluorescence was observed at the root of the conduit approximately 20 s after the injection. **(C)** The good perfusion zone was visualized within 60 s, and anastomosis was performed within the planned transection line (green arrow). **(D)** No vascular perfusion or perfusion times > 60 s were considered to indicate the poor perfusion zone (red arrow).

Statistical Analysis

Descriptive statistics were used to depict the demographic parameters of the patients. Measurement data are expressed as mean ± standard deviation. The independent sample t-test was used for comparison between groups, while Mann–Whitney U and Pearson's $\chi 2$ tests were performed to test the difference between the two groups. Statistical analysis was completed using SPSS® version 22 (IBM Corp. in Armonk, NY, USA), with $p < 0.05$ indicating a statistically significant difference.

RESULTS

Demographic Parameters

A total of 192 patients were included in this study. ICG-FA was performed in 86 cases (ICG-FA group) and was not performed in 106 cases (non-ICG-FA group). The patient and tumor characteristics of the entire cohort are shown in **Table 1**. The baseline characteristics were similar between the two groups, and there were no significant differences in age, sex, BMI, history of smoking, history of drinking, ASA, comorbidities, neoadjuvant chemotherapy, neoadjuvant radiotherapy, history of ESD, or tumor location. In both groups, squamous cell carcinoma was the most common pathological type. There were two patients with esophageal adenocarcinoma (2.3%) in the ICG-FA group and five patients with other pathological types (4.7%) in the non-ICG-FA group ($p = 0.038$), including two with sarcomatoid carcinomas, one with adenosquamous carcinoma, one with malignant melanoma, and one with neuroendocrine carcinoma.

Operative Outcomes and Pathological Characteristics

The operative outcomes and pathological characteristics are summarized in **Table 2**. The operative time was 249.77 ± 80.80 min for the ICG-FA group and 242.58 ± 57.92 min for the non-ICG-FA group. The intraoperative blood loss was 105.47 ± 57.12 ml for the ICG-FA group and 109.91 ± 76.13 ml for the non-ICG-FA group. There were no significant differences between the two groups in terms of postoperative hospital stay, fluid diet time, number of lymph node dissections, TNM stage, and vascular invasion. In addition, there were 20 patients with perineural invasion in the ICG-FA group, which was higher than that in the non-ICG-FA group (20 vs. 10, $p = 0.010$).

TABLE 1 | Demographic parameters and tumor characteristics of the patients.

	ICG-FA (n = 86)	Non-ICG-FA (n = 106)	*P*-value
Age (years)*	65.86 ± 6.54	64.94 ± 6.91	0.350
Sex, n (%)			0.252
Male	74(86.0)	97(91.5)	
Female	12(14.0)	9(8.5)	
BMI (kg/m^2)*	22.62 ± 2.97	22.05 ± 3.36	0.220
History of smoking, n (%)			0.404
No	49(57.0)	54(50.9)	
Yes	37(43.0)	52(49.1)	
History of drinking, n (%)			0.825
No	46(53.5)	55(51.9)	
Yes	40(46.5)	51(48.1)	
ASA, n (%)			0.224
II	79(91.9)	102(96.2)	
III	7(8.1)	4(3.8)	
Comorbidity, n (%)			
Hypertension	30(34.9)	31(29.2)	0.438
Diabetes mellitus	4(4.7)	4(3.8)	0.762
Cardiovascular disease	5(5.8)	4(3.8)	0.517
Obstructive lung disease	1(1.2)	5(4.7)	0.227
Cerebrovascular disease	3(3.5)	1(0.9)	0.327
Neoadjuvant chemotherapy, n (%)	13(15.1)	12(11.3)	0.519
Neoadjuvant radiotherapy, n (%)	1(1.2)	0(0)	0.448
Endoscopic submucosal dissection, n (%)	3(3.5)	0(0)	0.088
Histological type, n (%)			0.038[a]
Squamous cell carcinoma	84(97.7)	101(95.3)	
Adenocarcinoma	2(2.3)	0(0)	
Others	0(0)	5(4.7)	
Tumor location, n (%)			0.121
Upper	2(2.3)	8(7.5)	
Middle	35(40.7)	50(47.2)	
Lower	49(57)	48(45.3)	

ASA, American Society of Anesthesiologists; BMI, Body mass index.
**Values are expressed as mean ± SD.*
[a]statistically significant.

TABLE 2 | Operative and pathological outcomes of the ICG-FA group compared to the non-ICG-FA group.

	ICG-FA (n = 86)	Non-ICG-FA (n = 106)	*P*-value
Operation time (min)*	249.77 ± 80.80	242.58 ± 57.92	0.475
Intraoperative blood loss (ml)*	105.47 ± 57.12	109.91 ± 76.13	0.655
Restore fluid diet time (d)*	9.90 ± 3.64	12.30 ± 12.06	0.076
Postoperative hospital stay (d)*	13.85 ± 10.72	16.74 ± 17.24	0.177
Lymph node dissection (n)*	28.92 ± 13.86	30.07 ± 14.02	0.571
Pathological tumor category, n (%)			0.257
T1	20(23.3)	33(31.1)	
T2	20(23.3)	15(14.2)	
T3	46(53.5)	57(53.8)	
T4	0(0)	1(0.9)	
Pathological node category, n (%)			0.762
N0	46(53.5)	52(49.1)	
N1	25(29.1)	30(28.3)	
N2	13(15.1)	19(17.9)	
N3	2(2.3)	5(4.7)	
TNM stage, n (%)			0.712
Stage I	28(32.6)	32(30.2)	
Stage II	22(25.6)	26(24.5)	
Stage III	34(39.5)	42(39.6)	
Stage IV	2(2.3)	6(5.7)	
Vascular invasion, n (%)			0.506
No	74(86.0)	95(89.6)	
Yes	12(14.0)	11(10.4)	
Perineural invasion, n (%)			0.010[a]
No	66(76.7)	96(90.6)	
Yes	20(23.3)	10(9.4)	

**Values are expressed as mean ± SD.*
[a]Statistically significant difference.

TABLE 3 | Postoperative complications of the ICG-FA group compared to those of the non-ICG-FA[a] group.

	ICG-FA (n = 86)	Non-ICG-FA (n = 106)	*P*-value
Anastomosis leakage	1(1.2)	11(10.4)	0.009[b]
Vocal cord paralysis	1(1.2)	2(1.9)	0.687
Wound infection	3(3.5)	3(2.8)	0.794
Pleural effusion	11(12.8)	5(4.7)	0.064
Pneumonia	2(2.3)	5(4.7)	0.463
Chylothorax	1(1.2)	2(1.9)	0.687
Arrhythmia	0(0)	1(0.9)	0.366
Pneumothorax	1(1.2)	4(3.8)	0.259
ICU stay	1(1.2)	3(2.8)	0.421
Secondary surgery	0(0)	2(1.9)	0.200
Death	1(1.2)	0(0)	0.448

[a]Data are presented as n (%).
[b]Statistically significant difference.

Postoperative Complications

Details about the postoperative complications are presented in **Table 3**. One patient suffered from AL in the ICG-FA group and died of cancer progression and cachexia 105 days after surgery. The rate of AL was 1.2% in the ICG-FA group, which was significantly lower than the rate of 10.4% in the non-ICG-FA group ($p = 0.009$). According to the Clavien–Dindo classification, all of the patients in the non-ICG-FA group were classified as grade group IIIa. In addition to regular treatments, including fasting, total parenteral nutrition and anti-infection, they recovered after receiving endoscopic tube placement, irrigation or other non-surgical treatments. None of them underwent secondary surgery due to AL. The rate of vocal cord paralysis was not significantly different between the groups (1.2% vs. 1.9%, $p > 0.05$); all patients recovered with conservative treatment within 6 months after surgery. In the non-ICG-FA group, two patients underwent secondary surgery: One underwent a debridement suture due to a severe abdominal incision infection, and one case with chyle leak was recovered after secondary operation for thoracic duct ligation. There were no significant differences in the incidence of complications between the two groups, with the exception of the incidence of AL.

DISCUSSION

In this retrospective study, we found that ICG-FA is an effective strategy to prevent the occurrence of AL following McKeown MIE. Our results indicate that routine use of this method during operation could potentially improve the outcomes of McKeown MIE, and is a promising technology to evaluate the blood supply of the gastric conduit.

Previous studies have pointed out that many factors are likely to be associated with AL, including patient-related characteristics, intraoperative factors, and postoperative factors (8–10, 20). However, some factors, such as anastomotic tension, location of the anastomosis, and the surgical technique are modifiable. Blood perfusion remains the most important factor for performing anastomosis safely during esophagectomy, and it is essential to identify sufficient perfusion of the conduit if an appropriate method for assessing perfusion is available. Traditionally, perfusion of the conduit has been evaluated subjectively by surgeons based on several clinical signs, including the color of the conduit, palpable pulsation of the vessels, peristaltic movement, and active bleeding from marginal arteries (21). However, the above signs and characteristics might be inaccurate, as the assessment relies on the referral of the surgeon and tends to be inconsistent. Thus, an intraoperative tissue blood perfusion evaluation system needs to be established, in which the surgeon can receive objective and reliable information to select an appropriate anastomosis site.

Several previous techniques for assessing blood perfusion of the conduit include color Doppler ultrasound, laser Doppler flow meters, angiography, and oxygen spectroscopy. However, these technologies have not been widely accepted because of the cost of equipment, technical difficulties, and lack of reproducibility (11, 22). Recently, a near-infrared system named ICG-FA was used to perform intraoperative angiography and easily and objectively identify conduits with sufficient perfusion. Some papers have reported that ICG-FA might decrease the incidence of AL by assessing real-time blood flow during esophagectomy. However, these studies had certain limitations such as a small population under study and lack of a control group (10–17). Furthermore, due to the lack of standardization of the surgeon, technique, or conduit for evaluating ICG-FA, the consistency of the conclusions cannot be guaranteed. Thus, we conducted this research to overcome the limitations of previous studies. All patients underwent McKeown MIE with cervical anastomosis using a circular stapler by the same surgical team.

Takeuchi reported an AL rate of 13.3% in 5,354 patients undergoing radical esophageal cancer surgery (7). Karampinis (12) made all efforts to perform anastomosis in the zone of optimal perfusion and found a significant improvement in AL (18.2% vs. 3.0%) compared to the internal controls of the previous 55 patients who underwent esophagectomy. In our study, all patients in ICG-FA group were successful in fluorescence angiography. For 32 patients of them, we found that the whole conduit was well visualized within 60 s, which means that these conduits did not have poorly perfused areas. As for the remaining 54 patients, there is a poorly perfused area of various lengths at the distal end of the conduit according to the 60 s rule. In the ICG-FA group, anastomosis was operated in the site of conduit in which green fluorescence was observed within 60 s. The poorly perfused zone of conduit was removed after the anastomosis. The rate of AL for esophageal cancer resection was 10.4% in the non-ICG-FA group, and was significantly higher than the 1.2% in the ICG-FA group, suggesting that a reduction in the rate of AL of approximately 9% could be achieved by the use of ICG-FA. This evidence strongly demonstrates that sufficient blood perfusion of the gastric conduit is critical for thorough tissue healing at the anastomosis site.

Static blood perfusion of the gastric conduit by ICG-FA may not accurately display its perfusion. However, dynamic visualization of the conduit characterizes the perfusion by introducing a target time, which can better identify the optimal perfusion area. Kumagai (15) found that the leakage rate was 0% when the anastomosis was implemented in the area where the ICG perfusion was detected by the FA within 90 s. The rate of AL was a significantly lower than the 33% in the group that anastomosis was performed in areas where FA detected ICG perfusion after 90 s. Furthermore, Noma (23) recently reported that if perfusion was visualized within 20 s, the anastomosis was performed in this area, whereas if anastomotic areas were perfused within 30 s, further mobilization was performed prior to anastomosis implementation. The study found that the AL rates in patients who received the ICG protocol were significantly lower than in those assessed before protocol initiation (8.8% vs. 22%, $p = 0.03$). In our study, we chose 60 s after injection as a target time to identify the optimal zone for perfusion; this was because the study showed that 30% of the conduits were perfused in less than 60 s and this time was found to be clinically feasible (15). Second, in our previous clinical trials, we found that approximately 20 s after injection, blood flow was confirmed by ICG-FA, and vascular perfusion was well visualized within 60 s. After 60 s, the fluorescence imaging of the gastric wall was jagged and uneven, which was not suitable to identify anastomosis area. Therefore, we hypothesized that the risk of AL might be minimized if anastomosis was created in the area that was enhanced within 60 s; subsequently, we found that anastomosis in an area of the conduit where ICG perfusion was detected by FA within 60 s resulted in a lower leak rate.

There are some limitations to this study. First, this was a retrospective cohort study in a single institution, and the number of patients was limited in each group. To address this, we are now prospectively enrolling patients for randomized controlled assessment. Second, we did not evaluate blood perfusion of the conduit after anastomosis and did not understand the effect of anastomosis surgery on the regional blood supply. Third, ICG assessment was dependent on vascular perfusion via ICG-FA within 60 s; we need to establish an objective criterion for the speed of the ICG fluorescence stream in the gastric conduit. Lastly, ICG-FA requires highly specialized equipment that can be expensive and difficult to acquire.

In conclusion, for the assessment of esophageal conduits, ICG-FA has the potential to reduce the rate of AL in McKeown MIE. Further prospective studies are needed to confirm the usefulness of intraoperative ICG-FA for reducing the rate of AL.

ETHICS STATEMENT

The studies involving human participants were reviewed and approved by Research Ethics Committee of Sir Run Run Shaw

Hospital, School of Medicine, Zhejiang University. The patients/participants provided their written informed consent to participate in this study. Written informed consent was obtained from the individual(s) for the publication of any potentially identifiable images or data included in this article.

AUTHOR CONTRIBUTIONS

Collection of data: R-JL, Z-YZ, Z-FH, YX, Y-ZW, PC. Analysis of data: R-JL, PC. Writing of this paper: R-JL. General supervision of the research group: R-JL, Z-YZ. All authors contributed to the article and approved the submitted version.

REFERENCES

1. McGuire S. World Cancer Report 2014. Geneva, Switzerland: World Health Organization, International Agency for Research on Cancer, WHO Press. 2015. Advances in Nutrition. *Adv Nutr* (2016) 7(2):418–9. doi: 10.3945/an.116.012211
2. National Health Commission of The People's Republic Of China. Chinese guidelines for diagnosis and treatment of esophageal carcinoma 2018 (English version). *Chin J Cancer Res* (2019) 31(2):223–58. doi: 10.21147/j.issn.1000-9604.2019.02.01
3. Zheng RS, Sun KX, Zhang SW, Zeng HM, Zou XN, Chen R, et al. Report of cancer epidemiology in China, 2015. *Chin J Oncol* (2019) 41(1):19–28. doi: 10.3760/cma.j.issn.0253-3766.2019.01.005
4. Murakami Y, Takahashi I, Nishibuchi I, Doi Y, Okabe T, Kenjo M, et al. Long-term results of definitive concurrent chemoradiotherapy for patients with esophageal submucosal cancer (T1bN0M0). *Int J Clin Oncol* (2015) 20 (5):897–904. doi: 10.1007/s10147-015-0819-2
5. Low DE, Kuppusamy MK, Alderson D, Cecconello I, Chang AC, Darling G, et al. Benchmarking Complications Associated with Esophagectomy. *Ann Surg* (2019) 269(2):291–8. doi: 10.1097/SLA.0000000000002611
6. van der Werf LR, Busweiler LAD, van Sandick JW, van Berge Henegouwen MI, Wijnhoven BPL, Dutch Upper GI Cancer Audit (DUCA) group. Reporting National Outcomes After Esophagectomy and Gastrectomy According to the Esophageal Complications Consensus Group (ECCG). *Ann Surg* (2020) 271 (6):1095–101. doi: 10.1097/SLA.0000000000003210
7. Takeuchi H, Miyata H, Gotoh M, Kitagawa Y, Baba H, Kimura W, et al. A risk model for esophagectomy using data of 5354 patients included in a Japanese nationwide web-based database. *Ann Surg* (2014) 260(2):259–66. doi: 10.1097/SLA.0000000000000644
8. Walther B, Johansson J, Johnsson F, Von Holstein CS, Zilling T. Cervical or thoracic anastomosis after esophageal resection and gastric tube reconstruction: a prospective randomized trial comparing sutured neck anastomosis with stapled intrathoracic anastomosis. *Ann Surg* (2003) 238(6):803–12. doi: 10.1097/01.sla.0000098624.04100.b1 discussion 812-4.
9. Pham TH, Perry KA, Enestvedt CK, Gareau D, Dolan JP, Sheppard BC, et al. Decreased conduit perfusion measured by spectroscopy is associated with anastomotic complications. *Ann Thorac Surg* (2011) 91(2):380–5. doi: 10.1016/j.athoracsur.2010.10.006
10. Gooszen JAH, Goense L, Gisbertz SS, Ruurda JP, van Hillegersberg R, van Berge Henegouwen MI. Intrathoracic versus cervical anastomosis and predictors of anastomotic leakage after oesophagectomy for cancer. *Br J Surg* (2018) 105(5):552–60. doi: 10.1002/bjs.10728
11. Campbell C, Reames MK, Robinson M, Symanowski J, Salo JC. Conduit Vascular Evaluation is Associated with Reduction in Anastomotic Leak After Esophagectomy. *J Gastrointest Surg* (2015) 19(5):806–12. doi: 10.1007/s11605-015-2794-3
12. Karampinis I, Ronellenfitsch U, Mertens C, Gerken A, Hetjens S, Post S, et al. Indocyanine green tissue angiography affects anastomotic leakage after esophagectomy: A retrospective, case-control study. *Int J Surg* (2017) 48:210–4. doi: 10.1016/j.ijsu.2017.11.001
13. Zehetner J, DeMeester SR, Alicuben ET, Oh DS, Lipham JC, Hagen JA, et al. Intraoperative Assessment of Perfusion of the Gastric Graft and Correlation with Anastomotic Leaks after Esophagectomy. *Ann Surg* (2015) 262(1):74–8. doi: 10.1097/SLA.0000000000000811
14. Igari K, Kudo T, Toyofuku T, Jibiki M, Inoue Y, Kawano T. Quantitative evaluation of the outcomes of revascularization procedures for peripheral arterial disease using indocyanine green angiography. *Eur J Vasc Endovasc Surg* (2013) 46(4):460–5. doi: 10.1016/j.ejvs.2013.07.016
15. Kumagai Y, Hatano S, Sobajima J, Ishiguro T, Fukuchi M, Ishibashi KI, et al. Indocyanine green fluorescence angiography of the reconstructed gastric tube during esophagectomy: efficacy of the 90-second rule. *Dis Esophagus* (2018) 31 (12):1–4. doi: 10.1093/dote/doy052
16. Koyanagi K, Ozawa S, Oguma J, Kazuno A, Yamazaki Y, Ninomiya Y, et al. Blood flow speed of the gastric conduit assessed by indocyanine green fluorescence: New predictive evaluation of anastomotic leakage after esophagectomy. *Medicine (Baltimore)* (2016) 95(30):e4386. doi: 10.1097/MD.0000000000004386
17. Ohi M, Toiyama Y, Mohri Y, Saigusa S, Ichikawa T, Shimura T, et al. Prevalence of anastomotic leak and the impact of indocyanine green fluorescein imaging for evaluating blood flow in the gastric conduit following esophageal cancer surgery. *Esophagus* (2017) 14(4):351–9. doi: 10.1007/s10388-017-0585-5
18. Zhu ZY, Yong X, Luo RJ, Wang YZ. Clinical analysis of minimally invasive McKeown esophagectomy in a single center by a single medical group. *J Zhejiang Univ Sci B* (2018) 19(9):718–25. doi: 10.1631/jzus.B1800329
19. Luo R, He Z, Xu Y, Zhu Z. Comparison of the surgical outcomes of McKeown minimally invasive esophagectomy and Ivor-Lewis esophagectomy for the treatment of middle esophageal cancer: A single-center retrospective study. *Laparosc Endosc Robot Surg* (2020) 3(1):12–6. doi: 10.1016/j.lers.2020.01.001
20. Goense L, van Rossum PS, Tromp M, Joore HC, van Dijk D, Kroese AC, et al. Intraoperative and postoperative risk factors for anastomotic leakage and pneumonia after esophagectomy for cancer. *Dis Esophagus* (2017) 30(1):1–10. doi: 10.1111/dote.12517
21. Luketich JD, Pennathur A, Awais O, Levy RM, Keeley S, Shende M, et al. Outcomes after minimally invasive esophagectomy: review of over 1000 patients. *Ann Surg* (2012) 256(1):95–103. doi: 10.1097/SLA.0b013e3182590603
22. Son GM, Kwon MS, Kim Y, Kim J, Kim SH, Lee JW. Quantitative analysis of colon perfusion pattern using indocyanine green (ICG) angiography in laparoscopic colorectal surgery. *Surg Endosc* (2019) 33(5):1640–9. doi: 10.1007/s00464-018-6439-y
23. Noma K, Shirakawa Y, Kanaya N, Okada T, Maeda N, Ninomiya T, et al. Visualized Evaluation of Blood Flow to the Gastric Conduit and Complications in Esophageal Reconstruction. *J Am Coll Surg* (2018) 226 (3):241–51. doi: 10.1016/j.jamcollsurg.2017.11.007

18

Applications of Microscope-Integrated Indocyanine Green Videoangiography in Cerebral Revascularization Procedures

*Claudio Cavallo, Sirin Gandhi, Xiaochun Zhao, Evgenii Belykh, Daniel Valli, Peter Nakaji, Mark C. Preul and Michael T. Lawton**

Department of Neurosurgery, St. Joseph's Hospital and Medical Center, Barrow Neurological Institute, Phoenix, AZ, United States

Correspondence:
Michael T. Lawton
neuropub@barrowneuro.org

Indocyanine green videoangiography (ICG-VA) is a near-infrared range fluorescent marker used for intraoperative real-time assessment of flow in cerebrovascular surgery. Given its high spatial and temporal resolution, ICG-VA has been widely established as a useful technique to perform a qualitative analysis of the graft patency during revascularization procedures. In addition, this fluorescent modality can also provide valuable qualitative and quantitative information regarding the cerebral blood flow within the bypass graft and in the territories supplied. Digital subtraction angiography (DSA) is considered to be the gold standard diagnostic modality for postoperative bypass graft patency assessment. However, this technique is time and labor intensive and an expensive interventional procedure. In contrast, ICG-VA can be performed intraoperatively with no significant addition to the total operative time and, when used correctly, can accurately show acute occlusion. Such time-sensitive ischemic injury detection is critical for flow reestablishment through direct surgical management. In addition, ICG has an excellent safety profile, with few adverse events reported in the literature. This review outlines the chemical behavior, technical aspects, and clinical implications of this tool as an intraoperative adjunct in revascularization procedures.

Keywords: indocyanine green videoangiography, cerebral revascularization, extracranial-intracranial bypass, intracranial-intracranial bypass, graft patency

INTRODUCTION

Revascularization procedures are considered in the management of various cerebrovascular disorders, including complex intracranial aneurysms, moyamoya disease (MMD), symptomatic cerebral ischemia recalcitrant to standard medical therapy, and cranial base tumors that require a proximal major vessel sacrifice. MMD is a pathological condition that is characterized by a bilateral progressive narrowing at the terminal portion of the intracranial internal carotid arteries. This stenosis may lead to occlusion of the vessel lumen and a consequent abnormal, compensatory collateral neovascularization at the base of the brain. Superficial temporal artery (STA)-middle cerebral artery (MCA) bypass is the main direct revascularization procedure performed, and it is effective in reducing the risk of ischemic and hemorrhagic strokes as well as in improving cerebral ischemia (1–3).

Microscope-integrated indocyanine green videoangiography (ICG-VA) is a relatively recent technique used as an intraoperative adjunct for real-time assessment of anastomotic patency. Indocyanine green was approved by the US Food and Drug Administration (FDA) in 1956 for the evaluation of cardio-circulatory and liver functions. In addition, the FDA approved ICG for use in ophthalmic angiography in 1975 (4). Since then, ICG has been extensively used for retinal angiography (5, 6). Raabe et al. revived this technique to document intravascular flow in cerebral vessels to establish vascular patency (4). ICG-VA was also used for the intraoperative assessment of dural arteriovenous fistulas, for confirming complete aneurysm obliteration, and avoiding perforator or branch vessel compromise on microsurgical clipping (7). Over the years, ICG-VA has become an effective low-cost, non-invasive technique for confirming real-time intravascular flow in bypasses, with a good safety profile. The objective of our study was to present a focused review of the application of ICG-VA in cerebral bypass procedures and to describe the current diagnostic and therapeutic modalities of this technique.

CHEMICAL PROPERTIES, PHARMACOKINETICS, AND ADVERSE-EFFECT PROFILE OF ICG

ICG ($C_{43}H_{47}N_2NaO_6S_2$) is a tricarbocyanine dye with near-infrared fluorescent properties.

The absorption and emission peaks of ICG are 805 and 835 nm, respectively, which fall in the near-infrared (NIR) light range. The NIR peaks allow greater transmission of the fluorescence signal through the native tissue compared with the fluorophores, with peaks in the visible light range (6, 8–10). In theory, ICG fluorescence has a penetration depth of 10–20 mm in human tissues (11). This two-dimensional fluorescence imaging provides high spatial resolution and image quality compared with other intraoperative techniques.

On intravenous administration, ICG binds to alpha-1 lipoproteins, belonging to the globulin family, and remains intravascular as long as the vascular wall integrity is preserved. This fluorescent compound does not enter the enterohepatic circulation and is not metabolized in the body. It has a plasma half-life of 3–4 min and is excreted exclusively by the liver. Despite its relatively good safety profile, the ICG molecule or the 5% sodium iodine contained in the drug can potentially cause adverse reactions (4). Mild reactions, such as nausea, vomiting, pruritus, and sneezing, have been reported in ~0.15% of cases. Severe adverse reactions, including bronchospasm, laryngospasm, anaphylaxis, shock, myocardial infarction, cardiovascular arrest, and tonic clonic seizures have occurred in ~0.05% of cases (4). Overall, ICG is associated with a low rate of adverse reactions, comparable to other contrast media. Iodine allergy or prior adverse reactions to contrast media are contraindications for the administration of ICG.

TECHNICAL ASPECTS OF ICG-VA

Intraoperative technology for visualization of fluorescence is an integrated component of the currently available surgical microscopes. An excitation light in the NIR range is transmitted through the microscope optics to generate ICG fluorescence. This emitted electromagnetic radiation is invisible to the human eye and passes through the NIR optical filter (INFRARED 800. Zeiss AG, Oberkochen, Germany) that blocks both the excitation and the ambient light. An infrared-sensitive camera on the surgical microscope detects the ICG fluorescence and translates the signal into a real-time white image on a black background. Recently, an innovative dual-image videoangiography system was developed to overlay visible light and NIR fluorescence images and allow the simultaneous intraoperative visualization of both ICG fluorescence and surrounding anatomical structures (12).

Before activating the INFRARED 800 mode to perform ICG-VA, the focus distance and the magnification should be set at <300 mm and less than 5×, respectively. Afterward, the surgeon can adjust these two parameters during the INFRARED 800 recording to optimize the image. However, modern surgical microscopes usually assist the user with an automatic function that fine-tunes the settings to render the highest quality images. The KINEVO 900 (Carl Zeiss) provides an AutoZoom function that automatically adjusts the total magnification and diaphragm opening to the preconfigured values at the start of ICG-VA and an AutoGain function that automatically adjusts the camera gain to fit the NIR signal intensity within the dynamic range of the camera as the ICG-VA progresses. Chromatic aberration due to higher magnification and surgical field depth account for the inability of electromagnetic radiation of different wavelengths to focus on the same positions in the focal plane. Through the use of special lenses, apochromatic optics adjust light arrays of different colors to converge to the same focal point. This method achieves a variable degree of compensation that is more significant in the visible light spectrum (400–700 nm). Chromatic aberration of NIR light, like the ICG emission light (820–900 nm) can be compensated the most at working distances of <300 mm and at low magnification (<5×). The use of zoom and focal values other than those recommended can increase the focal point discrepancy between the NIR and visible light images and affect the quality of ICG-VA, resulting in a blurry NIR image.

The usual dose of ICG used is 0.2–0.5 mg/kg. At the time of administration, 25 mg of the dye is dissolved in 5 mL water and flushed with 10 mL of normal saline as a single intravenous bolus. Once the INFRARED 800 mode is activated, the ICG solution is injected through a peripheral line. ICG can cause lower values of peripheral oxygen saturation to be falsely displayed. The surgeon should manipulate and mobilize anatomical structures through the operating oculars of the surgical microscope to

Abbreviations: CBF, cerebral blood flow; CFI, cut flow index; CSF, Cerebrospinal fluid; DSA, Digital subtraction angiography; EC-IC, Extracranial-intracranial; FDA, US Food and Drug Administration; HP, hyperperfusion; ICG-VA, indocyanine green videoangiography; IC-IC, Intracranial-intracranial; MCA, Middle cerebral artery; MMD, Moyamoya disease; NIR, near infrared; PCA, Posterior cerebral artery; STA, Superficial temporal artery; TNE, transient neurological event.

ensure that the bypass graft is visible. Although NIR fluorescence has significantly greater penetration depth than visible light, the blood flow can be appreciated only in exposed blood vessels that are not obscured by anatomical structures, brain parenchyma, surgical instruments, or patties. The ICG fluorescence signal cannot be visualized directly through the operating oculars but is seen on the monitor of the surgical microscope following image processing (13, 14). The operating neurosurgeon can manipulate the vessels while the assistant reports the ICG-VA findings displayed on the screen with the ICG module activated.

An ICG-VA image takes ~10–30 s to appear on the screen. Once the recording is ended by the user, the automatic playback mode of the operating microscope allows the surgeon to assess the quality of the imaging in detail. ICG-VA can be repeated over time without any significant interference from the residual fluorescence of the previous injection. However, ICG should be reinjected after 20 min to guarantee adequate clearance of the tracer and optimize contrast enhancement (13, 14). Repeated administration of the dye should not exceed a total cumulative dose of 5 mg/kg.

ICG-VA can also analyze the intraluminal flow rate and flow velocity in selected regions of interest. In addition, a graph is generated to display the results of this quantitative analysis in a map delay time. The time characteristics of the graph allow the evaluation of the time to peak, defined as the interval from uprise of a wave to highest signal intensity, and washout time, represented by the interval from uprise of a wave to the time of rapid fall of signal intensity.

APPLICATION OF ICG-VA

Assessment of Graft Patency

During bypass surgery, the assessment of intravascular graft patency is essential to reduce the rate of graft failure. Early intraoperative identification of an occluded graft artery is critical for prompt surgical correction and for early restoration of blood flow to ensure a successful bypass. Several characteristics of the donor and graft vessels have been found to affect bypass function, including the graft diameters and the extent of focal atherosclerotic change (15). Other critical factors that play a role in intraoperative bypass patency include the cerebral blood flow demand of the downstream vascular territory and the direction of blood flow—antegrade vs. retrograde (15, 16). Technical aspects related to the surgical procedure or hypercoagulable states may also be responsible for the occurrence of a graft occlusion (17). Early intraoperative detection of an immediate bypass occlusion using ICG allows us to potentially identify and restore the patency of the bypass to prevent iatrogenic brain ischemia. Early detection may also impact the functional outcome for the patient and decrease the morbidity and mortality associated with revascularization procedures.

Direct intraoperative visual inspection of the anastomotic site cannot always accurately determine the patency of the graft vessel. The postoperative graft patency rate reported in the existing literature for an extracranial-intracranial (EC-IC) bypass is 87–96% (18–22). However, the aforementioned rate varies depending on the intraoperative diagnostic tool used to detect this complication. There are numerous intraoperative monitoring techniques for the evaluation of the graft patency. Among all of them, digital subtraction angiography (DSA) is considered to be the gold standard (23). Despite its diagnostic accuracy in identifying an intraoperative graft occlusion, this diagnostic imaging technique has several limitations, including its invasive nature and the associated risks; high procedural costs; the need for dedicated, trained personnel; and exposure of the patient to prolonged ionizing radiation (18). Moreover, DSA is time-consuming and detects the vessel occlusion in a delayed fashion, in contrast to ICG, which allows for an intraoperative diagnosis and immediate intervention. Other intraoperative monitoring techniques include Doppler ultrasonography (24) and thermal artery imaging (25). Intraoperative microvascular Doppler ultrasonography can be done directly on the bypass graft to assess its patency and quantitatively evaluate the blood flow metrics (26–28). The blood flow values can then be used to calculate the intraoperative cut flow index (CFI), which is the ratio of flow through the graft to the flow through the donor vessel prior to bypass (cut flow). CFI seems to be a sensitive parameter for postoperative bypass patency (29). Indeed, a previous study evaluating 51 bypass procedures for flow augmentation demonstrated that a CFI < 0.5 and CFI > 0.5 were associated with patency rates of 50 and 92%, respectively (28). Alternatively, an ultrasound system with a multifrequency linear probe can be used to perform a standard B-mode acquisition and a color Doppler evaluation with or without ultrasound contrast agents. This technique allows the intraoperative assessment of the arterial course and flow through the intracranial vessels present in the depth of the surgical field, which are deeper than the cortical surface in contact with the probe (30).

However, these techniques have major drawbacks in terms of spatial resolution and image quality, such that blood flow in small perforating arteries cannot be evaluated.

MR and CT angiography are effective non-invasive radiological modalities for evaluation of the patency of the bypass in the early postoperative period (18). Conventional DSA can be employed in the postoperative period to obtain valuable information regarding the graft patency and the dynamics of the bypass functionality (23). Other diagnostic adjuncts like functional cerebral blood flow (CBF) studies, SPECT, and Xe-enhanced CT are indicated to assess the postoperative cerebral perfusion.

As mentioned earlier, ICG-VA is a cost-effective and easy-to-use technique that provides real-time visualization of the fluorescent tracer inflow within cerebral vessels. ICG-VA is ideal for the intraoperative assessment of graft patency, and it seems to be superior to standard angiographic techniques (18). It consists of three different phases: arterial, capillary, and a combined arteriovenous phase generated by the recirculation of the dye. The early arterial phase is the most critical to detect delay or cessation of flow in the bypass graft, arterial branches, or perforators (4). Surgical microscope settings for fluorescence detection might differ substantially from the standard ones adopted for intraoperative visualization under conventional white light. Indeed, flow in perforating vessels is better visualized with a lower magnification and a shorter focus distance (4).

The remarkable spatial resolution of ICG-VA allows assessment of the morphology of graft patency and the hemodynamic of the bypass functioning (18). This diagnostic information is based on the pattern of filling of the graft with the fluorescent tracer compared with the contrast enhancement of the surrounding cerebral blood vessels. Moreover, this property allows the localization of the graft occlusion in real time in case of early bypass failure (13). Revision of the bypass graft might resolve this early intraoperative complication and improve surgical results related to revascularization procedures. Several clinical factors may influence the image quality with ICG-VA, such as the cardiovascular dynamics and cerebrospinal fluid (CSF) accumulation. The technical factors that qualitatively alter ICG-VA images include the speed of ICG injection and microscope settings, such as light intensity, working distance, magnification, and the diameter of the luminous field diaphragm opening. A previous study reported that ICG-VA image quality was notably affected by high magnification and depth of field based on chromatic aberration, as previously elaborated (13, 14).

In a previous series, Woitzik et al. reported bypass function in 31 of 35 (89%) STA-MCA bypasses, 2 of 2 (100%) STA-PCA bypasses, and 6 of 8 (75%) high-flow bypasses (18). Four STA-MCA bypasses had intraoperative occlusion, whereas 2 saphenous vein high-flow bypasses demonstrated moderate graft filling. In all these cases, ICG-VA localized the site of bypass failure at the anastomotic site, and timely surgical revision restored the flow through the bypass. Patency of the graft was subsequently documented by postoperative DSA or CT angiography.

Intraoperative Flow Analysis

Januszewski et al. described three different types of flow through a graft: Type I, robust anterograde flow; Type II, delayed anterograde flow; and Type III, anterograde delayed flow but with no continuity to the bypass site or no convincing flow. This study analyzed 36 EC-IC and intracranial-intracranial (IC-IC) bypasses performed in 33 ischemic patients with hemodynamic compromise despite maximal medical therapy (7). In their cohort, 8% of patients with Type II flow on ICG-VA had CTA findings indicating a graft occlusion within 72 h. Interestingly, none of the patients with Type II or Type III flow pattern had any clinical or radiological evidence of stroke in the postoperative period. This finding may be justified by the presence of competitive collateral flow leading to a lack of demand through the graft. Type III flow can also be caused by either technical surgical complications at the anastomosis or poor arterial graft quality and is associated with a higher probability of eventual graft failure (7). In contrast, failure in a Type II flow pattern is less likely to be related to the presence of competitive regional flow from collateral vessels. Therefore, the authors recommend reexploration of anastomoses in a Type II flow category to detect any early signs of bypass failure with the goal of immediate revision to salvage the bypass. If the quantitative flow characterization on ICG-VA images can be standardized for use across various medical centers, it would overcome a possible observer bias (7). Despite the results of this pilot study, a correlation between the flow characterization and the eventual clinical outcome is yet to be proven.

A quantitative analysis of flow was performed by Awano et al. using a specialized image analysis software (17). The ICG signal was quantified and the perfusion area of ICG was calculated at the point of maximal fluorescence intensity in specific regions of interest on the cortical surface (17). Awano et al. developed an innovative system based on visual light spectroscopy to continuously record hemodynamic changes of cortical blood flow during STA-MCA bypass surgery (17). Two groups of patients were included in this study, patients with and patients without MMD (with other indications for revascularization). The authors demonstrated that the ICG perfusion area was larger with a significant increase in cortical oxygen saturation in the MMD cohort. This could be attributable to the increase of blood flow demand and the larger pressure gradient between the anastomosed STA and the recipient vessels.

ICG-VA Role in Predicting Postoperative Neurological Complications

In recent years, several studies investigated the role of semi-quantitative and quantitative analysis of intraoperative ICG-VA findings in predicting the occurrence of postoperative neurological events after revascularization surgery in MMD. A variety of transient neurological events (TNEs) have been reported in the immediate postoperative period after STA-MCA bypass, which is most commonly employed in MMD treatment. TNEs occur in 14–77% of patients after MMD bypass surgery (3) and include extremity numbness, weakness, and episodic severe headaches (31–34), which could potentially have permanent neurological sequelae (31–34). The underlying causative mechanisms of TNEs are yet to be elucidated. However, the postoperative hemodynamic changes after revascularization procedures suggest that these complications might be related to local cerebral hyperperfusion (HP) (31, 35) or regional inflammation or due to a watershed shift (33, 36). In addition, extravasation of contrast materials in radiological imaging was found to be associated with cerebral HP after revascularization, suggesting a possible role for the breakdown of the blood-brain barrier (37, 38). Horie et al. described the diagnostic criteria for postoperative symptomatic HP as (1) the presence of focal neurologic deficits and/or severe headache, (2) confirmed graft patency by magnetic resonance angiography, (3) evident postoperative increase in CBF, and (4) absence of any ischemic changes and other pathologies (31, 32, 39–41). Postoperative HP occurs more frequently in adults than in pediatric patients in MMD (29, 31, 35). Postoperative radiological HP has been reported to occur in ~60% of the adult MMD population overall, and ~30% of the adult MMD population experiences symptomatic HP (35). Some diagnostic adjunct intraoperative laser Doppler or thermal diffusion probe (42) can detect an increase in intraoperative CBF in the anastomotic site, indicative of postoperative HP (43, 44). In addition, the use of infrared imaging, electromagnetic flowmetric, and Adobe Photoshop (Adobe Inc., San Jose, California) software have also been reported for the evaluation of hemodynamics (43–45). In patients undergoing a STA-MCA bypass for intracranial atherosclerotic disease or symptomatic carotid stenosis, a reduction in CBF and cerebrovascular reserve can be predictive of postoperative HP. However, this phenomenon does not apply to MMD patients (35, 41). In their prospective study, Horie et al. performed ICG-VA after STA-MCA anastomosis and compared cortical perfusion between the adult and pediatric populations with MMD as well as in adult patients with atherosclerotic disease (46). On evaluation of ICG intensity-time curves of the donor (STA), recipient (MCA), and the surrounding vessels, the postoperative HP was assumed to depend on the donor vessel caliber and on the poor integrity of the blood-brain barrier in the recipient. In this context, ICG-VA can be potentially utilized to predict postoperative HP in MMD patients. Similarly, a study by Uchino et al. suggested that semiquantitative analysis of ICG-VA is useful in predicting potential occurrence of HP after STA-MCA anastomosis in occlusive carotid artery disease (47). ICG-VA is effective in assessing intraoperative hemodynamic changes. Moreover, the blood flow index, calculated on the basis of the ICG intensity-time curve, can document the augmentation of cortical perfusion. A blood flow index increase greater than 3-fold from the baseline preoperative value may predict the occurrence of HP, whereas repeated SPECT is necessary to diagnose delayed postoperative HP.

Similarly, Uda et al. analyzed ICG-VA using specialized software (FlowInsight, Infocom Corporation, Shibuya, Tokyo, Japan) that allows the recording of several parameters in different regions of interest around the anastomotic site, including CBF, mean transit time, mean gradation time (Grad), and time to peak (TTP). Percentage change of these parameters after bypass was calculated using the formula ($\Delta X = (X_{after} - X_{before})/X_{before}$). They demonstrated that patients with $\Delta TTP \leq -12$, $\Delta CBF \geq 8$, or $\Delta Grad \geq 30$ have a higher risk of developing postoperative TNEs (3). Hemodynamic changes after bypass surgery, analyzed through ICG and FlowInsight, were predictive of postoperative TNE and correlated with their duration. Optimization of the clinical management of these patients may further reduce TNE-related complications after revascularization procedures. Despite several reports demonstrating the role of hemodynamic changes detected by ICG-VA image analysis in potentially predicting postoperative HP and TNEs, there is no current evidence showing a correlation with improved treatment outcomes. Moreover, the role of ICG-VA in predicting delayed postoperative HP several days after surgery remains uncertain (47). Larger studies are warranted to confirm these results and further elucidate the contribution of this fluorescent intraoperative technique.

Intraoperative Vessel Identification

EC-IC bypass surgery, in particular STA-MCA anastomosis, is the most common revascularization procedure for the treatment of cerebral ischemia. Designed and successfully performed for the first time by Yaşargil in 1967 (48–50), this surgery is aimed at providing alternative blood supply in patients with an underlying hemodynamic cerebrovascular insufficiency (51). Visualization of STA and its branches is critical, and an adequate donor artery can be selected preoperatively using different imaging modalities, including DSA, CTA, and magnetic resonance angiography (49). In addition, the course of STA from the underside of the frontotemporal skin flap can be mapped intraoperatively by light palpation, continuous Doppler ultrasound, or through the assistance of frameless electromagnetic neuronavigation to guarantee a safe dissection (49, 52). The parietal branch of STA is the more commonly used donor graft. However, in certain cases with a planned double-barrel STA-MCA bypass or with an atrophic or damaged parietal STA, the frontal branch of the artery is used. ICG-VA can aid in the intraoperative visualization of STA and assist in the identification of the donor artery, especially when the anterior frontal branch is selected. In addition, ICG-VA provided valuable intraoperative information for the mapping and preparation of the donor vessel (50).

Peña-Tapia et al. first described a new application of ICG-VA to identify a cortical target point and find an adequate recipient vessel (51). They used a rectangular template made of transparent plastic material that can be applied to both sides of the head and with a handle centered on the outer auditory canal. This template-based approach allows the preoperative identification of the end of the sylvian fissure, accurately relying on external landmarks (51). Two different highlighted lines are engraved on the surface of the plastic, and their overall orientation is aimed at identifying several M4 (segment of the MCA) branches emerging from the sylvian fissure, which can be selected as recipient vessels and marked on the patient's scalp.

Previous studies have shown that the application of ICG-VA is not limited to the identification or safe dissection of the STA in bypass procedures. In fact, this intraoperative technique has also been used to selectively target the most suitable cortical M4 recipient artery for flow-preserving bypass to trap complex MCA aneurysms (53). Alternatively, M2-M3 segments of the MCA could also be selected if the anatomy is favorable and the microsurgical dissection of the sylvian fissure is safe (53). However, M2-M3 segments may feed cortical M4 vessels and the STA-MCA anastomosis may redirect the blood supply to uninvolved vascular territories despite the use of anatomical landmarks, neuroimaging, and neuronavigation (52, 54). For this reason, a terminal branch of the MCA (M4) is preferred as a recipient vessel. Moreover, temporary ischemia is considered less invasive and is better tolerated in M4 superficial cortical arteries than in M2-M3 segments (54, 55). During intraoperative ICG-VA, the cortical surface in the surrounding area of the sylvian fissure is analyzed to detect the direction of the flow and possible delayed or reversed filling time of M4 branches during the arterial phase and other vascular structures during the capillary and venous phase (52, 54). Esposito et al. described a primary and a secondary identification in their surgical protocol for intraoperative ICG-VA (53). The primary identification consists of performing a baseline ICG-VA without any temporary occlusion of arterial vessels. On the contrary, the secondary identification consists of intraoperative ICG-VA with a "provocative" temporary occlusion. Delayed fluorescent filling of superficial M4 branches during either primary or secondary identification demarcates the cortical territory supplied, and any artery confined within this area can be selected as the recipient vessel (53). ICG-VA can be repeated

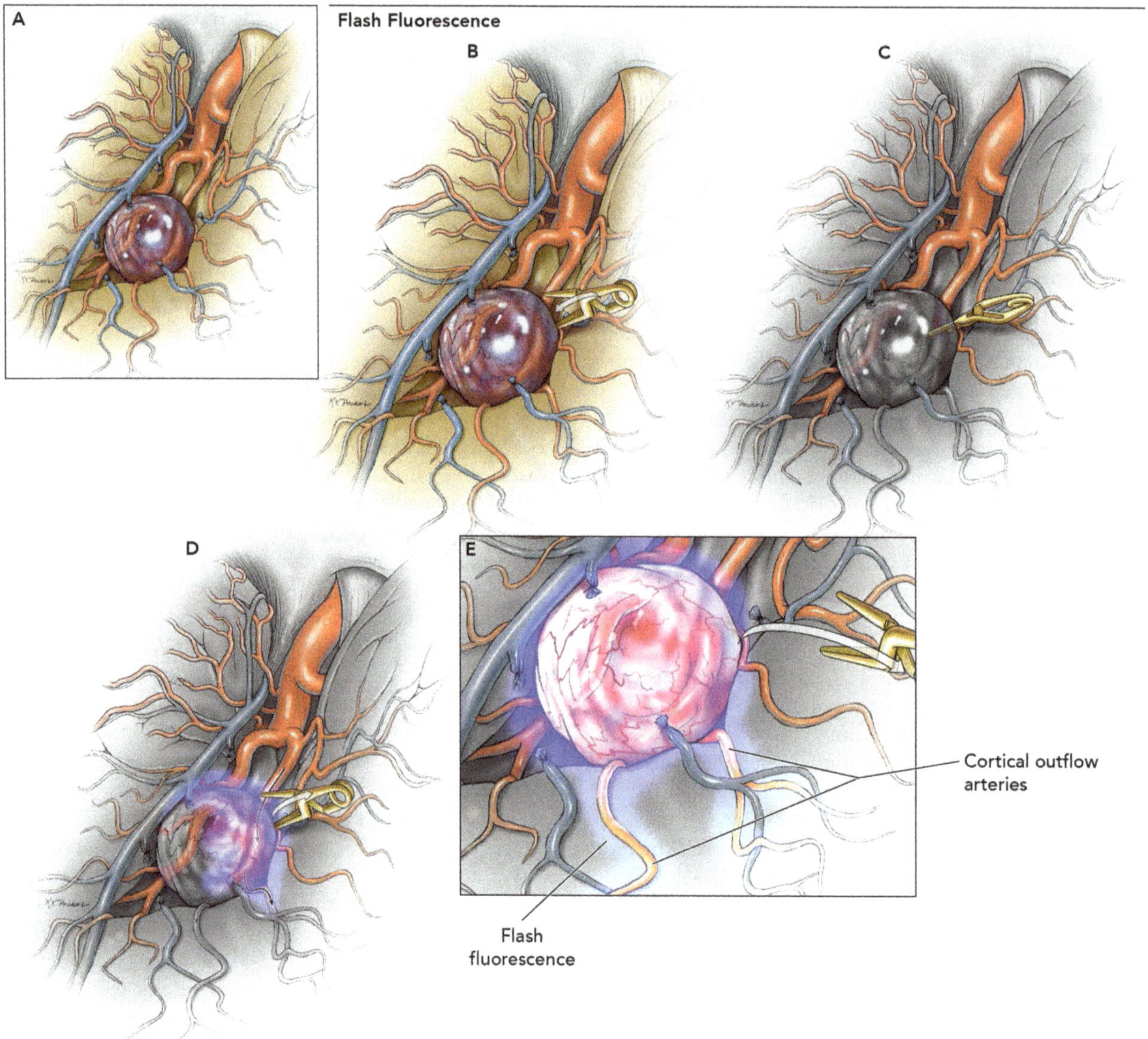

FIGURE 1 | Use of flash fluorescence technique to identify the efferent arteries of the aneurysm using ICG-VA. **(A)** Identification of candidate bypass recipient arteries among the surface M4 branches is difficult but could be improved using the following steps. **(B)** Temporary clip occlusion of the aneurysm inflow (afferent arteries) proximal to the aneurysm. **(C)** ICG-VA demonstrating initial fluorescence in uninvolved arterial branches. **(D)** Removal of temporary clip for aneurysm reperfusion. **(E)** Fluorescence seen in the efferent arteries to identify the most suitable recipient on the cortical surface for the bypass. Used with permission from Lawton (56).

after anastomosis to rule out any residual filling in the complex MCA aneurysm.

The senior author has previously introduced the "flash fluorescence" technique (**Figures 1, 2**) to select an adequate recipient artery for bypass. The application of this technique is summarized in the three following surgical steps: (1) proximal temporary occlusion of the afferent artery of the aneurysm, (2) ICG-VA to define the uninvolved cortical arteries, and (3) temporary clip removal for reperfusion of the afferent artery and concomitant flash fluorescence ICG run in efferent arteries on the cortical surface (57). The recipient artery is initially dark during the ICG-VA and flash fluorescence. This direct technique enables the selection of the distal recipient artery. An alternative, indirect technique has been described that relies on temporary occlusion of the uninvolved arteries adjacent to the aneurysm's afferent artery. In this case, the efferent arteries illuminate first and simultaneously flash fluorescence with temporary clip removal to highlight the arteries that should not be considered as recipients for the bypass. The direct technique is preferred, as it requires a more limited ischemia time and only one temporary clip. Flash fluorescence is especially valuable with distal MCA aneurysms that require bypass because the identification of a distal cortical recipient prevents unnecessary sylvian fissure dissection. Moreover, brain retraction is not

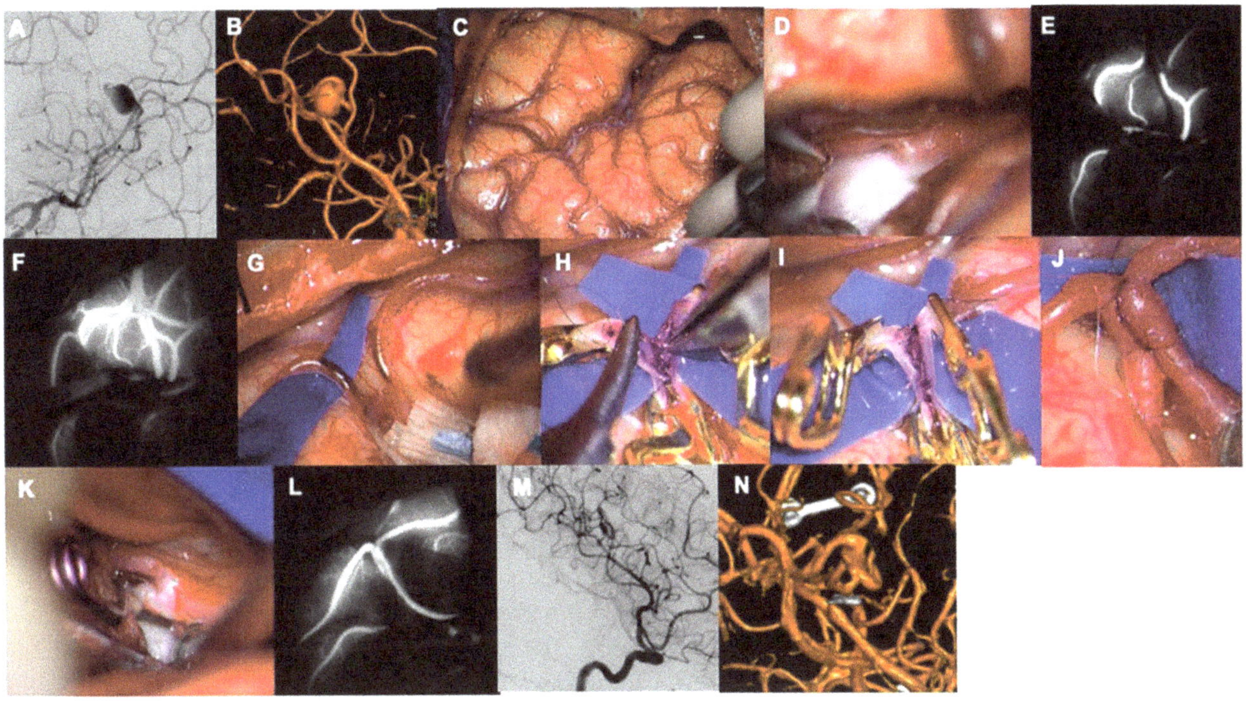

FIGURE 2 | A 47-year-old woman presented with a sudden headache suspicious for sentinel hemorrhage. **(A)** An aneurysm was found at the distal M2 segment with dolichoectatic morphology and two efferent branches (left ICA, AP view). **(B)** Left ICA, 3D reconstruction. **(C)** Sylvian fissure split to access the insular recess. **(D)** Aneurysm with parent artery. **(E)** Flash fluorescence technique was used to identify the efferent vessel to be used as a bypass recipient with proximal temporary clip occlusion. **(F)** Temporary clip removal led to flash ICG filling of this vascular territory and showed the angular artery as the outflow vessel. **(G)** *In situ* bypass of angular artery with posterior temporal artery was performed. **(H)** The intraluminal suture line was sewn with a single anchoring stitch to better visualize the walls. **(I,J)** The extraluminal suture line was sewn loosely, tightened, and tied. **(K)** Proximal aneurysm occlusion. **(L)** M3 MCA-M3 MCA *in situ* bypass perfused the donor angular artery as seen with ICG-VA. **(M)** Left ICA, lateral view. **(N)** Left ICA, 3D reconstruction. Used with permission from Lawton (56).

needed, and the anastomosis is more easily performed on the cortical surface than in the deep sylvian location. Compared with the conventional pterional craniotomy, the bone flap should be extended posteriorly to accommodate the more distal location of the anastomotic site. Other authors reported the use of transdural ICG-VA in STA-MCA bypass procedures to expose the appropriate cortical recipient distributing from the sylvian fissure and superficial vessels anatomy. The location of the recipient was then marked on the dura mater with pyoktanin blue to tailor the dural incision and prevent possible damage during dural opening and microsurgical dissection (58). ICG-VA has also been used to trace the course of the middle meningeal artery (MMA) for use in indirect bypass, encephalo-duro-myo-arterio-pericranial synangiosis for MMD (59). This MMA anterior branch provides collateral flow through the dura mater to the anterior cerebral artery territory both spontaneously and through indirect bypass (60, 61). The standard fronto-temporal craniotomy can damage the anterior branch of MMA given its course within the lesser wing of the sphenoid bone in 50–75% of patients (62, 63). Based on the ICG-VA findings, the craniotomy has been customized into a heart-shaped bone flap to prevent damage to the anterior MMA.

ICG-VA vs. FLUORESCEIN VIDEOANGIOGRAPHY

Fluorescence videoangiography has gained significant traction in the recent years in the practice of complex cerebrovascular neurosurgery. Despite the widespread acceptance of ICG-VA in neurosurgical procedures, the recent reemergence of fluorescein sodium as a fluorescent tracer has prompted authors to investigate and compare fluorescein videoangiography (FL-VA) with ICG-VA. An objective analysis was recently conducted by applying quantitative metrics to data derived from video capture images, which were subsequently elaborated by pixel intensity-analyzing software (62). In this fluorescence study, ICG-VA demonstrated a greater potential for allowing the robust visualization of the extracranial arteries, including the STA and thick intracranial vessels. On the contrary, FL-VA provided superior intraoperative information regarding perforating arteries, distal branches, and small vessels at high magnification deep in the surgical field (62). In addition, FL-VA allows the surgeon to perform a real-time flow assessment and manipulation of vessels of interest by direct intraoperative visualization through the operating microscope oculars.

The widespread acceptance of ICG-VA is attributable to its ease of use along with its diagnostic accuracy, low cost, and good safety profile (64). Another important advantage of ICG-VA is the ability to perform repeated injections with a short refractory period for intraoperative blood flow reassessment (64). The limitations of fluorescein in vascular neurosurgery are mainly related to its tendency to leak more readily into the extravascular space, resulting in a more persistent fluorescent signal in the surgical field that prevents repeated injections (64). Despite their differences, these two fluorescent modalities are complementary in nature, and their application should be based on the surgical procedure, the depth of the operative field, and the size of the vessels of interest.

FUTURE DIRECTION FOR APPLICATION OF ICG-VA

In recent years, a few novel techniques in the application of ICG-VA have been described. These techniques include the introduction of a "second window" ICG technique for glioblastoma resection that capitalizes on the inherent property of permeability of the tumor vasculature. A high dose of ICG is delivered ~24 h before surgery, leading to non-specific accumulation of the tracer within the tumor tissue. This technique may allow real-time intraoperative tumor identification to optimize surgical resection (65). Additionally, ICG-VA has been used to identify the venous drainage pattern and collateral circulations during tumor resection for possible venous sacrifice to predict and minimize the potential side effects (66). However, the role of these techniques in the setting of revascularization has yet to be elucidated.

Other Applications of ICG-VA

The contribution of ICG-VA has also been investigated for other types of revascularization procedures including coronary artery bypass. The calculated sensitivity and specificity of ICG in detecting 50% stenosis were 83.3 and 100%, respectively (67). However, ICG-VA is associated with several limitations that preclude its widespread acceptance and use in this subspecialty, in contrast to neurosurgery. ICG visualization of pedicle conduits is poorer when compared with skeletonized conduits, and each graft requires up to 4 min to be evaluated, resulting in a significant effect on the operative time (68). Moreover, the "semi-quantitative assessment" of graft patency with ICG-VA provides inadequate information on the distal coronary vasculature as well as competitive flow and transit times (69). Despite other studies showed promising results, the use of ICG for detecting coronary bypass patency has yet to be definitively proven (70).

CONCLUSION

ICG-VA has been widely established as a useful technique to perform qualitative analyses of graft patency and CBF during revascularization procedures. The widespread incorporation of ICG-VA is attributable to its ease of use, diagnostic accuracy, low cost, and excellent safety profile.

AUTHOR CONTRIBUTIONS

CC: literature review, manuscript draft, revision, and final draft approval. SG: manuscript draft, revision, and review of final manuscript. XZ and EB: manuscript draft and review of final draft. DV: literature review and final draft review. PN, MP, and ML: study supervision, review, and revision of the final draft.

ACKNOWLEDGMENTS

The authors thank the staff of Neuroscience Publications at Barrow Neurological Institute for assistance with manuscript preparation.

REFERENCES

1. Kuroda S, Kashiwazaki D, Hirata K, Shiga T, Houkin K, Tamaki N. Effects of surgical revascularization on cerebral oxygen metabolism in patients with Moyamoya disease: an 15O-gas positron emission tomographic study. *Stroke.* (2014) 45:2717–21. doi: 10.1161/strokeaha.114.006009
2. Miyamoto S, Yoshimoto T, Hashimoto N, Okada Y, Tsuji I, Tominaga T, et al. Effects of extracranial-intracranial bypass for patients with hemorrhagic moyamoya disease: results of the Japan Adult Moyamoya Trial. *Stroke.* (2014) 45:1415–21. doi: 10.1161/strokeaha.113.004386
3. Uda K, Araki Y, Muraoka S, Ota S, Wada K, Yokoyama K, et al. Intraoperative evaluation of local cerebral hemodynamic change by indocyanine green videoangiography: prediction of incidence and duration of postoperative transient neurological events in patients with moyamoya disease. *J Neurosurg.* (2019) 130:1367–75. doi: 10.3171/2017.10.JNS171523
4. Raabe A. *INFRARED 800 Video Angiography a Practical Guide for the Surgeon* Bern: University Clinic for Neurosurgery (2010).
5. Kogure K, David NJ, Yamanouchi U, Choromokos E. Infrared absorption angiography of the fundus circulation. *Arch Ophthalmol.* (1970) 83:209–14. doi: 10.1001/archopht.1970.00990030211015
6. Sakatani K, Kashiwasake-Jibu M, Taka Y, Wang S, Zuo H, Yamamoto K, et al. Noninvasive optical imaging of the subarachnoid space and cerebrospinal fluid pathways based on near-infrared fluorescence. *J Neurosurg.* (1997) 87:738–45. doi: 10.3171/jns.1997.87.5.0738
7. Januszewski J, Beecher JS, Chalif DJ, Dehdashti AR. Flow-based evaluation of cerebral revascularization using near-infrared indocyanine green videoangiography. *Neurosurg Focus.* (2014) 36:E14. doi: 10.3171/2013.12.Focus13473
8. Jobsis FF. Noninvasive, infrared monitoring of cerebral and myocardial oxygen sufficiency and circulatory parameters. *Science.* (1977) 198:1264–7. doi: 10.1126/science.929199
9. McCormick PW, Stewart M, Goetting MG, Balakrishnan G. Regional cerebrovascular oxygen saturation measured by optical spectroscopy in humans. *Stroke.* (1991) 22:596–602. doi: 10.1161/01.STR.22.5.596
10. Reynolds EO, McCormick DC, Roth SC, Edwards AD, Wyatt JS. New non-invasive methods for the investigation of cerebral oxidative metabolism and haemodynamics in newborn infants. *Ann Med.* (1991) 23:681–6. doi: 10.3109/07853899109148103
11. Miwa M. The principle of ICG fluorescence method. *Open Surg Oncol J.* (2010) 2:26–8. doi: 10.2174/1876504101002020026

12. Feletti A, Wang X, Tanaka R, Yamada Y, Suyama D, Kawase T, et al. Dual-image videoangiography during intracranial microvascular surgery. *World Neurosurg.* (2017) 99:572–9. doi: 10.1016/j.wneu.2016.12.070
13. Kim DL, Cohen-Gadol AA. Indocyanine-green videoangiogram to assess collateral circulation before arterial sacrifice for management of complex vascular and neoplastic lesions: technical note. *World Neurosurg.* (2013) 79:404.e1–6. doi: 10.1016/j.wneu.2012.07.028
14. Shah KJ, Cohen-Gadol AA. The application of FLOW 800 ICG videoangiography color maps for neurovascular surgery and intraoperative decision making. *World Neurosurg.* (2019) 122:e186–97. doi: 10.1016/j.wneu.2018.09.195
15. Vajkoczy P, Horn P, Schmiedek P. Standard superficial temporal artery-middle cerebral artery bypass surgery in hemodynamic cerebral ischemia: indication and technique. *Operat Techn Neurosurg.* (1999) 2:106–15. doi: 10.1016/S1092-440X(99)80002-4
16. Yoon S, Burkhardt JK, Lawton MT. Long-term patency in cerebral revascularization surgery: an analysis of a consecutive series of 430 bypasses. *J Neurosurg.* (2019) 131:86–7. doi: 10.3171/2018.3.Jns172158
17. Awano T, Sakatani K, Yokose N, Kondo Y, Igarashi T, Hoshino T, et al. Intraoperative EC-IC bypass blood flow assessment with indocyanine green angiography in moyamoya and non-moyamoya ischemic stroke. *World Neurosurg.* (2010) 73:668–74. doi: 10.1016/j.wneu.2010.03.027
18. Woitzik J, Horn P, Vajkoczy P, Schmiedek P. Intraoperative control of extracranial-intracranial bypass patency by near-infrared indocyanine green videoangiography. *J Neurosurg.* (2005) 102:692–8. doi: 10.3171/jns.2005.102.4.0692
19. EC/IC Bypass Study Group. Failure of extracranial-intracranial arterial bypass to reduce the risk of ischemic stroke. Results of an international randomized trial. *New Engl J Med.* (1985) 313:1191–200. doi: 10.1056/nejm198511073131904
20. Mendelowitsch A, Taussky P, Rem JA, Gratzl O. Clinical outcome of standard extracranial-intracranial bypass surgery in patients with symptomatic atherosclerotic occlusion of the internal carotid artery. *Acta Neurochir.* (2004) 146:95–101. doi: 10.1007/s00701-003-0154-7
21. Sundt TM Jr, Siekert RG, Piepgras DG, Sharbrough FW, Houser OW. Bypass surgery for vascular disease of the carotid system. *Mayo Clin Proc.* (1976) 51:677–92.
22. Schmiedek P, Piepgras A, Leinsinger G, Kirsch CM, Einhupl K. Improvement of cerebrovascular reserve capacity by EC-IC arterial bypass surgery in patients with ICA occlusion and hemodynamic cerebral ischemia. *J Neurosurg.* (1994) 81:236–44. doi: 10.3171/jns.1994.81.2.0236
23. Yanaka K, Fujita K, Noguchi S, Matsumaru Y, Asakawa H, Anno I, et al. Intraoperative angiographic assessment of graft patency during extracranial-intracranial bypass procedures. *Neurol Med Chir.* (2003) 43:509–12; discussion 13. doi: 10.2176/nmc.43.509
24. Badie B, Lee FT Jr, Pozniak MA, Strother CM. Intraoperative sonographic assessment of graft patency during extracranial-intracranial bypass. *AJNR Am J Neuroradiol.* (2000) 21:1457–9.
25. Nakagawa A, Hirano T, Uenohara H, Sato M, Kusaka Y, Shirane R, et al. Intraoperative thermal artery imaging of an EC-IC bypass in beagles with infrared camera with detectable wave-length band of 7-14 microm: possibilities as novel blood flow monitoring system. *Minim Invasive Neurosurg.* (2003) 46:231–4. doi: 10.1055/s-2003-42357
26. Charbel FT, Hoffman WE, Misra M, Ostergren L. Ultrasonic perivascular flow probe: technique and application in neurosurgery. *Neurol Res.* (1998) 20:439–42. doi: 10.1080/01616412.1998.11740545
27. Nakayama N, Kuroda S, Houkin K, Takikawa S, Abe H. Intraoperative measurement of arterial blood flow using a transit time flowmeter: monitoring of hemodynamic changes during cerebrovascular surgery. *Acta Neurochir.* (2001) 143:17–24. doi: 10.1007/s007010170133
28. Amin-Hanjani S, Du X, Mlinarevich N, Meglio G, Zhao M, Charbel FT. The cut flow index: an intraoperative predictor of the success of extracranial-intracranial bypass for occlusive cerebrovascular disease. *Neurosurgery.* (2005) 56(1 Suppl.):75–85; discussion 75–85. doi: 10.1227/01.neu.0000143032.35416.41
29. Fujimura M, Inoue T, Shimizu H, Saito A, Mugikura S, Tominaga T. Efficacy of prophylactic blood pressure lowering according to a standardized postoperative management protocol to prevent symptomatic cerebral hyperperfusion after direct revascularization surgery for moyamoya disease. *Cerebrovasc Dis.* (2012) 33:436–45. doi: 10.1159/000336765
30. Prada F, Del Bene M, Casali C, Saladino A, Legnani FG, Perin A, et al. Intraoperative navigated angiosonography for skull base tumor surgery. *World Neurosurg.* (2015) 84:1699–707. doi: 10.1016/j.wneu.2015.07.025
31. Fujimura M, Kaneta T, Mugikura S, Shimizu H, Tominaga T. Temporary neurologic deterioration due to cerebral hyperperfusion after superficial temporal artery-middle cerebral artery anastomosis in patients with adult-onset moyamoya disease. *Surg Neurol.* (2007) 67:273–82. doi: 10.1016/j.surneu.2006.07.017
32. Hayashi K, Horie N, Suyama K, Nagata I. Incidence and clinical features of symptomatic cerebral hyperperfusion syndrome after vascular reconstruction. *World Neurosurg.* (2012) 78:447–54. doi: 10.1016/j.wneu.2011.10.041
33. Hamano E, Kataoka H, Morita N, Maruyama D, Satow T, Iihara K, et al. Clinical implications of the cortical hyperintensity belt sign in fluid-attenuated inversion recovery images after bypass surgery for moyamoya disease. *J Neurosurg.* (2017) 126:1–7. doi: 10.3171/2015.10.Jns151022
34. Machida T, Nakano S, Ishige S, Ono J, Fujikawa A. Subcortical low-intensity lesions on fluid-attenuated inversion recovery images after revascularization surgery for moyamoya disease. *World Neurosurg.* (2017) 98:512–9. doi: 10.1016/j.wneu.2016.11.058
35. Uchino H, Kuroda S, Hirata K, Shiga T, Houkin K, Tamaki N. Predictors and clinical features of postoperative hyperperfusion after surgical revascularization for moyamoya disease: a serial single photon emission CT/positron emission tomography study. *Stroke.* (2012) 43:2610–6. doi: 10.1161/strokeaha.112.654723
36. Hayashi T, Shirane R, Fujimura M, Tominaga T. Postoperative neurological deterioration in pediatric moyamoya disease: watershed shift and hyperperfusion. *J Neurosurg Pediatr.* (2010) 6:73–81. doi: 10.3171/2010.4.Peds09478
37. Sharma P, Poppe AY, Eesa M, Steffanhagan N, Hudon M, Morrish W. Extravasating contrast material on angiography following carotid angioplasty and stenting: not necessarily subarachnoid hemorrhage. *J Neuroimaging.* (2010) 20:180–2. doi: 10.1111/j.1552-6569.2008.00316.x
38. Takayama K, Nakagawa H, Iwasaki S, Taoka T, Wada T, Myouchin K, et al. Cerebral hemorrhage with angiographic extravasation immediately after carotid artery stenting. *Radiat Med.* (2007) 25:359–63. doi: 10.1007/s11604-007-0147-1
39. Fujimura M, Mugikura S, Kaneta T, Shimizu H, Tominaga T. Incidence and risk factors for symptomatic cerebral hyperperfusion after superficial temporal artery-middle cerebral artery anastomosis in patients with moyamoya disease. *Surg Neurol.* (2009) 71:442–7. doi: 10.1016/j.surneu.2008.02.031
40. Fujimura M, Shimizu H, Inoue T, Mugikura S, Saito A, Tominaga T. Significance of focal cerebral hyperperfusion as a cause of transient neurologic deterioration after extracranial-intracranial bypass for moyamoya disease: comparative study with non-moyamoya patients using N-isopropyl-p-[(123)I]iodoamphetamine single-photon emission computed tomography. *Neurosurgery.* (2011) 68:957–64; discussion 64–5. doi: 10.1227/NEU.0b013e318208f1da
41. Kaku Y, Iihara K, Nakajima N, Kataoka H, Fukuda K, Masuoka J, et al. Cerebral blood flow and metabolism of hyperperfusion after cerebral revascularization in patients with moyamoya disease. *J Cereb Blood Flow Metab.* (2012) 32:2066–75. doi: 10.1038/jcbfm.2012.110
42. Mukerji N, Cook DJ, Steinberg GK. Is local hypoperfusion the reason for transient neurological deficits after STA-MCA bypass for moyamoya disease? *J Neurosurg.* (2015) 122:90–4. doi: 10.3171/2014.8.Jns132413
43. Nakagawa A, Fujimura M, Arafune T, Sakuma I, Tominaga T. Clinical implications of intraoperative infrared brain surface monitoring during superficial temporal artery-middle cerebral artery anastomosis in patients with moyamoya disease. *J Neurosurg.* (2009) 111:1158–64. doi: 10.3171/2009.4.Jns08585
44. Kawamata T, Kawashima A, Yamaguchi K, Hori T, Okada Y. Usefulness of intraoperative laser Doppler flowmetry and thermography to predict a risk of postoperative hyperperfusion after superficial temporal artery-middle cerebral artery bypass for moyamoya disease. *Neurosurg Rev.* (2011) 34:355–62; discussion 62. doi: 10.1007/s10143-011-0331-8

45. Mizumura S, Nakagawara J, Takahashi M, Kumita S, Cho K, Nakajo H, et al. Three-dimensional display in staging hemodynamic brain ischemia for JET study: objective evaluation using SEE analysis and 3D-SSP display. *Ann Nucl Med.* (2004) 18:13–21. doi: 10.1007/BF02985609
46. Horie N, Fukuda Y, Izumo T, Hayashi K, Suyama K, Nagata I. Indocyanine green videoangiography for assessment of postoperative hyperperfusion in moyamoya disease. *Acta Neurochir.* (2014) 156:919–26. doi: 10.1007/s00701-014-2054-4
47. Uchino H, Kazumata K, Ito M, Nakayama N, Kuroda S, Houkin K. Intraoperative assessment of cortical perfusion by indocyanine green videoangiography in surgical revascularization for moyamoya disease. *Acta Neurochir.* (2014) 156:1753–60. doi: 10.1007/s00701-014-2161-2
48. Yaşargil MG. *Microsurgery Applied to Neurosurgery.* Stuttgart: Georg Thieme Verlag (1969). Available online at: https://books.google.com/books?id=K_ogBQAAQBAJ&printsec=frontcover&dq=yasargil+microsurgery+applied+to+neurosurgery&hl=en&newbks=1&newbks_redir=0&sa=X&ved=2ahUKEwiE6bzxlKrlAhVDqJ4KHVLaCQEQuwUwAHoECAYQBQ#v=onepage&q=yasargil%20microsurgery%20applied%20to%20neurosurgery&f=false.
49. Newell DW, Vilela MD. Superficial temporal artery to middle cerebral artery bypass. *Neurosurgery.* (2004) 54:1441–8; discussion 8–9. doi: 10.1227/01.NEU.0000124754.84425.48
50. Esposito G, Burkhardt JK, Bozinov O, Regli L. Indocyanine green videoangiography for the identification of superficial temporal artery branches in EC-IC bypass surgery. *Acta Neurochir.* (2016) 158:565–70. doi: 10.1007/s00701-016-2703-x
51. Peña-Tapia PG, Kemmling A, Czabanka M, Vajkoczy P, Schmiedek P. Identification of the optimal cortical target point for extracranial-intracranial bypass surgery in patients with hemodynamic cerebrovascular insufficiency. *J Neurosurg.* (2008) 108:655–61. doi: 10.3171/jns/2008/108/4/0655
52. Esposito G, Durand A, Van Doormaal T, Regli L. Selective-targeted extra-intracranial bypass surgery in complex middle cerebral artery aneurysms: correctly identifying the recipient artery using indocyanine green videoangiography. *Neurosurgery.* (2012) 71(2 Suppl.):ons274–84; discussion ons84–5. doi: 10.1227/NEU.0b013e3182684c45
53. Esposito G, Dias S, Burkhardt JK, Bozinov O, Regli L. Role of indocyanine green videoangiography in identification of donor and recipient arteries in cerebral bypass surgery. *Acta Neurochir Suppl.* (2018) 129:85–9. doi: 10.1007/978-3-319-73739-3_12
54. Esposito G, Regli L. Selective Targeted cerebral revascularization via microscope integrated indocyanine green videoangiography technology. *Acta Neurochir Suppl.* (2014) 119:59–64. doi: 10.1007/978-3-319-02411-0_10
55. Kronenburg A, Esposito G, Fierstra J, Braun KP, Regli L. Combined bypass technique for contemporary revascularization of unilateral MCA and bilateral frontal territories in moyamoya vasculopathy. *Acta Neurochir Suppl.* (2014) 119:65–70. doi: 10.1007/978-3-319-02411-0_11
56. Lawton MT. Seven Bypasses: Tenets and Techniques for Revascularization. New York, NY: Thieme (2018).
57. Rodriguez-Hernandez A, Lawton MT. Flash fluorescence with indocyanine green videoangiography to identify the recipient artery for bypass with distal middle cerebral artery aneurysms: operative technique. *Neurosurgery.* (2012) 70(2 Suppl.):209–20. doi: 10.1227/NEU.0b013e31823158f3
58. Yokota H, Yonezawa T, Yamada T, Miyamae S, Kim T, Takamura Y, et al. Transdural indocyanine green videography for superficial temporal artery-to-middle cerebral artery bypass-technical note. *World Neurosurg.* (2017) 106:446–9. doi: 10.1016/j.wneu.2017.07.004
59. Tanabe N, Yamamoto S, Kashiwazaki D, Akioka N, Kuwayama N, Noguchi K, et al. Indocyanine green visualization of middle meningeal artery before craniotomy during surgical revascularization for moyamoya disease. *Acta Neurochir.* (2017) 159:567–75. doi: 10.1007/s00701-016-3060-5
60. Dusick JR, Gonzalez NR, Martin NA. Clinical and angiographic outcomes from indirect revascularization surgery for Moyamoya disease in adults and children: a review of 63 procedures. *Neurosurgery.* (2011) 68:34–43; discussion. doi: 10.1227/NEU.0b013e3181fc5ec2
61. Kuroda S, Houkin K. Bypass surgery for moyamoya disease: concept and essence of sugical techniques. *Neurol Med Chir.* (2012) 52:287–94. doi: 10.2176/nmc.52.287
62. Matano F, Mizunari T, Murai Y, Kubota A, Fujiki Y, Kobayashi S, et al. Quantitative comparison of the intraoperative utility of indocyanine green and fluorescein videoangiographies in cerebrovascular surgery. *Oper Neurosurg.* (2017) 13:361–6. doi: 10.1093/ons/opw020
63. Ma S, Baillie LJ, Stringer MD. Reappraising the surface anatomy of the pterion and its relationship to the middle meningeal artery. *Clin Anat.* (2012) 25:330–9. doi: 10.1002/ca.21232
64. Lane B, Bohnstedt BN, Cohen-Gadol AA. A prospective comparative study of microscope-integrated intraoperative fluorescein and indocyanine videoangiography for clip ligation of complex cerebral aneurysms. *J Neurosurg.* (2015) 122:618–26. doi: 10.3171/2014.10.Jns132766
65. Zeh R, Sheikh S, Xia L, Pierce J, Newton A, Predina J, et al. The second window ICG technique demonstrates a broad plateau period for near infrared fluorescence tumor contrast in glioblastoma. *PLoS ONE.* (2017) 12:e0182034. doi: 10.1371/journal.pone.0182034
66. Acerbi F, Vetrano IG, Sattin T, Falco J, de Laurentis C, Zattra CM, et al. Use of ICG videoangiography and FLOW 800 analysis to identify the patient-specific venous circulation and predict the effect of venous sacrifice: a retrospective study of 172 patients. *Neurosurg Focus.* (2018) 45:E7. doi: 10.3171/2018.4.Focus18120
67. Desai ND, Miwa S, Kodama D, Koyama T, Cohen G, Pelletier MP, et al. A randomized comparison of intraoperative indocyanine green angiography and transit-time flow measurement to detect technical errors in coronary bypass grafts. *J Thorac Cardiovasc Surg.* (2006) 132:585–94. doi: 10.1016/j.jtcvs.2005.09.061
68. Taggart DP, Choudhary B, Anastasiadis K, Abu-Omar Y, Balacumaraswami L, Pigott DW. Preliminary experience with a novel intraoperative fluorescence imaging technique to evaluate the patency of bypass grafts in total arterial revascularization. *Ann Thorac Surg.* (2003) 75:870–3. doi: 10.1016/s0003-4975(02)04669-6
69. Leacche M, Balaguer JM, Byrne JG. Intraoperative grafts assessment. *Semin Thorac Cardiovasc Surg.* (2009) 21:207–12. doi: 10.1053/j.semtcvs.2009.08.007
70. Ohmes LB, Di Franco A, Di Giammarco G, Rosati CM, Lau C, Girardi LN, et al. Techniques for intraoperative graft assessment in coronary artery bypass surgery. *J Thorac Dis.* (2017) 9(Suppl. 4):S327–32. doi: 10.21037/jtd.2017.03.77

19

Application of Fluorescein Fluorescence in Vascular Neurosurgery

Xiaochun Zhao[1]*, Evgenii Belykh*[1,2]*, Claudio Cavallo*[1]*, Daniel Valli*[1]*, Sirin Gandhi*[1]*, Mark C. Preul*[1]*, Peter Vajkoczy*[3]*, Michael T. Lawton*[1] *and Peter Nakaji*[1*]

[1] *Department of Neurosurgery, Barrow Neurological Institute, St. Joseph's Hospital and Medical Center, Phoenix, AZ, United States,* [2] *Department of Neurosurgery, Irkutsk State Medical University, Irkutsk, Russia,* [3] *Department of Neurosurgery, Charité – Universitätsmedizin Berlin, Berlin, Germany*

***Correspondence:**
Peter Nakaji
neuropub@barrowneuro.org

Background: Fluorescein sodium (FNa) is a fluorescent drug with a long history of use for assessing retinal blood flow in ophthalmology; however, its application in vascular neurosurgery is only now gaining popularity. This review summarizes the current knowledge about using FNa videoangiography in vascular neurosurgery.

Methods: We performed a literature review on the usage of FNa for fluorescent videoangiography procedures in neurosurgery. We analyzed methods of injection, dosages of FNa, visualizing platforms, and interpretation of FNa videoangiography. We also reviewed practical applications of FNa videoangiography during various vascular neurosurgeries.

Results: FNa videoangiography can be performed with intraarterial (intracarotid) or intravenous dye injections. Both methods provide excellent resolution with enhanced fluorescence that shows intravascular blood flow on top of visible surrounding anatomy, and both allow simultaneous purposeful microsurgical manipulations. Although it is invasive, an intracarotid FNa injection results in faster contrast appearance and higher-intensity fluorescence and requires a lower dose per injection (reported range, 1–50 mg) compared with peripheral intravenous FNa injection (reported range, 75–2,000 mg or 1–1.5 mg/kg body weight). Four optical excitation/detection tools for FNa videoangiography have been successfully used: conventional xenon-light operating microscope with a special filter set, pencil-type light-emitting diode probe with a filter set, laser-illumination operating microscope, and an endoscope with a filter set. FNa videoangiography was reported to be feasible and useful in various clinical scenarios, such as examining the feeders and drainers in arteriovenous malformation surgery, checking the patency of a microvascular anastomosis, and assessing blood flow during aneurysm clipping. FNa videoangiography can be repeated during the same procedure and used along with indocyanine green (ICG) videoangiography.

Conclusions: Compared with ICG videoangiography, FNa videoangiography has the advantages of enabling real-time inspection and better visualization at deep locations; however, thick vessel walls limit visualization of FNa in larger vessels. FNa videoangiography is a useful tool in multiple neurovascular scenarios and merits further studies to establish its clinical value.

Keywords: fluorescein angiography, fluorescein fluorescence, fluorescein sodium, vascular neurosurgery, aneurysm, arteriovenous malformation, arteriovenous fistula

INTRODUCTION

Techniques for evaluating blood flow are essential for successful neurosurgery on vascular lesions. Vascular lesions, such as cerebral aneurysms, arteriovenous malformations (AVMs), and dural arteriovenous fistulas (DAVFs), and other clinical scenarios requiring vascular anastomosis are characterized by unique flow alterations (e.g., aneurysmal turbulent flow). Clinical outcomes may be catastrophic if blood flow is severely compromised or if a vessel is ruptured during these procedures. Surgical intervention in such lesions includes blood flow monitoring to minimize the risk of rupture or to reestablish compromised normal circulation.

Multiple methods have been developed to examine circulation intraoperatively. These methods can be broadly classified on the basis of the principles of physics, drugs, and the devices used.

1. Observation and palpation, using the classic milking test, can assess patency of a dissected vessel. Pulsation waves and the color of blood (bright-red oxygenated vs. dark-red deoxygenated) are qualitative signs that are helpful in flow assessment but have multiple limitations (1).
2. Contact probe-based Doppler angiography can measure the volume and speed of the blood flow (2) using either a point-probe, which measures the target artery from one side, or an intracranial Charbel Micro-Flow probe (Transonic, Ithaca, NY), which measures the target artery from two sides.
3. Wide-field laser speckle imaging (785 nm, 50 mW laser) allows the generation of a real-time two-dimensional color-coded map of perfusion during open surgery and can be used as a noninvasive visualization and measurement of the relative cortical blood flow (3).
4. Digital subtraction angiography (DSA) is a robust but invasive imaging technique that remains the gold-standard examination for many vascular lesions. Intraoperative DSA requires a hybrid room setting (angiography setup in the operating room) and separate sterilization area (i.e., femoral area) (4–6).
5. Fluorescent videoangiography with various wide-field surgical microscopes with appropriate filters includes the use of indocyanine green (ICG) videoangiography and fluorescein sodium (FNa) videoangiography.
6. Confocal laser endomicroscopic angiography can employ FNa or ICG and assess brain microvasculature.

Abbreviations: AVM, arteriovenous malformation; CCA, common carotid artery; DAVF, dural arteriovenous fistula; DSA, digital subtraction angiography; FNa, fluorescein sodium; IA, intraarterial; ICG, indocyanine green; IV, intravenous; LED, light emitting diode.

This paper is a focused review of the history and current applications of FNa videoangiography for intraoperative neurovascular imaging.

HISTORY OF FNa VIDEOANGIOGRAPHY

According to Van Cader (7), the earliest study with FNa was conducted in 1881 by Ehrlich and colleagues, who analyzed the distribution of FNa after intravenous (IV) injection and demonstrated its presence in the anterior chamber of the eye. In ophthalmology, FNa has been extensively used to assess retinal blood flow (8, 9). In the late 1940s, FNa was adopted by Moore et al. to visualize neoplastic tissue in gastric adenocarcinomas and brain tumors (10, 11). Glial tumors were found to produce the most consistent positive fluorescence.

In 1967, FNa was first used to evaluate the intracranial circulation in animals and humans by Feindel et al. (12). A report of an AVM surgery by the same group in 1971 was the first record of FNa application in vascular neurosurgery (13). Since then, the number of studies reporting FNa videoangiography has been relatively limited, with the majority of studies published after 2013 (6, 14–23).

METABOLISM AND SAFETY OF FNa

Upon IV administration, FNa loosely binds to plasma proteins and exists as a protein-bound (80%) and free-salt (20%) substance. FNa is metabolized by glucuronidation in the liver. About 80% of IV FNa is converted to a monoglucuronide within 1 h, which is 95% less fluorescent. FNa is rapidly cleared by the kidneys through filtration and secretion and is almost completely excreted by 24 h (24).

FNa has been shown to be minimally toxic at a dose of 20 mg/kg body weight (1,500 mg for a 75-kg patient) (25). In ophthalmology, however, FNa is used extensively at dosages of 500 mg (26, 27) and as much as 30 mg/kg body weight. Median lethal doses of IV FNa are 2,200 mg/kg for mice, 600 to 1,000 mg/kg in rats, 1,000 mg/kg in dogs, and 350 mg/kg in rabbits (28). Complications such as cardiac effect, respiratory reaction, or seizure have been reported rarely, with the frequency of severe adverse effects reported as 1 in 1,900 and death as 1 in 222,000 (29). Patients injected with doses of more than 5 mg/kg body weight exhibit temporary yellow staining of skin, which disappears within 6 to 24 h as FNa is cleared (10). It was noted that patients with severe liver diseases may experience prolonged yellow skin staining (10). FNa administration for vascular neurosurgical applications requires a relatively low dose, and no complications related to FNa have been reported in the neurosurgical literature.

DOSAGES OF FNa FOR VASCULAR APPLICATIONS

IV and intraarterial (IA) injections of FNa require different dosages for optimal vascular imaging. IV administration usually requires a higher dosage than IA injection to achieve good contrast, as FNa dilutes during peripheral circulation, and 80% of the FNa binds to albumin and is deactivated in this process (30, 31). Wrobel et al. (32) reported a case of high-dose FNa videoangiography using 2,000 mg IV bolus. In other neurosurgical reports, IV doses range from 75 mg to 500 mg per bolus (6, 18–21, 30, 31, 33) or from 1 mg/kg to 1.5 mg/kg per body weight (16, 34).

Doses for IA injection are low, with 2 studies from the 1970s reporting 10 mg (13) and 50 mg (33) IV boluses, and more recent studies have used a dose as low as 10 ml of 0.01–0.02% FNa solution (0.001–0.002 mg) (20, 31) and 5 ml of 0.5–1% FNa solution (0.025–0.05 mg) (17). After investigating different dosages of FNa, Kuroda et al. reported 10 ml of 0.01–0.02% FNa bolus (0.001–0.002 mg) can be used to sufficiently detect the parent artery and perforating arteries of aneurysms without staining the vessel wall and without persistence in the vessel 5 min after IA injection (31).

SITE OF INJECTION: IV OR IA

IV routes can use central or peripheral venous access, which usually has not been specified in reports. IA injection, however, needs to be made directly into the carotid or vertebral circulation. Thus, the peripheral arterial accesses (radial artery) for blood pressure monitoring would be no different with an IV injection in terms of FNa mixing with blood. However, IA injection requires an additional vascular access site with associated risks, which is a drawback.

Catheterization of the common carotid artery (CCA) may be performed via a direct transcutaneous puncture or transfemoral retrograde catheterization. However, the detailed technique used to access the CCA for FNa injection was not specified in majority of the literature (13, 20, 31, 33). Ichikawa et al. inserted an IA catheter from the superficial temporal artery into the CCA for approximately 5 to 10 cm in a retrograde fashion and then successfully performed FNa videoangiography (17). Other potential retrograde injection sites, such as the occipital artery, merit future feasibility studies.

The major difference between IV injection and IA injection of FNa is the time period from the injection to different phases of FNa appearance in the field of view (**Figure 1**). The arterial phase of IA FNa injection appears immediately after injection (20, 31), usually no more than 2 s (13), and the venous phase fades out in <1 min (17). In comparison, the appearance takes longer in both phases with IV injection—it usually takes at least 10 s for the arterial phase and a minimum of 5 min until the fluorescence fades out (17, 31). The show-up and the fade-out of each phase after an IV injection are steep, and those in IV injection are delayed.

A shorter time period until fade-out is essential if repeated angiography is required, such as for evaluation of a DAVF before and after ligation or when accessing the patency of perforators during a series of clip adjustments in an aneurysm surgery (31). Kuroda et al. reported that IA FNa videoangiography can be repeated at least 5 times without staining the vessel wall in a short period of time, with the total dose significantly below the safety limits (31). However, the length of the period of intravascular stay was under debate; Kakucs et al. advocated that the longer time window of intravascular stay is one of the advantages of the IV injection, which provides more time of the angiography for use in analysis (15).

Because 80% of FNa molecules combine with albumin (30, 31), IV FNa injections usually require a higher dose than IA injections, which may lead to vessel wall staining and decrease the intravascular-extravascular contrast (31, 33). Furthermore, even with a higher IV dose administered, the observed fluorescence decreases as FNa dilutes with blood along the circulation. In IA injection, however, the FNa concentration in cerebral vasculature is high, providing higher contrast to the background anatomy. This is established for both FNa videoangiography (**Figure 1**) and ICG videoangiography (20, 31, 35). However, both IA and IV FNa administration routes can provide sufficient fluorescence intensity and sufficient information for interpretation (20).

In summary, compared with IV injection of FNa, IA injection has the advantage of better contrast, lower required dose, and the ability to be repeatedly performed in a limited time period without staining to the vessel wall. The disadvantage of IA injection is the necessity of additional vascular access to the CCA and its associated risks. Longer intravascular stay may be interpreted differently and can be advantageous or disadvantageous for both methods of administering FNa.

PHASES OF FNa VIDEOANGIOGRAPHY AND FACTORS THAT AFFECT PHASES

As with any angiography, FNa videoangiography has three main phases in which certain vessels are characteristically highlighted by fluorescence: the arterial, capillary, and venous phases. The duration of these phases (i.e., the duration of FNa fluorescence in arterial, capillary, and venous beds) depends on multiple factors. Mindful consideration of these factors is crucial for assessment and differentiation of normal and pathologic conditions. The interrelation of various factors, such as dosage and the route of administration, adds another level of complexity to assessments. Below, we briefly list these factors and discuss those particularly relevant to FNa in more details.

Site of Injection

With IV injections, FNa travels in the cardiopulmonary circulation and then appears in the systemic arterial circulation, which allows FNa to mix with large quantities of blood and thus provides a longer time to peak and less bright fluorescence compared with an IA injection. Additionally, the speed of

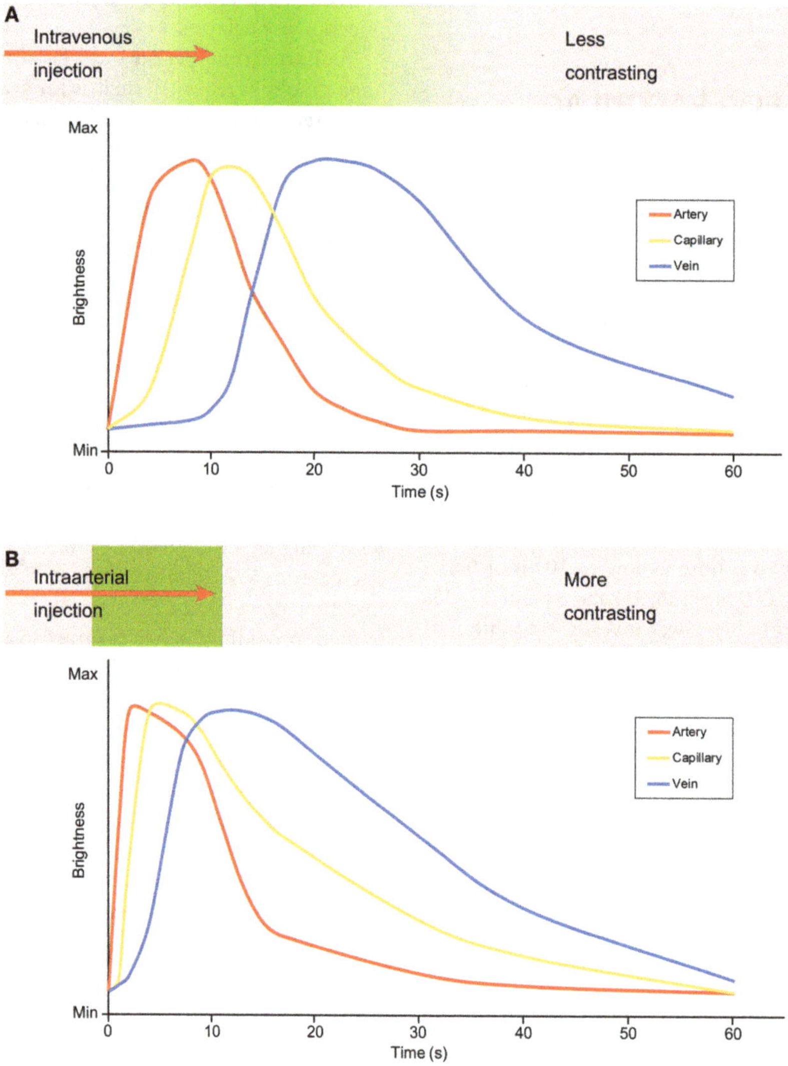

FIGURE 1 | Graphic demonstrating the contrast and brightness changes during angiography with an **(A)** intravenous and **(B)** intraarterial FNa injection. The green color embedded in the bar above the graph represents the flow of the fluorescein. With an intravenous injection, the fluorescein is diluted and contrasts less as shown in the less steep and delayed graph, compared with an intraarterial injection during which the fluorescein is more concentrated and contrasts better as shown by the steep and acute graph. Max, maximum; Min, minimum. Used with permission from Barrow Neurological Institute, Phoenix, Arizona.

injection plays a role in the fluorescence phases and should be standardized as a rapid bolus injection.

Dose

A large dose can prolong the intravascular stay of FNa but has the disadvantage of unspecific vessel wall staining. A dose of 2,000 mg of FNa was reported to remain detectable in the cerebral vessels for 60 min, and the authors suggested that using a lower dose may be better, as used with repetitive angiographies (32).

Vessel Wall Staining

Detected intravascular fluorescence can be due to FNa in the blood or due to the staining of the vessel wall. Stained vessel walls can lower the contrast effect and affect the interpretation of the videoangiography, especially given the impact on quality of subsequent angiographies.

Vascular Abnormalities

The arterial phase appears early when used in a patient with an abnormal connection between the venous and arterial circulations, such as a DAVF or AVM, where the blood flow is aberrantly fast. The arterial phase was reported to be 11 s in a case report of a DAVF (34) and 10–15 s in AVM surgeries (13, 16, 18, 23) after IV FNa injection. These durations are shorter than those reported during IV FNa videoangiography in aneurysm surgeries, in which the arterial phase typically appears for more than 20 s (20, 22, 31, 32).

The effect of a bypass can also influence the arterial phase appearance. Little et al. reported an average 1.7-s time decrease from the injection to the arterial phase in cortical arteries after superficial temporal artery–middle cerebral artery bypass. This change, along with visual transit of fluorescence signal through an anastomosis, can be used as an indicator of a successful bypass (33).

Cardiovascular Parameters

Cardiovascular parameters, such as arterial blood pressure and heart rate, may affect time-dependent angiographic parameters and should be taken into consideration.

Visualization Platform Parameters

The focus distance of the microscope, its angulation, position within the field of view, photobleaching properties, and irregularities of the surgical field increase the complexity when assessing fluorescence images (36).

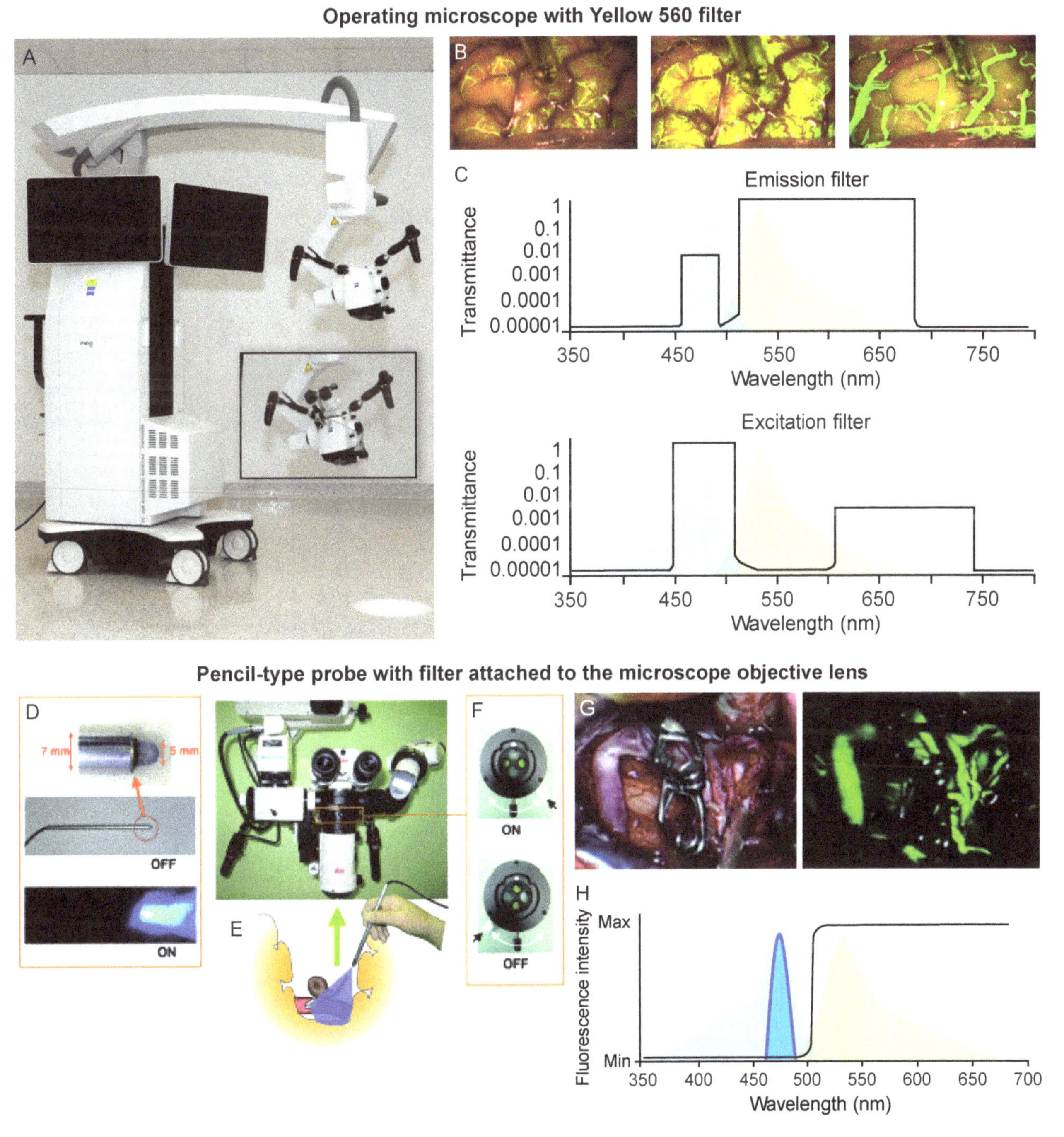

FIGURE 2 | Continued

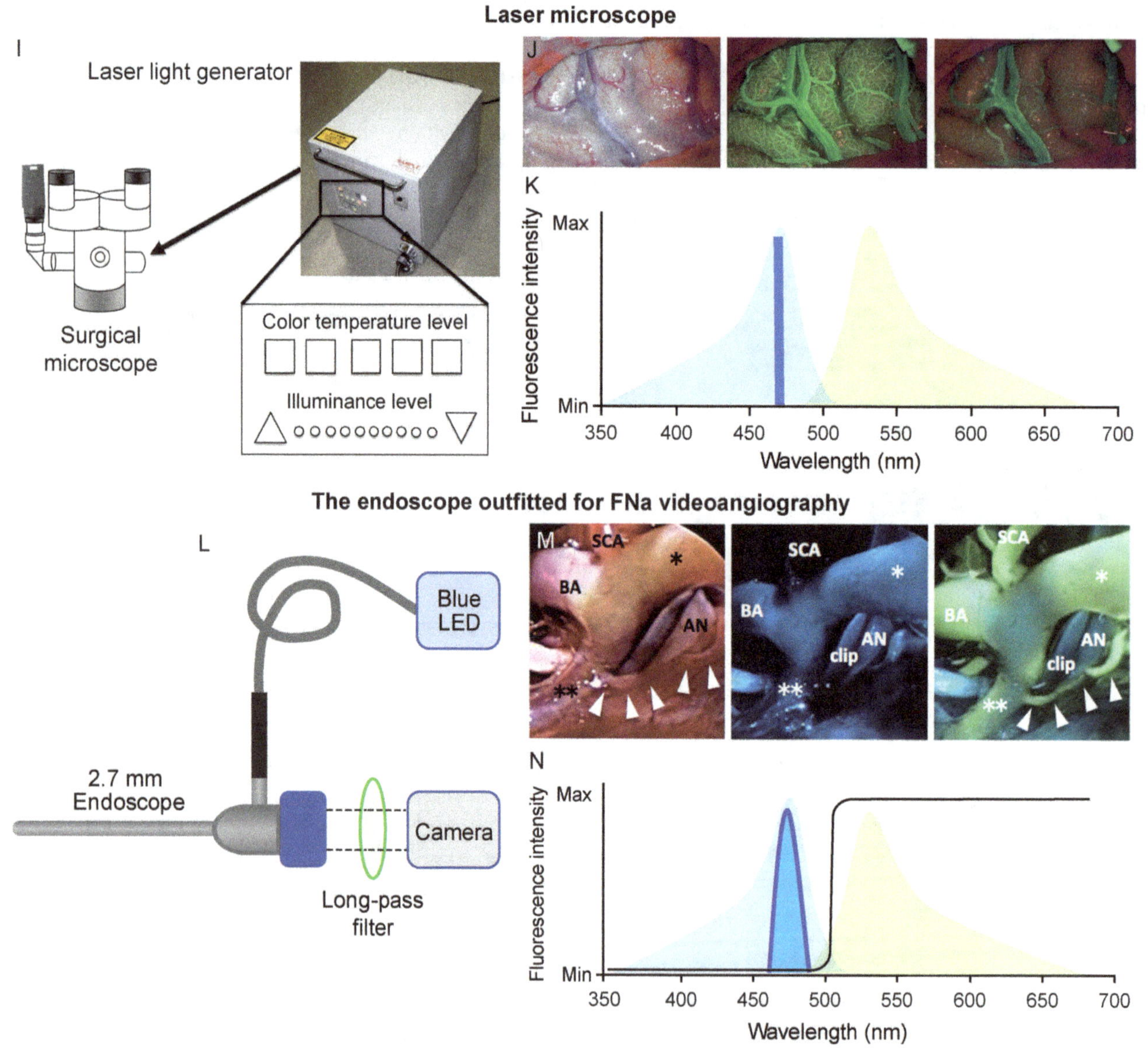

FIGURE 2 | Various platforms used for FNa videoangiography. **(A–C)** Operating microscope. **(A)** The operating microscope with Yellow 560 module (ZEISS KINEVO 900, Carl Zeiss AG, Oberkochen, Germany). **(B)** Intraoperative views of FNa videoangiography (left to right: arterial, capillary, and venous phases). **(C)** Patented filter combinations used in the operative microscope balances the intensities of narrow bands of excitation and emitted light to create a clear operating field view with yellow fluorescence of fluorescein. The excitation (bottom) and emission (top) profiles of fluorescein (peaks are 485 nm, blue; 514 nm, green, respectively) are shown on the background. The transmittance of filters at various wavelengths results in the uniform intensity of all bands, with a higher intensity of emitted yellow light. **(D-H)** Pencil-type probe with filter attached to the microscope objective lens. **(D)** The pencil-type probe with blue LED emission. **(E)** Sketch demonstrating the intraoperative usage of the probe. **(F)** The switch of the filter adapted to the operating microscope. **(G)** The intraoperative view using this device (left, fluorescence off; right, fluorescence on). **(H)** A diagram showing optical setup of the device. Blue LED light is concentrated around 465 nm, and a long-pass filter (black line) allows green emission light into the camera. **(I-K)** The laser microscope. **(I)** The illuminating device. **(J)** Images of the laser FNa videoangiography (left to right: intraoperative image under white light, capillary phase and venous phases of the FNa videoangiography). **(K)** Regular excitation (light blue) overlapping the emission (light green) laser light contains light only at 464 nm wavelength and does not interfere with the emission light; thus, the videoangiogram has good contrast. **(L–N)** An endoscope outfitted for FNa videoangiography. **(L)** A 2.7-mm straight endoscope is connected to a blue LED light source and a long-pass filter is inserted at the camera attachment. **(M)** The intraoperative view of endoscopic FNa videoangiography (left to right: under white light, under the blue LED before FNa injection, and after FNa injection). **(N)** The diagram showing optical setup of the device. Blue LED light is concentrated around 465 nm, and a long-pass filter (black line) allows green emission light into the camera. *, right posterior cerebral artery; **, left posterior cerebral artery; AN, aneurysm; BA, basilar artery; Max, maximum; Min, minimum; SCA, superior cerebellar artery. **(A–C,H,K,L,N)** are used with permission from Barrow Neurological Institute, Phoenix, Arizona.

VISUALIZING PLATFORMS

Different visualizing platforms that have been developed for FNa videoangiography are described briefly below (**Figure 2**).

Conventional Operating Microscopes With Fluorescein Filters (Figures 2A–C)

Unlike ICG videoangiography, which requires a separate infrared camera attached to the operating microscope to detect the infrared emission signal (39), the emission light of FNa requires only a filter for fluorescence to be visualized within the visible light spectrum. This may be the reason for the delayed application of ICG into the vascular field (39).

An FNa-specific filter set can be integrated into the surgical microscope to guarantee optimal intraoperative visualization of fluorescence and images superior in clarity. Novel microscopes have improved so much in fluorescence modality, and FNa fluorescence can offer such a brighter view that tumor resection can be performed in fluorescence mode throughout the whole surgery rather than switching between visualization modalities (40).

Pencil-Type Probe With Detachable Filter for the Microscope (Figures 2D–H)

Suzuki et al. used a pencil-type probe with a blue light-emitting diode (LED) at the tip (20, 30, 31); this setup can offer excitatory light while FNa fluorescence can be observed via a filter attached to the microscope (20, 30, 31). This pencil-type probe and filter represent an affordable option, and it enables surgeons to equip existing surgical microscopes with an FNa visualization mode.

A custom long-pass filter inset was designed to be manually installed at the bottom of the surgical microscope cylinder to visualize the FNa fluorescence (41). This device includes optical filters positioned across the three light pathways: two barrier filters for observation within the wavelength of FNa emitted fluorescence and one excitation filter.

Laser Illumination-Based Operating Microscope (Figures 2I–K)

Ito et al. reported the application of the laser microscope for intraoperative fluorescence cerebral angiography (22). Unlike traditional operating microscopes with a xenon lamp-generated light (wide wavelength spectrum), the laser microscope contains only three lasers of 640 nm (red), 532 nm (green), and 464 nm (blue) wavelengths. During illumination, these three wavelengths crosswire, resulting in white light that is similar to the regular xenon-generated light. During FNa videoangiography, the system turns off the green laser while leaving on the blue laser and low-intensity red laser. The peak emission wavelength of the FNa is 520 nm, which does not overlay with reflected blue and red laser lights. Therefore, such illumination offers better contrast. Furthermore, the laser illumination-based microscope produces significantly less tissue heat compared to xenon lamp illumination (38). Although this laser microscope is an early prototype, it provides well-controlled illumination that may benefit future developments of surgical microscopes.

FNa Videoangiography With an Endoscope (Figures 2L–N)

Hashimoto et al. reported their experience of FNa videoangiography visualized through the endoscope (20). A blue LED was adapted to the light source of the 2.7-mm endoscope to offer excitation light, and the emission light passed through a long-pass filter and was received by a camera.

In their detailed report, only three of 18 aneurysms could be completely inspected under the microscope after clipping, and no neck remnant was confirmed. Although microscopic FNa videoangiography showed that in all cases complete aneurysm occlusion had been achieved, subsequent inspection with the endoscopic FNa videoangiography allowed the investigators to detect and correct three of 18 cases with neck remnants and two of 18 cases with incomplete occlusion. Moreover, the perforator origin could be visualized only via endoscopic inspection and

TABLE 1 | Comparison of Advantages and Disadvantages of ICG- and FNa-Based Videoangiography.

Parameter	Fluorescent angiography	
	ICG	**FNa**
Thick vessel wall	Deeper penetration depth; can visualize STA, ICA, VA	Shallow penetration depth; cannot show flow in ICA or VA
Small vessels	Harder to visualize	Easier to visualize
Repeated IV injections or increased dose	Decreased intensity because of quenching	Can stain vessel wall resulting in false-positive fluorescence
Fluorescence detection	Infrared camera only	Eye, camera
Display	Always digital signal; separate LCD display or image injection into microscope eyepieces	Viewed through eyepieces or on any display
On-the-fly angiography	Requires image overlay; otherwise, need to review ICG video separately from natural light view	Can be in real time
View of surgical field	Two-dimensional	Three-dimensional in eyepieces/display
Contrast	Very high contrast	Average to high contrast

FNa, fluorescein sodium; ICA, internal carotid artery; ICG, indocyanine green; STA, superficial temporal artery; VA, vertebral artery.

TABLE 2 | Summary of clinical application of fluorescein videoangiography in the literature.

References	Injection method	Visualizing platform	Dose/concentration	Cases number	Lesion type	Time to arterial phase	Time to fade out	Comments
Feinde et al. (13)	IA	Stroboscopic light with Wratten 2B filter	1–2 ml/1% (10–20 mg)	1	AVM	Less than 2 s	N/A	First report in the literature
Little et al. (33)	IA (CCA)	Strobe light with Kodak-Wratten 47A filter	5 ml/1% (50 mg)	15	STA-MCA bypass	2.4 ± 0.4 s pre-bypass; 0.7 ± 0.3 s post-bypass	N/A	Bypass led to a 1.7 s decrease of the period from injection to arterial phase.
Wrobel et al. (32)	IV	ILC 302 and Oriel liquid light with Wratten 47A filter	20 ml/10% (2 g)	1	Aneurysm	30 s	60 min	2 g FNa caused long-time vessel wall staining
Suzuki et al. (30)	IV	A pencil-type probe with a blue LED/ filter attached to microscope	5 ml/10% (500 mg)	23	Aneurysm	15 s	N/A	The pencil-type probe is an affordable option for FNa videoangiography
Kuroda et al. (31)	IV and IA	A pencil-type probe with a blue LED filter attached to microscope	IV 5 ml/10% (500 mg); IA 10 ml/0.01–0.02% (1–2 mg)	IV, 5; IA, 13	Aneurysm	IV, 30 s; IA, immediately	IV, minimally 5 min; IA, 30 s	First study to report the advantage and disadvantage of IV and IA injections
Rey-Dios and Cohen-Gadol (16)	IV	OPMI Pentero 900	1 mg/kg	2	Aneurysm, 1; AVM, 1	20 s	N/A	
Ichikawa et al. (17)	IA (STA)	OPMI Pentero 900	5 ml/0.5–1%	10	Aneurysm	Immediately	Less than 1 min	3 F catheter inserted 5–10 cm into the STA
Lane and Cohen-Gadol (18)	IV	OPMI Pentero 900	75 mg	4	AVM	10–15 s	N/A	FNa videoangiography has the "real-time inspection" feature which is valuable in AVM surgery
Lane et al. (19)	IV	OPMI Pentero 900	75 mg	22	Aneurysm	20 s	20–30 min	Prospective comparison of FNa and ICG
Misra et al. (34)	IV	N/A	1.5 mg/kg	1	DAVF	11 s	N/A	First case report of use with a spinal AVM
Hashimoto et al. (20)	IV and IA	Olympus endoscope with long-pass filter; blue LED at the light source	IV 5 ml/10% (500 mg); IA 10 ml/0.01–0.02% (1–2 mg)	IV, 5; IA, 13	Aneurysm	IV, 30 s; IA, immediately	IV, N/A; IA 30 s	Endoscope can offer more information such as neck remnant and perforators preservation
Kakucs et al. (15)	IV	OPMI Pentero 900	5 ml/10% (500 mg)	10	Aneurysm	15 s	N/A	
Matano et al. (21)	IV	OPMI Pentero 900	250 mg	23	Aneurysm 18; bypass, 5	NA	N/A	Comparison of ICG and FNa in vascular surgery
Ito et al. (22)	IV	M500 OHS1 Laser microscope	2.5 ml/10% (250 mg)	1	Aneurysm	20 s	N/A	A novel laser microscope examining fluorescein angiography
Narducci et al. (6)	IV	OPMI Pentero 900	500 mg	11	Bypass	15–20 s	20–25 min	
Serrano-Rubio et al. (23)	IV	OPMI Pentero 900	75 mg	12	AVM	11.6 s	N/A	

AVM, arteriovenous malformation; CCA, common carotid artery; DAVF, dural arteriovenous fistula; FNa, fluorescein sodium; IA, intraarterial; ICG, indocyanine green; IV, intravenous; LED, light-emitting diode; MCA, middle cerebral artery; N/A, not applicable; STA, superficial temporal artery.

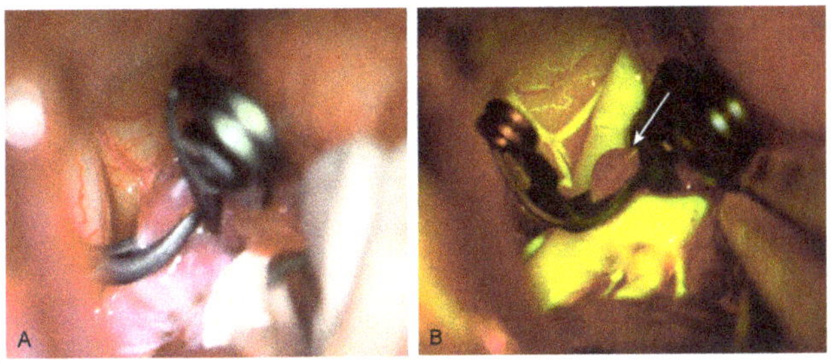

FIGURE 3 | Intraoperative images of an unruptured anterior communicating artery. **(A)** Intraoperative image under normal light. **(B)** Intraoperative image taken during FNa videoangiography; the aneurysm is not filling after being clipped (white arrow). Used with permission from Barrow Neurological Institute, Phoenix, Arizona.

not with the microscope, which allowed the identification and correction of two perforator occlusion events. The authors concluded that endoscopic FNa videoangiography had the same accuracy as DSA.

Although ICG videoangiography can also be obtained via endoscope, such ICG-infrared compatible endoscopes exceed 4 mm in diameter (42–44). Hashimoto et al. reported that in nine of 29 cases, a 4-mm endoscope was too large for visualization at deep locations (20). Therefore, thin endoscopes capable of FNa videoangiography represent a valuable adjunct to visualize blood flow in the vessels that are obscured during wide-field operations using microscope-based angiography.

COMPARISON OF ICG AND FNa VIDEOANGIOGRAPHIES

In vascular neurosurgery, intraoperative DSA remains the gold standard to assess the blood flow, but DSA requires a hybrid operating room and increases operating time (19).

Although ICG was applied to assess cerebral blood flow much later than FNa [ICG in 2003 (39), FNa in 1967 (12)], cerebral fluorescent videoangiography is currently more common with ICG than with FNa. ICG videoangiography can be repeated quickly and can demonstrate the vasculature clearly (45, 46); however, ICG still has several drawbacks. FNa and ICG both have features that can provide benefits in different scenarios—the features of both fluorophores are summarized in **Table 1**.

On one hand, unlike FNa, which can be observed in oculars, ICG requires a dedicated camera to detect the near-infrared signal and a separate display to present a pseudo-colored signal. The ICG signal does not interfere with visible spectral reflectance from the operating field and therefore provides a better contrast than FNa between surrounding structures (signal always = 0) and intravascular ICG (signal is high and always > 0), without the need to sacrifice any wavelength of the visible spectrum.

On the other hand, FNa can be seen as an orange color by the naked eye or as a bright yellow color when fluorescent. Because the excitation and emission wavelengths of FNa are within the visible spectrum, creation of a high contrast for FNa visualization requires the user to sacrifice some portion of the visible spectrum. Improvements with optical filter technologies have made it possible to selectively attenuate or block multiple spectral bands, allowing brighter overall images and making the consequential image demonstrate most of the reflected visible colors (brain, blood, and other tissues) and brighter FNa fluorescence simultaneously.

ICG is a fluorophore that can be visualized only by a near-infrared detector with a complete dark background (45), in which case the relationship of the surrounding anatomy and the vessels cannot be demonstrated. Furthermore, the ICG imaging can be visualized only via a separate infrared camera; therefore, the surgeon cannot change the view or perform real-time dissection on the basis of the information obtained from ICG videoangiography. Although these limitations were partially solved by live ICG-image overlay features on operating microscopes (47), such microscopes are not yet widely available.

FNa videoangiography provides less contrast than ICG but has the advantage of allowing visualization of the angiogram embedded in the thee-dimensional background anatomy within the ocular lens, which can enable real-time manipulation in situations of inadequate exposure, clip adjustment, and so on.

The second ICG injection can be less clear and less contrasting than the first because of quenching effects of dye remaining from the first injection (31). However, higher dosages of FNa with IV injection may stain the vessels for a substantial time, decreasing the specificity of FNa signal. Therefore, in terms of repeating fluorescent videoangiography quickly, ICG videoangiography may be preferred over IV FNa videoangiography (19, 21).

Another advantage of ICG is the longer wavelength emission that could penetrate thick vessel walls. It is reported that ICG is favorable in visualizing major arteries, such as the internal carotid artery and superficial temporal artery (21).

Lane et al. performed a prospective study comparing ICG and FNa videoangiographies in 22 patients and drew the conclusion that FNa can provide better visualization of vasculature at high magnification within deep operative fields (19). The limitation of ICG visualization at deep operative fields has been mentioned as its drawback in multiple studies (48–51). One study reported that inadvertent occlusion of small perforators was encountered in 6% (15/239) of the aneurysm clipping cases despite using ICG videoangiography (49).

ICG videoangiography and FNa videoangiography are valuable and mutually complementary tools in vascular neurosurgery, each with subtle advantages and disadvantages, and neither can yet replace intraoperative DSA as the gold standard. FNa and ICG could be used together sequentially as they do not interfere with each other. As technologies advance, the disadvantages of either modality are becoming less substantial (e.g., real-time ocular overlay of ICG videoangiography and laser illumination system).

CLINICAL APPLICATION OF FNa VIDEOANGIOGRAPHY IN VASCULAR NEUROSURGERY

The use of FNa videoangiography has been reported in many types of vascular neurosurgery, including treating aneurysms, AVMs, and DAVFs and bypass surgeries. A summary of clinical

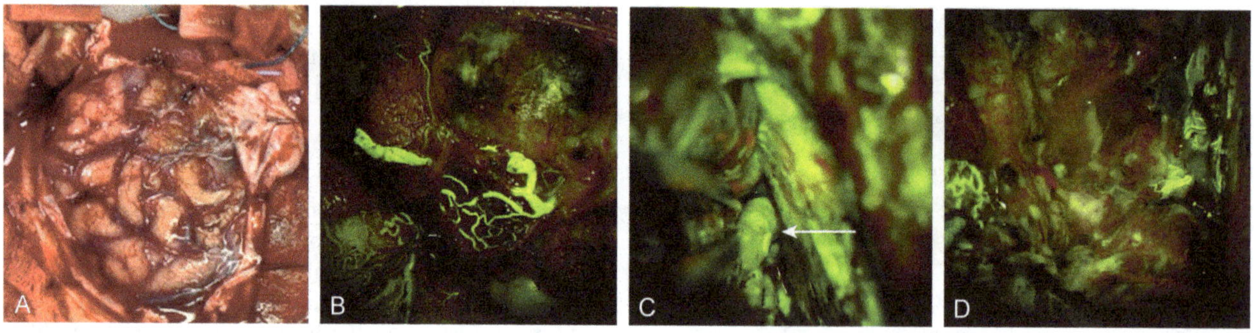

FIGURE 4 | Intraoperative images of a left frontal arteriovenous malformation **(A)** under normal light, **(B)** during FNa videoangiography, **(C)** during real-time inspection of the nidus and the deep feeders (white arrow) under FNa videoangiography during dissection, and **(D)** after total removal of the malformation. Used with permission from Barrow Neurological Institute, Phoenix, Arizona.

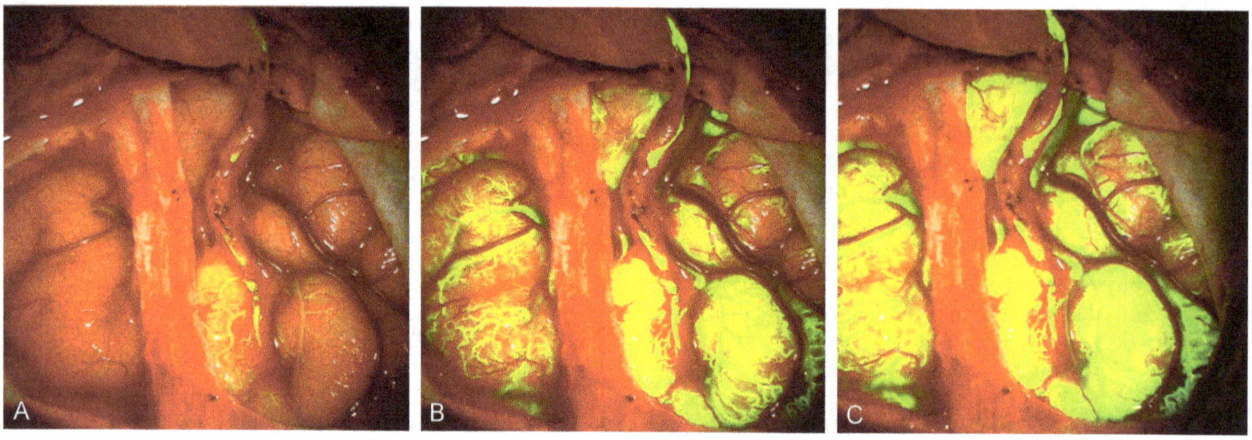

FIGURE 5 | FNa videoangiography images from a patient with moyamoya disease after a superficial temporal artery to middle cerebral artery bypass shows filling of **(A)** donor and recipient arteries, **(B)** cortical capillaries, and **(C)** all cortical vascular networks. Notice the filling starts at the bypass site and spreads around. Used with permission from Charite Universitätsmedizin Berlin, Berlin, Germany.

studies is presented in **Table 2** (6, 13, 15–23, 30–34), and clinical applications of FNa videoangiography are discussed below.

Cerebral Aneurysm Surgery (Figure 3)

For cerebral aneurysm surgery, it is of paramount importance to confirm the obliteration of the aneurysm neck as well as the patency of the parent vessels and small perforators intraoperatively (31). Lane et al. reported that FNa is preferable over ICG in terms of visualizing small perforators and aneurysm obliteration (19). For aneurysms at deep locations requiring a narrow corridor (i.e., anterior cerebral artery aneurysms through the lateral frontal approach), real-time manipulation of the surrounding anatomy under FNa videoangiography allows maximum exposure and inspection of the vessels of interest (19).

As discussed above, the endoscope can offer more information than FNa angiography, such as location of neck remnants and perforator preservation, as the endoscope provides a close and multi-angled inspection (20).

AVM Surgery (Figure 4)

AVMs are usually adhesive to the surrounding brain parenchyma. AVMs can be regarded as "intra-axial lesions" as most require subarachnoid and pial dissection. Numerous feeders can supply the nidus from the deep side, and these feeders may be blocked by brain parenchyma. Such a complex nature means that DSA remains the gold standard for evaluation (52), but it is not always available.

As mentioned above, fluorescence with traditional ICG videoangiography cannot be visualized via an ocular in real time. Deep feeders and the adhesive nature of AVMs make them challenging to operate on because thorough information usually cannot be obtained from a single angiography. Especially after circumferential dissection of the nidus or ligation of the superficial feeders, a premature venous filling indicates the presence of remaining deep feeders. Real-time dissection of the nidus and full inspection around it under videoangiography can facilitate localizing the rest of the feeders as well as provide a thorough examination of the lesion (16, 18). The real-time feature of FNa videoangiography is preferable over

ICG in such scenarios. In the only case of a spinal AVM reported as treated under FNa videoangiography (34), the vascular nidus was well visualized as being embedded in the background anatomy and the AVM was successfully resected.

DAVF Surgery

To date, there is no report of the application of FNa videoangiography for treating a DAVF. Unlike AVMs, DAVFs do not adhere to the surrounding parenchyma. The ligation of the fistula is concise and quick if the fistula can be accurately located; this feature of treating a DAVF requires repeated angiography in a short period of time. Even though IV injection of FNa for videoangiography has a relatively long intravascular stay, IA injection might be suitable in this scenario, and future investigation is merited.

Cerebrovascular Bypass Surgery (Figure 5)

FNa videoangiography can be used to evaluate the patency of the anastomosis and the improvement of the stenosis during cerebrovascular bypass surgery. The feature of real-time manipulation does not make FNa videoangiography differ from the ICG videoangiography in the bypass assessment (6). However, IA injection can be used to evaluate the effectiveness of the bypass apart from the evaluation of the patency. Little et al. carried out a study using IA injection in 1979 and reported that the duration from the injection to the arterial phase decreased from 2.4 ± 0.4 s to 0.7 ± 0.3 s (33). Such a decrease in time can help evaluate the improvement of the ischemic condition and offer another supplementary tool for evaluating the success of the bypass surgery.

CONCLUSION

The FNa-based fluorescent videoangiography techniques reviewed here represent an armamentarium of useful tools for various types of vascular neurosurgeries. Compared with ICG videoangiography, FNa videoangiography has the advantage of three-dimensional visualization of surrounding anatomy and allows real-time surgical manipulation, especially of small vessels in a narrow field. The disadvantages of FNa videoangiography are the incompetence in visualizing flow in thick-walled vessels and the staining of vessel walls at high doses. Advanced microscopy technologies, such as endoscopy and laser microscopy, have the potential to further improve the utility of FNa videoangiography. Finally, FNa videoangiography is affordable and may be complementary to ICG videoangiography for vascular neurosurgery.

AUTHOR CONTRIBUTIONS

PN and MP: conception and design. PN, ML, and PV: providing clinical cases. XZ: drafting the article. EB and CC: figures and graphs producing. EB, CC, DV, and SG: revising the article. PN: study supervision.

ACKNOWLEDGMENTS

The authors thank the staff of Neuroscience Publications at Barrow Neurological Institute for assistance with manuscript preparation.

REFERENCES

1. Acland R, Raja Sabapathy S. *Acland's Practice Manual for Microvascular Surgery*. 2nd Edn. Mumbai: Medknow (1989).
2. Amin-Hanjani S, Meglio G, Gatto R, Bauer A, Charbel FT. The utility of intraoperative blood flow measurement during aneurysm surgery using an ultrasonic perivascular flow probe. *Neurosurgery*. (2006) 58:ONS-305-ONS-312. doi: 10.1227/01.NEU.0000209339.47929.34
3. Hecht N, Woitzik J, König S, Horn P, Vajkoczy P. Laser speckle imaging allows real-time intraoperative blood flow assessment during neurosurgical procedures. *J Cereb Blood Flow Metab*. (2013) 33:1000-7. doi: 10.1038/jcbfm.2013.42
4. Woitzik J, Horn P, Vajkoczy P, Schmiedek P. Intraoperative control of extracranial—intracranial bypass patency by near-infrared indocyanine green videoangiography. *J Neurosurg*. (2005) 102:692–8. doi: 10.3171/jns.2005.102.4.0692
5. Yanaka K, Fujita K, Noguchi S, Matsumaru Y, Asakawa H, Anno I, et al. Intraoperative angiographic assessment of graft patency during extracranial-intracranial bypass procedures. *Neurol Medico Chir*. (2003) 43:509–13. doi: 10.2176/nmc.43.509
6. Narducci A, Onken J, Czabanka M, Hecht N, Vajkoczy P. Fluorescein videoangiography during extracranial-to-intracranial bypass surgery: preliminary results. *Acta Neurochir*. (2018) 160:767–74. doi: 10.1007/s00701-017-3453-0
7. Van Cader TC. History of ophthalmic photography. *J Ophthalmic Photogr*. (1978) 1:7–9.
8. Norton EW, Gutman F. Diabetic retinopathy studied by fluorescein angiography. *Ophthalmologica*. (1965) 150:5–17. doi: 10.1159/000304822
9. Russell RR, Ffytche T, Sanders M. A study of retinal vascular occlusion using fluorescein angiography. *Lancet*. (1966) 288:821–5. doi: 10.1016/S0140-6736(66)92254-9
10. Moore GE, Peyton WT, French LA, Walker WW. The clinical use of fluorescein in neurosurgery: the localization of brain tumors. *J Neurosurg*. (1948) 5:392–8. doi: 10.3171/jns.1948.5.4.0392
11. Moore GE. Fluorescein as an agent in the differentiation of normal and malignant tissues. *Science*. (1947) 106:130–1. doi: 10.1126/science.106.2745.130-a
12. Feindel W, Yamamoto YL, Hodge CP. Intracarotid fluorescein angiography: a new method for examination of the epicerebral circulation in man. *Can Med Assoc J*. (1967) 96:1.
13. Feindel W, Yamamoto YL, Hodge CP. Red cerebral veins and the cerebral steal syndrome: Evidence from fluorescein angiography and microregional blood flow by radioisotopes during excision of an angioma. *J Neurosurg*. (1971) 35:167–79. doi: 10.3171/jns.1971.35.2.0167
14. Zipfel GJ. Clipping of neurosurgical aneurysms: the dye is cast. *J Neurosurg*. (2015) 122:616–7. doi: 10.3171/2014.8.JNS14957
15. Kakucs C, Florian AI, Ungureanu G, Florian SI. Fluorescein angiography in intracranial aneurysm surgery: a helpful method to evaluate the security of clipping and observe blood flow. *World Neurosurg*. (2017) 105:406–11. doi: 10.1016/j.wneu.2017.05.172
16. Rey-Dios R, Cohen-Gadol AA. Technical principles and neurosurgical applications of fluorescein fluorescence using a microscope-integrated fluorescence module. *Acta Neurochir*. (2013) 155:701–6. doi: 10.1007/s00701-013-1635-y
17. Ichikawa T, Suzuki K, Watanabe Y. Intra-arterial fluorescence angiography with injection of fluorescein sodium from the superficial temporal artery during aneurysm surgery: technical notes. *Neurol Med Chir*. (2014) 54:490–496. doi: 10.2176/nmc.tn.2013-0232
18. Lane BC, Cohen-Gadol AA. A prospective study of microscope-integrated intraoperative fluorescein videoangiography during arteriovenous

malformation surgery: preliminary results. *Neurosurg Focus.* (2014) 36:E15. doi: 10.3171/2013.11.FOCUS13483
19. Lane B, Bohnstedt BN, Cohen-Gadol AA. A prospective comparative study of microscope-integrated intraoperative fluorescein and indocyanine videoangiography for clip ligation of complex cerebral aneurysms. *Neurosurg.* (2015) 122:618–26. doi: 10.3171/2014.10.JNS132766
20. Hashimoto K, Kinouchi H, Yoshioka H, Kanemaru K, Ogiwara M, Yagi T, et al. Efficacy of endoscopic fluorescein video angiography in aneurysm surgery—novel and innovative assessment of vascular blood flow in the dead angles of the microscope. *Operat Neurosurg.* (2017) 13:471–81. doi: 10.1093/ons/opw042
21. Matano F, Mizunari T, Murai Y, Kubota A, Fujiki Y, Kobayashi S, et al. Quantitative comparison of the intraoperative utility of indocyanine green and fluorescein videoangiographies in cerebrovascular surgery. *Operat Neurosurg.* (2017) 13:361–6. doi: 10.1093/ons/opw020
22. Ito Y, Suzuki K, Ichikawa T, Watanabe Y, Sato T, Sakuma J, Saito K. Intraoperative fluorescence cerebral angiography by laser surgical microscopy: comparison with xenon microscopy and simultaneous observation of cerebral blood flow and surrounding structures. *Operat Neurosurg.* (2018) 16:700–6. doi: 10.1093/ons/opy159
23. Serrano-Rubio A, Ruiz-Treviño AS, Orenday-Barraza JM, Vázquez-Gregorio R, Lee A, Nathal E. Sodium fluorescein videoangiography as an adjunct to resection of cerebral arteriovenous malformations. *World Neurosurg.* (2018) 117:e329–34. doi: 10.1016/j.wneu.2018.06.024
24. Dollery C. *Fluorescein, Therapeutic Drugs.* Edinburgh, Churchill Livingstone (1999).
25. Shinoda J, Yano H,Yoshimura SI, Okumura A, Kaku Y, Iwama T, Sakai N. Fluorescence-guided resection of glioblastoma multiforme by using high-dose fluorescein sodium. *J Neurosurg.* (2003) 99:597–603. doi: 10.3171/jns.2003.99.3.0597
26. Bennett TJ, Quillen DA, Coronica R. Fundamentals of fluorescein angiography. *Insight.* (2016) 41:5–11.
27. Kwan AS, Barry C, McAllister IL, Constable I. Fluorescein angiography and adverse drug reactions revisited: the Lions Eye experience. *Clin Exp Ophthalmol.* (2006) 34:33–8. doi: 10.1111/j.1442-9071.2006.01136.x
28. Alford R, Simpson HM, Duberman J, Hill GC, Ogawa M, Regino C, et al. Toxicity of organic fluorophores used in molecular imaging: literature review. *Mol Imaging.* (2009) 8:31. doi: 10.2310/7290.2009.00031
29. Yannuzzi LA, Rohrer KT, Tindel LJ, Sobel RS, Costanza MA, Shields W, et al. Fluorescein angiography complication survey. *Ophthalmology.* (1986) 93:611–7. doi: 10.1016/S0161-6420(86)33697-2
30. Suzuki K, Watanabe Y, Ichikawa T. Usefulness of intraoperative fluorescence cerebral angiography using fluorescein sodium. *Surg Cereb Stroke.* (2009) 37:240–5. doi: 10.2335/scs.37.240
31. Kuroda K, Kinouchi H, Kanemaru K, Nishiyama Y, Ogiwara M, Yoshioka H, et al. Intra-arterial injection fluorescein videoangiography in aneurysm surgery. *Operat Neurosurg.* (2012) 72:ons141–50. doi: 10.1227/NEU.0b013e3182752f32
32. Wrobel CJ, Meltzer H, Lamond R, Alksne JF. Intraoperative assessment of aneurysm clip placement by intravenous fluorescein angiography. *Neurosurgery.* (1994) 35:970–3. doi: 10.1097/00006123-199411000-00027
33. Little JR, Yamamoto YL, Feindel W, Meyer E, Hodge CP. Superficial temporal artery to middle cerebral artery anastomosis: intraoperative evaluation by fluorescein angiography and xenon-133 clearance. *J Neurosurg.* (1979) 50:560–9. doi: 10.3171/jns.1979.50.5.0560
34. Misra BK, Samantray SK, Churi ON. Application of fluorescein sodium videoangiography in surgery for spinal arteriovenous malformation. *J Clin Neurosci.* (2017) 38:59–62. doi: 10.1016/j.jocn.2016.12.004
35. Yamamoto S, Kim P, Kurokawa R, Itoki K, Kawamoto S. Selective intraarterial injection of ICG for fluorescence angiography as a guide to extirpate perimedullary arteriovenous fistulas. *Acta Neurochirurg.* (2012) 154:457–63. doi: 10.1007/s00701-011-1223-y
36. Belykh E, Miller EJ, Patel AA, Bozkurt B, Yagmurlu K, Robinson TR, Nakaji P, et al. Optical characterization of neurosurgical operating microscopes: quantitative fluorescence and assessment of PpIX photobleaching. *Sci Rep.* (2018) 8:12543. doi: 10.1038/s41598-018-30247-6
37. Suzuki K, Kodama N, Sasaki T, Matsumoto M, Ichikawa T, Munakata R, et al. Confirmation of blood flow in perforating arteries using fluorescein cerebral angiography during aneurysm surgery. *J Neurosurg.* (2007) 107:68–73. doi: 10.3171/JNS-07/07/0068
38. Sato T, Bakhit MS, Suzuki K, Sakuma J, Fujii M, Murakami Y, et al. Utility and safety of a novel surgical microscope laser light source. *PLoS ONE.* (2018) 13:e0192112. doi: 10.1371/journal.pone.0192112
39. Raabe A, Beck J, Gerlach R, Zimmermann M, Seifert V. Near-infrared indocyanine green video angiography: a new method for intraoperative assessment of vascular flow. *Neurosurgery.* (2003) 52:132–9. doi: 10.1227/00006123-200301000-00017
40. Belykh EG, Zhao X, Cavallo C, Bohl MA, Yagmurlu K, Aklinski JL, et al. Laboratory evaluation of a robotic operative microscope-visualization platform for neurosurgery. *Cureus.* (2018) 10:e3072. doi: 10.7759/cureus.3072
41. Ichikawa T, Suzuki K, Watanabe Y, Sato T, Sakuma J, Saito K. Development of and clinical experience with a simple device for performing intraoperative fluorescein fluorescence cerebral angiography: technical notes. *Neurol Med Chir.* (2016) 56:141–9. doi: 10.2176/nmc.tn.2015-0188
42. Nishiyama Y, Kinouchi H, Senbokuya N, Kato T, Kanemaru K, Yoshioka H, et al. Endoscopic indocyanine green video angiography in aneurysm surgery: an innovative method for intraoperative assessment of blood flow in vasculature hidden from microscopic view. *J Neurosurg.* (2012) 117:302–8. doi: 10.3171/2012.5.JNS112300
43. Bruneau M, Appelboom G, Rynkowski M, Van Cutsem N, Mine B, De Witte O. Endoscope-integrated ICG technology: first application during intracranial aneurysm surgery. *Neurosurg Rev.* (2013) 36:77–85. doi: 10.1007/s10143-012-0419-9
44. Mielke D, Malinova V, Rohde V. Comparison of intraoperative microscopic and endoscopic ICG angiography in aneurysm surgery. *Operat Neurosurg.* (2014) 10:418–25. doi: 10.1227/NEU.0000000000000345
45. Raabe A, Nakaji P, Beck J, Kim LJ, Hsu FP, Kamerman JD, Seifert V, Spetzler RF. Prospective evaluation of surgical microscope—integrated intraoperative near-infrared indocyanine green videoangiography during aneurysm surgery. *J Neurosurg.* (2005) 103:982–9. doi: 10.3171/jns.2005.103.6.0982
46. de Oliveira JG, Beck J, Seifert V, Teixeira MJ, Raabe A. Assessment of flow in perforating arteries during intracranial aneurysm surgery using intraoperative near-infrared indocyanine green videoangiography. *Operat Neurosurg.* (2007) 61:ONS-63–ONS-73. doi: 10.1227/01.neu.0000289715.18297.08
47. Martirosyan NL, Skoch J, Watson JR, Lemole GM Jr., Romanowski M, Anton R. Integration of indocyanine green videoangiography with operative microscope: augmented reality for interactive assessment of vascular structures and blood flow. *Operat Neurosurg.* (2015) 11:252–8. doi: 10.1227/NEU.0000000000000681
48. Dashti R, Laakso A, Niemelä M, Porras M, Hernesniemi J. Microscope integrated indocyanine green video-angiography in cerebrovascular surgery. *Acta Neurochir Suppl.* (2011) 109:247–50. doi: 10.1007/978-3-211-99651-5_39
49. Dashti R, Laakso A, Niemelä M, Porras M, Hernesniemi J, Microscope-integrated near-infrared indocyanine green videoangiography during surgery of intracranial aneurysms: the Helsinki experience. *Surg Neurol.* (2009) 71:543–50. doi: 10.1016/j.surneu.2009.01.027
50. Gruber A, Dorfer C, Standhardt H, Bavinzski G, Knosp E. Prospective comparison of intraoperative vascular monitoring technologies during cerebral aneurysm surgery. *Neurosurgery.* (2011) 68:657–73. doi: 10.1227/NEU.0b013e31820777ee
51. Washington CW, Zipfel GJ, Chicoine MR, Derdeyn CP, Rich KM, Moran CJ, et al. Comparing indocyanine green videoangiography to the gold standard of intraoperative digital subtraction angiography used in aneurysm surgery. *J Neurosurg.* (2013) 118:420–7. doi: 10.3171/2012.10.JNS11818
52. Yanaka K, Matsumaru Y, Okazaki M, Noguchi S, Asakawa H, Anno I, Nose T. Intraoperative angiography in the surgical treatment of cerebral arteriovenous malformations and fistulas. *Acta Neurochir.* (2003) 145:377–83. doi: 10.1007/s00701-003-0017-2

20

Optical Characterization of Sodium Fluorescein *In Vitro* and *Ex Vivo*

Ran Xu [1†], Wanda Teich [1†], Florian Frenzel [2], Katrin Hoffmann [2], Josefine Radke [3,4,5], Judith Rösler [1], Katharina Faust [1], Anne Blank [1], Susan Brandenburg [1], Martin Misch [1], Peter Vajkoczy [1], Julia Sophie Onken [1,4‡] and Ute Resch-Genger [2‡]*

[1] Department of Neurosurgery, Charité—Universitätsmedizin Berlin, Corporate Member of Freie Universität Berlin, and Humboldt-Universität zu Berlin, and Berlin Institute of Health, Berlin, Germany, [2] Division Biophotonics, Federal Institute for Materials Research and Testing (BAM), Berlin, Germany, [3] Department of Neuropathology, Charité—Universitätsmedizin Berlin, Corporate Member of Freie Universität Berlin, Humboldt-Universität zu Berlin, and Berlin Institute of Health, Berlin, Germany, [4] German Cancer Consortium (DKTK), Heidelberg, Germany, partner site Charité Berlin, Berlin, Germany, [5] Berlin Institute of Health (BIH), Berlin, Germany

***Correspondence:**
Ran Xu
ran.xu@charite.de

†These authors have contributed equally to this work and share first authorship

‡These authors share last authorship

Objective: The utilization of fluorescein-guided biopsies and resection has been recently discussed as a suitable strategy to improve and expedite operative techniques for the resection of central nervous system (CNS) tumors. However, little is known about the optical properties of sodium fluorescein (NaFl) in human tumor tissue and their potential impact on *ex vivo* analyses involving fluorescence-based methods.

Methods: Tumor tissue was obtained from a study cohort of an observational study on the utilization of fluorescein-guided biopsy and resection (n=5). The optical properties of fluorescein-stained tissue were compared to the optical features of the dye *in vitro* and in control samples consisting of tumor tissue of high-grade glioma patients (n=3) without intravenous (i.v.) application of NaFl. The dye-exposed tumor tissues were used for optical measurements to confirm the detectability of NaFl emission *ex vivo*. The tissue samples were fixed in 4%PFA, immersed in 30% sucrose, embedded in Tissue-Tek OCT compound, and cut to 10 μm cryosections. Spatially resolved emission spectra from tumor samples were recorded on representative slides with a Confocal Laser Scanning Microscope FV1000 (Olympus GmbH, Hamburg, Germany) upon excitation with λ_{exc} = 488 nm.

Results: Optical measurements of fluorescein in 0.9% sodium chloride (NaCl) under *in vitro* conditions showed an absorption maximum of $\lambda_{max\ abs}$ = 479 nm as detected with spectrophotometer Specord 200 and an emission peak at $\lambda_{max\ em}$ = 538 nm recorded with the emCCD detection system of a custom-made microscope-based single particle setup using a 500 nm long-pass filter. Further measurements revealed pH- and concentration-dependent emission spectra of NaFl. Under ex vivo conditions, confocal laser scanning microscopy of fluorescein tumor samples revealed a slight bathochromic shift and a broadening of the emission band.

Conclusion: Tumor uptake of NaFl leads to changes in the optical properties – a bathochromic shift and broadening of the emission band – possibly caused by the dye's high pH sensitivity and concentration-dependent reabsorption acting as an inner filter of the dye's emission, particularly in the short wavelength region of the emission spectrum where absorption and fluorescence overlap. Understanding the *ex vivo* optical properties of fluorescein is crucial for testing and validating its further applicability as an optical probe for intravital microscopy, immunofluorescence localization studies, and flow cytometry analysis.

Keywords: sodium fluorescein, spectroscopy, brain tumor, confocal, fluorescein-guided surgery, optical probe pH sensing, NaFl

INTRODUCTION

The utilization of fluorescein as an optical probe for guiding the resection and biopsy of central nervous system (CNS) tumors has been recently proposed as a powerful strategy to improve and expedite operative techniques (1–4). Sodium fluorescein (NaFl) is a fluorescent dye with a molecular weight of 376.3 g/mol that accumulates in tumor tissue where blood brain barrier (BBB) breakdown occurs and thus, enhances tumor visualization, contributing to the extent of resection which is in turn associated with a better overall survival rate (5–9). This dye has been successfully implemented in clinical applications in ophthalmology; in recent years, its implications for CNS tumor resection, as well as for vascular neurosurgery techniques have also been discussed (10–13).

However, little is known about the spectroscopic characteristics of fluorescein after its intravenous (i.v.) application, as it traverses the BBB and accumulates in tumor tissue. The tumor microenvironment is a complex compartment with spatiotemporal variability in tumor cells, acidity, hypoxia, secreted factors, and extracellular matrix proteins. Moreover, it is unknown how the dye is metabolized in this environment. This encouraged us to characterize the *in vitro* and *ex vivo* optical characteristics of NaFl to understand its spectroscopic features after biological tissue uptake with special emphasis on its potential further implications of fluorescent-based assays.

MATERIAL AND METHODS

Patients and Specimen Handling

The study was approved by the local Ethical Committee (EA1/284/20, EA4/219/17 and EA2/101/08) of the Charité University Hospital. All patients gave written consent for the off-label use of i.v. fluorescein-guided surgery or biopsy. All study patients had a contrast-enhancing lesion in which surgical resection was indicated, and their characteristics are listed in **Table 1**. The workflow of the experimental setup of human tissue is shown in **Figure 1**. Briefly, patients received intraoperatively a dosage of 5 mg/kg Fluorescein Alkon i.v. according to our standardized operating procedure for brain tumor surgery (n=5). Tumor surgery was performed in a standard fashion using the Pentero 900 microscope with Y560 filter, Carl Zeiss, Meditec, Oberkochen, Germany. The dye-exposed tumor tissue was brought to the laboratory on ice, and immediately fixed in 4% PFA overnight at 4°C, then immersed in 30% sucrose, and embedded in Tissue-Tek® O.C.T.™ compound. Cryosections were cut into slices of 10 μm thickness. Control samples (n=3) consisted of glioma tumor samples from patients who did not receive fluorescein-guided surgery due to contraindications. Hematoxylin & Eosin (H&E) staining was performed using a standard methodology and staining reagents. Images were collected using a Carl Zeiss Axio observer Z1 inverted immunofluorescence microscope equipped with standard DAPI (filter 49, excitation 365 nm, emission 445 ± 25nm), FITC (filter 38, excitation 470 ± 20nm, emission 525 ± 25nm nm), and Cy3 (filter 43, excitation 545 ± 12.5nm, emission 605 ± 35nm) filters, respectively.

Spectroscopy of NaFl *In Vitro*

The absorbance spectrum of fluorescein in 0.9% NaCl was measured in a cuvette with the spectrophotometer Specord 200. The emission spectrum of fluorescein in 0.9% NaCl under 488 nm laser excitation (Supercontinuum Laser Solea, PicoQuant) was recorded with a custom-made microscope-based single particle setup equipped with a 500 nm long-pass filter using the emCCD detection system (DU970P-BVF, Andor Ltd.).

Concentration- and pH-dependent emission spectra of NaFl *in vitro* were recorded using a spectral scanning Confocal Laser Scanning Microscope (CLSM) FluoView FV1000 (Olympus GmbH, Hamburg, Germany). The emission spectra were measured in droplets of the corresponding NaFl solutions, which were placed on standard microscopy coverslips #1.5 (0.170 mm). A multiline argon ion laser (30 mW) was used as excitation source (λ_{exc} = 488 nm), which was reflected by a beam splitter (BS 20/80) and focused onto the sample through an Olympus objective UPLSAPO 20x (numerical aperture N.A. 0.75). The emitted photons were collected with the same objective, focused onto a photomultiplier (PMT), and recorded in the wavelength range of 500 - 640 nm (spectral resolution of 2.0 nm, step sizes of 2.0 nm).

Spectroscopy of NaFl *Ex Vivo*

Spatially resolved emission spectra of tumor samples were recorded on representative tumor sections. Exemplarily chosen, but representative 10 regions of interests (ROIs) within the tumor tissue and one additional ROI as a blank or baseline control (recording background noise) were measured with the FV1000 (Olympus GmbH, Hamburg, Germany) upon excitation with λ_{exc} = 488 nm under almost the same experimental settings and conditions as described above. The *ex vivo* spectra, however, were measured in derogation through an objective UPLSAPO 20xW/0.75 in the range of 500 nm - 740 nm (spectral resolution of 5.0 nm and step sizes of 2.0 nm).

TABLE 1 | Patient characteristics.

	Age	Gender	Localization	Extent of resection	Histology
Fluorescein	50	M	Left temporolateral	Resection	Glioblastoma, IDH-wildtype (WHO grade IV), MGMT methylated
	58	M	Left temporopolar	Resection	Glioblastoma, IDH-wildtype (WHO grade IV), MGMT methylation
	87	M	Left temporolateral	Biopsy	Glioblastoma, IDH-wildtype (WHO grade IV), MGMT unmethylated
	71	F	Left temporomesial	Biopsy	Diffuse large B-cell lymphoma
	61	M	Left occipital	Resection	Post-transplant lymphoproliferative disorder (PTLD)
Control	24	F	Left temporomesial	Resection	Glioblastoma (WHO grade IV), MGMT unmethylated
	35	F	Right temporolateral	Resection	Glioblastoma (WHO grade IV), MGMT methylation
	64	F	Left frontal operculum	Resection	Glioblastoma (WHO grade IV), MGMT methylation

F, female; M, male.

Statistical Analysis and Figures

Values are generally presented as mean +/- SEM unless otherwise stated. Statistical significance was determined by Student t-test and statistical analysis was performed using Graphpad Prism software (Version 7.0). Elements of **Figures 1** and **5** were composed using BioRender.Com.

RESULTS

NaFl Tumor Samples Show Positive Signal in Both Green and Red Channels

To examine whether NaFl tumor tissue still showed measurable FITC signal after fixation, frozen sections were analyzed in the FITC channel of a fluorescent microscope. Indeed, all the samples exhibited a heterogeneous pattern of FITC signal (**Figure 2**). To clarify that the area of interest was in fact vital tumor tissue, consecutive sections were subjected to Hematoxylin & Eosin (H&E) staining and examined by a consultant neuropathologist to confirm the histopathological diagnosis of the rapid frozen sections (**Figure 2**). However, all samples showed also fluorescence signals in the CY3 channel (**Figure 2**). This observation was surprising since NaFl should not reveal a signal in the CY3 channel separated by the CY3 filter (covering the emission wavelength region of 605 ± 35nm by its transmission profile) under baseline *ex vivo* conditions. The observed changes in the spectroscopic features of NaFl might be of significant relevance in the future, e.g. for the in-depth analysis of *in vivo* tumor imaging using NaFl. To better

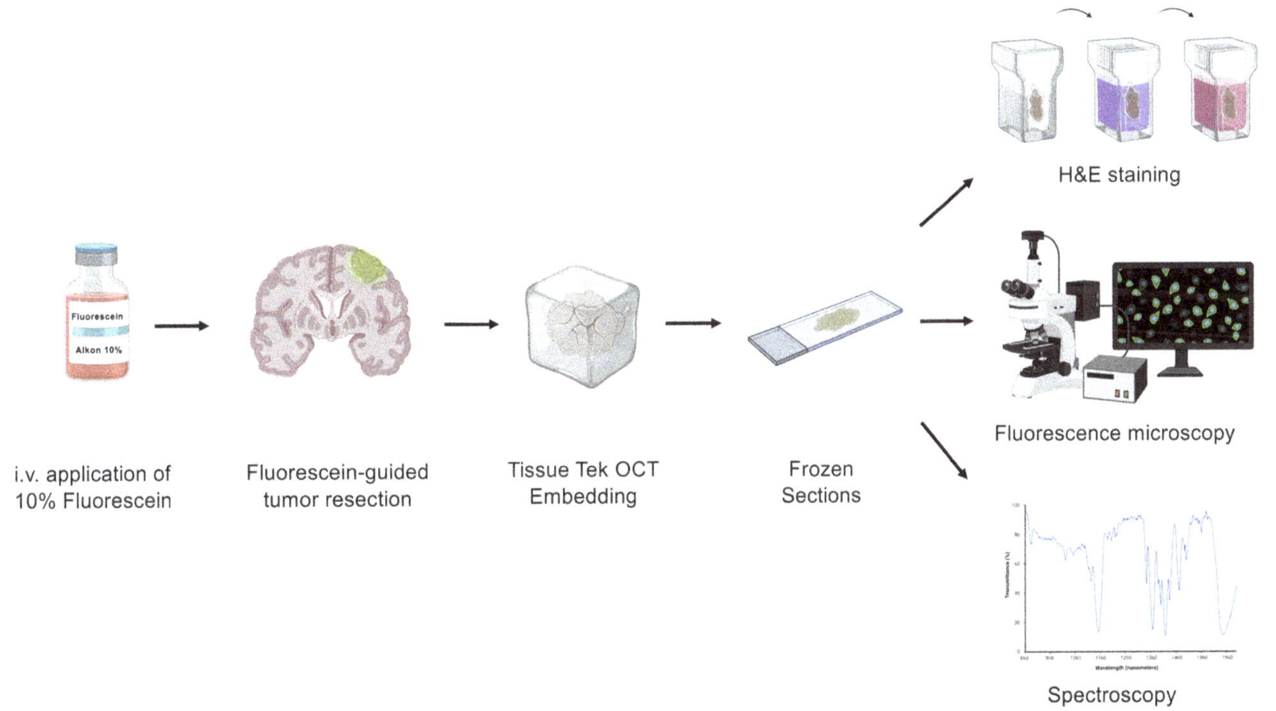

FIGURE 1 | Experimental workflow. Before tumor resection, patients received sodium fluorescein (NaFl) intravenously (i.v.). After fixation in 4% PFA and 30% sucrose immersion, the NaFl-stained tissue was embedded in Tissue-Tek OCT before cryosectioning. Frozen sections were then studied by fluorescence microscopy and spectroscopy measurements.

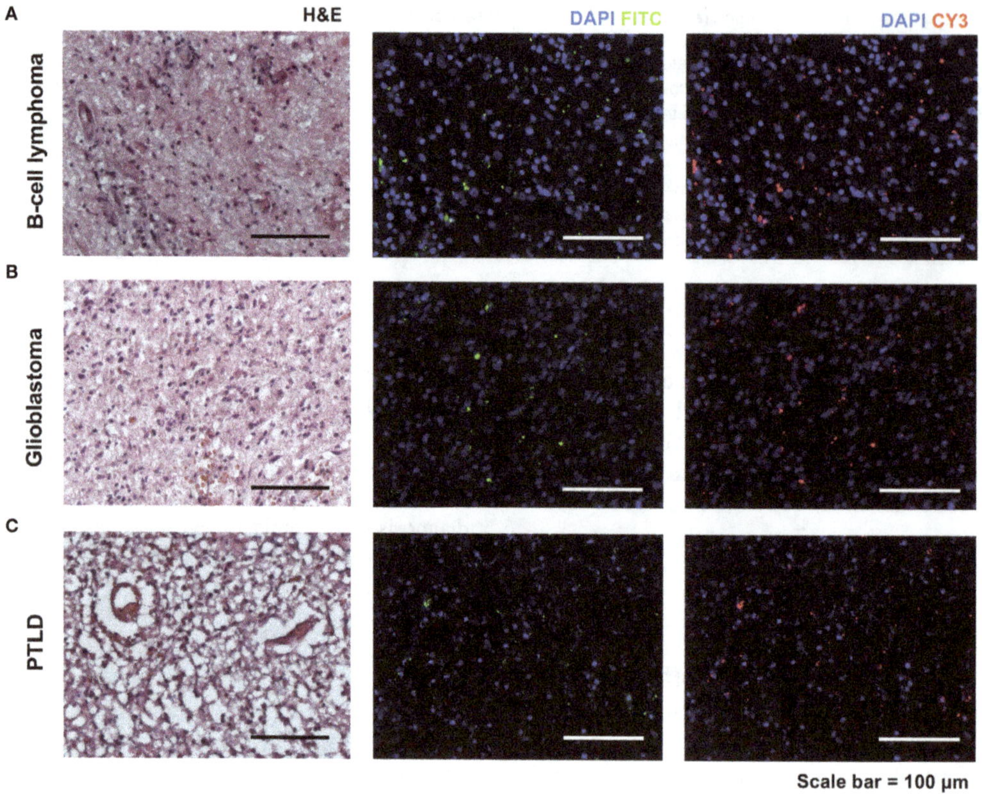

FIGURE 2 | Hematoxylin and eosin (H&E) staining of rapid sections in three different pathologies [**A**, B-cell lymphoma, **B**, glioblastoma, and **C**, posttransplant lymphoproliferative disorder (PTLD)] with consecutive slides using FITC and CY3 filters of an immunofluorescence microscope. All samples showed signals in the FITC channel, and unexpectedly, also in the CY3 channel (scale bar = 100 μm).

understand this shift in emission wavelength we performed a series of *in vitro* and *ex vivo* studies to characterize the optical properties of our optical probe.

Absorbance and Emission of NaFl *In Vitro*

Next, to elucidate the optical properties of NaFl *in vitro*, we measured absorbance and emission spectra of NaFl under *in vitro* conditions. Here, we observed a typical absorbance peak at $\lambda_{max\ abs}$ = 479 nm and an emission peak at $\lambda_{max\ em}$ = 538 nm (**Figure 3A**). These absorbance and emission maxima match well with the previously reported spectroscopic features of fluorescein (14).

Fluorescein-Stained Tumor Tissue Shows a Bathochromic Shift in Emission *Ex Vivo*

We next compared the *in vitro* emission spectra of NaFl to the corresponding emission spectra obtained *ex vivo* to better understand the optical behavior of this dye within the tumor core. Interestingly, in representative tumor samples, we observed a broadening of the dye's emission band and a slight, but significant spectral shift to longer wavelengths, also known as a bathochromic shift, compared to NaFl in buffer solution pH 8.04 *in vitro* (**Figure 3B**). The control samples showed a significantly lower emission intensity with a mean intensity of 530.6 (± 67.58) a.u. [= arbitrary (or relative) units] compared to 971.1 (± 146.1) a.u. at a wavelength of 540 nm in the NaFl tumor samples (p=0.0441) (**Figures 3C, D**).

pH-Dependent and Concentration-Dependent Emission

Since NaFl showed heterogeneous uptake in tumor tissue, we examined whether this finding could be explained by the characteristic pH-dependent emission features of the dye - also given that previous studies highlighted an acidic milieu of the tumor microenvironment contributing to a change in pH (15, 16). Therefore, we measured the absorbance spectra of NaFl in 0.9% NaCl solution and its emission spectra in different phosphate buffers (pH 5.54, pH 7.35, and pH 8.04). Our results reveal the well-known pH-dependence of the NaFl emission intensity that increases with increasing pH (**Figure 4A**) (17). Also, the heterogeneous uptake of the dye leading to different local NaFl concentrations could contribute to the spectroscopic effects observed *ex vivo*. Hence, we measured the spectra of NaFl *in vitro* at different dye concentrations. Thereby, we noticed not only a concentration-dependent emission intensity of the dye (**Figures 4B, C**), but also observed a red shift in the emission maxima with increasing NaFl concentrations (**Figure 4D**).

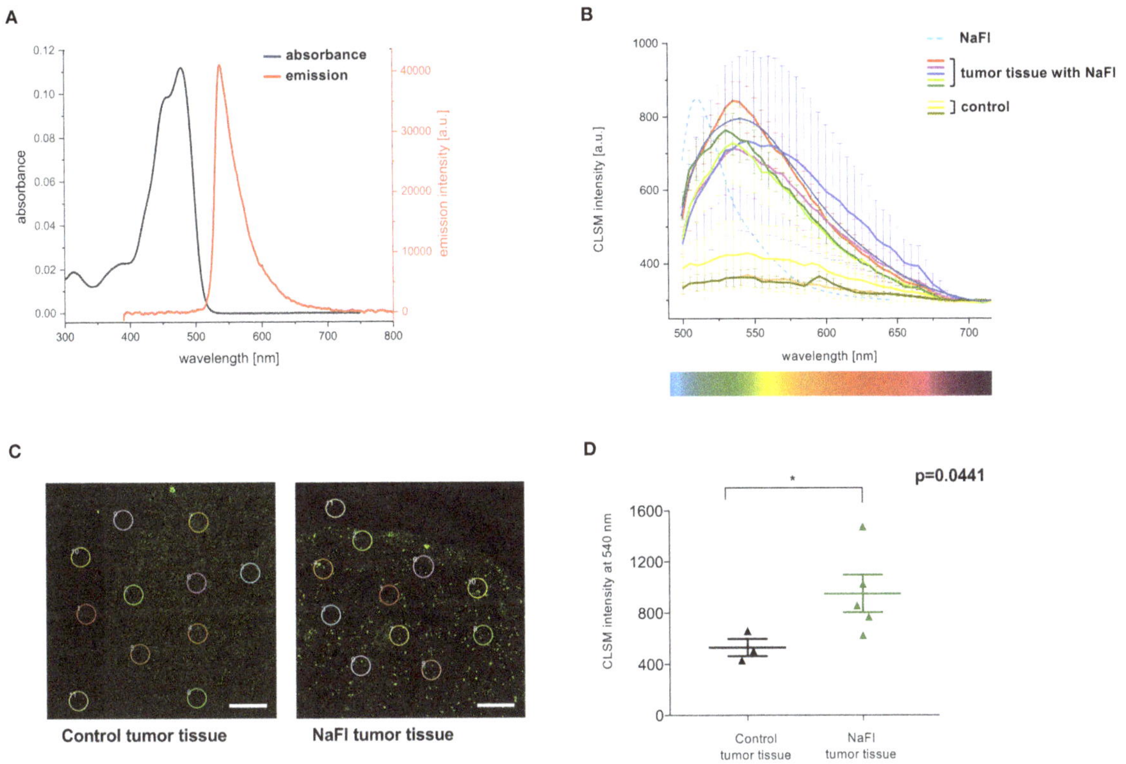

FIGURE 3 | Absorbance and emission of NaFl *in vitro* and *ex vivo*. **(A)** Absorbance (black line) and emission spectra (red line) under *in vitro* conditions show the typical maximum absorbance at $\lambda_{max\ abs}$ = 479 nm and an emission peak at $\lambda_{max\ em}$ = 538 nm. **(B)** Confocal Laser Scanning Microscopy (CLSM) emission spectra of NaFl in phosphate buffer solution at pH 8.04 *in vitro* (blue dashed line) and in *ex vivo* samples (colored solid lines). Exemplary, but representative *ex vivo* tumor samples with NaFl show a broadened, bathochromically shifted NaFl tumor emission (solid lines). A broad but very weak emission in the same wavelength region was also observed for the control samples. **(C, D)** Exemplary, but representative CLSM intensities of 10 regions of interests (ROIs) read out at 540 nm show a significantly higher signal in fluorescein tumor samples (971.1 ± 146.1 a.u.) versus control samples (530.6 ± 67.58 a.u.); p= 0.0441. Values are expressed in average ± S.E.M. (Scale bar = 100 µm).

DISCUSSION

Our results show that NaFl exhibits a significant broadening of its emission band together with a bathochromic shift after tissue uptake in CNS tumor samples. These changes could possibly be explained by the dye's high pH sensitivity and/or concentration-dependent reabsorption effects (**Figure 5**).

Furthermore, our data reveal a very heterogeneous distribution pattern of NaFl in tumor tissue on a microscopic level. This can also be observed intraoperatively by the neurosurgeon on a macroscopic scale. Traditionally, a heterogeneous uptake can be related to a variability in BBB properties and regionally distinct hyperpermeability. Our data show that this heterogeneous emission signal of the dye is also influenced by the dye's high pH sensitivity, potentially caused by the variability of the acidic milieu in the tumor microenvironment. This acidic milieu has also been discussed in the literature as a driver of cancer development (15). The fluorescein molecule can exist in different protonation states which all differ in their fluorescence features; only the dianion and monoanion of fluorescein emit a visible fluorescence of varying fluorescence efficiency or quantum yield while the neutral dye is non-emissive (17). A more acidic extracellular milieu should lead to the formation of the monoanion while a more basic environment favors the formation of the dye's dianion. This goes along with the pH-dependent emission spectra found for the dye in different buffer solutions. Moreover, the heterogeneous appearance of NaFl uptake in tumor tissue is likely caused by the high sensitivity of the NaFl emission behavior to its concentration. This corresponds with the observed decrease in fluorescence intensity with higher local dye concentration due to reabsorption effects. Our data confirm earlier reports that both the pH of the dye's local environment as well as dye concentration can affect the emission of NaFl, which could explain the findings of our *ex vivo* optical measurements, showing a red shift in fluorescence (18, 19).

The change in the intrinsic spectroscopic properties of fluorophores including spectral shifts and changes in the shape of fluorescence emission spectra caused by different environments have been reported before, and the tumor microenvironment is a complex system with a considerable variability in tumor cells, acidity, secretomes, and extracellular compartments that can likely cause changes in the dye's spectroscopic features (4). For example, another study also reported a bathochromic shift for fluorescein ligands bound to rabbit polyclonal anti-Fluorescein Fab fragments (20).

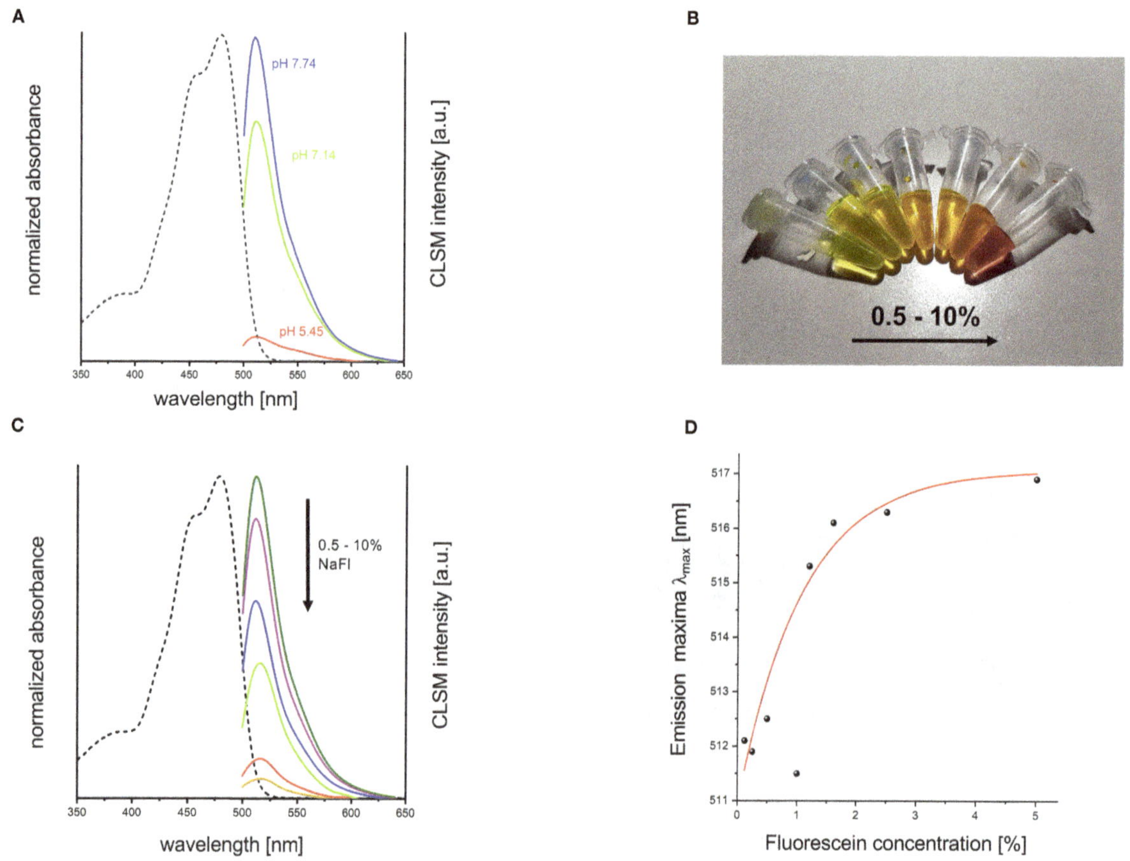

FIGURE 4 | pH- and concentration-dependent emission of NaFl. **(A)** Normalized absorbance (in 0.9% NaCl solution; dashed line) and pH dependent emission spectra of NaFl solutions in different phosphate buffers (phosphate buffer pH 5.54, pH 7.35, and pH 8.04) obtained with a confocal laser scanning microscope (CLSM). **(B)** Concentration series of Na-Fl solutions (in 0.9% NaCl), and **(C)** the corresponding absorbance (in 0.9% NaCl solution; dashed line), and concentration-dependent CLSM emission spectra (solid lines). **(D)** Emission maxima λ_{max} [nm] plotted against NaFl concentration [%] show a concentration-dependent red shift by about 5 nm.

Tumor tissue autofluorescence is a common phenomenon that should be considered, specifically when working with fluorescence-based assays. Some studies even suggest to utilize the spectral characteristics of the autofluorescence signals from glioma cells for diagnostic purposes (21, 22). To verify that autofluorescence signals do not potentially resemble or interfere with the NaFl signal, we measured the emission spectra of native tumor tissue without exposure to NaFl under the same conditions as used for the NaFl measurements. Although this experiment revealed a broad emission band in the green and red wavelength region, control tumor tissue showed only a very weak emission signal compared to the NaFl-stained tumor samples.

Since NaFl has been increasingly used for the guidance of brain tumor resection, it is crucial to understand its *ex vivo* optical properties, since they can impact further in-depth *in vivo* imaging analyses as well as fluorescence-based assays such as FACS analyses, immunofluorescence staining or *in vivo* microscopy (23, 24). The observation in our study that NaFl in tumor tissue revealed signals in the longer wavelength CY3 channel was surprising. The practical implication of these spectral changes is that if further fluorescence-based laboratory studies are conducted on CNS tumor tissue which were resected under fluorescein-guidance, labeling with secondary antibodies using dyes emitting in the FITC or Cy3 channel should be used with care as this can result in spectral interferences and crosstalk. Based on the broadening and bathochromic shift of the emission band, it seems to be more reasonable to switch to secondary antibodies labeled with dyes emitting in the blue (e.g. 350 – 408 nm) or preferably in the far red (630 – 647 nm) and near-IR channels (650 – 750 nm) in assays such as immunofluorescence microscopy and flow cytometry. The implications of the observed changes in optical properties are of relevant nature, especially if these fluorescent-based assays are used for further diagnostic purposes. Furthermore, in the clinical setting, the utilization of NaFl in combination with in-depth *in vivo* and *ex vivo* imaging techniques such as confocal laser endomicroscopy has also been discussed in recent studies in aiding histopathological diagnoses (25, 26). Hence, the increasing role of NaFl in such settings poses increasing interest on NaFl tumor kinetics, and further analysis of its spectroscopic features may help to distinguish its free form from fluorescein metabolites (fluorescein glucuronide).

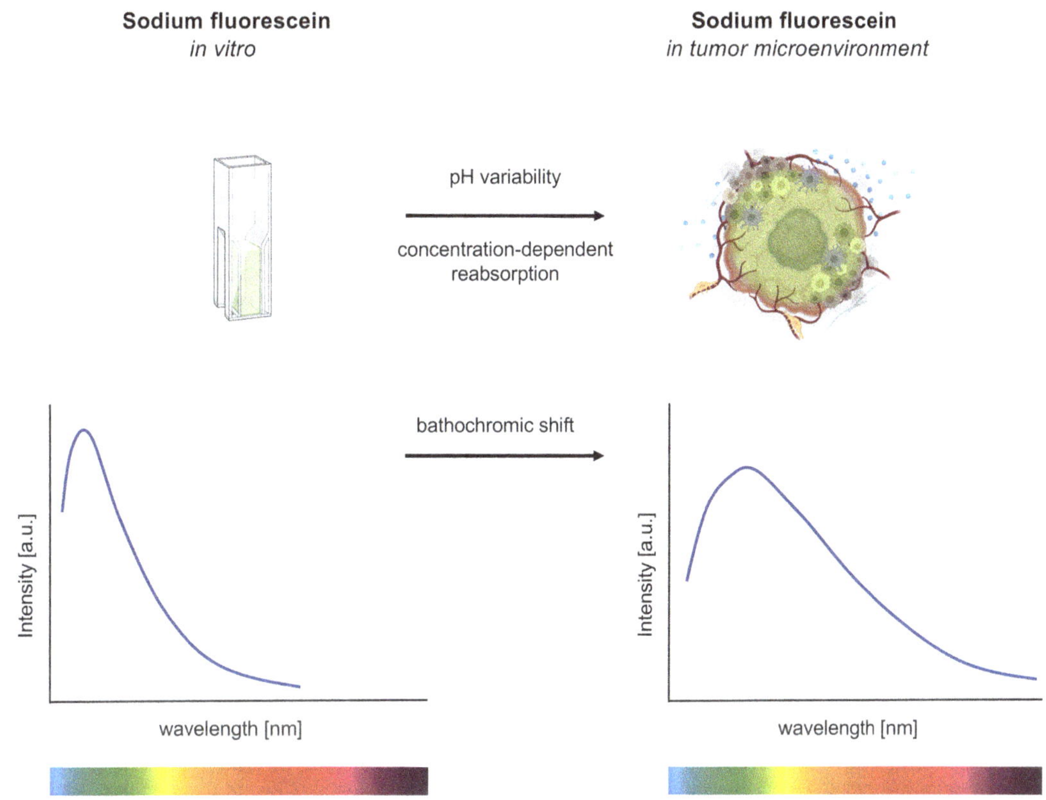

FIGURE 5 | Emission spectroscopy of sodium fluorescein (NaFl) under *in vitro* and *ex vivo* conditions. Exposure of NaFl to the tumor microenvironment shows a broadening and a bathochromic shift of the dye's emission spectrum. The pH sensitivity and the concentration-dependent reabsorption effect of the dye contribute to this red shift.

In summary, our data reveal changes of the spectroscopic properties of NaFl *ex vivo*, particularly a bathochromic shift in emission after tumor uptake, underpinning that the widespread use of fluorescein in neurosurgical procedures requires a detailed study of its optical properties in a clinical setting. Our study is, however, limited by a small sample size, heterogeneity in tumor histology, and the absence of *in vivo* pharmacokinetic properties of NaFl. Further studies are needed to fully understand the exact nature of the changes of the spectroscopic properties of NaFl *ex vivo* and related possible interference with other fluorescence-based assays in tumor tissue.

ETHICS STATEMENT

The studies involving human participants were reviewed and approved by Charité's Ethics Committee. The patients/participants provided their written informed consent to participate in this study.

AUTHOR CONTRIBUTIONS

WT, KH, FF, JoR, AB, SB, and RX conducted experiments and analyzed data. RX, JO, and UR-G designed the study. All authors contributed to writing and revising of the manuscript. All authors contributed to the article and approved the submitted version.

ACKNOWLEDGMENTS

We kindly thank Jimmy LaPrelle for proofreading the manuscript.

REFERENCES

1. Acerbi F, Broggi M, Schebesch KM, Hohne J, Cavallo C, De Laurentis C, et al. Fluorescein-Guided Surgery for Resection of High-Grade Gliomas: A Multicentric Prospective Phase II Study (FLUOGLIO). *Clin Cancer Res* (2018) 24:52–61. doi: 10.1158/1078-0432.CCR-17-1184
2. Rey-Dios R, Hattab EM, Cohen-Gadol AA. Use of Intraoperative Fluorescein Sodium Fluorescence to Improve the Accuracy of Tissue Diagnosis During Stereotactic Needle Biopsy of High-Grade Gliomas. *Acta Neurochir (Wien)* (2014) 156:1071–5. doi: 10.1007/s00701-014-2097-6
3. Stummer W, Novotny A, Stepp H, Goetz C, Bise K, Reulen HJ. Fluorescence-Guided Resection of Glioblastoma Multiforme by Using 5-Aminolevulinic Acid-Induced Porphyrins: A Prospective Study in 52 Consecutive Patients. *J Neurosurg* (2000) 93:1003–13. doi: 10.3171/jns.2000.93.6.1003

4. Hohne J, Acerbi F, Falco J, Akcakaya MO, Schmidt NO, Kiris T, et al. Lighting Up the Tumor-Fluorescein-Guided Resection of Gangliogliomas. *J Clin Med* (2020) 9:2405. doi: 10.3390/jcm9082405
5. Lacroix M, Abi-Said D, Fourney DR, Gokaslan ZL, Shi W, DeMonte F, et al. A Multivariate Analysis of 416 Patients With Glioblastoma Multiforme: Prognosis, Extent of Resection, and Survival. *J Neurosurg* (2001) 95:190–8. doi: 10.3171/jns.2001.95.2.0190
6. 2McGirt MJ, Chaichana KL, Gathinji M, Attenello FJ, Than K, Olivi A, et al. Independent Association of Extent of Resection With Survival in Patients With Malignant Brain Astrocytoma. *J Neurosurg* (2009) 110:156–62. doi: 10.3171/2008.4.17536
7. Brown TJ, Brennan MC, Li M, Church EW, Brandmeir NJ, Rakszawski KL, et al. Association of the Extent of Resection With Survival in Glioblastoma: A Systematic Review and Meta-Analysis. *JAMA Oncol* (2016) 2:1460–9. doi: 10.1001/jamaoncol.2016.1373
8. Stummer W, Reulen HJ, Meinel T, Pichlmeier U, Schumacher W, Tonn JC, et al. Extent of Resection and Survival in Glioblastoma Multiforme: Identification of and Adjustment for Bias. *Neurosurgery* (2008) 62:564–76; discussion 564-76. doi: 10.1227/01.neu.0000317304.31579.17
9. Diaz RJ, Dios RR, Hattab EM, Burrell K, Rakopoulos P, Sabha N, et al. Study of the Biodistribution of Fluorescein in Glioma-Infiltrated Mouse Brain and Histopathological Correlation of Intraoperative Findings in High-Grade Gliomas Resected Under Fluorescein Fluorescence Guidance. *J Neurosurg* (2015) 122:1360–9. doi: 10.3171/2015.2.JNS132507
10. Schebesch KM, Brawanski A, Hohenberger C, Hohne J. Fluorescein Sodium-Guided Surgery of Malignant Brain Tumors: History, Current Concepts, and Future Project. *Turk Neurosurg* (2016) 26:185–94. doi: 10.5137/1019-5149.JTN.16952-16.0
11. Zhao X, Belykh E, Cavallo C, Valli D, Gandhi S, Preul MC, et al. Application of Fluorescein Fluorescence in Vascular Neurosurgery. *Front Surg* (2019) 6:52. doi: 10.3389/fsurg.2019.00052
12. Ward KW. Superficial Punctate Fluorescein Staining of the Ocular Surface. *Optom Vis Sci* (2008) 85:8–16. doi: 10.1097/OPX.0b013e31815ed756
13. Desmettre T, Devoisselle JM, Mordon S. Fluorescence Properties and Metabolic Features of Indocyanine Green (ICG) as Related to Angiography. *Surv Ophthalmol* (2000) 45:15–27. doi: 10.1016/S0039-6257(00)00123-5
14. Sjoback R, Nygren J, Kubista M. Characterization of Fluorescein-Oligonucleotide Conjugates and Measurement of Local Electrostatic Potential. *Biopolymers* (1998) 46:445–53. doi: 10.1002/(SICI)1097-0282(199812)46:7<445::AID-BIP2>3.0.CO;2-5
15. Boedtkjer E, Pedersen SF. The Acidic Tumor Microenvironment as a Driver of Cancer. *Annu Rev Physiol* (2020) 82:103–26. doi: 10.1146/annurev-physiol-021119-034627
16. Petrova V, Annicchiarico-Petruzzelli M, Melino G, Amelio I. The Hypoxic Tumour Microenvironment. *Oncogenesis* (2018) 7:10. doi: 10.1038/s41389-017-0011-9
17. Sjöback R, Nygren J, Kubista M. Absorption and Fluorescence Properties of Fluorescein. *Spectrochim Acta A Mol Biomol Spectrosc* (1995) 51:L7–L21. doi: 10.1016/0584-8539(95)01421-P
18. Doughty MJ. pH Dependent Spectral Properties of Sodium Fluorescein Ophthalmic Solutions Revisited. *Ophthalmic Physiol Opt* (2010) 30:167–74. doi: 10.1111/j.1475-1313.2009.00703.x
19. McLoughlin CK, Kotroni E, Bregnhoj M, Rotas G, Vougioukalakis GC, Ogilby PR. Oxygen- and pH-Dependent Photophysics of Fluorinated Fluorescein Derivatives: Non-Symmetrical vs. Symmetrical Fluorination. *Sensors (Basel)* (2020) 20(18):5172. doi: 10.3390/s20185172
20. Voss EW Jr, Croney JC, Jameson DM. Discrete Bathochromic Shifts Exhibited by Fluorescein Ligand Bound to Rabbit Polyclonal Anti-Fluorescein Fab Fragments. *J Protein Chem* (2002) 21:231–41. doi: 10.1023/a:1019789118530
21. Croce AC, Fiorani S, Locatelli D, Nano R, Ceroni M, Tancioni F, et al. Diagnostic Potential of Autofluorescence for an Assisted Intraoperative Delineation of Glioblastoma Resection Margins. *Photochem Photobiol* (2003) 77:309–18. doi: 10.1562/0031-8655(2003)077<0309:DPOAFA>2.0.CO;2
22. Yuan Y, Yan Z, Miao J, Cai R, Zhang M, Wang Y, et al. Autofluorescence of NADH is a New Biomarker for Sorting and Characterizing Cancer Stem Cells in Human Glioma. *Stem Cell Res Ther* (2019) 10:330. doi: 10.1186/s13287-019-1467-7
23. Mazurek M, Kulesza B, Stoma F, Osuchowski J, Mandziuk S, Rola R. Characteristics of Fluorescent Intraoperative Dyes Helpful in Gross Total Resection of High-Grade Gliomas-a Systematic Review. *Diagnostics (Basel)* (2020) 10(12):1100. doi: 10.3390/diagnostics10121100
24. Stummer W, Koch R, Valle RD, Roberts DW, Sanai N, Kalkanis S, et al. Intraoperative Fluorescence Diagnosis in the Brain: A Systematic Review and Suggestions for Future Standards on Reporting Diagnostic Accuracy and Clinical Utility. *Acta Neurochir (Wien)* (2019) 161:2083–98. doi: 10.1007/s00701-019-04007-y
25. Acerbi F, Pollo B, De Laurentis C, Restelli F, Falco J, Vetrano IG, et al. Ex Vivo Fluorescein-Assisted Confocal Laser Endomicroscopy (Convivo(R) System) in Patients With Glioblastoma: Results From a Prospective Study. *Front Oncol* (2020) 10:606574. doi: 10.3389/fonc.2020.606574
26. Belykh E, Miller EJ, Carotenuto A, Patel AA, Cavallo C, Martirosyan NL, et al. Progress in Confocal Laser Endomicroscopy for Neurosurgery and Technical Nuances for Brain Tumor Imaging With Fluorescein. *Front Oncol* (2019) 9:554. doi: 10.3389/fonc.2019.00554

21

Intraoperative Confocal Laser Endomicroscopy *Ex Vivo* Examination of Tissue Microstructure During Fluorescence-Guided Brain Tumor Surgery

Evgenii Belykh[1], Xiaochun Zhao[1], Brandon Ngo[1], Dara S. Farhadi[1], Vadim A. Byvaltsev[2], Jennifer M. Eschbacher[3], Peter Nakaji[1] and Mark C. Preul[1]*

[1] Department of Neurosurgery, The Loyal and Edith Davis Neurosurgical Research Laboratory, Barrow Neurological Institute, St. Joseph's Hospital and Medical Center, Phoenix, AZ, United States, [2] Department of Neurosurgery and Innovative Medicine, Irkutsk State Medical University, Irkutsk, Russia, [3] Department of Neuropathology, Barrow Neurological Institute, St. Joseph's Hospital and Medical Center, Phoenix, AZ, United States

***Correspondence:**
Mark C. Preul
Neuropub@barrowneuro.org

Background: Noninvasive intraoperative optical biopsy that provides real-time imaging of histoarchitectural (cell resolution) features of brain tumors, especially at the margin of invasive tumors, would be of great value. To assess clinical-grade confocal laser endomicroscopy (CLE) and to prepare for its use intraoperatively *in vivo*, we performed an assessment of CLE *ex vivo* imaging in brain lesions.

Methods: Tissue samples from patients who underwent intracranial surgeries with fluorescein sodium (FNa)–based wide-field fluorescence guidance were acquired for immediate intraoperative *ex vivo* optical biopsies with CLE. Hematoxylin-eosin–stained frozen section analysis of the same specimens served as the gold standard for blinded neuropathology comparison. FNa 2 to 5 mg/kg was administered upon induction of anesthesia, and FNa 5 mg/kg was injected for CLE contrast improvement. Histologic features were identified, and the diagnostic accuracy of CLE was assessed.

Results: Of 77 eligible patients, 47 patients with 122 biopsies were enrolled, including 32 patients with gliomas and 15 patients with other intracranial lesions. The positive predictive value of CLE optical biopsies was 97% for all specimens and 98% for gliomas. The specificity of CLE was 90% for all specimens and 94% for gliomas. The second FNa injection in seven patients, a mean of 2.6 h after the first injection, improved image quality and increased the percentage of accurately diagnosed images from 67% to 93%. Diagnostic CLE features of lesional glioma biopsies and normal brain were identified. Seventeen histologic features were identified.

Conclusions: Results demonstrated high specificity and positive predictive value of *ex vivo* intraoperative CLE optical biopsies and justify an *in vivo* intraoperative trial. This new portable, noninvasive intraoperative imaging technique provides diagnostic features to discriminate lesional tissue with high specificity and is feasible for incorporation into the fluorescence-guided surgery workflow, particularly for patients with invasive brain tumors.

Keywords: brain histology, brain tumor, confocal laser endomicroscopy, fluorescein sodium, fluorescence, frozen section, optical biopsy

INTRODUCTION

Complete resection within the bounds of functional safety is the goal of neurosurgical treatment for most brain tumors, especially invasive tumors, such as high-grade glioma (HGG) (1, 2). Of particular importance are intraoperative tools that aid not only in the identification of abnormal brain tissue that should be resected but also in its differentiation from healthy brain tissue that should be preserved (3). Here we report an investigation of a relatively new handheld cellular resolution imaging tool that may prove valuable for intraoperative noninvasive optical biopsy.

Previous generations of the confocal laser endomicroscope (CLE) demonstrated initial feasibility in visualizing brain tumor microstructure with significant diagnostic accuracy (4). However, these designs were largely based on an imaging platform directly adapted from those used for gastrointestinal imaging. Thus, the US Food and Drug Administration (FDA) approved the use of these systems in the brain only for experimental purposes, and previous generations of CLE were used in only three limited trials that included *in vivo* and *ex vivo* intraoperative use (5–7). Disadvantages of the early designs included the necessity to sterilize the scanning probe between procedures; the wide 7-mm diameter of the probe, which limited the use of the CLE within narrow surgical corridors; and the straight profile of the probe as it fit into the surgeon's hand.

The novel-generation commercial clinical grade CLE was developed to address these shortcomings. The FDA-approved CLE system has a 5-mm-diameter probe that is curved like an aspiration instrument, and it has increased imaging resolution and is designed to work with a removable sterile sheet. Since the use of CLE for visualization of brain tumors was first reported, wide-field fluorescence guidance surgery has increased in popularity. Thus, fluorescein sodium (FNa) began to be administered as part of the standard neurosurgical procedure so that the bright glow of FNa fluorescence could be visualized with an operating microscope used in the Yellow560 mode.

To assess the clinical grade CLE and prepare for its intraoperative use *in vivo*, we designed an assessment of its *ex vivo* imaging performance in brain lesions, particularly invasive brain tumors. We studied CLE use during routine fluorescence-guided surgery (FGS) with the operating microscope to visualize and compare CLE tissue-imaging microstructure in *ex vivo* samples with frozen section biopsies of brain tumors. We assessed the feasibility and diagnostic accuracy of CLE optical biopsies of brain lesions to identify relevant practical and methodologic variables for future *in vivo* use in clinical studies.

Abbreviations: 5-ALA, 5-aminolevulinic acid; CI, confidence interval; CLE, confocal laser endomicroscope, confocal laser endomicroscopy; FDA, US Food and Drug Administration; FGS, fluorescence-guided surgery; FNa, fluorescein sodium; H&E, hematoxylin-eosin; HGG, high-grade glioma; ICG, indocyanine green.

MATERIALS AND METHODS

Study Design

This prospective study was conducted at St. Joseph's Hospital and Medical Center with approval from the Institutional Review Board for Human Research (IRB No, 10BN130). All participants gave informed voluntary consent for participation in this study and were recruited from patients who were operated on from August 2016 to May 2019. Patients eligible for inclusion were adults (>18 years old) scheduled at our institution for neurosurgical lesion removal involving FNa contrast administration. This convenience sample of patients with brain lesions, mostly tumors, were enrolled whenever there was availability of CLE for operations conducted by the neurosurgeons participating in the study. Standard intraoperative techniques were used during tumor resection, including neuronavigation, operating microscope, endoscopic assistance, and, in some patients, intraoperative functional mapping. Deidentified brain tumor samples were used for this study. Demographic characteristics were deemed irrelevant to the optical biopsy interpretation and quality-assessment aspects of this study and were not recorded.

FNa Administration

FNa was administered intravenously at the induction of anesthesia to create a contrast for wide-field fluorescence guidance using the Yellow560 mode of the operating microscope. The FNa dose was determined by the operating neurosurgeon. FNa 2 mg/kg was used in patients with gliomas and meningiomas, and FNa 5 mg/kg was used in patients with metastatic lesions. FNa was readministered at a 5-mg/kg dose if deemed necessary by the neurosurgeon. One patient received 40 mg/kg of FNa at the induction of anesthesia only.

Tissue Collection and Processing

Tissue samples that were removed as a part of the standard neurosurgical procedure were obtained during the tumor resection for examination. These samples were separate from those obtained for clinical care (i.e., frozen-section and permanent-section analyses). When possible, multiple biopsies of the tumor core and tumor bed area were acquired. The number of biopsies was determined by the operating neurosurgeon.

Samples were placed on a moisturized nonadherent surgical dressing, transferred to the CLE station (CONVIVO, Carl Zeiss Meditec, AG, Jena, Germany) in the same operating room, and imaged using the CLE probe affixed in a probe holder in an upright position. Tissue samples were imaged with CLE immediately after acquisition from the brain. The tissue samples were gently placed with microsurgical forceps to obtain optimal imaging. To obtain optimally balanced CLE images, we used a 488 nm excitation laser and a 517.5. to 572.5-nm bandpass filter at 1× zoom with automatic gain, resulting in resolution of 1920 × 1080 pixels and a 267 × 475 µm field of view.

The neurosurgeon was able to review the CLE images during the operation because they were displayed intraoperatively in real time on a large LED screen. When image brightness was not sufficient, the FNa was readministered according to the prescribed dosage at the request of the neurosurgeon.

After CLE imaging, tissue samples were placed on a piece of moistened absorbent cotton material in a plastic container. Samples were then submitted for histologic processing and hematoxylin-eosin (H&E) staining in the neuropathology department.

Image Analysis

The collected CLE images were processed using FIJI open-source software by applying the "despeckle" filter and creating short videos (3–20 frames in length) of select imaging locations. Deidentified CLE optical biopsies and H&E-stained sections were reviewed retrospectively in a blinded fashion by a board-certified neuropathologist (J.E.) competent in interpreting CLE images. The neuropathologist had no clinical information except that the biopsy had been performed during an intracranial procedure for removal of a lesion.

CLE optical biopsies were presented as multiple still images and video-like image loops. A CLE optical biopsy was graded as "lesional" when it was deemed representative of a tumor or necrotic tissue; as "normal" when it was representative of normal or reactive brain tissue; and as "nondiagnostic" when it was not representative of tumor or necrotic tissue (i.e., nondiagnostic of tumor). Seventeen histologic features were identified and assessed as "present" or "absent" in each CLE biopsy. The overall quality of CLE images for each optical biopsy was graded subjectively on a 6-point scale of zero to 5: 0 (not diagnostic or very bad), 1 (bad), 2 (poor), 3 (average), 4 (good), and 5 (very good). This quality assessment based on a subjective interpretation of clarity and brightness of tissue microstructure was performed by a neurosurgeon and a neuropathologist experienced in CLE and other fluorescence cell-imaging technologies.

H&E slides of biopsies were graded as "lesional" when they were representative of tumor tissue useful for diagnosis or interpretations and as "nonlesional" when they were representative of nontumor tissue, such as normal brain or gliotic reactive brain tissue. All H&E slides were useful for such interpretations. Each H&E slide was also labeled on the basis of the most likely diagnosis for a particular slide or as "nondiagnostic."

Image Interpretation

To assess how experience in working with CLE affects the interpretation of CLE images, we assigned two additional appraisers (both experienced senior neurosurgeons) to review a set of CLE images for interpretation. The first neurosurgeon (M.C.P.) was experienced in interpreting CLE images but was blinded to the image acquisition process. The second neurosurgeon (V.A.B.) had limited experience in interpreting CLE images but had assistance from a general pathologist who also lacked experience in interpreting CLE images. Prior to assessment, both neurosurgeons were instructed using a separate set of images on the key histologic features identifiable on CLE images. No information was provided to the neurosurgeons or general pathologist regarding case history, imaging, surgical information, or diagnosis.

Statistical Analysis

Statistical analysis was performed in Excel (Microsoft, Inc., Redmond, WA). The interpretation of CLE images and H&E histologic sections was compared. We also assessed CLE image quality and timing and dose of FNa injection. Exploratory diagnostic accuracy was calculated using a 2×2 table and standard formulas for the sensitivity, specificity, positive predictive value, and negative predictive value; results were reported according to the Standards for Reporting Diagnostic Accuracy Studies guidelines (8). For statistical analysis, CLE optical biopsies that were nondiagnostic of tumor tissue or that were labeled as normal tissue were used as a negative CLE test result. For the purpose of analysis, inconclusive H&E results were treated as "nonlesional."

RESULTS

Descriptive Analysis

Seventy-seven potentially eligible patients provided consent during the study period. CLE imaging was not performed for 13 patients because of surgery cancelation or CLE unavailability. Fourteen patients were excluded because their procedures were endoscopic transsphenoidal surgeries, and three patients were excluded because no biopsy samples were available for analysis. Thus, CLE imaging was available for 47 patients with 122 matched optical and histologic biopsies available for analysis (**Table 1**, **Figure 1**). Preliminary diagnoses by tumor type were as follows: 32 gliomas (19 primary glioblastomas, 5 recurrent glioblastomas, 5 infiltrating gliomas, 3 low-grade gliomas), 7 meningiomas, 4 metastatic brain lesions, 1 choroid plexus carcinoma, 1 craniopharyngioma, 1 schwannoma, and 1 arteriovenous malformation (reactive normal brain). All specimens were successfully analyzed *ex vivo* with CLE immediately after acquisition.

Second Dose of FNa

Resection of the lesion was completed in all patients under operating microscope visualization with and without Yellow560 mode irrespective of regard for *ex vivo* CLE analysis. In 7 cases (5 gliomas, 1 metastasis, and 1 choroid plexus carcinoma), FNa (5 mg/kg) was subsequently administered after the initial resection to evaluate the edge with subsequent biopsy acquisition for CLE analysis. FNa was readministered at a mean (SD) of 157 (52) min after the first administration. Analysis of these specimens showed improved brightness and contrast and improved overall image quality. For the cases in which the reinjection was performed, the percentage of images with an accurate diagnosis increased from 67% (18 of 27) to 93% (14 of 15), and the percentage of nondiagnostic CLE

TABLE 1 | General characteristics on confocal laser endomicroscopy of 122 biopsy specimens from 47 cases.

Final diagnosis	Cases	Biopsies	Biopsies per case, mean	Diagnosis on the basis of H&E staining (no. of biopsies)
GBM	19	52	2.7	HGG (30); infiltrating glioma (12); reactive gliotic brain (5); normal brain (3); necrosis (1); inconclusive (1)
Recurrent GBM	5	24	4.8	HGG (11); infiltrating glioma (10); necrosis (1); reactive gliotic brain (1); inconclusive (1)
Infiltrating glioma	5	13	2.6	Infiltrating glioma (11); reactive gliotic brain (1); normal brain (1)
LGG	3	8	2.7	Infiltrating glioma (4); normal brain (4)
Metastasis	4	9	2.3	Metastasis (8); reactive gliotic brain (1)
Meningioma	7	9	1.3	Meningioma (9)
Choroid plexus carcinoma	1	4	4	Choroid plexus carcinoma (4)
Craniopharyngioma	1	1	1	Craniopharyngioma (1)
Schwannoma	1	1	1	Schwannoma (1)
AVM	1	1	1	Reactive gliotic brain (1)

AVM, arteriovenous malformation; GBM, glioblastoma multiforme; H&E, hematoxylin-eosin; HGG, high-grade glioma; LGG, low-grade glioma.

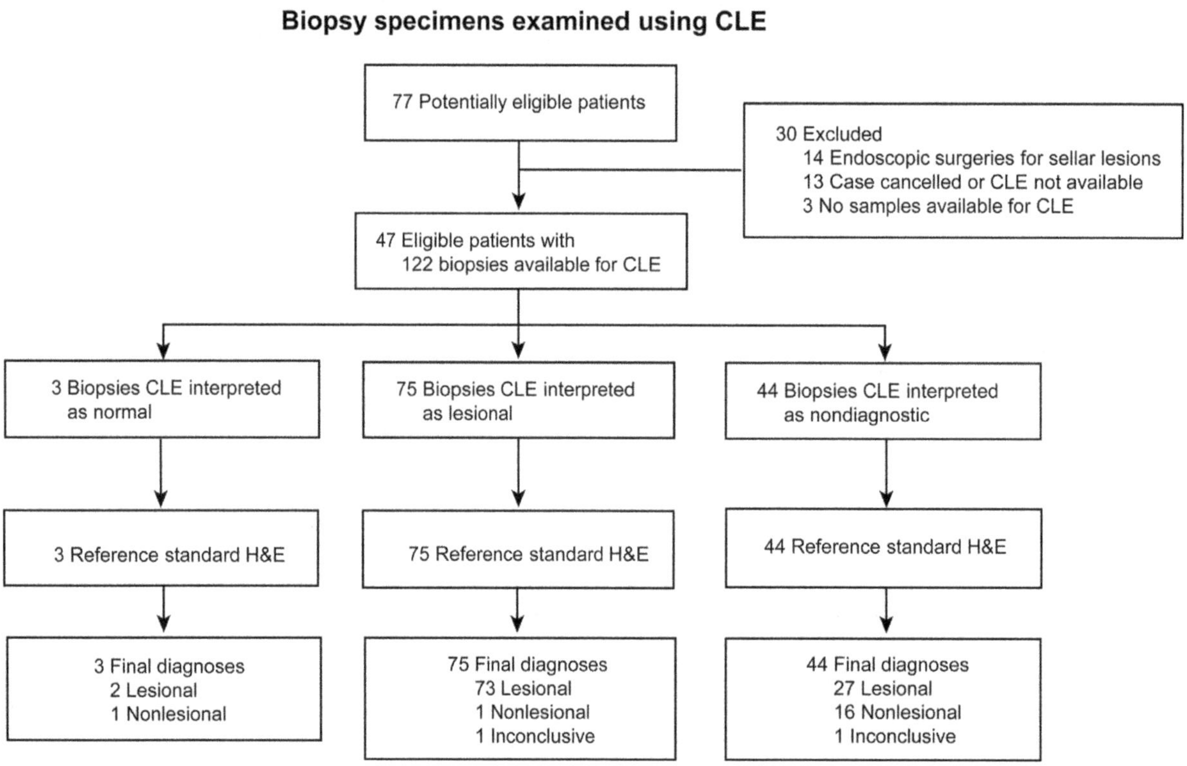

FIGURE 1 | Flowchart of 122 biopsy specimens from 47 patients with brain tumors examined using confocal laser endomicroscopy (CLE). H&E, hematoxylin-eosin. *Used with permission from Barrow Neurological Institute, Phoenix, Arizona.*

decreased from 26% (7 of 27) to 13% (2 of 15), although our study was not powered to detect differences in these subgroups (P=0.11 and P=0.31, respectively, by χ^2 analysis).

Timing of FNa Injection

In many cases, biopsy acquisition occurs more than 90 min after the first FNa administration, which results in suboptimal contrast in CLE images (7). This decrease in image quality was also found for biopsies in the current study when the FNa was injected 1 to 5 min before imaging. However, the analysis of all biopsies, as well as the glioma-only biopsies obtained at different time points after FNa injection, showed no correlation between the timing of FNa administration and image quality (r=−0.14, P>0.05) or with the probability of the CLE optical biopsy being used to diagnose specimens as either lesional or nondiagnostic (logistic regression P=0.93).

CLE Histologic Features

Various histologic features were assessed to elucidate characteristics of diagnostic and nondiagnostic CLE optical biopsies (**Figure 2**).

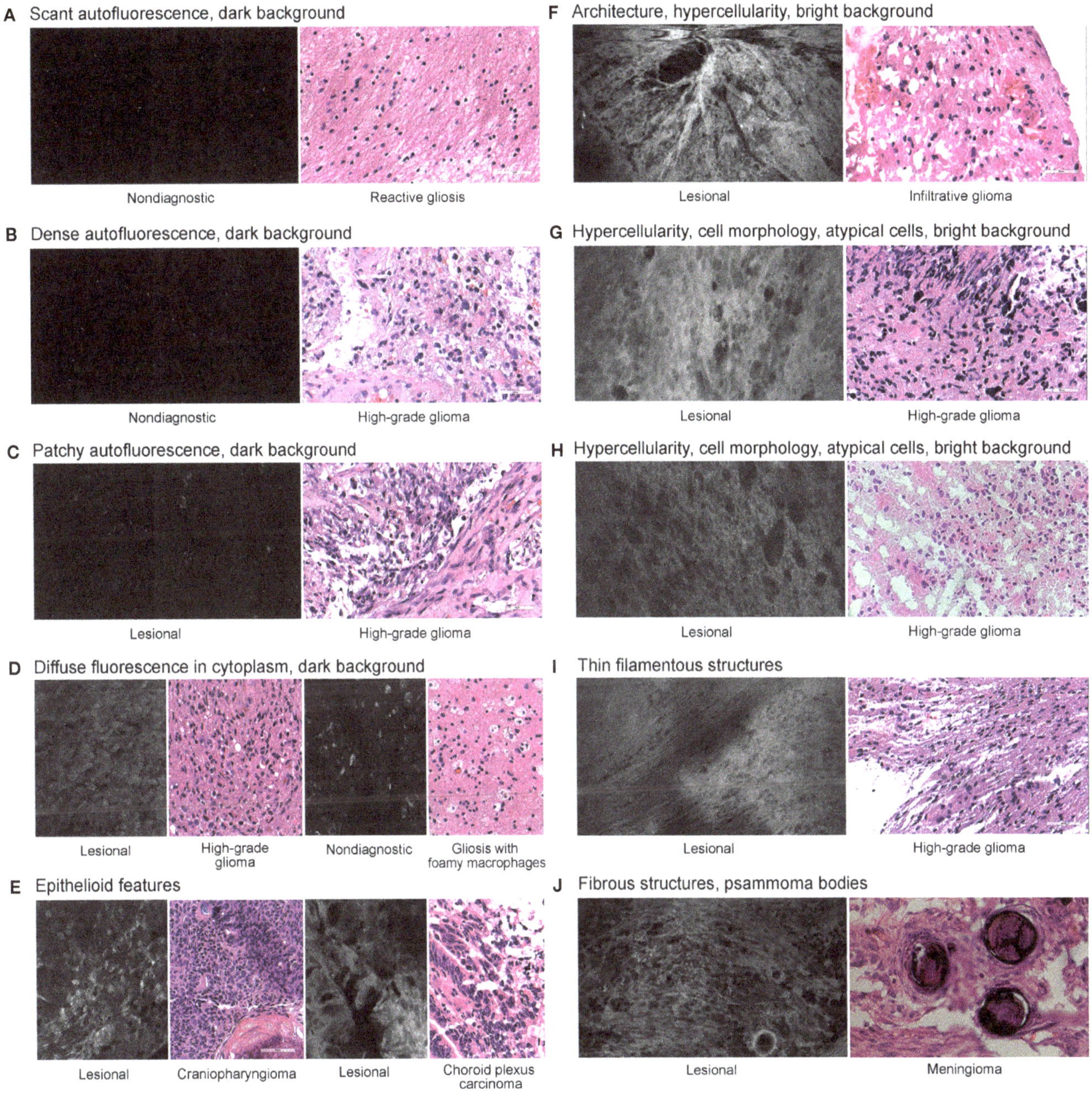

FIGURE 2 | Histologic features identified on confocal laser endomicroscopy images of various brain tumors and matching hematoxylin-eosin images. We identified three types of autofluorescence: scant **(A)**, dense **(B)**, and patchy **(C)**. We also identified the following image characteristics as separate histologic features: diffuse intracytoplasmic fluorescence **(D)**, epithelioid features **(E)**, hypercellularity **(F–H)**, filamentous structures **(I)**, and fibrous structures **(J)**. An example of characteristic identifiable tissue architecture as a histologic feature is shown in **(F)**. Examples of characteristic identifiable features of cell morphology and atypical cells are shown in **(G)** and **(H)**. An example of psammoma bodies is presented in **(J)**. We classified the brightness of background (extracellular space) as dark **(A–D)** or bright **(F–I)**. *Used with permission from Barrow Neurological Institute, Phoenix, Arizona.*

The prevalence of identifiable histologic features on CLE imaging was specifically studied in select biopsies of glioma, reactive gliosis, and normal brain samples (**Figure 3**).

Autofluorescence

Three types of autofluorescence were distinguished: scant, patchy, and dense. Scant autofluorescence was frequently observed in nonglioma samples that were deemed nondiagnostic by CLE ($P<0.001$), but there were no significant differences in the frequencies of patchy and dense fluorescence.

Diffuse Intracellular Fluorescence

In some CLE optical biopsies, cells exhibited diffuse accumulation of FNa in the cytoplasm. This accumulation was

Feature		CLE Lesional				CLE Nondiagnostic				CLE Normal				P Value	
		Glioma (n=53)		Nonglioma (n=0)		Glioma (n=23)		Nonglioma (n=15)		Glioma (n=0)		Nonglioma (n=1)			
		Inf. Glioma (22)	HGG (31)	Gliosis (0)	Normal (0)	Inf. Glioma (14)	HGG (9)	Gliosis (8)	Normal (7)	Inf. Glioma (0)	HGG (0)	Gliosis (1)	Normal (0)	Lesional Glioma vs. Nondiagnostic Glioma	Lesional Glioma vs. Nondiagnostic Nonglioma
Autofluorescence	Scant	5%	19%			14%	22%	63%	57%			0%		0.90	**<.001**
	Dense	27%	26%			43%	44%	25%	14%			0%		0.14	0.87
	Patchy	23%	29%			57%	44%	63%	29%			0%		**0.03**	0.24
Fluorescence diffusely in cytoplasm		32%	10%			7%	22%	25%	14%			100%		0.54	0.78
Background	Dark	14%	26%			57%	78%	100%	86%			100%		**<.001**	**<.001**
	Bright (extravasation)	86%	77%			43%	33%	13%	0%			0%		**0.001**	**<.001**
Architecture		95%	77%			36%	22%	38%	14%			100%		**<.001**	**<.001**
Cell morphology		73%	74%			0%	0%	38%	14%			100%		**<.001**	**<.001**
Atypical cells		38%	48%			0%	0%	0%	0%			0%		**<.001**	**0.004**
Hypercellularity		77%	65%			0%	22%	13%	0%			0%		**<.001**	**<.001**
Epithelial features		0%	0%			0%	0%	0%	0%			0%		NA	NA
Vessels		23%	16%			0%	11%	0%	29%			100%		0.19	0.91
Fibrous structures	Collagen fibers	5%	0%			0%	0%	0%	0%			0%		0.67	0.50
	Thin filamentous structures	0%	3%			7%	0%	0%	0%			100%		0.87	0.50
	Abundant fibrous structures	14%	6%			7%	22%	0%	14%			0%		0.95	0.86
Psammoma bodies		0%	0%			0%	0%	0%	0%			0%		NA	NA
RBC artifacts prevalent		14%	13%			50%	22%	13%	43%			100%		**0.03**	0.39

FIGURE 3 | Prevalence of histologic features among gliomas and normal or reactive brain tissue specimens. This analysis excluded 2 confocal laser endomicroscopy (CLE) optical biopsies with false-positive results, 2 CLE optical biopsies with false-negative results, and 1 nondiagnostic sample stained with hematoxylin-eosin. Table cells are shaded to reflect the prevalence of the specified feature among each group of specimens on a spectrum from red (0%) to green (100%). Boldface type indicates statistical significance. HGG, high-grade glioma; NA, not available; RBC, red blood cell. *Used with permission from Barrow Neurological Institute, Phoenix, Arizona.*

especially noticeable in tissue from carcinomas. In gliomas, however, the frequency of this pattern was not significantly different among nontumor and glioma biopsies.

Background Color

The pattern of CLE images in which the extracellular space was dark, and usually darker than the cells, was significantly more prevalent in nonglioma specimens (P<0.001) and in glioma specimens that were rated nondiagnostic (P<0.001). However, bright background was observed in most glioma samples diagnosed as lesional, and it was almost absent in biopsies from normal and reactive brain (P<0.001).

Cellular Features

Features such as tissue architecture, cell morphology, atypical cells, and hypercellularity were more prevalent in lesional glioma biopsies than in normal and reactive brain (P<0.001 for all). These features were also more prevalent in lesional glioma biopsies than in glioma biopsies that were labeled nondiagnostic on CLE (P<0.001 for all).

Epithelial Features

The pattern of hypercellular areas with cells contacting each other and having glandular or epithelial arrangement was observed in all three metastases, in one choroid carcinoma, and in the epithelial portion of the craniopharyngioma specimen. This feature was not observed in gliomas.

Vessels

Vessels were not frequently identified, most likely because of the lack of blood flow in *ex vivo* samples, which hampered detection. No differences were observed in their frequency of occurrence in the diagnostic, nondiagnostic, and normal brain samples. However, normal capillaries with FNa-stained vessel walls were deemed more characteristic of normal brain, or possibly of invasive glioma, than of cellular tumor.

Fibrous Structures

Various acellular fibrous structures were encountered, mostly in meningiomas, but were rarely seen in gliomas. However, some thin filamentous structures representing myelinated cell processes could be seen in gliomas. Psammoma bodies were identified in meningiomas as large, round, contrast-impermeable structures.

Red Blood Cell Artifacts

Although red blood cell artifacts are inevitable during CLE imaging, an abundance of blood was encountered significantly more often in nondiagnostic CLE biopsies of gliomas than in lesional CLE biopsies of gliomas (P=0.02).

Blinded Review by Trained Neuropathologist

The overall diagnostic accuracy for all biopsies analyzed by a trained neuropathologist was 75%. Lesional CLE biopsies were used as positive CLE test results; nonlesional CLE, which included nondiagnostic and true negative normal or reactive brain CLE, were used as negative CLE test results (**Table 2**). Diagnostic accuracy in various tumor types was elucidated by performing subgroup analyses in glioma, metastases, and meningioma samples, which confirmed high positive predictive value of CLE optical biopsies (98%, 91%, and 83%, respectively) (**Table 3**). Notably, two CLE optical biopsies that were labeled as lesional had nonlesional H&E labeling such that they might have been true positives, which would further improve specificity and positive predictive value to 100% for all specimens and for gliomas (**Figure 4**).

Blinded Review by Trained and Untrained Appraisers

Overall diagnostic accuracy for all biopsies blinded for analysis by a neurosurgeon with experience interpreting CLE images was 78% vs 71% for the neurosurgeon without CLE image-reading experience. The comparative diagnostic accuracy data are presented in **Figure 5** and **Table 4**. Both the experienced neuropathologist and the experienced neurosurgeon demonstrated higher specificity and positive predictive value for gliomas.

TABLE 2 | Confocal laser endomicroscopy interpretation of 122 biopsy specimens from 47 patients.

H&E Diagnosis	Specimens	Confocal Laser Endomicroscopy Interpretation				
		Lesional		Nonlesional		
				Normal		Nondiagnostic
		TP	FP	TN	FN	
Choroid plexus carcinoma	4	3				1
Craniopharyngioma	1	1				
HGG	41	31			1	9
Infiltrating glioma	37	22			1	14
Meningioma	9	6				3
Metastasis	8	7				1
Necrosis	2	2				
Normal brain	8		1			7
Reactive gliotic brain	9			1		8
Schwannoma	1	1				
Inconclusive	2	1				1

H&E, hematoxylin-eosin; HGG, high-grade glioma: FN, false negative; FP, false positive; TN, true negative; TP, true positive.

TABLE 3 | Diagnostic accuracy of *ex vivo* confocal laser endomicroscopy (CLE) analyzed by a neuropathologist experienced in CLE image interpretation.

Value	All samples	Gliomas	Carcinomas[a]	Meningiomas
Sensitivity	72 (62–80)	66 (55–76)	83 (51–97)	63 (26–90)
Specificity	90 (67–98)	94 (69–100)	94 (69–100)	94 (69–100)
Positive predictive value	97 (90–100)	98 (89–100)	91 (57–100)	83 (36–99)
Negative predictive value	38 (25–54)	37 (23–53)	89 (64–98)	84 (60–96)

Data are reported as percentage (95% confidence interval).
[a]Carcinomas included metastatic lesions and choroid plexus carcinomas.

Adverse Effects

No adverse effects due to biopsy acquisition or FNa administration were noted. One patient was inadvertently administered 40 mg/kg of FNa at the induction of anesthesia, resulting in yellowish skin discoloration that resolved uneventfully within 48 h. No other adverse reactions were observed.

DISCUSSION

The projected clinical applications for the use of CLE in neurosurgery are to guide biopsy acquisition, to provide preliminary diagnosis in a manner similar to that of frozen section, and to perform screening for tumor detection during resection. In this study, we evaluated CLE optical biopsies of 122 *ex vivo* brain samples from 47 patients. The results demonstrated high sensitivity for this diagnostic technology in detecting cellular brain tumor tissue, which has significantly informative clinical value.

Image Interpretation

Our results demonstrated that a neuropathologist and neurosurgeons experienced in reading CLE images interpreted images of gliomas with greater specificity than an inexperienced neurosurgeon, even in consultation with an inexperienced pathologist. Previous reports have indicated that special training and experience are necessary to interpret the gray scale confocal images of intravital microscopy (9–13). However, in our study, the scores are not greatly dissimilar among the experienced neuropathologist, the experienced neurosurgeon, and the inexperienced neurosurgeon assisted by a general pathologist. The interpretative accuracy of these scores is surprising, given that no information was provided to the personnel about the clinical or historical nature of the cases. In the normal surgery-pathology workflow, such additional contextual information would be a requisite part of the

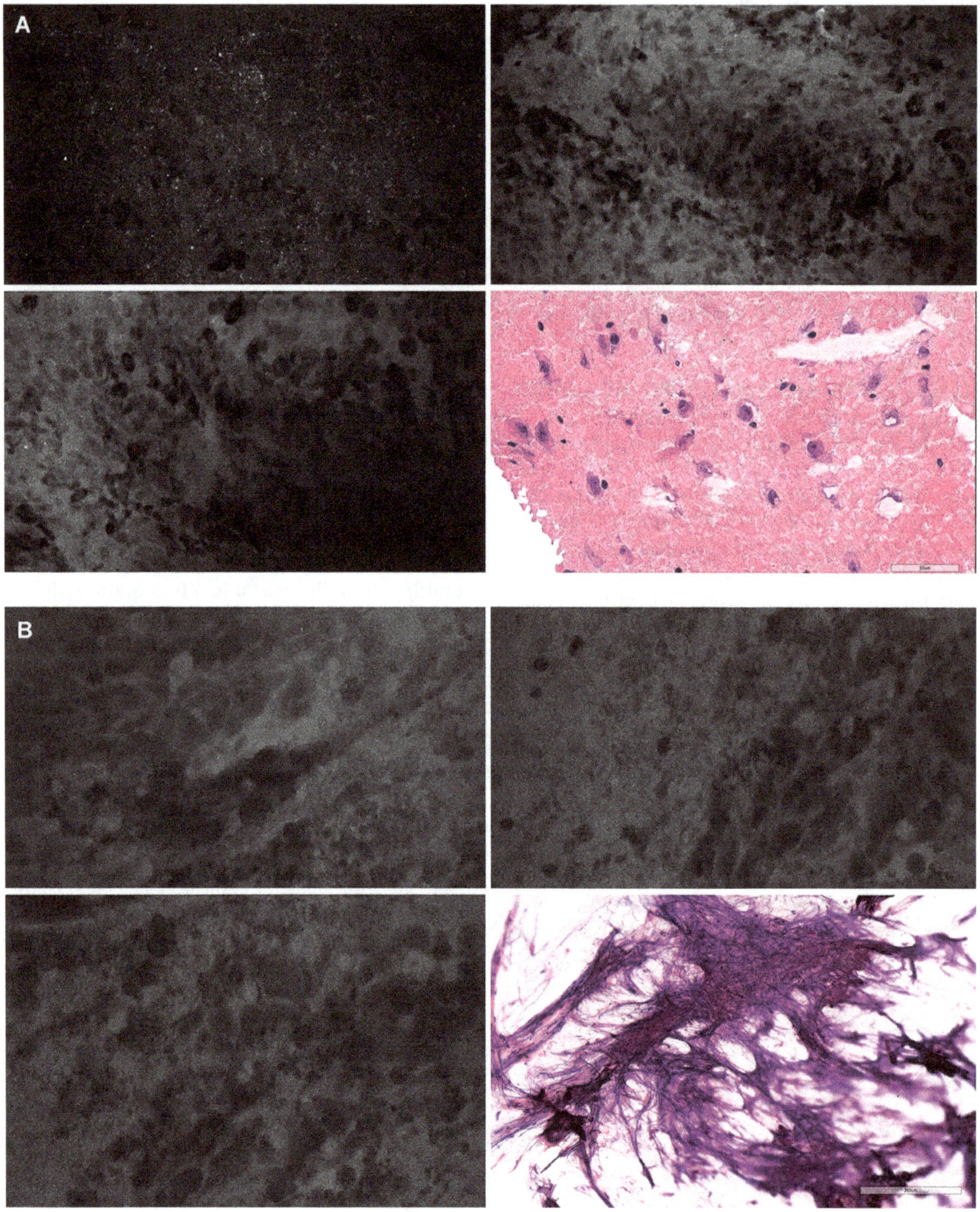

FIGURE 4 | Positive confocal laser endomicroscopy (CLE) optical biopsies with negative hematoxylin-eosin (H&E) stain results. **(A)** In one optical biopsy, extravasation of FNa highlighted the background and revealed hypercellular areas of atypical large cells. Overall, this CLE optical biopsy was thought to be highly representative of a lesional tissue. However, the H&E-stained specimen was read as normal cortex without a tumor. We hypothesized that there might be a sampling error and that the specimen contained a tumor area that had been missed during histologic sectioning. **(B)** This optical biopsy demonstrated extravasation of FNa with hypercellular areas containing large atypical cells highly suggestive of a cellular tumor. However, because of the scant tissue available for histologic processing, the H&E stain results were inconclusive. Both H&E-stained specimens were treated as nonlesional for diagnostic accuracy analysis. However, if these two H&E biopsy specimens had been treated as lesional, then both specificity and positive predictive value would be 100%. *Used with permission from Barrow Neurological Institute, Phoenix, Arizona.*

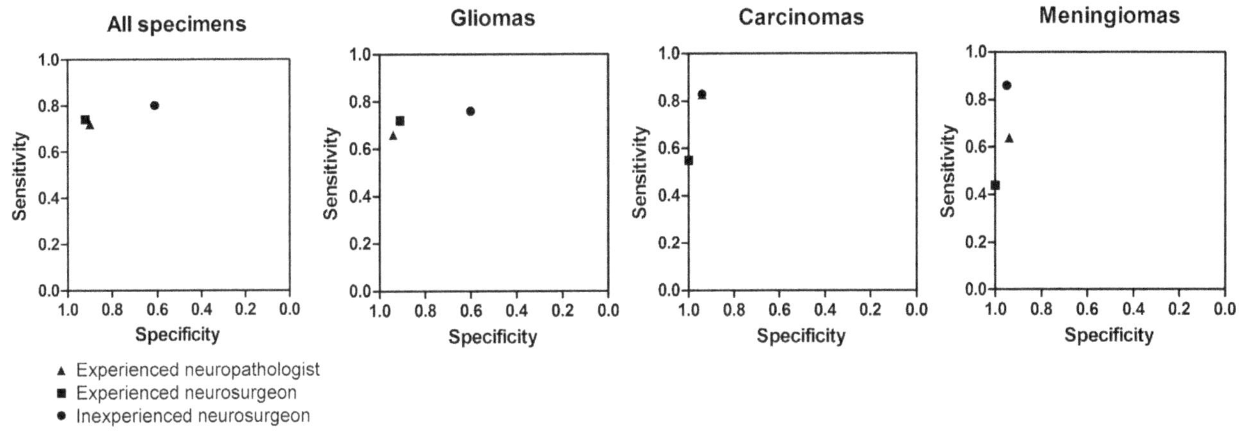

FIGURE 5 | Diagnostic accuracy diagrams for all specimens together and for gliomas, carcinomas, and meningiomas analyzed separately, as assessed by an experienced neuropathologist, an experienced neurosurgeon, and an inexperienced neurosurgeon using confocal laser endomicroscopy. *Used with permission from Barrow Neurological Institute, Phoenix, Arizona.*

TABLE 4 | Diagnostic accuracy of *ex vivo* confocal laser endomicroscopy analyzed by an experienced neuropathologist, an experienced neurosurgeon, and an inexperienced neurosurgeon.

Tissue type, diagnostic parameter	Experienced neuropathologist	Experienced neurosurgeon	Inexperienced neurosurgeon
All samples			
Sensitivity	72 (62–80)	74 (65–83)	80 (70–90)
Specificity	90 (67–98)	92 (69–98)	61 (44–72)
Positive predictive value	97 (90–100)	97 (90–100)	71 (59–80)
Negative predictive value	38 (25–54)	47 (31–61)	72 (56–84)
Glioma			
Sensitivity	66 (55–76)	72 (61–82)	76 (62–87)
Specificity	94 (69–100)	91 (67–98)	60 (42–72)
Positive predictive value	98 (89–100)	96 (87–99)	66 (52–78)
Negative predictive value	37 (23–53)	49 (31–69)	71 (53–84)
Carcinoma[a]			
Sensitivity	83 (51–97)	55 (32–76)	83 (51–97)
Specificity	94 (69–100)	100 (60–100)	94 (68–100)
Positive predictive value	91 (57–100)	100 (68–100)	91 (57–100)
Negative predictive value	89 (64–98)	50 (24–71)	89 (62–98)
Meningioma			
Sensitivity	63 (26–90)	44 (21–69)	86 (42–99)
Specificity	94 (69–100)	100 (63–100)	95 (71–100)
Positive predictive value	83 (36–99)	100 (56–100)	86 (42–99)
Negative predictive value	84 (60–96)	53 (27–73)	95 (71–100)

Data are reported as percentage (95% confidence interval).
[a]*Includes metastatic lesions and choroid plexus carcinoma.*

interpretation of CLE images for diagnosis and surgical guidance (7).

In the future, CLE image interpretation could be augmented by robust automated computer image analysis, which would allow for rapid identification of useful information from among the hundreds to thousands of images that may be acquired from one patient (14–16) and by digital telepathology consultation provided by an expert (17). In addition to confirming the diagnostic value of the new-generation CLE system, this study addresses the implementation of CLE into the surgery-pathology operating room workflow during FGS of the brain. As discussed below, the results provide data that will be helpful in planning future *in vivo* CLE studies in various tumor types.

Implications for Practice: Incorporation of CLE into the Workflow of Fluorescence-Guided Brain Surgery

Building on a previous study in which FNa was administered approximately 5 min before CLE imaging (7), this study demonstrated the feasibility of using CLE in Yellow560 mode during FGS when FNa is administered upon induction of anesthesia. This timing of FNa injection favors navigation using the wide-field fluorescence operative microscope (18, 19), and it has been studied in several clinical trials (20, 21). However, after early administration of FNa, we found that the contrast in CLE images was insufficient in some cases, thus requiring readministration of FNa. Readministration of FNa resulted in improved CLE image quality. Interestingly, we found no correlation between the time of contrast injection and overall image quality, which may be related to the heterogeneity of the tumor tissue or blood artifacts and to the *ex vivo* nature of the study.

Reinjection of FNa showed important benefits for image quality and interpretation. Analysis of these specimens showed improved brightness, contrast, and improved overall image quality. For the cases in which the reinjection was performed, the percentage of images with an accurate diagnosis increased by 50%, and the percentage of nondiagnostic CLE decreased by 50%. In some cases, reinjection allowed us to obtain meaningful interpretation where with only a single injection at the start of the case, this would not have been possible. Although reinjection of FNa improved CLE image quality, the diffusion of FNa at the resection cavity can hamper the selectivity of Yellow560 wide-field fluorescence guidance, but this hindrance was not a major problem for us. However, there are some relevant considerations for reinjection of FNa. When administered later during surgery FNa extravasates at the regions of surgical injury creating false-positive fluorescence, which was the major critique of FNa as a contrast agent for wide-field fluorescence guidance (22). Future *in vivo* studies should address this problem. Most likely, CLE could best be used after resection under Yellow560 guidance to facilitate inspection of the surgical resection bed at the conclusion of surgery (i.e., to interrogate suspected tumor invasion into eloquent or surrounding cortex). Interestingly, when 40 mg/kg FNa was administered, CLE demonstrated high-quality images with excellent contrast in visualizing tumor cells, further supporting our approach to reinject FNa to increase image contrast and clarity.

Alternatively, FNa could be used for CLE optical biopsy during or at the completion of resection under 5-aminolevulinic acid (5-ALA) guidance. Simultaneous use of 5-ALA and FNa has been reported previously (23). Our experience with the new operating microscope in Blue400 and Yellow560 modes demonstrates that the two channels can be alternated without compromising image quality. Concurrent FNa-contrasted CLE may be advantageous during surgeries performed using near-infrared guidance (e.g., using indocyanine green [ICG]) because of the absence of spectral overlap with FNa (24, 25). Confocal-assisted fluorescence microscopy with ICG as a contrast has also been reported (26, 27). In view of future incorporation of CLE into the workflow of FGS, diagnostic accuracy using CLE should be compared to wide-field fluorescence imaging technology using various diagnostic fluorophore agents, such as FNa, 5-ALA, and ICG.

For safe maximal resection, other techniques should also be considered, particularly intraoperative stimulation and awake brain mapping using fluorescence (28). These and other functional methods are designed to be highly sensitive for eloquent brain areas that should be preserved, whereas the goal of FGS and CLE is to specifically detect and reveal tumor regions for the surgical decision on whether to resect. These two methods can therefore provide mutually complementary information.

The use of CLE requires coordination with the anesthesiologist for timely and accurate administration of the FNa dose. Importantly, we believe that close association with a neuropathologist, either remotely or in the operating room, is necessary, especially at the initial adoption stage of the CLE technology, as was the case for this *ex vivo* application. Coordination and communication between the neurosurgeon in the operating room using the CLE and the neuropathologist providing rapid examination of the images acquired on the fly is fully supported by this CLE technology, and this will be especially advantageous for *in vivo* use. The images can be ported to any computer workstation or even handheld computing device (e.g., "smart phone") supporting image display. CLE systems will require and foster a close partnership and collaboration between the neurosurgeon and neuropathologist.

Diagnostic Accuracy in Different Tumor Types

Because glioma tissue is often challenging to distinguish from normal brain tissue without special or enhanced imaging techniques, *in vivo* CLE optical biopsy of gliomas is of particular interest because it yields histopathologic imaging results immediately. With our experience from experimental animal studies and early clinical studies, we have identified characteristic CLE patterns and have developed confidence in our interpretation of CLE images and in our successful identification of hypercellular HGG samples (5, 29, 30). In contrast to previous studies, this study assessed multiple matched biopsies from the same patient, including multiple samples that were read as gliotic brain without tumor.

CLE images from within a tumor mass may readily display characteristic cellular features that are unique to and therefore diagnostic of the tumor type. However, although imaging within a main tumor mass may be useful for rapid histologic recognition and confirmation, the main purpose and advantage of the CLE is to recognize abnormal histologic features at the marginal regions of tumor to identify regions that can be surgically optimized. Such an imaging situation occurs within the surgical resection bed when assessing whether to extend the tumor removal. The CLE field of view is small (267 × 475 μm), and thus the concentration on identifiable histologic features at the tumor or pathological margins may not include readily visible diagnostic features that inform an exact tumor type. Instead, the focus should be on distinguishing abnormal histoarchitectural features, such as those described in the results.

Coupled with our previous studies on the differentiation of glioma tissue from injured normal brain in the murine model (31), the current work deepens our understanding of the CLE features of nontumor normal and gliotic brain tissue in humans. Most of the specimens of gliotic and normal brain tissue were labeled as nondiagnostic of brain tumor because they lacked typical cellular features and high cellularity, although most of them had dark extracellular backgrounds and some autofluorescent speckles. Normal cells were not clearly visible on these images, which impeded a definitive conclusion that the optical biopsy was representative of normal brain tissue. Interestingly, increased speckles on CLE images obtained with a similar device have previously been observed in low-grade gliomas after administration of 5-ALA (32), but they most likely represented autofluorescence (33). Whether this observation indicates the normal appearance of brain tissue using CLE imaging with FNa contrast is not clear. We believe that future *in vivo* studies should focus on the assessment of marginal tissue to better distinguish normal brain tissue when interpreting a dark CLE optical biopsy with autofluorescence in the absence of cellular architecture features (**Figure 6**).

With respect to metastatic lesions and choroid plexus carcinomas, CLE provides high-contrast, clear, and reliable images of cellular features that are highly diagnostic of cellular tumor. Most nondiagnostic CLE optical biopsies are attributable to blood artifacts that hide the actual tissue or the FNa contrast redistribution over time, which diminishes contrast among cells and among their nuclei, cytoplasm, and extracellular compartments.

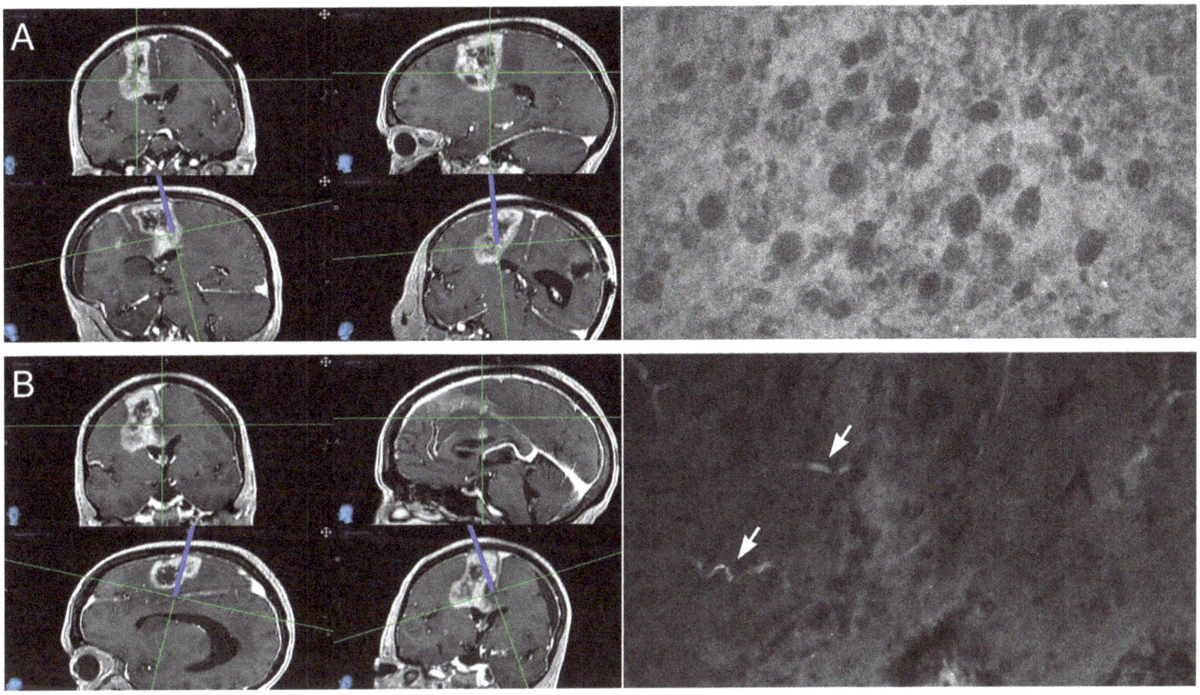

FIGURE 6 | Illustrative example of confocal laser endomicroscopy (CLE) (*right*) used in combination with intraoperative navigation (*left*). Multiple biopsies were performed during resection of a high-grade glioma; two biopsies are shown. **(A)** A biopsy specimen obtained from a deep posterior contrast-enhancing tumor margin. CLE findings were positive for tumor showing atypical cellular features and hypercellularity. A diagnosis of high-grade glioma was made on the basis of hematoxylin-eosin (H&E) staining of this biopsy specimen. Resection was extended further and deeper. **(B)** A biopsy specimen was obtained from a deep noncontrast-enhancing posteromedial tumor margin. CLE had findings negative for tumor and showed normal-appearing vessels (*arrows*). This biopsy specimen was identified as normal cortex with focal vessels on H&E staining. *Used with permission from Barrow Neurological Institute, Phoenix, Arizona.*

In all available meningioma samples, including one composed of 80% dura and 20% invasive meningioma tissue, CLE provided clear high-contrast images of hypercellular tissue with fibrous structures and psammoma bodies, when present. Because normal marginal nonmeningioma samples were not available for CLE assessment, we used normal and gliotic brain tissue as negative controls for calculating the diagnostic accuracy in meningiomas. However, for future *in vivo* studies of meningiomas, multiple biopsies of the dura at the edge of the tumor should be obtained, similar to the tissue acquisition workflow in gliomas. We have thoroughly examined features of normal dura with FNa in a pig model (unpublished data), but its appearance at the marginal tumor regions should be better characterized in future studies.

Study Power Considerations

In this study, the prevalence of lesional samples was 84% (102 of 122) among all samples and 82% (80 of 97) among the glioma samples. The Buderer formula (34), with accuracy set at 0.05, prevalence of disease in the tested population set at 84%, and a sample size of 122, resulted in z=1.127 and confidence interval (CI) within 0.70 to 0.75 for sensitivity and z=1.687 and CI of 0.90 to 0.92 for specificity. For gliomas, the power analysis resulted in z=0.594 with CI of <50% for sensitivity and z=1.307 and CI of 0.80 to 0.85 for specificity. Although our study was underpowered for sensitivity, it is the first feasibility study to provide prevalence and diagnostic accuracy values for the planning of future diagnostic accuracy studies using CLE. For example, assuming 82% prevalence of tumor-positive samples, 94% specificity, and 66% sensitivity, the study size should be 419 for calculation of sensitivity and 103 for specificity to obtain a 95% CI and 0.05 accuracy.

Study Limitations

Factors such as biopsy location, tumor type, the experience of the CLE user, and the extent of the scanned region of interest may have introduced biases and should be controlled for in future studies. This study is limited to *ex vivo* analyses because of the unavailability of the sterile CLE probe sheaths during the time the study was conducted; thus, human *in vivo* use was precluded. However, this situation may be viewed as advantageous because it may have decreased sampling error compared with *in vivo* acquisition for methodologic reasons, as it is more certain that the CLE images were obtained from and directly correlated with the same biopsy region, which is often difficult to accomplish intraoperatively.

Nevertheless, we acknowledge that sampling error is unavoidable with the small field of view of the imaging probe. H&E slides of multiple samples were inhomogeneous when viewed under the microscope: some had areas of necrosis encompassing up to 75% of the whole section, and some had infiltrating tumor in only 20% of their area, with the remaining regions consisting of vessels and hemorrhage. Use of CLE may identify and distinguish tumor cellular areas that are later missed on standard histologic examination (**Figure 4**). Two CLE optical biopsies that were classified as having normal results (i.e., false-negative results) had dark backgrounds and normal-appearing vessels suggestive of normal brain; however, few regions of interest were imaged with CLE for this sort of optical biopsy, and therefore the infiltrative tumor areas detected on H&E slides may have been missed. To minimize the sampling error, we moved the probe across specimens to visualize larger areas and to identify locations with high-quality confocal images bearing diagnostic features, but the area that is scanned is subject to user bias.

CONCLUSION

Our results demonstrate the feasibility of incorporating CLE assessment of tissue microarchitecture in FGS. CLE optical biopsies showed high specificity and positive predictive value in fresh *ex vivo* glioma samples. These results reinforce the utility of CLE in providing real-time intraoperative cell resolution imaging to the neurosurgeon that is comparable to and faster than conventional histologic analysis from tissue biopsies in the operating room. These results also provide background data for planning future *in vivo* clinical studies.

ETHICS STATEMENT

The studies involving human participants were reviewed and approved by St. Joseph's Hospital and Medical Center with approval from the Institutional Review Board for Human Research. The patients/participants provided their written informed consent to participate in this study.

AUTHOR CONTRIBUTIONS

Study planning and coordination: PN, MP, JE, EB. Acquisition of surgical biopsies and patient recruitment: PN. Acquisition of confocal images: EB, XZ. Processing and organizing of the data and confocal images: BN, DF, EB. Assessment of confocal images: EB, MP, VB, JE. Histology processing: EB. Histology reading: JE. Statistical analysis: EB, BN, DF. Writing a draft: BN, DF, EB. Review of the draft: EB, BN, DF, VB, MP, PN. All authors contributed to the article and approved the submitted version.

ACKNOWLEDGMENTS

The authors thank the Neuroscience Publications staff at Barrow Neurological Institute for assistance with manuscript preparation. We also thank Thomas Chastain and the staff of the pathology department for excellent technical assistance. This work is a part of the doctoral dissertation of EB. Part of this work was presented at the 2019 AANS meeting on April 13 to 17, 2019, in San Diego, California.

REFERENCES

1. D'Amico RS, Englander ZK, Canoll P, Bruce JN. Extent of Resection in Glioma-A Review of the Cutting Edge. *World Neurosurg* (2017) 103:538–49. doi: 10.1016/j.wneu.2017.04.041
2. Sanai N, Berger MS. Glioma extent of resection and its impact on patient outcome. *Neurosurgery* (2008) 62(4):753–64; discussion 264-6. doi: 10.1227/01.neu.0000318159.21731.cf
3. Barbosa BJ, Mariano ED, Batista CM, Marie SK, Teixeira MJ, Pereira CU, et al. Intraoperative assistive technologies and extent of resection in glioma surgery: a systematic review of prospective controlled studies. *Neurosurg Rev* (2015) 38(2):217–26; discussion 26-7. doi: 10.1007/s10143-014-0592-0
4. Belykh E, Cavallo C, Gandhi S, Zhao X, Veljanoski D, Izady Yazdanabadi M, et al. Utilization of intraoperative confocal laser endomicroscopy in brain tumor surgery. *J Neurosurg Sci* (2018) 62(6):704–17. doi: 10.23736/S0390-5616.18.04553-8
5. Sanai N, Eschbacher J, Hattendorf G, Coons SW, Preul MC, Smith KA, et al. Intraoperative confocal microscopy for brain tumors: a feasibility analysis in humans. *Neurosurgery* (2011) 68(2 Suppl Operative):282–90; discussion 90. doi: 10.1227/NEU.0b013e318212464e
6. Eschbacher J, Martirosyan NL, Nakaji P, Sanai N, Preul MC, Smith KA, et al. *In vivo* intraoperative confocal microscopy for real-time histopathological imaging of brain tumors. *J Neurosurg* (2012) 116(4):854–60. doi: 10.3171/2011.12.JNS11696
7. Martirosyan NL, Eschbacher JM, Kalani MY, Turner JD, Belykh E, Spetzler RF, et al. Prospective evaluation of the utility of intraoperative confocal laser endomicroscopy in patients with brain neoplasms using fluorescein sodium: experience with 74 cases. *Neurosurg Focus* (2016) 40(3):E11. doi: 10.3171/2016.1.FOCUS15559
8. Bossuyt PM, Reitsma JB, Bruns DE, Gatsonis CA, Glasziou PP, Irwig L, et al. STARD 2015: an updated list of essential items for reporting diagnostic accuracy studies. *BMJ* (2015) 351:h5527. doi: 10.1136/bmj.h5527
9. Liu JT, Loewke NO, Mandella MJ, Leigh SY, Levenson RM, Crawford JM, et al. Real-time pathology through *in vivo* microscopy. *Stud Health Technol Inform* (2013) 185:235–64. doi: 10.3233/978-1-61499-234-9-235
10. Farnetani F, Scope A, Braun RP, Gonzalez S, Guitera P, Malvehy J, et al. Skin Cancer Diagnosis With Reflectance Confocal Microscopy: Reproducibility of Feature Recognition and Accuracy of Diagnosis. *JAMA Dermatol* (2015) 151 (10):1075–80. doi: 10.1001/jamadermatol.2015.0810
11. Rao BK, Mateus R, Wassef C, Pellacani G. *in vivo* confocal microscopy in clinical practice: comparison of bedside diagnostic accuracy of a trained physician and distant diagnosis of an expert reader. *J Am Acad Dermatol* (2013) 69(6):e295–300. doi: 10.1016/j.jaad.2013.07.022
12. Rajadhyaksha M, Marghoob A, Rossi A, Halpern AC, Nehal KS. Reflectance confocal microscopy of skin *in vivo*: From bench to bedside. *Lasers Surg Med* (2017) 49(1):7–19. doi: 10.1002/lsm.22600
13. Wells WA, Thrall M, Sorokina A, Fine J, Krishnamurthy S, Haroon A, et al. *in vivo* and *Ex Vivo* Microscopy: Moving Toward the Integration of Optical Imaging Technologies Into Pathology Practice. *Arch Pathol Lab Med* (2019) 143(3):288–98. doi: 10.5858/arpa.2018-0298-RA
14. Izadyyazdanabadi M, Belykh E, Mooney MA, Eschbacher JM, Nakaji P, Yang Y, et al. Prospects for Theranostics in Neurosurgical Imaging: Empowering Confocal Laser Endomicroscopy Diagnostics via Deep Learning. *Front Oncol* (2018) 8:240. doi: 10.3389/fonc.2018.00240
15. Izadyyazdanabadi M, Belykh E, Mooney M, Martirosyan N, Eschbacher J, Nakaji P, et al. Convolutional neural networks: Ensemble modeling, fine-tuning and unsupervised semantic localization for neurosurgical CLE images. *J Visual Commun Image Represent* (2018) 54:10–20. doi: 10.1016/j.jvcir.2018.04.004
16. Izadyyazdanabadi M, Belykh E, Zhao X, Moreira LB, Gandhi S, Cavallo C, et al. Fluorescence Image Histology Pattern Transformation Using Image Style Transfer. *Front Oncol* (2019) 9:1–7. doi: 10.3389/fonc.2019.00519
17. Fuks D, Pierangelo A, Validire P, Lefevre M, Benali A, Trebuchet G, et al. Intraoperative confocal laser endomicroscopy for real-time *in vivo* characterization during surgical procedures. *Surg Endosc* (2019) 33(5):1544 52. doi: 10.1007/s00464-018-6442-3

18. Acerbi F, Broggi M, Eoli M, Anghileri E, Cavallo C, Boffano C, et al. Is fluorescein-guided technique able to help in resection of high-grade gliomas? *Neurosurg Focus* (2014) 36(2):E5. doi: 10.3171/2013.11.FOCUS13487
19. Acerbi F, Broggi M, Broggi G, Ferroli P. What is the best timing for fluorescein injection during surgical removal of high-grade gliomas? *Acta Neurochir (Wien)* (2015) 157(8):1377–8. doi: 10.1007/s00701-015-2455-z
20. Acerbi F, Broggi M, Schebesch KM, Hohne J, Cavallo C, De Laurentis C, et al. Fluorescein-Guided Surgery for Resection of High-Grade Gliomas: A Multicentric Prospective Phase II Study (FLUOGLIO). *Clin Cancer Res* (2018) 24(1):52–61. doi: 10.1158/1078-0432.CCR-17-1184
21. Falco J, Cavallo C, Vetrano IG, de Laurentis C, Siozos L, Schiariti M, et al. Fluorescein Application in Cranial and Spinal Tumors Enhancing at Preoperative MRI and Operated With a Dedicated Filter on the Surgical Microscope: Preliminary Results in 279 Patients Enrolled in the FLUOCERTUM Prospective Study. *Front Surg* (2019) 6:49. doi: 10.3389/fsurg.2019.00049
22. Stummer W. Poor man's fluorescence? *Acta Neurochirurgica* (2015) 157 (8):1379–81. doi: 10.1007/s00701-015-2471-z
23. Schwake M, Stummer W, Suero Molina EJ, Wolfer J. Simultaneous fluorescein sodium and 5-ALA in fluorescence-guided glioma surgery. *Acta Neurochir (Wien)* (2015) 157(5):877–9. doi: 10.1007/s00701-015-2401-0
24. Cho SS, Salinas R, Lee JYK. Indocyanine-Green for Fluorescence-Guided Surgery of Brain Tumors: Evidence, Techniques, and Practical Experience. *Front Surg* (2019) 6:11. doi: 10.3389/fsurg.2019.00011
25. Cho SS, Salinas R, De Ravin E, Teng CW, Li C, Abdullah KG, et al. Near-Infrared Imaging with Second-Window Indocyanine Green in Newly Diagnosed High-Grade Gliomas Predicts Gadolinium Enhancement on Postoperative Magnetic Resonance Imaging. *Mol Imaging Biol* (2019) 22:1427–37. doi: 10.1007/s11307-019-01455-x
26. Charalampaki P, Nakamura M, Athanasopoulos D, Heimann A. Confocal-Assisted Multispectral Fluorescent Microscopy for Brain Tumor Surgery. *Front Oncol* (2019) 9:583:583. doi: 10.3389/fonc.2019.00583
27. Martirosyan NL, Cavalcanti DD, Eschbacher JM, Delaney PM, Scheck AC, Abdelwahab MG, et al. Use of *in vivo* near-infrared laser confocal endomicroscopy with indocyanine green to detect the boundary of infiltrative tumor. *J Neurosurg* (2011) 115(6):1131–8. doi: 10.3171/2011.8.Jns11559
28. Duffau H. Surgery for Malignant Brain Gliomas: Fluorescence-Guided Resection or Functional-Based Resection? *Front Surg* (2019) 6:21:21. doi: 10.3389/fsurg.2019.00021
29. Sankar T, Delaney PM, Ryan RW, Eschbacher J, Abdelwahab M, Nakaji P, et al. Miniaturized handheld confocal microscopy for neurosurgery: results in an experimental glioblastoma model. *Neurosurgery* (2010) 66(2):410–7; discussion 7-8. doi: 10.1227/01.NEU.0000365772.66324.6F
30. Martirosyan NL, Georges J, Kalani MY, Nakaji P, Spetzler RF, Feuerstein BG, et al. Handheld confocal laser endomicroscopic imaging utilizing tumor-specific fluorescent labeling to identify experimental glioma cells *in vivo*. *Surg Neurol Int* (2016) 7(Suppl 40):S995–S1003. doi: 10.4103/2152-7806.195577
31. Belykh E, Miller EJ, Patel AA, Yazdanabadi MI, Martirosyan NL, Yagmurlu K, et al. Diagnostic Accuracy of a Confocal Laser Endomicroscope for *in vivo* Differentiation Between Normal Injured And Tumor Tissue During Fluorescein-Guided Glioma Resection: Laboratory Investigation. *World Neurosurg* (2018) 115:e337–e48. doi: 10.1016/j.wneu.2018.04.048
32. Sanai N, Snyder LA, Honea NJ, Coons SW, Eschbacher JM, Smith KA, et al. Intraoperative confocal microscopy in the visualization of 5-aminolevulinic acid fluorescence in low-grade gliomas. *J Neurosurg* (2011) 115(4):740–8. doi: 10.3171/2011.6.JNS11252
33. Cavallo C, Gandhi S, Zhao X, Belykh E, Valli D, Nakaji P, et al. Applications of Microscope-Integrated Indocyanine Green Videoangiography in Cerebral Revascularization Procedures. *Front Surg* (2019) 6:1–10. doi: 10.3389/fsurg.2019.00059
34. Buderer NM. Statistical methodology: I. Incorporating the prevalence of disease into the sample size calculation for sensitivity and specificity. *Acad Emerg Med* (1996) 3(9):895–900. doi: 10.1111/j.1553-2712.1996.tb03538.x

Permissions

All chapters in this book were first published by Frontiers; hereby published with permission under the Creative Commons Attribution License or equivalent. Every chapter published in this book has been scrutinized by our experts. Their significance has been extensively debated. The topics covered herein carry significant findings which will fuel the growth of the discipline. They may even be implemented as practical applications or may be referred to as a beginning point for another development.

The contributors of this book come from diverse backgrounds, making this book a truly international effort. This book will bring forth new frontiers with its revolutionizing research information and detailed analysis of the nascent developments around the world.

We would like to thank all the contributing authors for lending their expertise to make the book truly unique. They have played a crucial role in the development of this book. Without their invaluable contributions this book wouldn't have been possible. They have made vital efforts to compile up to date information on the varied aspects of this subject to make this book a valuable addition to the collection of many professionals and students.

This book was conceptualized with the vision of imparting up-to-date information and advanced data in this field. To ensure the same, a matchless editorial board was set up. Every individual on the board went through rigorous rounds of assessment to prove their worth. After which they invested a large part of their time researching and compiling the most relevant data for our readers.

The editorial board has been involved in producing this book since its inception. They have spent rigorous hours researching and exploring the diverse topics which have resulted in the successful publishing of this book. They have passed on their knowledge of decades through this book. To expedite this challenging task, the publisher supported the team at every step. A small team of assistant editors was also appointed to further simplify the editing procedure and attain best results for the readers.

Apart from the editorial board, the designing team has also invested a significant amount of their time in understanding the subject and creating the most relevant covers. They scrutinized every image to scout for the most suitable representation of the subject and create an appropriate cover for the book.

The publishing team has been an ardent support to the editorial, designing and production team. Their endless efforts to recruit the best for this project, has resulted in the accomplishment of this book. They are a veteran in the field of academics and their pool of knowledge is as vast as their experience in printing. Their expertise and guidance has proved useful at every step. Their uncompromising quality standards have made this book an exceptional effort. Their encouragement from time to time has been an inspiration for everyone.

The publisher and the editorial board hope that this book will prove to be a valuable piece of knowledge for researchers, students, practitioners and scholars across the globe.

List of Contributors

Yuki Nakamura, Masahiro Takada, Akane Higami, He Jiaxi, Makoto Fujino, Rie Nakagawa, Yukiko Inagaki, Yoshiaki Matsumoto, Kosuke Kawaguchi, Masahiro Kawashima, Eiji Suzuki and Masakazu Toi
Department of Surgery (Breast Surgery), Kyoto University Hospital, Kyoto, Japan

Michiko Imamura
Department of Breast and Endocrine Surgery, Hyogo College of Medicine, Hyogo, Japan

Phileas Johannes Proskynitopoulos
Department of Neurosurgery, Cologne Medical Center, Cologne, Germany

Patra Charalampaki and Makoto Nakamura
Department of Neurosurgery, Cologne Medical Center, University Witten-Herdecke, Witten, Germany
Witten-Herdecke University, Witten, Germany

Axel Heimann
Institute for Neurosurgical Pathophysiology, Medical University Mainz, Mainz, German

Yosuke Kitagawa, Shota Tanaka, Takahide Nejo, Reiko Matsuura, Tsukasa Koike, Satoshi Takahashi, Masashi Nomura, Shunsaku Takayanagi and Nobuhito Saito
Department of Neurosurgery, Graduate School of Medicine, The University of Tokyo, Tokyo, Japan

Yugo Kuriki and Akira Ogasawara
Laboratory of Chemistry and Biology, Graduate School of Pharmaceutical Sciences, The University of Tokyo, Tokyo, Japan

Yasuteru Urano
Laboratory of Chemistry and Biology, Graduate School of Pharmaceutical Sciences, The University of Tokyo, Tokyo, Japan
Laboratory of Chemical Biology and Molecular Imaging, Graduate School of Medicine, The University of Tokyo, Tokyo, Japan

Kyoko Yamamoto and Mako Kamiya
Laboratory of Chemical Biology and Molecular Imaging, Graduate School of Medicine, The University of Tokyo, Tokyo, Japan

Taijun Hana
Department of Neurosurgery, Graduate School of Medicine, The University of Tokyo, Tokyo, Japan
Genome Science Division, Research Center for Advanced Science and Technology, The University of Tokyo, Tokyo, Japan

Akitake Mukasa
Department of Neurosurgery, Graduate School of Medical Sciences, Kumamoto University, Kumamoto, Japan

Michael Reinert
Laboratory for Biomedical Neurosciences, Neurocenter of Southern Switzerland, Ente Ospedaliero Cantonale, Torricella-Taverne, Switzerland
Department of Neurosurgery, Neurocenter of Southern Switzerland, Ente Ospedaliero Cantonale, Lugano, Switzerland
Faculty of Biomedical Neurosciences, Università Della Svizzera Italiana, Lugano, Switzerland
Medical Faculty, University of Bern, Bern, Switzerland

Deborah Piffaretti
Laboratory for Biomedical Neurosciences, Neurocenter of Southern Switzerland, Ente Ospedaliero Cantonale, Torricella-Taverne, Switzerland
Faculty of Medicine, Graduate School for Cellular and Biomedical Sciences, University of Bern, Bern, Switzerland

Marco Wilzbach, Christian Hauger and Roland Guckler
Carl Zeiss Meditec AG, Oberkochen, Germany

Maria Luisa D'Angelo
Laboratory for Biomedical Neurosciences, Neurocenter of Southern Switzerland, Ente Ospedaliero Cantonale, Torricella-Taverne, Switzerland

Francesco Marchi
Laboratory for Biomedical Neurosciences, Neurocenter of Southern Switzerland, Ente Ospedaliero Cantonale, Torricella-Taverne, Switzerland
Department of Neurosurgery, Neurocenter of Southern Switzerland, Ente Ospedaliero Cantonale, Lugano, Switzerland

Zeping Yu, Wenli Zhang, Xiang Fang, Chongqi Tu and Hong Duan
West China School of Medicine/West China Hospital, Sichuan University, Chengdu, China

Serik K. Akshulakov, Talgat T. Kerimbayev and Yermek A. Urunbayev
Department of Neurosurgery, JSC "National Center for Neurosurgery", Nur-Sultan, Kazakhstan

Michael Y. Biryuchkov
Department of Neurosurgery and Traumatology, West Kazakhstan Marat Ospanov State Medical University, Aktobe, Kazakhstan

Dimitrios Athanasopoulos
Department of Neurosurgery, Cologne Medical Center, University Witten-Herdecke, Witten, Germany

Solmaz AghaAmiri and Sukhen C. Ghosh
The Brown Foundation Institute of Molecular Medicine, McGovern Medical School, The University of Texas Health Science Center at Houston, Houston, TX, United States

Servando Hernandez Vargas and Ali Azhdarinia
The Brown Foundation Institute of Molecular Medicine, McGovern Medical School, The University of Texas Health Science Center at Houston, Houston, TX, United States
Therapeutics & Pharmacology Program, The University of Texas MD Anderson UTHealth Graduate School of Biomedical Sciences, Houston, TX, United States

Christie Lin and Adam J. Uselmann
OnLume, Inc., Madison,WI, United States

Hop S. Tran Cao and Naruhiko Ikoma
Department of Surgical Oncology, Division of Surgery, The University of Texas MD Anderson Cancer Center, Houston, TX, United States

Kurt V. Shaffer
Department of Neurosurgery, Barrow Neurological Institute, St. Joseph's Hospital and Medical Center, Phoenix, AZ, United States

Chaoqun Lin
Department of Neurosurgery, School of Medicine, Southeast University, Nanjing, China

Lukui Chen
Department of Neurosurgery, Neuroscience Center, Cancer Center, Integrated Hospital of Traditional Chinese Medicine, Southern Medical University, Guangzhou, China

Masood Pasha Syed
Department of Medicine, Saint Vincent Hospital, Worcester, MA, United States

Chunjie Li
State Key Laboratory of Oral Diseases, National Clinical Research Center for Oral Diseases, West China School of Stomatology, Sichuan University, Chengdu, China
Department of Head and Neck Oncology, West China Hospital of Stomatology, Sichuan University, Chengdu, China
Department of Medical Affairs, West China Hospital of Stomatology, Sichuan University, Chengdu, China

Lingyun Zhou
Center of Infectious Diseases, West China Hospital of Sichuan University, Chengdu, China

Honglin Li, Pingchuan Ma and Zhongkai Ma
State Key Laboratory of Oral Diseases, National Clinical Research Center for Oral Diseases, West China School of Stomatology, Sichuan University, Chengdu, China
Department of Head and Neck Oncology, West China Hospital of Stomatology, Sichuan University, Chengdu, China

Yubin Cao
State Key Laboratory of Oral Diseases, National Clinical Research Center for Oral Diseases, West China School of Stomatology, Sichuan University, Chengdu, China
Department of Oral and Maxillofacial Surgery, West China Hospital of Stomatology, Sichuan University, Chengdu, China

Wenbin Yang
State Key Laboratory of Oral Diseases, National Clinical Research Center for Oral Diseases, West China School of Stomatology, Sichuan University, Chengdu, China
Department of Oral and Maxillofacial Surgery, West China Hospital of Stomatology, Sichuan University, Chengdu, China
Department of Medical Affairs, West China Hospital of Stomatology, Sichuan University, Chengdu, China

Samuel W. Cramer and Clark C. Chen
Department of Neurosurgery, University of Minnesota, Minneapolis, MN, United States

Masaki Kaibori, Hisashi Kosaka, Kosuke Matsui, Morihiko Ishizaki, Hideyuki Matsushima, Takumi Tsuda, Hidehiko Hishikawa, Tadayoshi Okumura and Mitsugu Sekimoto
Department of Surgery, Kansai Medical University, Osaka, Japan

Liudmila A. Bardonova, Roman A. Polkin, Sergey V. Ochkal, Valerij V. Shepelev and Marat A. Aliyev
Neurosurgery and Innovative Medicine Department, Irkutsk State Medical University, Irkutsk, Russia

Naomi R. Onaka
University of Arizona College of Medicine, Phoenix, AZ, United States

Alexander A. Potapov
Federal State Autonomous Institution "N. N. Burdenko National Scientific and Practical Center for Neurosurgery" of the Ministry of Healthcare of the Russian Federation, Moscow, Russia

Chase H. Foster
Department of Neurological Surgery, George Washington University Hospital, Washington, DC, United States

Peter J. Morone
Department of Neurological Surgery, Vanderbilt University Medical Center, Vanderbilt University, Nashville, TN, United States

Samuel B. Tomlinson
School of Medicine and Dentistry, University of Rochester Medical Center, Rochester, NY, United States

Aaron A. Cohen-Gadol
Goodman Campbell Brain and Spine, Department of Neurological Surgery, Indiana University, Indianapolis, IN, United States

Rao-Jun Luo, Zi-Yi Zhu, Zheng-Fu He, Yong Xu and Yun-Zheng Wang
Department of Thoracic Surgery, Sir Run Run Shaw Hospital, School of Medicine, Zhejiang University, Hangzhou, China

Ping Chen
Zhejiang Provincial Key Laboratory of Laparoscopic Technology, Sir Run Run Shaw Hospital, School of Medicine, Zhejiang University, Hangzhou, China

Daniel Valli
Department of Neurosurgery, Barrow Neurological Institute, St. Joseph's Hospital and Medical Center, Phoenix, AZ, United States

Ran Xu, Wanda Teich, Judith Rösler, Katharina Faust, Anne Blank, Susan Brandenburg, Martin Misch and Peter Vajkoczy
Department of Neurosurgery, Charite´ – Universitätsmedizin Berlin, Corporate Member of Freie Universität Berlin, and Humboldt-Universität zu Berlin, and Berlin Institute of Health, Berlin, Germany

Julia Sophie Onken
Department of Neurosurgery, Charite´ – Universitätsmedizin Berlin, Corporate Member of Freie Universität Berlin, and Humboldt-Universität zu Berlin, and Berlin Institute of Health, Berlin, Germany
German Cancer Consortium (DKTK), Heidelberg, Germany, partner site Charite´ Berlin, Berlin, Germany

Florian Frenzel, Katrin Hoffmann and Ute Resch-Genger
Division Biophotonics, Federal Institutxe for Materials Research and Testing (BAM), Berlin, Germany

Evgenii Belykh
Department of Neurosurgery, Barrow Neurological Institute, St. Joseph's Hospital and Medical Center, Phoenix, AZ, United States
Department of Neurosurgery, Irkutsk State Medical University, Irkutsk, Russia

Sirin Gandhi, Ali Tayebi Meybodi, Claudio Cavallo, Xiaochun Zhao, Leandro Borba Moreira, Michael T. Lawton, Peter Nakaji and Mark C. Preul
Department of Neurosurgery, St. Joseph's Hospital and Medical Center, Barrow Neurological Institute, Phoenix, AZ, United States

Vadim A. Byvaltsev
Department of Neurosurgery, JSC "National Center for Neurosurgery", Nur-Sultan, Kazakhstan
Department of Neurosurgery and Innovative Medicine, Irkutsk State Medical University, Irkutsk, Russia

Dara S. Farhadi
University of Arizona College of Medicine, Phoenix, AZ, United States
Department of Neurosurgery, The Loyal and Edith Davis Neurosurgical Research Laboratory, Barrow Neurological Institute, St. Joseph's Hospital and Medical Center, Phoenix, AZ, United States

Brandon Ngo
Department of Neurosurgery, The Loyal and Edith Davis Neurosurgical Research Laboratory, Barrow Neurological Institute, St. Joseph's Hospital and Medical Center, Phoenix, AZ, United States

Jennifer M. Eschbacher
Department of Neuropathology, Barrow Neurological Institute, St. Joseph's Hospital and Medical Center, Phoenix, AZ, United States

Index

A

Acoustic Neurinoma, 8, 15

Acridine Orange, 101, 162-165, 167-168

Anaplastic Astrocytoma, 8, 11, 13

Aneurysm, 61, 171, 184, 188-189, 193-196, 198-204

Arteriovenous Fistula, 194, 200

Arteriovenous Malformation, 169-170, 175-176, 193-194, 200, 202, 204, 215-216

Autofluorescence, 24, 46-47, 127, 210, 212, 217, 222

B

Biliary Excretion, 64, 152

Bladder Cancer, 102, 118-119, 126-128, 159, 166, 168

Blood-brain Barrier, 78-81, 86-88, 90, 97-103, 114, 133, 142-143, 149, 170, 187

Brain Biopsy, 45-47, 49-52, 139

Brain Tissue, 7, 10, 13, 15, 18, 23-24, 46-47, 52-53, 58-59, 72, 88, 92, 132, 143-144, 148, 165, 214-215, 218, 222-223

Brain Tumor, 7-8, 11, 15-19, 28-29, 50-54, 62, 68, 75, 78-79, 82-84, 86, 91-93, 95-98, 100-103, 115, 117, 130, 132, 136-140, 147-148, 150, 165-166, 168, 206, 210, 212-214, 219, 222, 225

Breast Cancer, 1-2, 5-6, 20, 59, 89, 99, 103, 139, 161

Bypass Graft, 159, 183, 185-186

C

Cancer Imaging, 71, 76, 101, 159, 162-163

Cell Surface, 148

Central Nervous System, 55, 78-79, 81, 83, 87, 96, 116, 139-140, 205-206

Chemotherapy, 6-7, 31, 34, 37, 82, 97-98, 100-101, 105-106, 125, 131, 136, 140, 144-146, 149-150, 152, 159, 178-180

Cholangiocarcinoma, 164, 166

Confocal Endomicroscopy, 59, 61, 103, 106, 129, 134, 137-138, 165

Cytoplasm, 56, 58, 90, 165, 217, 222

D

Deep Brain Stimulation, 49-50, 52

Diagnostic Accuracy, 45, 50-51, 64-65, 67, 70, 73, 76, 82, 113, 117, 130, 190, 212-215, 219-225

Drug Delivery, 78-79, 83-84, 86-89, 94, 96-98, 100-101, 103, 148, 150-152

E

Emission Light, 184, 198-199

Endoscope, 28-29, 46-48, 50, 52, 56-57, 93, 103, 113, 117, 167, 193, 198-202, 204

Esophageal Cancer, 177-178, 181-182

Extracellular Space, 60, 84, 89, 217-218

Extravasation, 56, 59, 79, 83-86, 92, 94-95, 98-99, 178, 186, 191, 220

F

Fluorescein Sodium, 17-18, 45, 50, 52-53, 70, 78, 80, 86, 92, 102-103, 106, 114, 117, 129-130, 133, 139, 165-166, 193-194, 199-200, 203-204, 212-214, 224

Fluorescence Imaging, 2, 19, 29, 45, 55, 62, 66, 72, 74-76, 96, 99, 115-116, 139, 151-152, 158-161, 168, 175, 181, 184, 192, 222

Fluorescence Intensity, 15, 72, 90, 93, 169, 172, 186, 209

Fluorescence-guided Surgery, 7-8, 16-19, 29, 50, 52, 54, 61, 63, 74-79, 84, 86, 96, 99, 102, 106, 111, 114, 116, 126, 129-130, 138, 149, 214

Fluorescent Signal, 16, 55-56, 58, 70, 72, 190

G

Gastric Adenocarcinomas, 66, 75, 194

Glioblastoma, 7-9, 11-12, 15-16, 21, 26-27, 29, 53, 61, 66-68, 70-72, 75, 79, 82, 89, 95-102, 106-107, 115-117, 130, 133, 135, 139-146, 148-150, 164, 166, 168, 190, 192, 204, 207-208, 211-212, 216, 225

Glioma, 16-22, 28-29, 46, 50-52, 56, 61-62, 67-69, 74-76, 78-79, 82-83, 85-86, 88-117, 129-130, 133, 139, 148-150, 165-168, 205-206, 210, 212-214, 216-219, 221-225

Glioma Tissue, 18-19, 50, 82, 165, 222

Graft Patency, 159, 183, 185-186, 190-191, 203

Gross Total Resection, 16, 105-107, 109-110, 116

H

Heme Biosynthetic Pathway, 90-91

Hepatectomy, 151-154, 156, 159-160

High-grade Glioma, 16, 22, 82, 89, 92-93, 95-96, 101, 105-106, 108-109, 111-113, 115-116, 139, 205, 214, 216, 218-219, 223

I

Indocyanine Green, 1-2, 5-6, 13, 16-17, 46-48, 52-56, 61, 64, 74, 78-80, 86, 90, 92, 99, 103, 106, 111-112, 134, 150-152, 165, 169-170, 175-178, 182-184, 190-194, 199-200, 203-204, 212, 214, 222, 225

Intraoperative Fluorescence, 19, 29, 52, 62, 75-76, 99, 102, 114-115, 117, 139, 159, 162-163, 168, 175, 199, 204, 212

L

Lesional Tissue, 50, 213, 220

Light Spectrum, 24, 184, 199

Lipid, 84-85, 89, 95, 99, 101, 144, 165

Lipoproteins, 93, 101, 103, 153, 184

Lymphoma, 19, 84, 116, 139, 207-208

M

Malignant Tumor, 8

Meta-analysis, 2, 6, 76, 96, 105-112, 114-116, 118-120, 123, 126-127, 212
Molecular Weight, 63-64, 73, 84, 89, 92, 94, 97, 163, 170, 206
Mortality Rate, 46, 147, 177

N
Nanoparticle Technology, 89, 148
Necrotic Tissue, 50, 113, 215
Neoplastic Tissue, 58, 136, 143, 194
Neovascularization, 56, 97, 152, 183
Neurosurgery, 7-8, 11, 15-17, 21, 29, 31, 45, 47, 52-55, 59, 61, 67, 72, 78, 98-103, 105, 115-117, 129, 139-140, 149-150, 153, 160, 162, 167, 173, 175-176, 183, 189-194, 201, 203-206, 212-213, 219, 224-225
Neurosurgical Treatment, 8, 214

O
Operative Time, 38, 41, 72, 113, 178-179, 183, 190
Optical Biopsy, 52-53, 61, 213-216, 220, 222, 224
Osteosarcomas, 37, 66-67, 75, 166

P
Pancreatic Cancer, 91, 166
Passive Delivery, 75, 84, 99
Pelvic Tumor, 30, 44
Pharmacokinetics, 75, 89, 92-93, 95, 99, 102-103, 142, 148, 168, 184
Photodynamic Therapy, 16, 22, 28-29, 86, 89, 91, 99-101, 106, 111, 114-117, 126, 140-141, 144, 148-152, 156, 161-163, 167-168
Photosensitizer, 114, 119, 141-145, 147-150, 153, 168
Plasma Protein, 93

R
Radiodynamic Therapy, 162, 167-168
Radioisotope, 1-4
Radiotherapy, 7, 15, 31, 79, 101, 105-106, 110, 115, 125, 140, 146, 149, 164-168, 178-180

S
Sacroiliac Joint, 30-31, 35, 39, 42-44
Sentinel Lymph Node, 1-2, 4-6
Sonodynamic Therapy, 117, 162, 165, 168
Surgical Management, 75, 171, 175, 183
Surgical Oncology, 54, 60, 63-64, 73, 76, 162-163
Surgical Resection, 14, 21-22, 27-28, 31, 54-55, 66, 72, 95, 105-107, 109-113, 116, 139-140, 143, 145, 149, 166, 172, 174, 190, 206, 222
Survival Outcome, 105-106

T
Tumor Extension, 114, 129
Tumor Segmentation, 129, 132-133, 137-139
Tumor Tissues, 17, 84-85, 91, 94, 96, 100, 132, 163, 205
Tumor Vasculature, 84-85, 94, 114, 190
Tumor Visualization, 64, 67, 86, 113, 121, 152, 206

V
Vascular Neurosurgery, 16, 47, 61, 190, 193-194, 201, 203, 206, 212
Videoangiography, 16, 52, 61, 169-171, 174-176, 183-184, 189-196, 198-204, 225

www.ingramcontent.com/pod-product-compliance
Lightning Source LLC
LaVergne TN
LVHW082203200926
848484LV00008B/2206